Anaerobic Infections

INFECTIOUS DISEASE AND THERAPY

Series Editor

Burke A. Cunha

Winthrop-University Hospital
Mineola, and
State University of New York School of Medicine
Stony Brook, New York

The book is dedicated to my wife, Joyce,
my children Dafna, Tammy, Yoni, and Sara, and
my granddaughter Darly.

Preface

Since the publication of the first edition of the book entitled *Pediatric Anaerobic Infections*, much has changed in our understanding and knowledge of the role of anaerobic bacteria in infections in children and adults. More clinical studies were performed describing their activity in a variety of infections, including head and neck infections, skin and soft tissue infections, abdominal and visceral abscesses, and infections after trauma. With increased awareness and early recognition, patient care improved those infections caused by these organisms.

In the past three decades, resistance of anaerobic bacteria increased to many of the antimicrobials used for their therapy. During this period, newer antimicrobial agents effective against these organisms were introduced. Methods for their identification were improved and simplified, as their taxonomy has changed.

As the field has expanded we felt the need to expand the scope of *Pediatric Anaerobic Infections* to include infections affecting the pediatric and adult populations. This volume does just that by covering the entire spectrum of adult and pediatric infections. Chapters include all age groups, while presenting illnesses unique to the neonatal age. The current volume updates our knowledge of diagnosis and therapy, resistance to antimicrobials, and the newer agents, indications and contraindications for surgery, and the therapy of complications. Newer diagnostic tests are included, and the nomenclature of the organisms is updated and newer and current references are included.

Each chapter is set up to present the information in the most user-friendly way and emphasis has been given to treatment of various infections for ready use by all clinicians, including internists, pediatricians, ear, nose, and throat surgeons, general surgeons, and family practitioners. I am hopeful that the practicing physicians will continue to find this reference work useful in delivering care for their patients.

Itzhak Brook

Acknowledgments

I am most grateful to those who have made this book possible.

I would like to express my deepest gratitude to my parents, Haya and Baruch, who worked so hard to ensure that I would have a proper education. They have always encouraged the development of my scientific curiosity and capabilities. I would also like to thank my children and especially my wife, Joyce, for her patience, support, and understanding.

I am indebted to many of my teachers in the Hareali Haivri High School of Haifa, Israel, for their devotion and enthusiastic teaching, which were instrumental in promoting my scientific, professional, and ethical development. I am especially grateful to my biology teacher, Mr Z. Zilberstein, for his enthusiastic recognition of nature's role in human life, and to my physics teacher, Mr. L. Green, for teaching me an analytical and scientific approach to my studies. I am grateful to many of my teachers in the Hebrew University Hadassah School of Medicine in Jerusalem and especially to the late Professor H. Berenkoff, who introduced me to the wonders of microbiology; to Dr. T. Sacks, who taught me clinical microbiology; and to Dr. S. Levine from Kaplan Hospital, Rehovot, Israel, who taught me general pediatrics.

I owe special gratitude to my teacher and mentor at UCLA, Dr. S. M. Finegold, for sharing his knowledge of anaerobic microbiology and clinical infectious diseases. Dr. Finegold has served over the years as a constant source of support and encouragement. Other teachers who provided invaluable help are Drs. W. J. Martin and V. L. Sutter from UCLA, and Drs. C. V. Sumaya, G. D. Overturf, and P. Wherle, who taught me about pediatric infectious diseases.

I am also grateful to my friends and collaborators who assisted in many of the clinical and laboratory studies: K. S. Bricknel for his excellent gas liquid chromatography work, and L. Calhoun, P. Yocurn and D. E. Giraldo for their dedication and laboratory support.

Finally, I would like to thank the many medical students, house officers, infectious diseases fellows, and faculty members of the University of California, Los Angeles; University of California, Irvine; George Washington University and Georgetown University, Washington, DC; and the National Naval Medical Center in Bethesda, Maryland, for their collaboration in clinical studies. I am especially grateful to Drs. J. C. Coolbaugh and R. I. Walker from the Naval Medical Research Institute and Drs. T. B. Elliott and G. D. Ledney of the Armed Forces Radiobiology Research Institute in Bethesda, Maryland for their outstanding support of my research efforts. I am very grateful to Diane Citron for her helpful review and comments of the book.

Contents

1 | Introduction to Anaerobes

ANAEROBES AS PATHOGENS

Anaerobic bacteria differ in their pathogenicity. Not all of them are believed to be clinically significant, while others are known to be highly pathogenic. Table 1 lists the major anaerobes that are most frequently encountered clinically. The taxonomy of anaerobic bacteria has changed in recent years because of their improved characterization using genetic studies (1). The ability to differentiate between similar strains enables better characterization of type of infection and predicted antimicrobial susceptibility. The species of anaerobes most frequently isolated from clinical infections are in decreasing frequency: the clinically important anaerobes are of gram-negative rods (*Bacteroides*, *Prevotella*, *Porphyromonas*, *Fusobacterium*, *Bilophila* and *Sutterella*), gram-positive cocci (primarily *Peptostreptococcus*), gram-positive spore-forming (*Clostridium*) and non-spore-forming bacilli (*Actinomyces*, *Propionibacterium*, *Eubacterium*, *Lactobacillus*, and *Bifidobacterium*), and gram-negative cocci (mainly Veillonella) (2). About 95% of the anaerobes isolated from clinical infections are members of these genera. The remaining isolates belong to species not yet described, but these usually can be assigned to the appropriate genus on the basis of morphologic characteristics and fermentation products. The frequency of recovery of the different anaerobic strains differs in various infectious sites. The 12 years experience in recovering anaerobic bacteria from adults and children at two medical centers is presented in Table 2 (3). The main isolates were anaerobic gram-negative bacilli (*Bacteroids*, *Prevotella*, and *Porphyromonas*; 43% of anaerobic isolates), anaerobic gram-positive cocci (26%), *Clostridium* spp. (7%), and *Fusobacterium* spp. (5%). This chapter discusses the main anaerobic species and their role in infectious processes.

CLASSIFICATION OF ANAEROBES

Anaerobes do not multiply in oxygen but have different susceptibility to oxygen. Most normal flora anaerobes are extremely oxygen sensitive, while those that cause infections are more aero-tolerant. The aero-tolerance of several anaerobes is through the production of superoxide dismutase, they produce on exposure to oxygen. The negative oxidation–reduction potential (Eh) of the environment is a critical factor in the survival of anaerobic bacteria.

Anaerobes do not grow on solid media in room air (10% CO_2, 18% O_2); facultative anaerobes grow both in the presence and absence of air, and microaerophilic bacteria grow poorly or not at all aerobically but grow better under 10% CO_2 or anaerobically. Anaerobes are divided into "strict anaerobes" that are unable to grow in the presence of more than 0.5% O_2 or "moderate anaerobes" that are capable of growing at between 2% and 8% O_2.

GRAM-POSITIVE SPORE-FORMING BACILLI

Anaerobic spore-forming bacilli belong to the genus *Clostridium*. Morphologically, the clostridia are highly pleomorphic, ranging from short, thick bacilli to long filamentous forms, and are either ramrod straight or slightly curved. The clostridia found most frequently in clinical infections are *Clostridium perfringens* (Fig. 1), *Clostridium septicum*, *Clostridium butyricum*, *Clostridium sordellii*, *Clostridium ramosum*, and *Clostridium innocuum*.

C. perfringens is an inhabitant of soil and of intestinal contents of humans and animals and is the most frequently encountered histotoxic clostridial species (4). This microorganism, which

TABLE 1 Anaerobic Bacteria Most Frequently Encountered in Clinical Specimens

Organism	Infectious site
Gram-positive cocci	
Peptostreptococcus spp.	Respiratory tract, intra-abdominal and subcutaneous infections
Microaerophilic streptococci[a]	Sinusitis, brain abscesses
Gram-positive bacilli	
Non-spore-forming Actinomyces spp.	Intracranial abscesses, chronic mastoiditis, aspiration pneumonia, head and neck infections
Propionibacterium acnes	Shunt infections (cardiac, intracranial)
Bifidobacterium spp.	Chronic otitis media, cervical lymphadenitis
Spore-forming	
Clostridium spp.	
C. perfringens	Wounds and abscesses, sepsis
C. septicum	Sepsis
C. sordellii	Necrotizing infections
C. difficile	Diarrheal disease, colitis
C. botulinum	Botulism
C. tetani	Tetanus
Gram-negative bacilli	
Bacteroides fragilis group (B. fragilis, B. thetaiotamicron)	Intra-abdominal and female genital tract infections, sepsis, neonatal infection
Pigmental Prevotella and Porphyromonas spp.	Orofacial infections, aspiration pneumonia, periodontitis
Prevotella oralis	Orofacial infections
Prevotella B. oris-buccae	Orofacial infections, intra-abdominal infections
P. bivia, P. disiens	Female genital tract infections
Fusobacterium spp.	
F. nucleatum	Orofacial and respiratory tract infections, brain abscesses, bacteremia
F. necrophorum	Aspiration pneumonia, bacteremia

[a] Not obligate anaerobes.

elaborates a number of necrotizing extracellular toxins, is easily isolated and identified in the clinical laboratory. *C. perfringens* seldom produces spores in vivo. It can be characterized in direct smears of a purulent exudate by the presence of stout gram-variable rods of varying length, frequently surrounded by a capsule. *C. perfringens* can cause a devastating illness with high mortality. Clostridial bacteremia is associated with extensive tissue necrosis, hemolytic anemia, and renal failure. The incidence of clostridial endometritis, a common event following septic abortions, has decreased as medically supervised abortions have increased (2).

    C. perfringens accounted for 48% of all clostridial isolates in our hospitals (Table 2) and was primarily isolated from wounds (26% of *C. perfringens*) isolates, blood (16%), abdomen (14%), and obstetrical and gynecological infections (13%).

    C. septicum, long known as an animal pathogen, has been found in humans within the last decade, often associated with malignancy. The intestinal tract is thought to be the source of the organism, and most of the isolates are recovered from the blood.

    C. sordellii causes life threatening infections after trauma, childbirth, gynecological procedures, medically induced abortions, surgery and injection of elicit drugs. It can cause rapid progressive tissue necrosis, shock, multiorgan failure and death in about 3/4 of patients (4a).

    Although *Clostridium botulinum* usually is associated with food poisoning, wound infections caused by this organism are being recognized with increasing frequency. Proteolytic strains of types A and B have been reported from wound infections. Disease caused by *C. botulinum* usually is an intoxication produced by ingestion of contaminated food (uncooked meat, poorly processed fish, improperly canned vegetables), containing a highly potent neurotoxin. Such food may not necessarily seem spoiled, nor may gas production be evident. The polypeptide neurotoxin is relatively heat labile, and food containing this toxin may be rendered innocuous by exposure to 100°C for 10 minutes.

TABLE 2 Percentage of Recovery of Anaerobes in Each Infection Site at Walter Reed Army Medical and Naval Medical Centers 1973–1985

Specimen source	Total number of specimens	Total number of anaerobic isolates	Number anaerobic isolates/ specimen	Bacteroides spp.	Fusobacterium spp.	Clostridium spp.	Lactobacillus spp.	Eubacterium spp.	Propionibacterium spp.	Bifidobacterium spp.	Actinomyces spp.	Veillonella spp.	Peptostreptococcus spp.
Abdomen	359	550	1.53	299 (55)[a]	43 (8)	71 (13)	4 (1)	31 (6)	23 (4)			8 (1)	71 (13)
Abscess	820	1416	1.73	725 (51)	97 (7)	71 (5)	7 (0.5)	44 (3)	54 (4)	5 (0.5)	2 (0.2)	28 (2)	383 (27)
Bile	66	75	1.14	29 (39)	1 (1)	27 (36)			9 (12)				9 (12)
Bites	9	12	1.33	5 (42)	1 (8)				2 (17)				4 (33)
Blood	587	634	1.08	222 (35)	24 (4)	70 (11)	1 (0.2)	13 (2)	229 (36)	1 (0.2)		7 (1)	67 (11)
Bone	37	69	1.86	24 (35)	4 (6)	2 (3)			1 (1)	9 (13)		2 (3)	27 (39)
Central nervous system	220	225	1.02	16 (7)	2 (1)	4 (2)			163 (72)		1 (0.5)		39 (17)
Chest	191	283	1.48	101 (37)	31 (11)	18 (6)	1 (0.4)	9 (3)	51 (18)	4 (1)		9 (3)	59 (21)
Cysts	206	348	1.69	153 (44)	5 (1)	6 (2)	4 (1)	6 (2)	24 (7)	1 (0.3)		10 (3)	139 (40)
Ear	25	47	1.88	12 (26)	1 (2)	1 (2)			7 (15)			1 (2)	25 (53)
Eye	55	66	1.20	8 (12)	3 (5)	11 (17)			36 (55)			4 (6)	4 (6)
Genitourinary	30	52	1.73	29 (56)	2 (4)	1 (2)	1 (2)	3 (6)	3 (6)			2 (4)	11 (21)
Grafts	13	15	1.15	4 (27)		1 (7)			5 (33)				5 (33)
Joints	63	69	1.10	9 (13)		1 (1)			39 (57)				13 (19)
Lymph glands	70	76	1.09	11 (15)	3 (4)	8 (12)	1 (1)		48 (63)	1 (1)			10 (13)
Obstetric/ gynecologic	871	1328	1.52	654 (49)	42 (3)	50 (4)	15 (1)	28 (2)	28 (2)	12 (1)	1 (1)	28 (2)	470 (35)
Sinuses	102	159	1.56	53 (33)	11 (7)	2 (1)		2 (1)	36 (23)	1 (1)		7 (4)	47 (30)
Tumors	61	79	1.30	33 (42)	1 (1)	1 (1)		1 (1)	22 (28)	1 (0.1)	1 (1)	1 (1)	19 (24)
Wounds	622	987	1.59	425 (43)	20 (2)	124 (13)	6 (1)	18 (2)	66 (7)	1 (1)		14 (1)	313 (31)
Miscellaneous	51	67	1.31	23 (34)	3 (4)	3 (4)		2 (3)	20 (30)	1 (1)		2 (3)	13 (19)
Total	4458	6557	1.47	2835 (43)	294 (5)	471 (7)	40 (1)	158 (2)	874 (13)	27 (0.4)	5 (0.1)	125 (2)	1728 (26)

[a] In parentheses: percentage of all anaerobic bacteria isolated from source indicated.
Source: From Ref. 3.

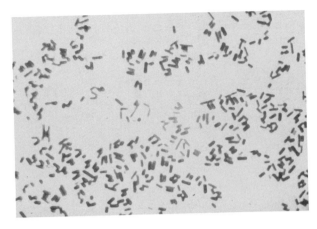

FIGURE 1 Gram stain of *Clostridium perfringens*.

C. botulinum is usually associated with food poisoning (2); botulism is an intoxication caused by ingestion of contaminated food containing its highly potent neurotoxin. However, wound infections caused by proteolytic strains of types A and B has been reported with increasing frequency and can also produce botulism.

C. botulinum has also been associated with newborns presenting with hypotonia, respiratory arrest, areflexia, ptosis, and poorly responding pupils. Botulism in infants is caused by toxin from the germination of ingested spores and *C. botulinum* in the bowel lumen. *C. butyricum* can also be recovered from infection of the abdomen, abscesses, bile, wounds, and blood.

Clostridium difficile has been incriminated as the causative agent of antibiotic-associated and spontaneous diarrhea and colitis (5). A formerly infrequently isolated strain of *C. difficile* known as BI/NAP1 has recently been implicated in geographically diverse outbreaks of *C. difficile*-associated disease which have severe clinical presentations and poor outcomes (5).

Clostridium tetani is rarely isolated from human feces. Infections caused by this bacillus are a result of contamination of wounds with soil containing *C. tetani* spores. The spores will germinate in devitalized tissue and produce the neurotoxin that is responsible for the clinical findings of tetanus. *C. tetani* has been recovered from patients presenting with otogenous tetanus (6).

Clostridia can be isolated from various infectious sites. These organisms are especially prevalent in abscesses (mostly abdominal, rectal area, and oropharyngeal), and peritonitis (1). The distribution of clostridia in these infections is explained by their prevalence in the normal gastrointestinal and cervical flora from where they may originate (7).

Clostridia strains (*C. perfringens*, *C. butyricum*, and *C. difficile*) have been recovered from blood and peritoneal cultures of necrotizing enterocolitis and from infants with sudden death syndrome (8–10). Strains of *Clostridium* were recovered from children with bacteremia of gastrointestinal origin (11) and with sickle cell disease (12). Clostridial strains have been recovered from specimens obtained from patients with acute (13) and chronic (14) otitis media, chronic sinusitis and mastoiditis (15,16), peritonsillar abscesses (17), peritonitis (18,19), liver and spleen abscesses (20), abdominal abscesses (21), and neonatal conjunctivitis (22,23).

GRAM-POSITIVE NON-SPORE-FORMING BACILLI

Anaerobic, gram-positive, non-spore-forming rods comprise part of the microflora of the gingival crevices, the gastrointestinal tract, the vagina, and the skin. Since many of them appear to be morphologically similar, they have been difficult to separate by the usual bacteriologic tests. Several distinct genera are recognized: *Actinomyces*, *Arachnia*, *Bifidobacterium*, *Eubacterium*, *Lactobacillus*, and *Propionibacterium*.

The *Actinomyces*, *Arachnia*, and *Bifidobacterium* of the family *Actinomycetaceae* are gram-positive, pleomorphic, anaerobic to microaerophilic bacilli. Species of the genus *Bifidobacterium* are part of the commensal flora of the mouth gastrointestinal tract and female genital tract and constitute a high proportion of the normal intestinal flora in humans, especially in breast-fed infants (24). Although some infections caused by these organisms have been reported (25–28), little is known about their pathogenic potential.

Eubacterium spp. are part of the flora of the mouth and the bowel. They have been recognized as pathogens in chronic periodontal disease (29) and in infections associated with intra-uterine devices (30), and have been isolated from patients with bacteraemia associated with malignancy (31) and from female genital tract infection (32). *Lactobacillus* spp. are ubiquitous inhabitants of the human oral cavity, the vagina, and the gastrointestinal tract (33). They have been implicated in various serious deep-seated infections, amnionitis (33) and bacteraemia (34). *Eubacterium, Lactobacillus,* and *Bifidobacterium* spp. have been isolated in pure culture in only a few instances and are usually isolated in mixed culture from clinical specimens (1). The infections where they have been found most often are chronic otitis media and sinusitis, aspiration pneumonia, and intra-abdominal, obstetric and gynecological and skin, and soft-tissue infections (1,35,36).

Actinomyces israelii and *Actinomyces naeslundii* are normal inhabitants of the human mouth and throat (particularly gingival crypts, dental calculus, and tonsillar crypts) and are the most frequently isolated pathogenic actinomycetes. These organisms have been recovered from intracranial abscesses (37), chronic mastoiditis (16), aspiration pneumonia (38), and peritonitis (18). Although actinomycetes often are present in mixed culture, they are clearly pathogenic in their own right and may produce widespread devastating disease anywhere in the body (39). The lesions of actinomycosis occur most commonly in the tissues of the face and neck, lungs, pleura, and ileocecal regions. Bone, pericardial, and anorectal lesions are less common, but virtually any tissue may be invaded; a disseminated, bacteremic form has been described.

Propionibacterium spp. are part of the normal bacterial flora that colonize the skin (40), conjunctiva (41), oropharynx, and gastrointestinal tract (42). These non-spore-forming, anaerobic, gram-positive bacilli are frequent contaminants of specimens of blood and other sterile body fluids and have been generally considered to play little or no pathogenic role in humans.

Propionibacterium acnes and other *Propionibacterium* spp. have, however, been recovered with or without other aerobic or anaerobic organisms as etiologic agents of multiple infection sites (43–54). These include conjunctivitis (43), intracranial abscesses (44,45), peritonitis (46), and dental, parotid (47,48), pulmonary (47,48), and other serious infections (49). They have often been recovered as a sole isolate in specimens obtained from patients with infections associated with a foreign body (such as an artificial valve), endocarditis (50,51), and central nervous system shunt infections (50,52). The possible role of *P. acnes* in the pathogenesis of acne vulgaris was suggested. The data that support this are based on the recovery of this organism in large numbers from sebaceous follicles, especially in patients with acne, on its ability to elaborate enzymes such as lipase, protease, and hyaluronidase, and on its ability to activate the complement system and enhance chemotactic activity of neutrophils (53).

GRAM-NEGATIVE BACILLI

The anaerobic gram-negative rods are differentiated into genera on the basis of the fermentation acids they produce. The family *Bacteroidaceae* contains several genera of medical importance: *Bacteroides fragilis* group, *Prevotella, Porphyromonas, Bacteroides,* and *Fusobacterium.*

Bacteroides fragilis Group

B. fragilis group is the most prevalent bacteriodaceae isolated. *B. fragilis* is the most prevalent organism in the *B. fragilis* group, accounting for 41% to 78% of the isolates of the group. However, it should be remembered that the other members of the group account for the rest of the *B. fragilis* group isolates. The relative distribution of the different *B. fragilis* group has important clinical implications in the management of infections involving anaerobic bacteria. This is because of the different antimicrobial susceptibility of various *B. fragilis* group members. Although members of *fragilis* group produce beta-lactamase and resist

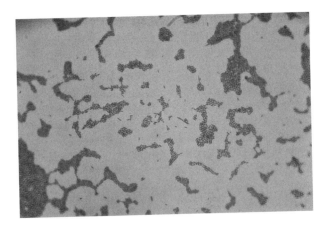

FIGURE 2   Gram stain of *Bacteroides fragilis.*

penicillin, their susceptibility to cephalosporins is variable (2) but predictable. Other *B. fragilis* group also has variable resistance to penicillins and cephalosporins.

The *B. fragilis* group is the species of Bacteroidaceae that occur with greatest frequency in clinical specimens. These organisms are resistant to penicillin by virtue of production of beta-lactamase and by other unknown factors (55). This organism was formerly classified as subspecies of *B. fragilis* (i.e., ss. *fragilis*, ss. *distasonis*, ss. *ovatus*, ss. *thetaiotaomicron*, and ss. *vulgatus*). They have been reclassified into distinct species on the basis of DNA homology studies (1,56). *B. fragilis* (formerly known as *B. fragilis* ss. *fragilis*, one of the subspecies of *B. fragilis*) is the anaerobe most frequently isolated from infections (Fig. 2).

Although *B. fragilis* group is the most common species found in clinical specimens, it is the least common *Bacteroides* present in fecal flora, comprising only 0.5% of the bacteria present in stool. The pathogenicity of this group of organisms probably results from its ability to produce capsular material, which is protective against phagocytosis (57). Because of its presence in normal flora of the gastrointestinal tract, this organism is predominant in bacteremia associated with intra-abdominal infections (2,32), peritonitis and abscesses following rupture of viscus (18,19), and subcutaneous abscesses or burns near the anus (58,59). Although *B. fragilis* is not generally found as part of the normal oral flora, it can colonize the oral cavity of patients with poor oral hygiene or of those who previously received antimicrobial therapy, especially penicillin. Following the colonization of the oropharyngeal cavity, these organisms also can be recovered from infections that originate in this area such as aspiration pneumonia (38,60), lung abscess (60,61), chronic otitis media (14), brain abscess (37), and subcutaneous abscess or burns near the oral cavity (58,59).

B. fragilis can be recovered from infectious processes in the newborn. The newborn infant is at risk of developing these infections when born to a mother with amnionitis, experienced premature rupture of membranes, or acquire the infection during the newborn's passage through the birth canal, where *B. fragilis* is part of the normal flora (62). *B. fragilis* was recovered from newborns with aspiration pneumonia (63), bacteremia (11), omphalitis (64), and subcutaneous abscesses and occipital osteomylitis following fetal monitoring (65). *Bilophila wadsworthia* and *Centipeda periodontii* are new genuses and species found in abdominal and endodontic infections respectedly (66).

Prevotella oralis is part of the normal flora of the mouth and vagina. Unlike *B. fragilis*, however, strains of *P. oralis* generally are susceptible to penicillin and the cephalosporins, although more strains of *P. oralis* have shown resistance to these drugs. *P. oralis* almost never is found in pure culture in clinical infection. This organism can possess a capsule (67). It has been recovered from almost all types of respiratory tract and subcutaneous infections, including aspiration pneumonia (38), lung abscess (61), chronic otitis media (14), and sinusitis (15), and subcutaneous abscesses around the oral cavity (58).

Pigmented *Prevotella* and *Porphyromonas* require the presence of both hemin and vitamin K_1 for growth. The requirement for vitamin K_1 in vivo often is met by coexistence with organisms that are capable of supplying this need Pigmented *Prevotella* and *Porphyromonas* are part of the normal oral and vaginal flora and are the predominant anaerobic gram negative bacilli isolated from respiratory infections. These include aspiration pneumonia (38), lung abscess (61), chronic otitis media (14), and chronic sinusitis (15). These organisms have been recovered also from abscesses and burns around the oral cavity (58), human bites (68), paronychia (69), urinary tract infection (70), brain abscesses (37), and osteomyelitis (71). Also, they have been isolated from patients with bacteremia associated with infections of the upper respiratory tract (11). Pigmented *Prevotella* and *Porphyromonas* play a major role in the pathogenesis of periodontal disease (72) and periodontal abscesses (73).

Of the pigmented *Prevotella* and *Porphyromonas, Porphyromonas asaccharolytica* is generally the most frequent clinical isolate. *Prevotella intermedia* is identified less frequently, and *Prevotella melaninogenica* is the least common. The presence of capsular material suppresses phagocytosis and is therefore an important factor influencing the pathogenicity of the pigmented *Prevotella* and *Porphyromonas* (67,74,75). *Porphyromonas gingivalis* is very similar to *P. asaccharolytica* and only the production of phenylacetic acid by *P. gingivalis* will differentiate them (76). *P. gingivalis* is an important isolate in periodontitis (76).

Bacteroides ruminicola ss. *brevis* also has been recovered from these sites (38,61) as well as from peritonsillar abscesses (17), chronic sinusitis (15), mastoiditis (16), and peritonitis (18). *B. ruminicola* has recently been divided into *Prevotella buccae* and *Prevotella oris* according to their beta-glucosidase activity (76). *P. oris* strains are generally more resistant to penicillin than *P. buccae*.

B. bivia and *B. disiens* are important isolates in obstetrical and gynecological infections. They account for 9% and 1% of all anaerobic gram-negative bacilli isolates.

Bacteroides ureolyticus (formerly called *Bacteroides corrodens* and related to Campylobacter) characteristically forms small colonies with a zone around or under the colony that has been described as "pitting" of the agar: thus its former name "corrodens." *B. ureolyticus* is part of the normal flora of the mouth and has been isolated from blood cultures shortly after dental surgery, periodontal abscesses, aspiration pneumonia (38,60), and lung abscesses (60,61).

Fusobacterium Species

Cells of *Fusobacterium* spp. are moderately long and thin with tapered ends and have typical fusiform morphology. The species of *Fusobacterium* seen most often in clinical infections are *Fusobacterium nucleatum, Fusobacterium necrophorum, Fusobacterium mortiferum,* and *Fusobacterium varium. F. nucleatum* is the predominant *Fusobacterium* from clinical specimens, often associated with infections of the mouth, lung (38,60), and brain (37). They are often isolated from abscesses, obstetrical and gynecological infections, chest infections, blood, and wounds (77).

Since these organisms are part of the normal flora of the oral and gastrointestinal flora, they are found in almost all types of infections in children. These include bacteremia (11,32), meningitis associated with otologic diseases (37,44,45), peritonitis following rupture of viscus (18), and subcutaneous abscesses and burns near the oral or anal orifices (Fig. 3) (58,59).

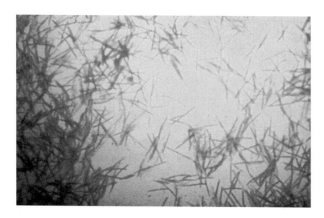

FIGURE 3 Gram stain of *Fusobacterium nucleatum.*

A growing resistance of anaerobic gram-negative bacilli previously susceptible to penicillins has been noticed in the last three decades (78,79). Resistance grew among members of the pigmented *Prevotella* and *Porphyromonas, Fusobacterium* spp., *P. oralis, P. disiens, P. bivia,* and *P. oris-buccae*. The main mechanism of resistance is through the production of the enzyme beta-lactamase. Complete identification and susceptibility testing and ability to produce beta-lactamase of members of the *B. fragilis* group as well as other anaerobic gram-negative bacilli are factors of practical importance when making choices between antimicrobials for the therapy of infections involving these organisms.

The recovery rate of the different anaerobic gram-negative bacilli in infected sites is similar to their distribution in the normal flora (1,7). While *B. fragilis* group were more often isolated in sites proximal to the gastrointestinal tract (abdomen, bile), pigmented *Prevotella* and *Porphyromonas* and *Fusobacterium* spp. were more prevalent in infections proximal to the oral cavity (bones, sinuses, chest), and *P. bivia* and *P. disiens* were more often isolated in obstetric and gynecologic infections. Knowledge of this common mode of distribution allows for logical choice of antimicrobials adequate for the therapy of infections in these sites.

GRAM-POSITIVE COCCI

Anaerobic cocci have been most often reported either as "anaerobic streptococci" or "anaerobic gram-positive cocci." These organisms were previously divided into *Peptococcus* spp. and *Peptostreptococcus* sp. However, they are currently all named *Peptostreptococcus* spp. and further divided according to species primarily on the basis of their metabolic products (76). The species most commonly isolated are *Peptostreptococcus magnus* (18% of all anaerobic gram-positive cocci isolated in Table 2), *Peptostreptococcus asaccharolyticus* (17%), *Peptostrepto-coccus anaerobius* (16%), *Peptostreptococcus prevotii* (13%), and *Peptostreptococcus micros* (4%) (2,3,76).

The infectious sites where anaerobic cocci predominate are in descending order of frequency: ear, bone, cysts, obstetric and gynecologic, abscesses, and sinuses. These organisms are part of the normal flora of the mouth, upper respiratory tract, intestinal tract, vagina, and skin (7). Their presence has been documented in adults in a variety of syndromes, including endocarditis, brain abscesses, puerperal sepsis, traumatic wounds, and postoperative necro-tizing fasciitis (2,3). They have been recovered in children in subcutaneous abscesses and burns around the oral and anal areas, intra-abdominal infections (18), decubitus ulcers (80), and also have been isolated as causes of bacteremia (11), and brain abscesses (37,81). These organisms are predominant isolates also in all types of respiratory infections in children and adults including chronic sinusitis (15), mastoiditis (16), acute (82,83) and chronic (14) otitis media, aspiration pneumonia (38,60), and lung abscess (60,61). They generally are recovered mixed with other aerobic or anaerobic organisms but in many cases, they are the only pathogens recovered. This may be of particular significance in cases of bacteremia (11,32,82) or acute otitis media (83).

Microaerophilic streptococci are not true anaerobes as they can become also tolerant after subculture, however they grow better anaerobically, and are often grouped under anaerobes in many studies. These organisms include the *Streptococcus anginosus* group (previously called *Streptococcus milleri* group, that include *Streptococcus constellatus* and *S. intermedius*), and *Gemella morbillorum* (previously called *Streptococcus morbillorum*) (84). Microaerophilic streptococci are of particular importance in chronic sinusitis (14) and brain abscess (37,81,85,86). They were also recovered from obstetric and gynecologic infections and abscesses(85,86).

GRAM-NEGATIVE COCCI

There are three species described as anaerobic gram-negative cocci: *Veillonella, Acidaminococcus,* and *Megasphaera*. There are two described species of *Veillonella* and only one each of the other two genera. The veillonellae are the most frequently involved of the three species and are part of the normal flora of the mouth, vagina, and the small intestine of some persons (7). Although they rarely are isolated from clinical infections, these organisms have been recovered occasionally from almost every type of infection mostly mixed with other bacteria (3,87,88). *Veillonella* spp. were recovered from abscesses, aspiration pneumonias, endocarditis, meningitis, burns, bites, and sinuses.

CONCLUSION

Many infectious diseases can be produced by anaerobic bacteria. Anaerobes of major clinical importance tend to follow certain predictable patterns according to anatomic sites and their virulence. In the upper respiratory passages and lung, the major anaerobic pathogens are *Peptostreptococcus* spp., pigmental *Prevotella* and *Porphyromonas* spp., and *Fusobacterium* spp. In intra-abdominal infections and female genital infections, the most frequent isolates are of the *B. fragilis* group followed by anaerobic gram-positive cocci and *Clostridium* species.

Recognition of the pathogenic features of these organisms enables prompt identification and initiation of appropriate management of the infections that they cause.

REFERENCES

1. Jousimies H, Summanen P. Recent taxonomic changes and terminology update of clinically significant anaerobic gram-negative bacteria (excluding spirochetes). Clin Infect Dis 2002; 35(Suppl. 1):S17–21.
2. Finegold SM. Anaerobic Bacteria in Human Disease. New York: Academic Press, 1977.
3. Brook I. Recovery of anaerobic bacteria from clinical specimens in 12 years at two military hospitals. J Clin Microbiol 1988; 26:1181–8.
4. Hatheway CL. Toxogenic clostridia. Clin Microbiol Rev 1990; 3:66–98.
4a. Aldape MJ, Bryant AE, Stevens DL. *Clostridium Sordellii*: epidemiology, clinical findings, and current perspectives in diagnosis and treatment. Clin Infect Dis 2006; 43:1436–46.
5. Sunenshine RH, McDonald LC. *Clostridium difficile*-associated disease: new challenges from an established pathogen. Cleve Clin J Med 2006; 73:187–97.
6. Bhatia R, Prabhakar S, Grover VK. Tetanus. Neurol India 2002; 50:398–407.
7. Rosebury T. Microorganisms Indigenous to Man. New York: McGraw-Hill Book Company, 1966.
8. Cashore WJ, Peter G, Lauermann M, Stonestreet BS, Oh W. *Clostridium* colonization and clostridial toxin in neonatal necrotizing enterocolitis. J Pediatr 1981; 98:308–11.
9. Sturm R, Staneck JL, Stauffer LR, Neblett WW, III. Neonatal necrotizing enterocolitis associated with penicillin resistant *Clostridium butyricum*. Pediatrics 1980; 66:928–31.
10. Cooperstock MS, Steffen E, Yolken R, Onderdonk A. *Clostridium difficile* in normal infants and sudden infant death syndrome: an association with infant formula feeding. Pediatrics 1982; 70:91–5.
11. Brook I, Controni G, Rodriguez W, Martin WJ. Anaerobic bacteremia in children. Am J Dis Child 1980; 134:1052–6.
12. Brook I, Gluck RS. *Clostridium paraputrificum* sepsis in sickle cell disease: a report of a case. South Med J 1980; 73:1644–5.
13. Brook I, Schwartz RH, Controni G. *Clostridium ramosum* isolation in acute otitis media. Clin Pediatr 1979; 18:699–700.
14. Brook I. Microbiology of chronic otitis media with perforation in children. Am J Dis Child 1980; 130:564–6.
15. Brook I. Bacteriological features of chronic sinusitis in children. JAMA 1981; 246:967–9.
16. Brook I. Aerobic and anaerobic bacteriology of chronic mastoiditis in children. Am J Dis Child 1981; 135:478–9.
17. Brook I. Aerobic and anaerobic bacteriology of peritonsillar abscess in children. Acta Pediatr Scand 1981; 70:831–5.
18. Brook I. Bacterial studies of peritoneal cavity and postoperative surgical wound drainage following perforated appendix in children. Ann Surg 1980; 192:208–12.
19. Brook I. A 12 year study of aerobic and anaerobic bacteria in intra-abdominal and postsurgical abdominal wound infections. Surg Gynecol Obstet 1989; 169:387–92.
20. Brook I, Frazier E. Microbiology of liver and spleen abscesses. J Med Microbiol 1998; 47:1075–80.
21. Brook I, Frazier E. Aerobic and anaerobic microbiology of retroperitoneal abscesses. Clin Infect Dis 1998; 26:938–41.
22. Brook I, Martin WJ, Finegold SM. Effect of silver nitrate application on the conjunctival flora of the newborn and the occurrence of clostridial conjunctivitis. J Pediatr Ophthalmol Strabismus 1978; 15:173–83.
23. Brook I. Clostridial infection in children. J Med Microbiol 1995; 42:78–82.
24. Sato J, Mochizuki K, Homma N. Affinity of the *Bifidobacterium* to intestinal mucosal epithelial cells. Bifidobacteria Microflora 1982; 1:51–4.

25. Gorbach SL, Thadepalli H. Clindamycin in pure and mixed anaerobic infections. Arch Intern Med 1974; 134:87–92.
26. O'Connor J, MacCormick DE. Mixed organism peritonitis complicating continuous ambulatory peritoneal dialysis. N Z Med J 1982; 95:811–2.
27. Thomas AV, Sodeman TH, Bentz RR. *Bifidobacterium (Actinomyces) eriksonii* infection. Am Rev Respir Dis 1974; 110:663–8.
28. Hata D, Yoshida A, Ohkubo H, et al. Meningitis caused by *Bifidobacterium* in an infant. Pediatr Infect Dis J 1988; 7:669–71.
29. Vincent JW, Falkler WA, Suzuki JB. Systemic antibody response of clinically characterized patients with antigens of *Eubacterium brachy* initially and following periodontal therapy. J Periodontol 1986; 57:625–31.
30. Hill GB, Ayers OM, Kohan AP. Characteristics and sites and infection of *Eubacterium nodatum, Eubacterium timidum, Eubacterium brachy,* and other asaccharolytic eubacteria. J Clin Microbiol 1987; 25:1540–5.
31. Fainstein V, Elting LS, Bodey GP. Bacteremia caused by non-sporulating anaerobes in cancer patients. A 12-year experience. Medicine (Baltimore) 1989; 68:151–62.
32. Brook I. Anaerobic bacterial bacteremia: 12-year experience in two military hospitals. J Infect Dis 1989; 160:1071–5.
33. Cox SM, Phillips LE, Mercer LJ, Stager CE, Waller S, Faro S. Lactobacillemia of amniotic fluid origin. Obstet Gynecol 1986; 68:134–5.
34. Sherman ME, Albrecht M, DeGirolami PC, et al. *Lactobacillus*: an unusual case of splenic abscess and sepsis in an immunocompromised host. Am J Clin Pathol 1987; 88:659–62.
35. Brook I, Frazier EH. Significant recovery of nonsporulating anaerobic rods from clinical specimens. Clin Infect Dis 1993; 16:476–80.
36. Brook I. Isolation of non-sporing anaerobic rods from infections in children. J Med Microbiol 1996; 45:21–6.
37. Brook I. Microbiology and management of brain abscess in children. J Pediatr Neurol 2004; 2:125–30.
38. Brook I, Finegold SM. Bacteriology of aspiration pneumonia in children. Pediatrics 1980; 65:1115–20.
39. Brook I. Actinomycosis. In: Goldman L, Ausiello D, eds. Cecil Textbook of Medicine. 22nd ed. Philadelphia, PA: Saunders, 2004:1883–5 (chap. 337).
40. Mourelatos K, Eady EA, Cunliffe WJ, Clark SM, Cove JH. Temporal changes in sebum excretion and propionibacterial colonization in preadolescent children with and without acne. Br J Dermatol 2007; 156:22–31.
41. Brook I, Pettit TH, Martin WJ, Finegold SM. Aerobic and anaerobic bacteriology of acute conjunctivitis. Ann Ophthalmol 1978; 11:13–6.
42. Elsner P. Antimicrobials and the skin physiological and pathological flora. Curr Probl Dermatol 2006; 33:35–41.
43. Brook I. Presence of anaerobic bacteria in conjunctivitis associated with wearing contact lenses. Ann Ophthalmol 1988; 20:397–9.
44. Heineman HS, Braude AI. Anaerobic infection of the brain. Observations on eighteen consecutive cases of brain abscess. Am J Med 1963; 35:682–97.
45. Mathisen GE, Meyer RD, George WL, et al. Brain abscess and cerebritis. Rev Infect Dis 1984; 6:101–6.
46. Dunkle LM, Brotherton TJ, Feigin RD. Anaerobic infections in children: a prospective study. Pediatrics 1976; 57:311–20.
47. Goldberg MH. *Corynebacterium*: an oral-systemic pathogen. Report of cases. J Oral Surg 1971; 29:349–51.
48. Finegold SM, Bartlett JG. Anaerobic pleuropulmonary infections. Cleve Clin J Med 1975; 42:101–11.
49. Kaplan K, Weinstein L. Diptheroid infections of man. Ann Intern Med 1969; 70:919–29.
50. Steinbok P, Cochrane DD, Kestle JR. The significance of bacteriologically positive ventriculoperitoneal shunt components in the absence of other signs of shunt infection. J Neurosurg 1996; 84:617–23.
51. Brook I, Frazier EH. Infections caused by *Propionibacterium* species. Rev Infect Dis 1991; 13:819–22.
52. Beeler BA, Crowder JG, Smith JW, White A. *Propionibacterium acnes*: pathogen in central nervous system shunt infection. Report of three cases including immune complex glomerulo-nephritis. Am J Med 1976; 61:935–8.
53. Purdy S, deBerker D. Acnes. BMJ 2006; 333:949–53.
54. Brook I. Infection caused by *Propionibacterium* in children. Clin Pediatr 1994; 33:486–90.
55. Nakano V, Padilla G, do Valle Marques M, Avila-Campos MJ. Plasmid-related beta-lactamase production in *Bacteroides fragilis* strains. Res Microbiol 2004; 155:843–6.
56. Holdeman LV, Cato EP, Moore WE. Taxonomy of anaerobes: present state of the art. Rev Infect Dis 1984; 6(Suppl. 1):S3–10.
57. Botta GA, Arzese A, Minisini R, Trani G. Role of structural and extracellular virulence factors in gram-negative anaerobic bacteria. Clin Infect Dis 1994; 18:S260–4.

58. Brook I, Frazier EH. Aerobic and anaerobic bacteriology of wounds and cutaneous abscesses. Arch Surg; 1990; 125:1445-51.
59. Mousa HA. Aerobic, anaerobic and fungal burn wound infections. J Hosp Infect 1997; 37:317–23.
60. Bartlett JG. Anaerobic bacterial infections of the lung and pleural space. Clin Infect Dis 1993; 16(Suppl. 4):S248–55.
61. Brook I, Finegold SM. The bacteriology and therapy of lung abscess in children. J Pediatr 1979; 94:10–4.
62. Brook I, Barrett CT, Brinkman CR, III, Martin WJ, Finegold SM. Aerobic and anaerobic flora of maternal cervix and newborn's conjunctiva and gastric fluid: a prospective study. Pediatrics 1979; 63:451–5.
63. Brook I, Martin WJ, Finegold SM. Neonatal pneumonia caused by members of the *Bacteroides fragilis* group. Clin Pediatr 1980; 19:541–4.
64. Brook I. Bacteriology of neonatal omphalitis. J Infect 1982; 5:127–31.
65. Brook I. Osteomyelitis and bacteremia caused by *Bacteroides fragilis*: a complication of fetal monitoring. Clin Pediatr 1980; 19:639–40.
66. Finegold SM, Jousimies-Somer H. Recently described clinically important anaerobic bacteria: medical aspects. Clin Infect Dis 1997; 25(Suppl. 2):S88–93.
67. Brook I, Gillmore JD, Coolbaugh JC, Walker RI. Pathogenicity of encapsulated *Bacteroides melanino-genicus* group, *Bacteroides oralis*, and *Bacteroides ruminicola* in abscesses in mice. J Infect 1983; 7:218–26.
68. Brook I. Microbiology of human and animal bite wounds. Pediatr Infect Dis J 1987; 6:29–32.
69. Brook I. Paronychia: a mixed infection. Microbiology and management. J Hand Surg [Br] 1993; 18:358–9.
70. Brook I. Urinary tract infection caused by anaerobic bacteria in children. Urology 1980; 16:596–8.
71. Brook I, Frazier EH. Anaerobic osteomyelitis and arthritis in a military hospital: a 10-year experience. Am J Med 1993; 94:21–8.
72. Kilian M, Frandsen EV, Haubek D, Poulsen K. The etiology of periodontal disease revisited by population genetic analysis. Periodontol 2000 2006; 42:158–79.
73. Brook I, Frazier EH, Gher ME. Aerobic and anaerobic microbiology of periapical abscess. Oral Microbiol Immunol 1991; 6:123–5.
74. Okuda K, Takazoe I. Antiphagocytic effects of the capsular structure of a pathogenic strain of *Bacteroides melaninogenicus*. Bull Tokyo Med Dent Univ 1973; 14:99–104.
75. Brook I. *Prevotella* and *Porphyromonas* infections in children. J Med Microbiol 1995; 42:340–7.
76. Jousimies-Somer HR, Summanen P, Baron EJ, Citron DM, Wexler HM, Finegold SM. Wadsworth-KTL Anaerobic Bacteriology Manual. 6th ed. Belmont, CA: Star Publishing, 2002.
77. Brook I. Fusobacterial infections in children. J Infect 1994; 28:155.
78. Brook I, Calhoun L, Yocum P. Beta lactamase producing isolates of *Bacteroides* species from children. Antimicrob Agents Chemother 1980; 18:164–6.
79. Brook I. Infections caused by beta-lactamase-producing *Fusobacterium* spp. in children. Pediatr Infect Dis J 1993; 12:532–4.
80. Montgomerie JZ, Chan E, Gilmore DS, Canawati HN, Sapico FL. Low mortality among patients with spinal cord injury and bacteremia. Rev Infect Dis 1991; 13:867–71.
81. Brook I, Friedman E, Rodriguez WJ, Controni G. Complications of sinusitis in children. Pediatrics 1980; 66:568–72.
82. Brook I. Peptostreptococcal infection in children. Scand J Infect Dis 1994; 26:503–10.
83. Brook I, Anthony BF, Finegold SM. Aerobic and anaerobic bacteriology of acute otitis media in children. J Pediatr 1978; 92:13–6.
84. Belko J, Godmann DA, Macone A, Zaidi AK. Clinical significant infections with organisms of *Streptococcus milleri* group. Pediatr Infect. Dis J 2002; 21:715–23.
85. Brook I. Microaerophilic streptococcal infection in children. J Infect 1994; 28:241–9.
86. Brook I, Frazier EH. Microaerophilic streptococci as a significant pathogen: a twelve-year review. J Med 1994; 25:129–44.
87. Brook I. Veillonella infections in children. J Clin Microbiol 1996; 34:1283–5.
88. Brook I, Frazier E. Infections caused by *Veillonella* species. Infect Dis Clin Prac 1992; 1:377–81.

2 | Anaerobes as Part of the Human Indigenous Microbial Flora

The human mucous and epithelial surfaces are colonized with aerobic and anaerobic microorganisms (1). These surfaces are the skin, conjunctiva, mouth, nose, throat, lower intestinal tract, vagina, and the urethra. The trachea, bronchi, esophagus, stomach, and upper urinary tract are not normally colonized by indigenous flora. However, a limited number of transient organisms may by present at these locations. Differences in the environment, such as oxygen tension and pH and variations in bacterial adherence, account for the changing patterns of bacterial colonization. The microflora also varies within the different body sites; in the oral cavity, for example, the organisms in the buccal folds vary in their concentration and types from those from the tongue or gingival sulci. However, the bacteria that prevail in a system generally belong to certain major bacterial species. The relative and total bacterial counts can be influenced by various factors, such as age, diet, anatomic variations, illness, hospitalization, and antimicrobial therapy.

Anaerobes outnumber aerobes in all mucous surfaces, and certain types predominate in the different sites (Tables 1 and 2). Their recovery is inversely related to the oxygen tension. Their predominance in the skin, mouth, nose, and throat which are exposed to oxygen is explained by the anaerobic microenvironment generated by the facultative bacteria that consume oxygen.

Recognizing the unique composition of the flora at certain sites is useful for predicting which organisms may be involved in an adjacent infection and can assist in the selection of empiric antimicrobial therapy. It can also be useful in determining the source and significance of microorganisms recovered from body sites. For example, bacterial endocarditis caused by *Enterococcus faecalis* is more often associated with urinary tract infection, while alpha hemolytic streptococcal endocarditis is more often observed in patients with poor dental hygiene and tooth extraction.

Knowledge of the indigenous microflora is helpful in determining the consequence of overgrowth of one microorganism by another. Antimicrobials that suppress the intestinal anaerobes may select for the over growth of *Clostridium difficile* which can result in the production of a potent enterotoxin inducing colitis. Recognition of the normal flora can also help the microbiology laboratory to select proper selective culture media inhibiting certain organisms regarded as contaminants. Furthermore, proper media can enhance the growth of expected pathogens. The recovery of certain organisms from the blood can suggest a possible port of entry (i.e., *Clostridium* and *Bacteroides fragilis* usually originate from the gastrointestinal tract) (2).

The normal flora is not exclusively a potential hazard for the host. It can also serve as a beneficial partner. An example of such a benefit is the development of vitamin K deficiency following antimicrobial therapy, which suppresses the gut flora that produces this vitamin.

The normal flora also serves as protector from colonization and subsequent invasion by potential pathogens. Bacterial interference (BI) may play a major role in the maintenance of the normal flora of skin and mucous membranes, by preventing colonization and subsequent invasion by exogenous bacteria (Fig. 1). BI is expressed through several mechanisms. These includes the production of antagonistic substances, changes in the microenvironment and reduction of needed nutritional substances (3). The mediators of BI include the production of

TABLE 1 Normal Aerobic and Anaerobic Flora

	Aerobes	Anaerobes	Predominant anaerobic organisms
Skin			*Propionbacterium acnes*, *Peptostreptococcus* spp.
Oral cavity	10^{8-9}	10^{9-11}	Pigmented *Prevotella*, and *Porphyromonas*, *Fusobacterium* spp.
Upper GI[a]	10^{2-5}	10^{3-7}	*Bacteroides fragilis* group
Lower GI[b]	10^{5-9}	10^{10-12}	*Clostridium* spp.
Vagina	10^{8}	10^{9}	*Prevotella bivia*, *Prevotella disiens*

Number of organisms per 1 g secretion or contents.
[a] The small intestine and accending colon.
[b] The transverse, descending colon, and rectum.

bacteriocins, bacteriophages, or bacteriolytic enzymes, and molecules such as hydrogen peroxide, lactic or fatty acids and ammonia (3).

THE SKIN

The commonest members of the cutaneous microflora are *Staphylococcus*, *Micrococcus*, *Corynebacterium*, *Propionibacterium*, *Brevibacterium*, and *Acinetobacter* and the yeast *Pityrosporum* (Table 2). The skin flora varies depending on the skin site and its characteristics.

Several potential pathogens are only transient residents around orifices. The oral region or sites that can be in contact with the oropharyngeal flora (i.e., nipples, fingers, genitalia) can become colonized with oral flora organisms (4). These include *Haemophilus*, *Peptostreptococcus*, *Fusobacterium*, and pigmented *Prevotella* and *Porphyromonas* spp. Similarly the rectal, vulvovaginal areas, and lower extremities may become colonized with colonic and vaginal organisms. These include *B. fragilis* group, *Clostridium* spp., (of rectal origin), or *Neisseria gonorrheae*, group B Streptococci, and *Prevotella* (of vaginal origin). These can cause local (i.e., wounds, abrasions, infected burns, decubitus ulcers) or serious infections including bacteremia (2).

The anaerobic microflora of the skin generally is made up of the genus *Propionibacterium* (5). *Propionibacterium acnes* predominates, while *Propionibacterium granulosum* and *Propionibacterium*

TABLE 2 Predominant Human Microbial Flora at Body Sites

Type of bacteria	Skin	Conjunctiva	Nasopharynx	Oral cavity	Lower gastro-intestinal tract	Genitourinary tract
Aerobic and facultative						
Staphylococcus spp.	+	+	+			
Streptococcus spp.	+	+	+	+	+[a]	+
Haempohilus spp.				+		
Moraxella catarrhalis				+		
Enterobacteriaceae					+	+
Anaerobic						
Veillonella sp.				+	+	+
Peptostreptococcus spp.		+	+	+	+	+
Actinomyces spp.				+		+
Bifidobacterium spp.				+	+	+
Eubacterium spp.				+	+	+
Lactobacillus spp.					+	+
Propionibacterium spp.	+	+	+		+	
Clostridium spp.					+	
Fusobacterium spp.					+	
Bacteriodes spp.					+	+
Prevotella spp.			+[b]			+[c]
Porphyromonas spp			+[b]			

[a] *Enterococcus* spp.
[b] Pigmented species.
[c] *Prevotella bivia* and *Prevotella disiens*.

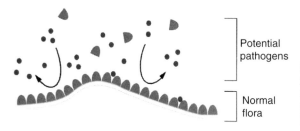

Potential
pathogens

Normal
flora

FIGURE 1 Normal flora organisms prevent colonization by potential pathogens by physically competing with them on colonization sites and essential nutrients, and by production of bacteriocins.

avidum are rare. *P. acnes* and *P. granulosum* are found on skin with a high sebum content; *P. acnes* is found in all postpubertal individuals; whereas *P. granulosum* is found in 10% and 20% of individuals in numbers about 100 to 1000 fold fewer than *P. acnes*. *Eubacterium* and *Peptostreptococcus* may also be encountered.

These microorganisms grow within the sebaceous glands openings and consequently their distribution is proportional to the number of glands, the amount of sebum, and the composition of skin surface lipids (6).

Propionibacteria produce free fatty acids from triglycerides by generating lipase (7). These acids are antibacterial and antifungal and interfere with the growth of nonindigenous microorganism such as *Staphylococcus* spp., *Streptococcus pyogenes*, and aerobic gram negative bacilli. These fatty acids may, however, play a deleterious role in the development of acne by causing inflammation (8). The numbers of *P. acnes* are higher in adults than in young children. Because of their prevalence in the skin and the ear canal, they can contaminate blood cultures and aspirates of cerebrospinal fluid, abscesses, and middle ear fluid.

THE ORAL CAVITY

The establishment of the normal oral flora is initiated at birth. Lactobacilli and Peptostreptococci, reach high numbers within a few days. *Actinomyces*, *Fusobacterium*, and *Nocardia* are acquired by six months. Following that time, *Prevotella*, *Porphyromonas*, *Leptotrichia*, *Propionibacterium*, and *Candida* also are established (9). *Fusobacterium* populations attain high numbers after dentition.

The predominant facultative organisms are the alpha-hemolytic streptococci (the species *mitis*, *milleri*, *sanguis*, *intermedius*, and *salivarius*) (10). Other organisms are *Moraxella catarrhalis* and *Haemophillus influenzae*, which may cause otitis, sinusitis, or bronchitis. Encapsulated *H. influenzae* can cause meningitis and bacteremia. The oropharynx also contains *Staphylococcus aureus* and *Staphylococcus epidermidis* that can cause chronic infections.

The oropharynx is seldom colonized by Enterobacteriaceae. In contrast, hospitalized patients are often colonized with these organisms. This may be due to selection following the administration of antimicrobials (11) and can contribute to the development of anaerobic gram negative bacilli (AGNB) pneumonia.

Oropharyngeal selective decontamination using topical polymyxin B, neomycin, and vancomycin is effective in reducing colonization and pneumonia with *S. aureus* and AGNB, without suppression of anaerobes organisms (12).

Anaerobes are present in large numbers in the mouth and the oropharynx, particularly in patients with poor dental hygiene, caries, or periodontal disease (Fig. 2). They outnumber the aerobes 10:1 to 100:1. The predominant anaerobes are *Peptostreptococcus*, *Veillonella*, *Bacteroides*, pigmented *Prevotella* and *Porphyromonas*, and *Fusobacterium* spp., *Porphyromonas gingivalis*, *Bacteroides ureolyticus*. *Actinomyces* spp., treponemas, *Leptotrichia buccalis*, *Bifidobacterium*, *Eubacterium*, and *Propionibacterium* spp., (1). Some of these organisms are a potential source of chronic infections such as otitis, sinusitis, aspiration pneumonia and lung abscesses, and oropharyngeal and dental abscesses.

Anaerobes can adhere to dental surfaces and contribute through the elaboration of metabolic products to the production of both caries and periodontal disease ranging from gingivitis to periodontitis (10).

Oropharyngeal Flora

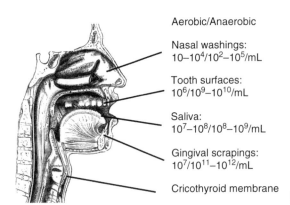

Aerobic/Anaerobic

Nasal washings:
$10-10^4/10^2-10^5$/mL

Tooth surfaces:
$10^6/10^9-10^{10}$/mL

Saliva:
$10^7-10^8/10^8-10^9$/mL

Gingival scrapings:
$10^7/10^{11}-10^{12}$/mL

Cricothyroid membrane

FIGURE 2   The microbiology of the oral flora.

The oral cavity is an open ecosystem, with a dynamic balance between the entrance of organisms, colonization, and the host defenses directed at their removal. To avoid elimination, bacteria adhere to either hard dental surfaces or epithelial surfaces and form a biofilm. Biofilm is defined as a community of bacteria intimately associated with each other and included within an exopolymer matrix: this biological unit exhibits its own properties. The oral biofilm formation and development have been correlated with all common oral and otolaryngological pathologies, such as dental caries, periodontal disease peri-implantitis otitis, sinusilitis and tonsillitis (13) (Fig. 3) (9).

The recovery rate of aerobic (*H. influenzae*, *M. catarrhalis*, and *S. aureus*) and anaerobic (*Prevotella*, *Porphyromonas*, and *Fusobacterium*) beta-lactamase producing bacteria (BLPB) in the oropharynx has increased in recent years, and these organisms were isolated in over half of the patients with head and neck infections (14). BLPB can protect not only themselves from the activity of penicillin but also penicillin-susceptible organisms as the enzyme is released into the infected tissue or abscess fluid (15). The high incidence of isolation of BLPB may be due to their selection following penicillin therapy (16).

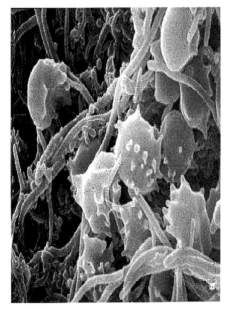

FIGURE 3   Scanning electron micrograph of dental plaque biofilm.

THE GASTROINTESTINAL TRACT

Gastrointestinal tract colonization is initiated during delivery as the newborn aspirates cervical canal material (17). The development of the flora is a gradual, and is determined by factors such as composition of the maternal gut micro flora, environmental, and genetic aspects. Variables such as, dietary constituents, gestational age, degree of hygiene, mode of delivery, use of antibiotics or other medication and a need for nursing in incubators, can all effect the microbial colonization (18).

Streptococci, enterococci, and staphylococci usually are present in the first days of life. At the end of one week the fecal flora is predominately anaerobic and contains *Bifidobacterium*, *Bacteroides*, and *Clostridium* spp. The commonest facultative fecal flora is *Escherichia coli* and *E. faecalis* (19). Both prematurity and breast feeding were less frequently associated with colonization by anaerobes, *B. fragilis* was less likely to be recovered in breast-fed infants than in their formula-fed counterparts, and *Bifidobacterium* predominates in breast-fed infants (20). After weaning the numbers of *Bifidobacterium* decrease, while *Bacteroides* increases.

The gut flora plays an essential role in the development of the gut immunity. Intestinal micro-organisms can down-regulate an allergic inflammation by counterbalancing type 2 T-helper cell responses and by enhancing antigen exclusion through an immunoglobulin (Ig)A response (21).

The gastrointestinal flora is dynamic and varies at different locations and levels. These changes depend on factors such as anatomical changes, diet, state of health, and ingestion of medication that alter the stomach acidity, secretory Igs, intestinal motility, and BI (22). Factors that interfere with colonization are active peristalsis, gastric acidity, and high oxidation–reduction potential.

The esophagus, stomach, duodenum, jejunum, and proximal ileum normally contain relatively few bacteria. However, the flora becomes more complex and the number of different bacterial species increases in the distal portions.

Even though the stomach is constantly seeded with oropharyngeal organisms (22), the gastric acidity decreases their number. Those who receive acid reducing medications, or suffer from gastric bleeding have a higher pH, and subsequently more surviving bacteria (23). The bacterial counts in the small intestine are relatively low, with total counts of 10^2 to 10^5 aerobic and anaerobic organisms per milliliter. The predominate organisms up to the ileocecal valve are gram-positive facultatives, while *Bacteroides* (mostly *B. fragilis* group), *Bifidobacterium*, *Lactobacillus*, and coliform predominate below that structure (24). The colon is colonized by the largest numbers of microorganisms of any inhabited region of the human body; 300 to 400 different species and 10^{12} bacteria per gram fecal material. Approximately 99.9% of these bacteria are anaerobic (ratio aerobes to anaerobes; 1 to 1000 or 10,000) (Fig. 4).

Bacteroides is the predominant bacterial genus in the intestine, present at approximately 10^{11} organisms per gram dry weight (24). The most frequently isolated are *Bacteroides vulgatus*, *B. thetaiotaomicron*, *B. distasonis*, *B. fragilis*, and *B. ovatus*. Among the gram-positive rods, *Bifidobacterium adolescents*, *Eubacterium aerofaciens*, *Eubacterium lentum*, and *C. ramosum* predominate (24).

B. fragilis group and other AGNB undergoes morphological changes as it transforms itself to become a pathogen (25). About 80% of AGNB recovered from blood and abscesses were encapsulated, while only 10% of stool or pharynx isolates were encapsulated ($p < 0.001$). Pili were observed in 6% of blood, 75% of abscesses, and 69% of normal flora isolates ($p < 0.001$).

AGNB expresses different morphological features at different sites as some structures are advantageous or detrimental (25). Pili enables mucosal adherence to those who colonize. Because they are not exposed to macrophages, capsules do not provide them with any advantage. In abscesses, capsules provide protection from macrophages, and pili enable attachment. In contrast, the presence of pili may interfere with systemic spread, since piliated organisms may be more easily phagocytosed (26). The gut harbors numerous AGNB but only those that can adapt to the changing environment can cause illness.

Anatomic and physiologic derangement in the gut can lead to bacterial overgrowth in the upper small bowel (22). This was demonstrated in patients with hypochlorydia, atropic

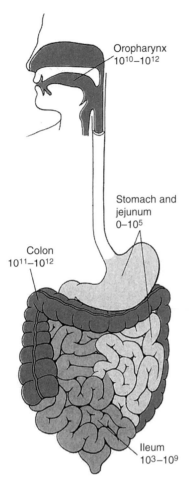

Oropharynx
10^{10}–10^{12}

Stomach and
jejunum
0–10^5

Colon
10^{11}–10^{12}

Ileum
10^3–10^9

FIGURE 4 The number of endogenous anaerobic organisms in the gastrointestinal tract.

gastritis, intake of antacids or cimetidine, ineffective peristalsis, multiple diverticula, cirrhosis, chronic malnutrition, excessive small bowel resection, and abdominal irradiation (22). Proliferation of a colonic-type flora in the small intestine can cause a variety of metabolic disturbances, including steatorrhea, vitamin B_{12} deficiencies, and carbohydrate malabsorption.

Acute diarrhea produces profound alterations in the gut flora. Under certain conditions the resident microflora is eclipsed by a pathogen (27). The rapid transit of diarrheal stool results in a marked reduction in the large bowel anaerobic population. Resolution of diarrhea is accompanied by rapid restitution of the normal flora.

The normal colonic flora is relatively constant and constitutes a defense mechanism against infections by pathogens. Suppression of the anaerobic flora by antimicrobials effective against most anaerobic bacteria except *C. difficile*, can cause pseudomembranous colitis (28). The ability of colonic flora to interfere with the establishment of pathogens is termed "colonization resistance" (29). Antibiotics effective against anaerobes increase the gut population and subsequently the potentials for translocation of Enterobacteriaceae (30).

Numerous studies utilized selective gut decontamination in an attempt to eradicate only the Enterobacteriaceae and preserve the anaerobes by using antimicrobials that are only effective against Enterobacteriaceae (31). The subjects of these studies were generally immunosupressed individuals and those prone to infections. The antimicrobials were either nonabsorbable (i.e., polymyxin, neomycin, bacitracin) or absorbable (i.e., trimethoprim/sulfamethoxazole, quinolones) (31). However, there is no consensus yet regarding the practical implications of using selective decontamination.

VAGINAL AND CERVICAL FLORA

The vagina contains a complex microbial flora (32). Lactobacilli colonize the vagina shortly after birth, because of the mother's hormonal stimulation. As this effect wanes, lactobacilli are replaced with aerobic gram-positive cocci. At puberty the cyclic hormonal stimulation ensues, the squamous epithelium glycogen content increases and lactobacilli returns. Lactobacilli metabolize glycogen, producing lactic acid, which contributes to a low vaginal pH (4.5–5.5) in adults. The low pH select for certain microorganisms, such as Candida and anaerobes, but inhibits the growth of fastidious bacteria including Enterobacteriaceae.

The mean bacterial counts in the vagina and cervix are approximately 10^8 organisms/ml. About 50% of these are anaerobic (32). The cervical canal contains mixed aerobic and anaerobic flora. The aerobic components consist of lactobacilli, group B streptococci, *Enterococcus* spp., *S. epidermidis*, *S. aureus*, and Enterobacteriaceae.

The anaerobic component consists predominately of lactobacillus and peptostreptococci. *Clostridium* spp. include *bifermentans, perfringens, ramosum*, and *difficile*. The predominant gram negative bacilli are *P. disiens, P. bivia*, pigmented *Prevotella* and *Porphyromonas, B. fragilis*, and *Prevotella oralis*. Veillonella, bifidobacteria, and eubacteria are also present.

Variations in cervical-vaginal flora are related to the effects of age, pregnancy, and menstrual cycle. Estrogen can increase the bacterial population of the female genital tract, while progesterone decreases it (33). The flora before puberty, during childbearing years, pregnancy, and after menopause is not uniform. Colonization with lactobacilli is low in children and in postclimactic years, and is high in pregnancy and the reproductive years.

The influence of pregnancy on the vaginal flora is important because the newborn is exposed to it during delivery or through exposure to infected amniotic fluid (17). The major change during pregnancy is an increase in the colonization by lactobacilli (17,32). This increase in the number of non-virulent lactobacilli at the expense of the more virulent microorganisms may serve to protect the fetus from exposure to pathogens.

COLONIZATION OF GASTROINTESTINAL TRACT IN THE NORMAL INFANT

The developing fetus is protected from the bacterial flora of the maternal genital tract. Initial colonization of the newborn and of the placenta usually occurs after rupture of the maternal membranes. During a vaginal delivery the neonate is exposed to the cervical birth canal flora, which includes many aerobic and anaerobic bacteria (34,35).

The predominant aerobic bacteria present in the cervical flora are staphylococci, diphtheroids, alpha-hemolytic streptococci, *Gardnerella vaginalis*, lactobacilli, and *E. coli*. The most common anaerobic organisms are *Prevotella bivia, Prevotella disiens, B. fragilis* group, *P. acnes*, Peptostreptococci, pigmented prevotella and porphyromonas, clostridia, and lactobacilli (36).

The newborn is colonized initially on the skin and mucosa of the nasopharynx, oropharynx, conjunctivae, umbilical cord, and the external genitalia. In most infants, the organisms colonize these sites without causing any inflammatory changes.

The colonization of the gastrointestinal tract by bacteria begins immediately after delivery. Conjunctival and gastric contents of vaginally delivered infants contain many aerobic and anaerobic bacteria that are identical to the maternal genital flora (17,37). As the newborn infant's birth weight and duration of pregnancy increased, more potentially pathogenic aerobic (such as *E. coli* and *S. aureus*) and anaerobic bacteria (such as the *B. fragilis* group) were found in gastric contents; also prolongation of labor brought about increased numbers of anaerobes. These organisms represent a transient load of bacteria acquired during delivery (38). The only organism whose recovery from gastric aspirates has clinical importance is Group B streptococci (39). This has particular importance in newborns with signs of infection.

The bacterial flora is usually heterogeneous during the first few days of life, independently of feeding habits. After the first week of life, a stable bacterial flora is usually established (40). In full-term infants a diet of breast milk induces the development of a flora rich in *Bifidobacterium* spp. Other obligate anaerobes, such as *Clostridium* spp. and *Bacteroides* spp., are rarely isolated and also Enterobacteriaceae and enterococci are relatively few. During the corresponding period, formula-fed babies are often colonized by other anaerobes in addition to bifidobacteria and by facultatively anaerobic bacteria.

The initially sterile meconium becomes colonized in most instances within 24 hours with aerobic and anaerobic bacteria, predominantly micrococci, *E. coli*, *Clostridium* spp., and streptococci (41). The presence of various types of clostridia can be demonstrated at that age (18,42,43). Facultatively anaerobic bacteria colonize from the first days of life followed closely by bifidobacteria. The number of facultative bacteria fall by the third day, and the suppression is attributed to the establishment of an acetate and acetic acid buffer of low pH in the intestinal lumen (44). Bifidobacteria reach high levels to become the predominant organisms, although other anaerobes such as *Bacteroides* spp., clostridia, and anaerobic streptococci are also present.

Several factors influence the composition of the fecal bacterial flora. These include the type of feeding (breast or formula), the route of delivery, gestational age term and exposure to antimicrobials. Anaerobes other than bifidobacteria tend not to persist in breast-fed infants during the period of exclusive breast feeding (45). Formula-fed neonates harbor higher number of facultative anaerobes, and colonization by bifidobacteria generally is slower compared to breast-fed infants (46). Anaerobic bacteria other than bifidobacteria are also found in the feces of formula-fed infants during the first week of life, and these persist beyond the neonatal period. The isolation rates of *B. fragilis* and other anaerobic bacteria in term babies approach that of adults within a week. The percentage of stools containing anaerobic bacteria increased with age and by four or six days of age 96% of infants were colonized with anaerobic bacteria, and 61% were colonized with *B. fragilis*. *E. coli*, *Klebsiella* spp., *Enterobacter* spp., and *Proteus* spp. were the most frequently colonizing aerobic gram-negative bacilli.

Mode of Delivery

Almost three-fourths of term infants delivered vaginally, whether formula-fed or breast-fed, are colonized with at least one aerobic gram-negative bacilli by 48 hours of age. In contrast, isolation rates before 48 hours was lower in term infants delivered by cesarean section and in premature infants delivered by the vaginal route. There are no differences in recovery of species of *Clostridium*, *Bifidobacterium*, *Eubacterium*, *Fusobacterium*, *Propionibacterium*, *Lactobacillus*, *Peptostreptococcus*, and *Veillonella*. *Bifidobacterium* isolates are recovered more frequently from breast-fed infants, while *Veillonella* isolates are isolated more frequently from infants delivered by cesarean section (18,43).

Gronlund et al. (47) found that fecal colonization of infants born by cesarean delivery is delayed and their gut flora may be disturbed for up to six months after the birth. Colonization rates by *Bifidobacterium* and *Lactobacillus* spp. reached the rates of vaginally delivered infants at 30 and 10 days, respectively. Infants born by cesarean delivery are less often colonized with bacteria of the *B. fragilis* group than were vaginally delivered infants: At six months the rates were 36% and 76%, respectively ($p=0.009$). The clinical relevance of these changes is, however, unknown.

Bennet and Nord (48) illustrated that there are no major differences in the gut flora of normal full-term newborn infants and preterm infants during intensive or intermediate care. However, caesarean section leads to a lower isolation rate of *Bifidobacteria* and *Bacteroides* spp. During antibiotic treatment anaerobic bacteria are isolated only from only 10% of the infants. After treatment, there is a slow regrowth of *Bifidobacterium* spp., but *Bacteroides* spp. are not usually reestablished.

Neut et al. (49) found that colonization of the gastrointestinal tract in newborns delivered by cesarean section occurs during the first days of life by environmental bacteria. It is more rapid in breast-fed than in bottle-fed infants. The intestinal flora is more diversified in the formula-fed infants. The first bacteria encountered are facultative anaerobes; they remain predominant during the first two weeks of life. In comparison to vaginal delivery, there are low levels of strict anaerobes after cesarean section; members of the *B. fragilis* group can be absent after 14 days of life and *Bifidobacterium* spp. are only isolated sporadically.

Cesarean section, low gestational age, and low birth weight were significantly associated with increased recovery of *C. perfringens* in stools (50).

Feeding Mode

The influence of breast-feeding on the predominance of the *Bifidobacterium* spp. in the newborn also was studied (51). Specific growth promoting factors for this organism were found in human milk, while other milks, including cow's milk, sheep's milk, and infant formulas, did not promote the growth of this species. Other investigators believe that *Bifidobacterium* spp. inhibits the growth of *E. coli* (52) by producing large amounts of acetic acid. Furthermore, because of the small buffering capacity of human milk, the infant gut is maintained at acid levels that inhibit the growth of *Bacteroides*, *Clostridium*, and *E. coli*. It is postulated that these conditions grant the breast-fed infant resistance to gastroenteritis.

The prevalence and counts of *C. difficile* as well as *E. coli* are significantly lower in the gut of breast-fed infants than in that of formula-fed infants, whereas the prevalence and counts of *Bifidobacterium* spp. is similar among both groups (53).

The Newborn's Maturity

Preterm babies are also colonized by facultatively anaerobic bacteria from the first days of life, and these remained at high levels resembling the full-term formula-fed babies. However, the intestinal colonization of preterm infants differed from that in full-term, breast-fed infants in the high counts of facultatively anaerobic bacteria and late appearance of bifidobacteria and from both groups of full-term infants in the early stable colonization by *Bacteroides* spp. (54). It is postulated that the composition of intestinal microflora of preterm low birth weight babies contributes to their predisposition to neonatal necrotizing enterocolitis. The gut of extremely low birth weight infants is colonized by a paucity of aerobic and anaerobic bacterial species. Breast feeding and reduction of antibiotic exposure increased the number of these organisms and fecal microbial diversity (55).

Effect of Antimicrobial Therapy

Bennet et al. evaluated the microflora of newborns during intensive care therapy and treatment with five antibiotic regimens (56). Aerobic and anaerobic fecal bacterial flora of normal newborns, preterm newborn infants without other health problems, and five groups of newborn infants treated with combinations of benzylpenicillin, cloxacillin, flucloxacillin, ampicillin, cefuroxime, cefoxitin, and gentamicin were compared. Preterm birth alone was associated with growth of Klebsiella which could be attributed to a higher rate of cesarean section in preterm than in term infants. All antibiotic regimens led to a pronounced suppression of anaerobic flora and overgrowth of Klebsiella but not with other aerobic gram negative bacilli. Minimal colonization with *C. difficile* and *C. perfringens* occurred. The authors concluded that disturbances of the intestinal microbial ecology can be expected in newborn infants after preterm birth by cesarean section and/or treatment with antibiotics, including some penicillins that are usually regarded as relatively harmless in this respect in adults.

Treatment with antibiotics was not associated with occurrence of *C. perfringens*. However, in infants with *C. perfringens*, intrapartum antibiotics were associated with increased appearance of abdominal distension ($p < 0.05$).

Effect of Iron Supplements

The iron content of the formula influences the number of *Clostridium* spp. in the large intestine of infants (57). *Clostridium tertium* is more often isolated from breast-fed infants than from either group of bottle-fed infants, and *Clostridium butyricum* is more frequently recovered from infants bottle fed with iron supplement than from breast-fed infants or infants bottle fed without iron supplement. Enhancement of bacterial growth by iron has been recognized for some *Clostridium* spp. (58) *C. difficile* and *Clostridium paraputrificum* were not isolated from breast-fed infants but were recovered from the stools of healthy bottle-fed infants. *C. butyricum*, *C. paraputrificum*, *Clostridium perfringens*, and the toxin of *C. difficile* have been implicated in the pathogenesis of necrotizing enteritis (59). Whether these organisms are primary pathogens or secondary invaders of an otherwise damaged intestinal mucosa remains unclear. However, it can be postulated that bottle-fed infants, especially those receiving an iron supplement, are at a greater risk for developing necrotizing enteritis caused by *C. butyricum*, *C. difficile*, and *C. paraputrificum* than are breast-fed infants in cases of damaged intestinal mucosa.

REFERENCES

1. Socransky SS, Manganiello SD. The oral microflora of man from birth to senility. J Periodontol 1971; 42:485–96.
2. Brook I. Bacteremia caused by anaerobic bacteria in children. Crit Care 2002; 6:205–11.
3. Brook I. Bacterial interference. Crit Rev Microbiol 1999; 25:155–72.
4. Brook I, Frazier EH. Aerobic and anaerobic bacteriology of wounds and cutaneous abscesses. Arch Surg 1990; 125:1445–51.
5. Evans CA, Smith WM, Johnson EA, Gilbert ER. Bacterial flora of the normal human skin. J Invest Dermatol 1950; 15:305–24.
6. McGinley KJ, Webster GF, Ruggieri MR, Leyden JJ. Regional variation in density of cutaneous *Propionibacterium*: correlation of *Propionbacterium acnes* populations with sebaceous secretions. J Clin Microbiol 1980; 12:672–5.
7. Till AE, Goulden V, Cunliffe WJ, Holland KT. The cutaneous microflora of adolescent, persistent and late-onset acne patients does not differ. Br J Dermatol 2000; 142:885–92.
8. Pawin H, Beylot C, Chivot M, et al. Physiopathology of acne vulgaris: recent data, new understanding of the treatments. Eur J Dermatol 2004; 14:4–12.
9. Sbordone L, Bortolaia C. Oral microbial biofilms and plaque-related diseases: microbial communities and their role in the shift from oral health to disease. Clin Oral Investig 2003; 7:181–8.
10. Lovegrove JM. Dental plaque revisited: bacteria associated with periodontal disease. J NZ Soc Periodontol 2004; 87:7–21.
11. Hiar I, Tande D, Gentric A, Garre M. Oropharyngeal colonization by gram-negative bacteria in elderly hospitalized patients: incidence and risk factors. Rev Med Interne 2002; 23:4–8.
12. Bergmans DC, Bonten MJ, Gaillard CA, et al. Prevention of ventilator-associated pneumonia by oral decontamination: a prospective, randomized, double-blind, placebo-controlled study. Am J Respir Crit Care Med 2001; 164:382–8.
13. Morris DP. Bacterial biofilm in upper respiratory tract infection. Curr Infect Dis Rep 2007; 9:186–92.
14. Brook I. Beta-lactamase producing bacteria in head and neck infection. Larynscope 1988; 98:428–31.
15. Brook I. The role of beta-lactamase-producing bacterial in the persistence of streptococcal tonsillar infection. Rev Infect Dis 1984; 6:601–7.
16. Brook I, Gober AE. Emergence of beta-lactamase-producing aerobic and anaerobic bacteria in the oropharynx of children following penicillin chemotherapy. Clin Pediatr 1984; 23:338–41.
17. Brook I, Barrett CT, Brinkman CR, III, Martin WJ, Finegold SM. Aerobic and anaerobic bacterial flora of the maternal cervix and newborn gastric fluid and conjunctiva: a prospective study. Pediatrics 1979; 63:451–5.
18. Long SS, Swenson RM. Development of anaerobic fecal flora in healthy newborn infants. J Pediatr 1977; 91:298–301.
19. Orrhage K, Nord CE. Factors controlling the bacterial colonization of the intestine in breastfed infants. Acta Paediatr 1999; 88:47–57.
20. Harmsen HJ, Wildeboer-Veloo AC, Raangs GC, et al. Analysis of intestinal flora development in breast-fed and formula-fed infants by using molecular identification and detection methods. J Pediatr Gastroenterol Nutr 2000; 30:61–7.
21. Kirjavainen PV, Gibson GR. Healthy gut microflora and allergy: factors influencing development of the microbiota. Ann Med 1999; 31:288–92.
22. Hao WL, Lee YK. Microflora of the gastrointestinal tract: a review. Methods Mol Biol 2004; 268:491–502.
23. Howden CW, Hunt RH. Relationship between gastric secretion and infection. Gut 1987; 28:96–107.
24. Finegold SM, Sutter VL, Mathisen GE. Normal indigenous intestinal flora 1983. In: Hentges DJ. (Ed) Human Intestinal Microflora in Health and Disease. New York: Academic Press, 3–31.
25. Brook I, Myhal LA, Dorsey CH. Encapsulation and pilus formation of *Bacteroides* spp. in normal flora abscesses and blood. J Infect 1992; 25:251–7.
26. Beachey EH. Bacterial adherence: adhesion receptor interactions mediating the attachment of bacteria to mucosal surfaces. J Infect Dis 1981; 143:325–44.
27. Gorbach SL, Banwell JG, Jacobs B, et al. Intestinal microflora in Asiatic cholera: I "Rice Water" (Stockholm). J Infect Dis 1970; 121:32–7.
28. Hurley BW, Nguyen CC. The spectrum of pseudomembranous enterocolitis and antibiotic-associated diarrhea. Arch Intern Med 2002; 162:2177–84.
29. van der Waaij D, Berghuis de Vries JM, Lekkerkerk van der Wees JEC. Colonization resistance of the digestive tract in conventional and antibiotic-treated mice. J Hyg 1971; 69:405–11.

30. Berg RD. Promotion of the translocation of enteric bacteria from the gastrointestinal tracts of mice by oral treatment with penicillin, clindamycin, or metronidazole. Infect Immun 1981; 33:854–61.
31. Klustersky J. A review of chemoprophylaxis and therapy of bacterial infection in neutropenic patients. Diag Microl Inf Dis 1989; 12:201s–7.
32. Larsen B. Vaginal flora in health and disease. Clin Obstet Gynecol 1993; 36:107–21.
33. Singh KB, Mahajan DK, Tewari RP. Hormonal modulation of the vaginal bacterial flora in experimental polycystic ovarian disease. J Clin Lab Anal 1996; 10:233–8.
34. Garland SM, Ni Chuileannain F, Satzke C, Robins-Browne R. Mechanisms, organisms and markers of infection in pregnancy. J Reprod Immunol 2002; 57:169–83.
35. Coplerud CP, Ohm MJ, Galask RP. Aerobic and anaerobic flora of the cervix during pregnancy and puerperium. Am J Obstet Gynecol 1976; 126:858–68.
36. Larsen B, Galask RP. Vaginal microbial flora: practical and theoretic relevance. Obstet Gynecol 1980; 55(Suppl.):100s–13.
37. Brook I, Martin WJ. Bacterial colonization in intubated newborns. Respiration 1980; 40:323–8.
38. Mims LC, Medawar MS, Perkins JR, Grubb WR. Predicting neonatal infections by evaluation of the gastric aspirate: a study in 207 patients. Am J Obstet Gynecol 1972; 114:232–8.
39. Puopolo KM, Madoff LC, Eichenwald EC. Early-onset group B streptococcal disease in the era of maternal screening. Pediatrics 2005; 115:1240–6.
40. Fanaro S, Chierici R, Guerrini P, Vigi V. Intestinal microflora in early infancy: composition and development. Acta Paediatr 2003; 91:48–55.
41. Hanson LA, Adlerberth I, Carlsson B, et al. Host defense of the neonate and the intestinal flora. Acta Paediatr Scand 1989; 351:122–5.
42. Hopkins MJ, Macfarlane GT, Furrie E, Fite A, Macfarlane S. Characterisation of intestinal bacteria in infant stools using real-time PCR and northern hybridisation analyses. FEMS Microbiol Ecol 2005; 54:77–85.
43. Rotimi VO, Cuerden BI. The development of the bacterial flora in normal neonates. J Med Microbiol 1981; 14:51–62.
44. Bullen CL, Tearle PV. Bifidobacteria in the intestinal tract of infants: an in vitro study. J Med Microbiol 1976; 9:335–44.
45. Stark PL, Lee A. The microbial ecology of the large bowel of breast and formula-fed infants during the first year of life. J Med Microbiol 1982; 15:189–203.
46. Hewitt JH, Rigby J. Effect of various milk feeds on numbers of *Escherichia coli* and *Bifodobacterium* in the stools of new-born infants. J Hyg (Camb) 1976; 77:129–39.
47. Gronlund MM, Lehtonen OP, Eerola E, Kero P. Fecal microflora in healthy infants born by different methods of delivery: permanent changes in intestinal flora after cesarean delivery. J Pediatr Gastroenterol Nutr 1999; 28:19–25.
48. Bennet R, Nord CE. Development of the faecal anaerobic microflora after caesarean section and treatment with antibiotics in newborn infants. Infection 1987; 15:332–6.
49. Neut C, Bezirtzoglou E, Romond C, Beerens H, Delcroix M, Noel AM. Bacterial colonization of the large intestine in newborns delivered by cesarean section. Zentralbl Bakteriol Mikrobiol Hyg [A] 1987; 266:330–7.
50. Ahtonen P, Lehtonen OP, Kero P, Eerola E, Hartiala K. *Clostridium perfringens* in stool, intrapartum antibiotics and gastrointestinal signs in a neonatal intensive care unit. Acta Paediatr 1994; 83:389–90.
51. Simhon A, Douglas JR, Drasar BS, Soothill JF. Effect of feeding on infant's faecal flora. Arch Dis Child 1982; 57:54–8.
52. Kim SH, Yang SJ, Koo HC, et al. Inhibitory activity of *Bifidobacterium longum* Hy8001 against vero cytotoxin of *Escherichia coli* 0157:H7. J Food Prot 2001; 64:1667–73.
53. Penders J, Vink C, Driessen C, London N, Thijs C, Stobberingh EE. Quantification of *Bifidobacterium* spp., *Escherichia coli* and *Clostridium difficile* in faecal samples of breast-fed and formula-fed infants by real-time PCR. FEMS Microbiol Lett 2005; 243:141–7.
54. Stark PL, Lee A. The bacterial colonization of the large bowel of pre-term low birth weight neonates. J Hyg (Camb) 1982; 89:59–67.
55. Gewolb IH, Schwalbe RS, Taciak VL, Harrison TS, Panigrahi P. Stool microflora in extremely low birthweight infants. Arch Dis Child Fetal Neonatal Ed 1999; 80:F167–73.
56. Bennet R, Eriksson M, Nord CE, Zetterstrom R. Fecal bacterial microflora of newborn infants during intensive care management and treatment with five antibiotic regimens. Pediatr Infect Dis 1986; 5:533–9.
57. Mevissen-Verhage EAE, Marcelis JH, de Vos MN, Harmsen-van Amerongen WC, Verhoef J. *Bifidobacterium*, *Bacteroides*, and *Clostridium* spp. in fecal samples from breast-fed infants with and without iron supplement. J Clin Microbiol 1987; 25:285–9.
58. de Jong AE, Eijhusen GP, Brouwer-Post EJ, et al. Comparison of media for enumeration of *Clostridium perfringens* from food. J Microbiol Methods 2003; 54:359–66.
59. de la Cochetiere MF, Piloquet H, des Robert C, et al. Early intestinal bacterial colonization and necrotizing enterocolitis in premature infants: the putative role of Clostridium. Pediatr Res 2004; 56:366–70.

3 | Collection, Transportation, and Processing of Specimens for Culture

The perception that anaerobes have little or no role in many infections originates from the fact that many past studies did not attempt to identify such a role or used improper methods for collecting specimens for anaerobes. Therefore, carefully assessing studies for methodological properties before judging their ability to determine the role of anaerobes in an infectious process is essential. Multiple examples of differences in the rate of recovery of anaerobic bacteria between studies that used proper techniques and those that used improper techniques can be found.

Earlier studies of chronic otitis media (1) and human and animal bites (2), which did not employ methods for anaerobes found these organisms in a small number of cases. However, when better techniques were used, anaerobes were recovered in the majority of the cases (3,4). Because anaerobes may invade any body site, and they have been recovered in a variety of infections in children, anaerobes' potential role in an infectious site should be assessed individually. The prevalence of anaerobic bacteria in an infection is a major factor in deciding which clinical specimens should be processed for anaerobes.

The proper management of anaerobic infection depends on appropriate documentation of the bacteria causing the infection. Without such an approach, the patient may be exposed to inappropriate, costly, and undesirable antimicrobial agents and their adverse side effects.

Anaerobic infections present special bacteriologic problems not encountered in other types of infections, and such problems may make the therapeutic approach even more difficult. Generally, bacteriologic results will not be available so quickly as in aerobic infections, particularly if the infection is mixed (as are more than one-half of the cases). Some laboratories may fail to recover certain or all of the anaerobes present in a specimen. This situation can occur particularly when the specimen is not promptly put under anaerobic conditions for transport to the laboratory. If care is not taken to avoid contamination of the specimen with normal flora, anaerobes may be recovered which have little to do with the patient's illness. As all laboratories are not equipped to identify anaerobes accurately, presumptive results may be very misleading.

Appropriate cultures for anaerobic bacteria are especially important in mixed aerobic and anaerobic infections. Techniques or media that are inadequate for isolation of anaerobic bacteria, either because of a lack of an anaerobic environment or because of an overgrowth of aerobic organisms, can mislead the clinician to assume that the aerobic organisms recovered are the only pathogens present in an infected site, therefore causing the clinician to direct therapy toward only those aerobic organisms.

The nature of the various organisms in a mixed infection will also influence the choice of drugs. Drugs active against anaerobic bacteria may be quite inactive against the accompanying aerobic or facultative organisms. When mixed infections involve several organisms, two or more drugs may be required to provide effective coverage for each of the organisms in the mixture.

Because anaerobic bacteria frequently can be involved in various infections, ideally, all properly collected specimens should be cultured for these organisms. The physician should make special efforts to isolate anaerobic organisms in infections in which these organisms are frequently recovered, such as abscesses, wounds in and around the oral and anal cavities, chronic otitis media and sinusitis, aspiration pneumonia, and intraabdominal and obstetrical and gynecological infections among others.

TABLE 1   Methods for Collection of Specimen for Anaerobic Bacteria

Infection site	Methods
Abscess or body cavity	Aspiration by syringe and needle
	Incised abscesses—syringe or swab (less desirable); specimen obtained during surgery after cleansing the skin
	Aspirates obtained under computed tomography or ultrasound guidance (e.g., abdominal abscesses)
Tissue or bone	Surgical specimen using tissue biopsy scraping or curette
Sinuses or mucus surface abscesses	Aspiration after decontamination or surgical specimen
Ear	Aspiration after decontamination of ear canal and membrane; in perforation: cleanse ear canal and aspirate through perforation
Pulmonary	Transtracheal aspiration, lung puncture or bronchial lavage,[a] and bronchial brushing[a]
Pleural	Thoracentesis
Urinary tract	Suprapubic bladder aspiration
Female genital tract	Culdocentesis following decontamination, surgical specimen, transabdominal needle aspirate of uterus, and intrauterine brush[a]

[a] Using double-lumen catheter and quantitative culture.

The most acceptable documentation of an anaerobic infection is through culture of anaerobic microorganisms from the infected site. Three elements requiring the cooperation of the physician and the microbiology laboratory are essential for appropriate documentation of anaerobic infection: collection of appropriate specimens, expeditious transportation of the specimen, and careful laboratory processing.

COLLECTION OF SPECIMENS

Specimens must be obtained free of contamination so that saprophytic organisms or normal flora are excluded, and culture results can be interpreted correctly (Table 1). Because indigenous anaerobes often are present on the surfaces of skin and mucous membranes in large numbers, even minimal contamination of a specimen with the normal flora can give misleading results. On this basis, specimens can be designated according to their acceptability for anaerobic culture to either the acceptable or unacceptable category. Materials that are appropriate for anaerobic cultures should be obtained using a technique that bypasses the normal flora. Unacceptable or inappropriate specimens can be expected to yield normal flora also and therefore have no diagnostic value. Sites that are normally inhabited by a rich indigenous flora, such as the oral cavity, intestinal tract, or vagina, should not be cultured for anaerobes except under specific circumstances. Unacceptable specimens include coughed sputum, bronchoscopy aspirates, gingival, and throat swabs, feces, gastric aspirates, voided urine, and vaginal swabs (Table 2). Exceptions to these guidelines can be made when the clinical condition warrants such a culture. For example, selective media may be used to detect only a possible pathogen, such as *Clostridium difficile*, in stool obtained from a patient with colitis.

Acceptable specimens include blood specimens, aspirates of body fluids (pleural, pericardial, cerebrospinal, peritoneal, and joint fluids), urine collected by percutaneous suprapubic bladder aspiration, abscess contents, deep aspirates of wounds, and specimens collected by special techniques, such as transtracheal aspirates (TTA), direct lung puncture,

TABLE 2   Specimens that Should Not Be Cultured for Anaerobes

Feces or rectal swabs
Throat or nasopharyngeal swabs
Sputum or bronchoscopic specimens
Routine or catheterized urine
Vaginal or cervical swabs
Material from superficial wound or abscesses not collected properly to exclude surface contaminations
Material from abdominal wounds obviously contaminated with feces, such as an open fistula

TABLE 3 Specimens Appropriate for Anaerobic Culture

All normally sterile body fluids other than urine, such as blood, pleural, and joint fluids
Urine obtained by suprapubic bladder aspiration
Percutaneous transtracheal aspiration, direct lung puncture, or double-lumen catheter bronchial brushing and bronchoalveolar lavage (both cultured quantitatively)
Culdocentesis fluid obtained after decontamination of the vagina
Material obtained from closed abscesses
Material obtained from sinus tracts or draining wounds

or double-lumen catheter bronchial brushing and bronchoalveolar lavage (Table 3). Direct needle aspiration is probably the best method of obtaining a culture, while use of swabs is much less desirable. Specimens obtained from sites that normally are sterile may be collected after thorough skin decontamination, as is for the collection of blood, spinal joint, or peritoneal fluids.

Cultures of coughed sputum and specimens obtained from bronchial brushing or bronchoscopy except for those done via a protective double-lumen catheter generally are contaminated with normal oral and nasal aerobic and anaerobic flora and are therefore unsuitable for culture. Acceptable respiratory specimens include: percutaneous or TTA, bronchial brushing collected via a double-lumen protected catheter, "protected" bronchoalveolar lavage, direct lung puncture, thoracentesis fluid, and lung tissue. Because the trachea below the thyroglossal area is sterile in the absence of pulmonary infection, TTA, which is done below this site, is a reliable procedure for obtaining suitable culture material for the diagnosis of pulmonary infection (5,6). TTA is usually not recommended in patients with severe hypoxia, hemorrhagic diathesis, or severe cough (7). Rare complications, such as hypoxia, bleeding, subsequent emphysema, or arrhythmia, have been reported in adult patients (8). In children, side effects of this procedure included mild hemoptysis and, in rare instances, subcutaneous emphysema. TTA has been used successfully also for the diagnosis of aspiration pneumonia and lung abscess in children (6). Cultures obtained by TTA contained fewer pathogens than did cultures of expectorated sputum.

Some clinical situations may present the clinician with difficult issues regarding obtaining an adequate culture, such as a tracheal culture of an intubated patient with tracheobronchitis, endometrial culture in patients with suspected endometritis after delivery, or a tonsillar surface culture searching for beta-lactamase–producing bacteria. In all these instances, the cultures from surrounding areas of the infected sites show similar isolates to those isolated from the infectious condition. Therefore, selective search for virulent organisms only, such as anaerobic gram negative bacilli (AGNB) or beta-lactamase–producing bacteria, may be helpful.

Diagnosis and Cultures

Cultures are helpful but nonessential for diagnosis in some infections such as tetanus, botulism, and gas gangrene. In some infections, such as minor skin and soft-tissue infections or ruptured appendix anaerobes are part of the infectious flora, but their presence does not need to be documented. However, their identification may be necessary when complication occurs (i.e., generalized peritonitis, bacteremia) in very young or very old patients with underlying serious illnesses, in those who require prolonged therapy, or in infections that failed to respond to empirical therapy. Even in these instances, it is not always necessary to identify all isolates, and it may be sufficient to search for antibiotic-resistant ones such as the *Bacteroides fragilis* group.

Even though it is important to obtain cultures prior to therapy, it may be still important to get them after the patient has been treated for a while. Since it may take at least several days and sometimes even longer to obtain definite bacterial information, generation of interim reports may assist in the management of seriously ill patients.

TRANSPORTATION OF SPECIMENS

The ability to recover anaerobes is influenced by the care applied to transportation and laboratory processing of specimens. Unless proper precautionary measures are taken during collection, transport, and laboratory processing, pronounced changes can occur in the aerobic and anaerobic microbial population of a clinical specimen (9). Sensitivity to oxygen causes some obligate anaerobes to die rapidly when exposed to air. In clinical samples, obligate anaerobes can be overgrown by facultative anaerobes unless the sample is processed rapidly after collection. The organisms must be protected, therefore, from the deleterious effects of oxygen during the time between the collection of the specimen and the inoculation of that specimen into the proper anaerobic medium in the microbiology laboratory. Failure to take proper precautions may result in misleading data, which may be detrimental to the patient (9–13).

Anaerobes vary in the conditions they require for survival. In accordance with their oxygen sensitivity, some organisms are classified as "moderate" and some as "fastidious." The moderate group is capable of growing in a 2% to 8% oxygen concentration. *B. fragilis*, *Prevotella oralis*, *Prevotella melaninogenica*, *Fusobacterium nucleatum*, and *Clostridium perfringens* belong to this group. Some fastidious anaerobes will grow at 0.5% oxygen levels, and some are extremely oxygen sensitive, such as some strains of *B. fragilis* and peptostreptococci (14). Low oxidation–reduction potential is another basic requirement for growth of certain anaerobic bacteria, as for *Bacteroides vulgatus* and *Clostridium sporogenes* (15). Such conditions usually exist in areas where anaerobes are present as part of the normal flora and at infected sites. The implication of these observations is that specimens must be carefully and rapidly handled in both transporting and processing to ensure good recovery of anaerobes.

The specimens should be placed into an anaerobic transporter containing anaerobic transport medium with an oxidation–reduction indicator as soon as possible after their collection. Aspirates of liquid specimen or tissue are always preferred to swabs, although systems for the collection of all three culture forms are commercially available (Fig. 1). Several versions of the anaerobic transport media also are commercially available (Baltimore Biological Laboratories, Cockeysville, Maryland, U.S.A.; Anaerobe Systems, Morgan Hill, California, U.S.A.).

These transport media are very helpful in preserving the anaerobes until the time of inoculation. Liquid specimen is best aspirated into a syringe through a needle and injected

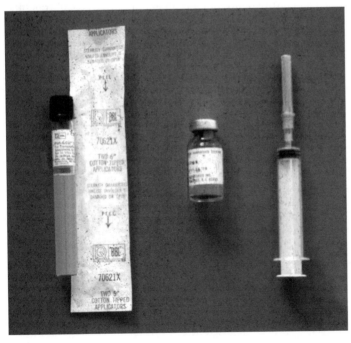

FIGURE 1   Commercial transport media used for the transportation of anaerobic specimens. *Left*, swab; *middle*, vial; *right*, syringe and needle.

into the anaerobic (oxygen-free) transport vial containing an oxidation–reduction indicator. Contrary to past recommendations, syringes used for aspiration should not be utilized for transportation because spillage of their contents could be hazardous, there is a potential danger of needle stick injuries, and because oxygen diffuses into plastic syringes (within 30 minutes). Body fluids can be transported in sterile tubes, especially if they contain more than 1 mL, with as small an airspace above the fluid level as possible, and kept upright to avoid mixing with air.

Swabs may be placed in the sterilized tubes containing carbon dioxide or prereduced, anaerobically sterile Carey and Blair semisolid media. A preferred method is to use a swab that has been prepared in a prereduced anaerobic tube. However, this is not commercially available.

Tissue specimens or swabs can be transported anaerobically in a Petri dish placed in a sealed plastic bag that can be rendered anaerobic by use of an anaerobic generator (BBL Microbiological Systems, Cockeysville, Maryland, U.S.A.) (Fig. 2). Alternatively, small pieces of tissue may be placed into the anaerobic transporter by removing the cap and pushing the tissue into the agar. Most of the common and clinically important anaerobic bacteria are moderate anaerobes, as shown by the examination of various types of clinical specimens for anaerobes (14,15).

Syed and Loesche (16) studied the survival of human dental plaque flora in various transport media and concluded that because numbers and kinds of microorganisms in clinical materials vary widely, no transport device should be expected to give optimal protection for all anaerobes that may be encountered in specimens. Even though some of the transport systems can support the viability of anaerobic organisms for up to 24 hours (17,18), all specimens should be transported and processed as rapidly as possible after collection to avoid loss of fastidious oxygen-sensitive anaerobes and overgrowth of facultative bacteria.

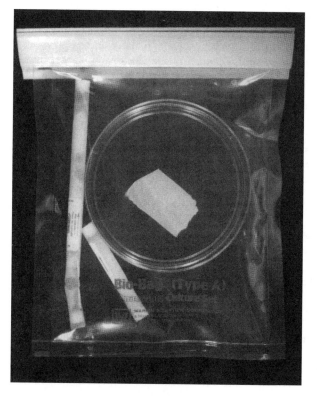

FIGURE 2   Commercial anaerobic bag system used for transportation of tissue or other specimens.

When delay in transportation is expected, specimen should be kept at room temperature, as cold temperature enhances oxygen diffusion, and incubator temperature cause loss of some bacterial strains and overgrowth of others.

We have observed significant differences in the recovery rate of anaerobic bacteria from abscesses when we compared two commercially available transport media. One system was far superior to the other, although both were licensed for use (19). Because many studies that document the efficacy of transport systems for anaerobes use stock cultures (18) and not clinical specimens, the clinical microbiology laboratory should evaluate the performance of each system in clinical specimen before accepting the system for clinical use.

PROCESSING OF SPECIMENS IN THE LABORATORY

Laboratory diagnosis of anaerobic infections begins with observing the gross appearance (necrosis, pus) and odor, as well as the examination of a Gram-stained smear of the specimen. Putrid or fetid smell in a clinical sample is almost always associated with the presence of anaerobes and is due to the production of volatile short-chain fatty acids and amines by these organisms. The appearance and relative number of the Gram-stained organisms will give important preliminary information regarding types of organisms present, suggest the need for special selective media, suggest appropriate initial therapy, preserve the relative proportions of organisms present at the time of specimen collection, and serve as a quality control on the final culture analysis. The laboratory should be able to recover all of the morphological types in the approximate ratio in which they are seen.

When necessary, phase-contrast or dark-field microscopy can help detect the presence of motile organisms, spores, and morphotypes (i.e., spirochetes) that do not grow on ordinary media.

Immunofluorescence staining can assist in detecting special organisms such as *Actinomyces* spp. and *Propionibacterium propionicus*. Unfortunately, this method is not specific enough for *B. fragilis* group and other AGNB.

The techniques for cultivation of anaerobes should provide optimal anaerobic conditions throughout processing. Detailed procedures of these methods can be found in microbiology manuals (12,13). Briefly, these methods could be the prereduced tube method (i.e., the VPI roll tube method) or the anaerobic glove box technique, which provides an anaerobic environment throughout processing, or the GasPak system (Becton Dickinson Co., Cockeysville, Maryland, U.S.A.) or the Bio-Bag system (Pfizer Diagnostics Division, Groton, Connecticut, U.S.A.), which is a more simplified method.

As a minimum requirement for the recovery of anaerobes, specimens should be inoculated onto enriched nonselective blood agar medium (containing vitamin K_1 and hemin) such as Brucella, trypticase soy, or schaedler agar; for anaerobic gram-negative bacilli, a selective medium such as laked sheep blood agar with kanamycin and vancomycin. Bacteroides bile esculin agar allows the growth of *B. fragilis* group and *Bilophila wadsworthia*; phenylethylalcohol agar excludes swarming *Proteus* spp. and other aerobic gram-negative bacilli. For *Clostridium*, egg yolk–neomycin agar may be used.

Although vitamin K_1-enriched thioglycolate broth (steamed before use) is generally used as a backup culture, this media alone should never be used as a substitute for a solid media. Interestingly, however, many clinical laboratories still use liquid media. The major limitation of such media is the probability of overgrowth of slow-growing strict anaerobes by rapid-growing aerobic and facultative organisms.

Cultures should be placed immediately under anaerobic conditions and incubated for 48 hours or longer. Plates should then be examined for approximate number and types of colonies present. Each colony type should be isolated, tested for aero-tolerance, and identified.

An additional period of 36 to 48 hours is generally required to completely identify the anaerobic bacteria to a species or genus level, using biochemical tests. Kits containing these biochemical tests are commercially available (Pfizer Diagnostics Division, Groton, Connecticut, U.S.A.). Rapid kits that detect preformed enzymes are commercially available. They require a heavy inoculum, take a short incubation period (four hours in air), and have a 60–90% identification capability (20). Other rapid tests that have potential use and can also be used directly on clinical isolates are the direct fluorescent microscopy and direct gas liquid chromatography. Gas liquid chromatography has been used to assist in the identification of anaerobes (13) and has also been used for presumptive rapid and direct identification of these organisms in pus specimens (21). Nucleic acid probes have been developed for identification of indicator bacteria of periodontal disease. Currently, polymerase chain reaction methods with sequencing of the 16S RNA gene has become the new "gold standard" for identification of anaerobes (22,23).

Blood Cultures

It is advisable to inoculate two bottles in a ratio of 1 mL of blood to 10 mL of media; one bottle should be vented to optimize recovery of strict aerobes and the other unvented for the isolation of anaerobes. Care should be taken not to introduce air to the anaerobic bottle when inoculating with the blood, and avoid shaking the bottle to avoid further aeration. Bottles showing growth should be subcultured anaerobically, and negative culture bottles should be held for a week.

There are several commercially available blood culture media that are adequate for recovery of anaerobes (13). Automated system enabling detection of anaerobes in blood culture bottles that detect released radioactive CO_2 (13).

Identification of an anaerobe to a species level is often cumbersome, expensive, and time-consuming, taking up to 72 hours. The decision of what level of testing is necessary for identifying an anaerobic organism is often a controversial issue. Usually, the clinician has to make such a decision. Occasionally, species identification of an organism will provide the diagnosis, as is the case with *C. difficile* in a patient with colitis or *Clostridium botulinum* in infants with botulism (11). However, because the origin of most anaerobes is endogenous, there are rarely epidemiological reasons to obtain their complete identification. Identifying the *B. fragilis* group that is more often causing bacteremia and septic complications has significant prognostic value.

Identification of an anaerobe is most helpful in determining what antibiotic to use in these species whose antibiotic susceptibility is predictable. Until the late 1970s, most clinically significant anaerobes except *B. fragilis* group were susceptible to penicillin (11). Therefore, extensive identification and antibiotic susceptibility testing were unnecessary. In the last decade, however, there have been significant changes, and now there is more variability in antimicrobial susceptibility patterns (see chapters 37 & 38). These changes have necessitated more extensive identification as well as antimicrobial susceptibility testing for some anaerobic bacteria. Organisms that should be identified include the following:

1. Isolates from sterile body sites (i.e., blood, cerebrospinal fluid, joint).
2. An organism with particular epidemiological or prognostic significance (e.g., *C. difficile*).
3. An organism with known variable or unique susceptibility.

ANTIMICROBIAL SUSCEPTIBILITY OF ANAEROBIC BACTERIA (SEE ALSO CHAPTERS 37 & 38)

The susceptibility of anaerobic bacteria to antimicrobial agents has become less predictable. Resistance to several antimicrobial agents by *B. fragilis* group and other AGNB has increased over the past decade (24). A decrease in susceptibility to penicillin of *C. perfringens* has been noted (25). And the susceptibility of *Clostridium* species (other than *C. perfringens*) is variable and often unpredictable. Anaerobic organisms to be selected for susceptibility testing should include these organisms.

The tests most useful for individual isolates are the Etest (AB Biodisk, Solna, Sweden) which is relatively expensive and the microbroth dilution test (these commercial trays do not always contain all the appropriate antimicrobials) (26). In addition to susceptibility testing, screening of anaerobic isolates (particularly *Bacteroides* species) for beta-lactamase activity may

TABLE 4   Anaerobic Infections for which Susceptibility Testing Is Indicated

Serious or life-threatening infections (e.g., brain abscess, bacteremia, or endocarditis)
Infections that failed to respond to empiric therapy
Infections that relapsed after initially responding to empiric therapy
Infections where an antimicrobial will have a special role in the patients outcome
When an empirical decision is difficult because of absence of precedent
When there are few susceptibility data available on a bacterial species
When the isolate(s) is often resistant to antimicrobial
When the patient requires prolonged therapy (e.g., septic arthritis, osteomyelitis, undrained abscess, or infection of
  a graft or a prosthesis)

be helpful. We routinely screen AGNB for beta-lactamase production using the nitrocefin disc. Such beta-lactamase screening of these isolates rapidly provides information regarding their penicillin susceptibility. It should be borne in mind that a longer-than-usual period (up to one hour) may be required for some organisms to show a positive reaction. Occasional bacterial strains may resist beta-lactamase antibiotics through mechanisms other than the production of beta-lactamase.

It is important to perform susceptibility testing to isolates recovered from sterile body sites, those that are recovered in pure culture or those that are clinically important and have variable or unique susceptibility.

The fact that routine susceptibility testing of all anaerobic isolates is time-consuming and in many cases unnecessary must be recognized. Therefore, susceptibility testing should be limited to selected anaerobic isolates (Table 4) (27). Antibiotics tested should include penicillin, a broad-spectrum penicillin, a penicillin plus a beta-lactamase inhibitor, clindamycin, chloramphenicol, cefoxitin, a third-generation cephalosporin, metronidazole, tigecycline, a carbapenem (i.e., imipenem), and an extended spectrum quinolone (i.e., moxifloxacin) (28).

Correlation of the results of in vitro susceptibility and clinical and bacteriological response is not always possible. This discrepancy occurs because of a variety of reasons: individuals may improve without antimicrobial or surgical therapy, infections vary in duration, severity, and extent; failure can occur because of lack of needed surgical drainage; response depends on individual patients status such as underlying condition, age, and nutritional status; and the antimicrobial may not be effective because of enzymatic inactivation or a low Eh or pH at the infection site, low concentration at the site of infection; and because of variations or imperfections in the susceptibility testing. It is not necessary to eliminate all of the infecting organisms because reduction in counts or modification of the metabolism of certain isolates alone may be sufficient to achieve a good clinical response. Synergy between two or more infecting organisms, which is a common event in anaerobic infections, may confuse the clinical picture.

CONCLUSION

The physician treating a patient with suspected anaerobic infection must use appropriate methods of obtaining samples of the infected site. Proper procedure allows the physician to bypass areas of the normal flora and assures appropriate and rapid transportation of the sample. Reliable microbiological data can be obtained only when proper procedures are followed.

REFERENCES

1. Liu YS, Lim DJ, Lang R, et al. Microorganisms in chronic otitis media with effusion. Ann Otol Rhinol Laryngol 1976; 85:145–51.
2. Mann RJ, Hoffeld TA, Farmer CB. Human bite infection of hand: twenty years of experience. J Hand Surg 1977; 2:97–104.
3. Brook I, Finegold SM. Bacteriology of chronic otitis media. JAMA 1979; 241:487–8.
4. Merriam CV, Fernandez HT, Citron DM, Tyrrel KL, Warren YA, Goldstein EJ. Bacteriology of human bite wound infections. Anaerobe 2006; 9:83–6.
5. Pecora DV. A method of securing uncontaminated tracheal secretions for bacterial examination. J Thorac Surg 1959; 37:653–4.

6. Brook I. Percutaneous transtracheal aspiration in the diagnosis and treatment of aspiration pneumonia in children. J Pediatr 1980; 90:1000–4.
7. Bartlett JG, Rosenblatt JE, Finegold SM. Percutaneous transtracheal aspiration in the diagnosis of anaerobic pulmonary infection. Ann Intern Med 1973; 22:535–40.
8. Spencer CD, Beaty HN. Complications of transtracheal aspiration. N Engl J Med 1972; 286:304–6.
9. Dowell VR, Jr. Anaerobic infections. In: Bodily HL, Updyke EL, Mason JO, eds. Diagnostic Procedures for Bacterial, Mycotic and Parasitic Infections. 5th ed. New York: American Public Health Association, 1970:494–543.
10. Dowell VR, Jr., Hawkins TM. Laboratory methods in anaerobic bacteriology, CDC laboratory manual. U.S. Department of Health, Education, and Welfare. Atlanta: Center for Disease Control (publ. no. (CDC) 74-8272).
11. Finegold SM. Anaerobic Bacteria in Human Disease. New York: Academic Press, 1977.
12. Holdeman LV, Cato EP, Moore WEC, eds. Anaerobe Laboratory Manual. 4th ed. Blacksburg, VA: Virginia Polytechnic Institute and State University, 1977.
13. Jousimies-Somer HR, Summanen P, Baron EJ, Citron DM, Wexler HM, Finegold SM. Wadsworth-KTL Anaerobic Bacteriology Manual. 6th ed. Belmont, CA: Star Publishing, 2002.
14. Thomas SJ, Eleazer PD. Aerotolerance of an endodontic pathogen. J Endod 2003; 29:644–5.
15. Imlay JA. How oxygen damages microbes: oxygen tolerance and obligate anaerobiosis. Adv Microb Physiol 2002; 46:111–53.
16. Syed SA, Loesche WJ. Survival of human dental plaque flora in various transport media. Appl Microbiol 1972; 24:638–44.
17. Citron DM, Warren YA, Hudspeth MK, Goldstein EJ. Survival of aerobic and anaerobic bacteria in purulent clinical specimens maintained in the Copan Venturi Transystem and Becton Dickinson Port-a-Cul transport systems. J Clin Microbiol 2000; 38:892–4.
18. Hindiyeh M, Acevedo V, Carroll KC. Comparison of three transport systems (Starplex StarSwab II, the new Copan Vi-Pak Amies Agar Gel collection and transport swabs, and BBL Port-A-Cul) for maintenance of anaerobic and fastidious aerobic organisms. J Clin Microbiol 2001; 39:377–80.
19. Brook I. Comparison of two transport systems for recovery of aerobic and anaerobic bacteria from abscesses. J Clin Microbiol 1987; 25:2020–2.
20. Dellinger CA, Moore LVA. Use of the rapid ID-ANA System to screen for enzyme activities that differ among species of bile-inhibited *Bacteroides*. J Clin Microbiol 1986; 23:289–93.
21. Gorbach SL, Mayhew JW, Bartlett JG. Rapid diagnosis of anaerobic infections by direct gas–liquid chromatography of clinical specimens. J Clin Invest 1976; 57:478–84.
22. Nagy E, Urban E, Soki J, Terhes G, Nagy K. The place of molecular genetic methods in the diagnostics of human pathogenic anaerobic bacteria. A minireview. Acta Microbiol Immunol Hung 2006; 53:183–94.
23. Song Y. PCR-based diagnostics for anaerobic infections. Anaerobe 2005; 11:79–91.
24. Aldridge KE, Sanders CV. Susceptibility trending of blood isolates of the *Bacteroides fragilis* group over a 12-year period to clindamycin, ampicillin-sulbactam, cefoxitin, imipenem, and metronidazole. Anaerobe 2002; 8:301–5.
25. Roberts SA, Shore KP, Paviour SD, Holland D, Morris AJ. Antimicrobial susceptibility of anaerobic bacteria in New Zealand: 1999–2003. J Antimicrob Chemother 2006; 57:992–8.
26. Rosenblatt JE, Gustafson DR. Evaluation of the Etest for susceptibility testing of anaerobic bacteria. Diagnostic Microbiol Infect Dis 1995; 22:279–84.
27. Finegold SM. Perspective on susceptibility testing of anaerobic bacteria. Clin Infect Dis 1997; 25(Suppl. 2):s251–3.
28. Clinical and Laboratory Standards Institute (CLSI) [formerly National Committee for Clinical Laboratory Standards (NCCLS)]. Methods for Antimicrobial Susceptibility Testing of Anaerobic Bacteria. 6th ed., Vol. 24. Wayne, PA: CLSI, January 2004 (approved standard, CLSI document M11-A6).

4 | Clinical Clues to Diagnosis of Anaerobic Infections

Infections caused by anaerobic bacteria are common and may be serious and life-threatening. Anaerobes are the predominant components of the bacterial flora of normal human skin and mucous membranes, and are therefore a common cause of bacterial infections of endogenous origin. Infections due to anaerobic bacteria can evolve all body systems and sites (1). The predominant ones include: abdominal, pelvic, respiratory, and skin and soft tissues infections. Because of their fastidious nature, they are difficult to isolate from infectious sites and are often overlooked. Failure to direct therapy against these organisms often leads to clinical failures. Their isolation requires appropriate methods of collection, transportation, and cultivation of specimens. Treatment of anaerobic bacterial infection is complicated by the slow growth of these organisms, which makes diagnosis in the laboratory possible only after several days, by their often polymicrobial nature and by the growing resistance of anaerobic bacteria to antimicrobial agents.

The diagnosis of anaerobic infections may be difficult, but is expedited by recognition of certain clinical signs. These signs are summarized in Table 1. Even though many of the clues are not specific, the presence of several of them in a patient can be still suggestive of an anaerobic infection.

Predisposing conditions and bacteriologic hints should alert the clinician, who may apply diagnostic procedures to ascertain the nature of the pathogens and the extent of the infection. Bacteriologic findings suggestive of anaerobic infection are listed in Table 2.

Almost all anaerobic infections originate from the patient's own microflora. Poor blood supply and tissue necrosis lower the oxidation–reduction potential and favor the growth of anaerobes. Any condition that lowers the blood supply to an affected area can predispose to anaerobic infection. Therefore, foreign body, malignancy, surgery, edema, shock, trauma, colitis, and vascular disease may predispose to anaerobic infection. Previous infection with aerobic or facultative organisms also may make the local tissue conditions more favorable for the growth of anaerobic organisms. The human defense mechanisms also may be impaired by anaerobic conditions (2).

ASSOCIATION OF INFECTIONS WITH MUCOSAL SURFACES

The source of bacteria involved in most of the anaerobic infections is the normal indigenous flora of an individual. The mucous surfaces of the child becomes colonized with aerobic and anaerobic flora within a short time after birth (3,4). Anaerobic bacteria are the most common residents of the skin and mucous membrane surfaces (5) and outnumber aerobic bacteria in the normal oral cavity and gastrointestinal tract at a ratio of 10:1 and 1000:1, respectively (6). Examples of these mucous and skin surfaces are the oral, and nasal cavities, the gastrointestinal lumen and the conjunctiva, the skin surfaces of different locations, and the sebaceous glands. It is not surprising, therefore, that a large proportion of anaerobic bacteria that are part of the normal mucous membrane flora can be recovered from infection in proximity to these sites.

The inoculum of organisms that may penetrate into an infectious site such as human bite, or perforated gut, usually is complex and contains a mixture of aerobic or anaerobic flora. Although the inoculum of certain organisms that possess greater pathogenicity such as

TABLE 1 Clues to Diagnosis of an Anaerobic Infection

Infection adjacent to a mucosal surface
Foul-smelling lesion or discharge
Classic presentation of an anaerobic infection (e.g., Necrotic gangrenous tissue, gas gangrene, abscess formation)
Free gas in tissue or discharges
Bacteremia or endocarditis with no growth on aerobic blood cultures
Infection related to the use of antibiotics effective against aerobes only (e.g., ceftazidime, old quinolones, aminoglycosides,
    trimethoprim–sulfamethoxazole)
Infection related to tumors or other destructive processes
Septic thrombophlebitis
Infection following animal or human bite
Black discoloration of exudates containing Pigmented *Prevotella* or *Porphyromonas* which may fluoresce under ultraviolet light
"Sulfur granules" in discharges caused by actinomycosis
Clinical condition predisposing to anaerobic infection (following maternal amnionitis, perforation of bowel, etc.)

Source: From Ref. 1.

Bacteroides fragilis can be initially small, they may become the predominant isolates as the infection progresses.

Anaerobes belonging to the indigenous flora of the oral cavity can be recovered from various infections adjacent to that area such as cervical lymphadenitis (7,8); subcutaneous abscesses (9) and burns (10) in proximity to the oral cavity; human and animal bites (11); paronychia (12); tonsillar and retropharyngeal abscesses (13); chronic sinusitis (14); chronic otitis media (15); periodontal abscess (16); thyroiditis (17); aspiration pneumonia (18); empyema (19), and bacteremia associated with one of the above infections (20). The predominant anaerobes recovered in these infections are species of anaerobic gram-negative bacilli including pigmented *Prevotella* and *Porphyromonas*, *Prevotella oralis*, *Fusobacterium*, and gram-positive anaerobic cocci (*Peptostreptococcus* spp.) which are all part of the normal flora, the mucous surfaces of the oral, pharyngeal, and sinus flora (Table 3).

A similar correlation exists in infections associated with the gastrointestinal tract. Such infections include peritonitis that develops after rupture of appendix (21), liver and spleen abscesses (22), abscesses and burns (10) near the anus, intra-abdominal abscess (23), and bacteremia associated with any of these infections (20). The anaerobes that predominate in these infections are *Bacteroides* spp. (predominantly *B. fragilis* group), clostridia (including *Clostridium perfringens*), and *Peptostreptococcus* spp.

Another site where a correlation exists between the normal flora and the anaerobic bacteria isolated from infected sites is the genitourinary tract. These infections include amnionitis, septic abortion, and other pelvic inflammations (24). The anaerobes usually isolated from these sites are species of *Prevotella* and *Fusobacterium* and *Peptostreptococcus* spp. Organisms belonging to the vaginal–cervical flora are also important pathogens of neonatal infections.

TABLE 2 Bacteriological Finding Suggestive of Anaerobic Infection

Inability to grow in aerobic cultures, organisms seen on Gram stain of the original material
Typical morphology for anaerobes on Gram stain
Anaerobic growth on proper media containing antibiotic-suppressing aerobes
No growth or routine bacterial culture ("sterile-pus")
Growth in anaerobic zone of fluid or agar media
Growth anaerobically on media containing paromomycin, kanamycin, neomycin, or vancomycin
Gas, foul-smelling odor in specimen or bacterial culture
Characteristic colonies on anaerobic plates
Young colonies of pigmented *Prevotella* and *Porphyromonas* may fluoresce red under ultraviolet light, and older colonies
    produce a typical dark pigment
Characteristic colonies on agar plates under anaerobic conditions (e.g., *Clostridium perfringens*, *Fusobacterium nucleatum*)

Source: From Ref. 1.

TABLE 3 Recovery of Anaerobic Bacteria in Patients[a]

Infection	Peptostrepto-coccus spp.	Clostridium spp.	Bacteroides fragilis group	Pigmented Prevotella and Porphyromonas, Prevotella oralis	P. bivia and P. disien	Fusobac-terium spp.
Bacteremia	1	1	2	1	0	1
Central nervous system	2	1	1	2	0	1
Head and neck	3	1	1	3	0	3
Thoracic	2	1	1	3	0	3
Abdominal	3	3	3	1	1	3
Obstetric-gynecology	3	2	1	1	2	1
Skin and soft tissue	2	1	2	2	1	1

[a] Frequency of recovery in anaerobic infections: 0 = none, 1 = rare (1–33%), 2 = common (34–66%), 3 = very common (67–100%).

FOUL-SMELLING SPECIMEN OR DISCHARGE FROM AN INFECTED AREA

The presence of putrid smell is the most specific clue for anaerobic infection and is caused by-products of metabolic end products of the anaerobic organisms, which are mostly organic acids. However, the absence of a foul-smelling discharge does not exclude anaerobic infection as not all anaerobic bacteria produce it. In deep-seated infections, these odors cannot always be appreciated.

THE PRESENCE OF GANGRENOUS NECROTIC TISSUE

The presence of anoxic conditions can result in the formation of gangrenous necrotic tissue. This anoxic condition predisposes for anaerobic infection, because anaerobes benefit and proliferate under such conditions.

FREE GAS IN TISSUES

Gas formation is caused by the metabolic end products such as amines and organic acids that are released by the multiplying anaerobic organism and is enhanced by anoxic conditions. However, some aerobic organisms, such as *Escherichia coli*, also can produce gas in infected tissues. The formation of gas can be detected by palpation or by radiographic examination of the involved area.

THE ABSENCE OF GROWTH IN AEROBIC CULTURES OF INFECTED AREAS

The lack of bacterial growth in aerobic cultures is of particular significance in putrid specimens obtained before administration of antimicrobial therapy. This also can occur in anaerobic bacteremia, in which aerobic blood cultures do not reveal the infecting organisms. An additional clue to the presence of anaerobes could be the presence of bacterial forms in properly performed Gram stain preparations in which the aerobic bacterial cultures show no growth. Many laboratories assume that failure to cultivate anaerobes in thioglycolate broth excludes anaerobes from the infection, but thioglycolate broth inoculated in room air would not provide adequate anaerobic conditions. Furthermore, overgrowth of rapid-growing aerobic organisms, which often are present in many mixed infections, may mask the presence of slower growing anaerobes.

INFECTION THAT PERSISTS AFTER ADMINISTRATION OF ANTIBIOTICS

Most anaerobes are susceptible to penicillins, although many anaerobic gram-negative bacilli are resistant to that drug (25). Other commonly used antibiotics to which almost all anaerobes are resistant are the aminoglycosides and the "older" quinolones (i.e. ciprofloxacin). Therefore, persistence or recurrence of an infection in the face of either of these, or other antimicrobial agents to which anaerobes are resistant, should arouse suspicion to the presence of anaerobic bacteria in the infection.

CLINICAL SITUATIONS PREDISPOSING TO ANAEROBIC INFECTION

Any exposure of the sterile body cavity to indigenous mucous surface flora can result in infection. Anaerobes are especially common in chronic infections. Certain infections are very likely to involve anaerobes as important pathogens and their presence should always be assumed. Such infections include brain abscess, oral or dental infections, human or animal bites, aspiration pneumonia and lung abscesses, peritonitis following perforation of viscus, amnionitis, endometritis, septic abortions, tubo-ovarian abscess, abscesses in and around the oral and rectal areas, and pus forming necrotizing infections of soft tissue or muscle. Conditions that decrease the redox potential predispose to anaerobic conditions. The list of these and other general conditions that predispose to anaerobic infection is presented in Table 4. Certain malignant tumors such as colonic, uterine and bronchogenic carcinomas, and necrotic tumors of the head and neck have the tendency to become infected with anaerobic bacteria (26). The anoxic conditions in the tumor and exposure to the endogenous adjacent mucous flora may predispose for these infections.

The newborn, and especially those suffering from fetal distress or are delivered following maternal amniotic infection, are prone to anaerobic infection. Examples of such infections are the occurrence of neonatal pneumonia after aspiration of infected amniotic fluid (27) or the introduction of anaerobic bacteria indigenous to the vaginal–cervical area into the insertion site of the fetal-monitoring needle, an event that can cause scalp abscess and osteomyelitis (28).

ANAEROBIC INFECTIONS AS A CLUE TO MEDICAL CONDITIONS

An anaerobic infection can provide a clue and a warning to the presence of an underlying medical problem. Brain abscess may be due to an underlying dental infection such as

TABLE 4   Clinical Conditions that Predispose to Anaerobic Infection

Reduced redox potential
  Anoxia or destruction of tissue
  Foreign body
  Obstruction and stasis
  Vascular insufficiency
  Burns
  Infection caused by aerobic bacteria or mycobacteria
  Tumor
Neonatal conditions
  Maternal aminionitis
  Fetal distress
  Fetal monitoring
General conditions
  Collagen vascular disease
  Corticosteroids
  Diabetes mellitus
  Hypogammaglobulinemia
  Neutropenia
  Immunosuppression
  Cytotoxic drug
  Splenectomy
  Malignancy (colon, lung, leukemia, uterus)
  Surgery or trauma of oral, gastrointestinal or urogenital areas
  Bites
  Aspiration of oral secretions
  Therapy with antibiotics ineffective against anaerobes

periodontitis or periopical abscess and lung abscess can be a clue to underlying bronchogenic malignancy. Malignant disease can be first detected because of an anaerobic infection. Malignancy or other process in the colon can induce sepsis with *Clostridium* spp. (especially *Clostridium septicum*) (29) or arthritis caused by *Eubacterium lentum* (30) or emerge first as abdominal wall myonecrosis (31). *Capnocytophaga* which is member of the oral microflora can cause sepsis in patients with leukemia (32).

Malignancy is often associated with the development of local or systemic anaerobic infection (26). Systemic infections may reflect compromises in host defenses at several levels. Infections may be due to alterations in local conditions at the site of the neoplasm, allowing bacteria to gain access to the blood. The humural immunity, the bactericidal plasma action, and the intracellular killing properties of neutrophils, monocytes, and macrophages may be compromised (33–36).

Local conditions at the neoplasm site can also predispose to infection. The condition in the tumor may predispose for an anaerobic–aerobic infection. Tumors may outgrow their blood supply and become necrotic. The lowered oxygen tension may, therefore, favor the growth of anaerobic organisms. A tumor can extend into surrounding tissues, causing barrier break-through onto mucosal and epithelial surfaces. Alimentary tract inflammatory and focal necrosis can be found in the colonic mucosa in leukemia (37–39) and after cancer chemotherapy (40). Another factor underlying the increased susceptibility of patients with cancer to infection and bacteremia is their overall poor nutritional status (34).

Insufficient blood supply of rapidly growing solid tumors can lead to the presence of tissue hypoxia. Vaupel (41) demonstrated that tumor oxygenation powerfully predicts the prognosis of patients receiving radiotherapy for intermediate and advanced stage cancer of the uterine cervix. Hypoxia is also known to decrease the efficiency of the currently used anticancer modalities like surgery, chemotherapy, and radiotherapy. Therefore, hypoxia seems to be a major limitation in current anticancer therapy.

Clostridium spp. possesses a selective colonization ability of hypoxic/necrotic areas within the tumor. The anaerobic environment within the tumor provided this oxygen sensitive organism with adequate conditions for proliferation. The use of non-pathogenic *Clostridium* spp. to deliver toxic agents to the tumor cells is under investigation takes advantage of this unique phenomena (42).

Anaerobic glycolysis is significantly increased in tumor tissue, with a resulting accumulation of lactic acid in this tissue and its environment. Spores of non-pathogenic *Clostridium* spp. can localize and germinate in neoplasms and produce extensive lysis of tumors without concomitant effect on normal tissue (43). *Clostridium* septicemia originating from an infection within tumor lesions has been reported (44–47). *C. septicum* infection is highly associated with the presence of a malignancy, either known or occult at the time infection occurs. Occult tumors are mostly situated in the cecal area of the bowel. Predisposing conditions for this type of infection are hematologic malignancies, colon carcinoma, neutropenia, diabetes mellitus, and disruption of the bowel mucosa (48,49).

Bacteremia due to gram-negative anaerobic bacilli is also common in patients with solid tumors (47). Felner and Dowell (50) reported that 57 of 250 (23%) of patients with "Bacteroides" (*B. fragilis* group, *Fusobacterium* spp., and pigmented *Prevotella* spp.) bacteremia had malignancy as a predisposing condition. The most common one were adenocarcinoma of the colon and uterine or cervical tumors.

Many bacterial infections in adults and children with malignancies are polymicrobial in nature (47). The bacteria isolated from many of these patients originated from the normal flora of the skin or the mucous membrane at or adjacent to the site of the infection.

CONCLUSIONS

The diagnosis of anaerobic infections can be expedited by the early recognition of certain clinical signs. Predisposing conditions and microbiological hints can alert the physician to the presence of anaerobic infection. Most anaerobic infections originate from the patient's own endogenous microflora. Poor blood supply and tissue necrosis lower the oxidation–reduction potential and can favor the growth of anaerobic bacteria. Conditions that lower the local blood supply can predispose to anaerobic infection at that site. These conditions include: trauma, foreign body, malignancy, surgery, edema, shock, colitis, and vascular disease. An anaerobic infection can provide a clue and a warning to the presence of an underlying medical problem.

REFERENCES

1. Finegold SM. Anaerobic Bacteria in Human Disease. New York: Academic Press, 1977.
2. Ingham HR, Sisson PR, Middleton RL, Narang HK, Codd AA, Selkon JB. Killing of gram-negative bacteria by polymorphonuclear leukocytes: role of an O_2-independent bactericidal system. J Clin Invest 1982; 69:959–70.
3. Brook I, Barrett CT, Brinkman CR, III, Martin WJ, Finegold SM. Aerobic and anaerobic flora of maternal cervix and newborn gastric fluid and conjunctiva: a prospective study. Pediatrics 1979; 63:451–5.
4. Gronlund MM, Arvilommi H, Kero P, Lehtonen OP, Isolauri E. Importance of intestinal colonisation in the maturation of humoral immunity in early infancy: a prospective follow up study of healthy infants aged 0–6 months. Arch Dis Child Fetal Neonatal Ed 2000; 83:F186–92.
5. Gibbons RJ. Aspects of the pathogenicity and ecology of the indigenous oral flora of man. In: Ballow A, et al. ed. Anaerobic Bacteria: Role in Disease. Springfield, IL: Charles C Thomas, 1974:267–85.
6. Mai V, Morris JG, Jr. Colonic bacterial flora: changing understandings in the molecular age. J Nutr 2004; 134:459–64.
7. Brook I. Aerobic and anaerobic bacteriology of cervical adenitis in children. Clin Pediatr 1980; 19:693–6.
8. Brook I, Frazier EH. Microbiology of cervical lymphadenitis in adults. Acta Otolaryngol 1998; 118:443–6.
9. Brook I, Frazier EH. Aerobic and anaerobic bacteriology of wounds and cutaneous abscesses. Arch Surg 1990; 125:1445–51.
10. Brook I, Randolph JG. Aerobic and anaerobic flora of burns in children. J Trauma 1981; 21:313–8.
11. Goldstein EJC. Current concepts on animal bites: bacteriology and therapy. Curr Clin Top Infect Dis 1999; 19:99–111.
12. Brook I. Aerobic and anaerobic microbiology of paronychia. Ann Emerg Med 1990; 19:994–6.
13. Brook I, Frazier EH, Thompson DH. Aerobic and anaerobic microbiology of peritonsillar abscess. Laryngoscope 1991; 101:289–92.
14. Brook I, Frazier EH. Correlation between microbiology and previous sinus surgery in patients with chronic maxillary sinusitis. Ann Otol Rhinol Laryngol 2001; 110:148–51.
15. Brook I. Microbiology and management of chronic suppurative otitis media in children. J Trop Pediatr 2003; 49:196–9.
16. Brook I, Frazier EH, Gher ME. Aerobic and anaerobic microbiology of periapical abscess. Oral Microbiol Immunol 1991; 6:123–5.
17. Brook I. Microbiology and management of acute suppurative thyroiditis in children. Int J Pediatr Otorhinolaryngol 2003; 67:447–51.
18. Bartlett JG. Anaerobic bacterial infections of the lung and pleural space. Clin Infect Dis 1993; 16(Suppl. 4):S248–55.
19. Brook I, Frazier EH. Aerobic and anaerobic microbiology of empyema. A retrospective review in two military hospitals. Chest 1993; 103:1502–7.
20. Brook I. Anaerobic bacterial bacteremia: 12-year experience in two military hospitals. J Infect Dis 1989; 160:1071–5.
21. Brook I, Frazier EH. A 12 year study of aerobic and anaerobic bacteria in intra-abdominal and postsurgical abdominal wound infections. Surg Gynecol Obstet 1989; 169:387–92.
22. Brook I, Frazier EH. Microbiology of liver and spleen abscesses. J Med Microbiol 1998; 47:1075–80.
23. Brook I, Frazier EH. Aerobic and anaerobic microbiology of retroperitoneal abscesses. Clin Infect Dis 1998; 26:938–41.
24. Walker CK, Workowski KA, Washington AE, Soper D, Sweet RL. Anaerobes in pelvic inflammatory disease: implications for the centers for disease control and prevention's guidelines for treatment of sexually transmitted diseases. Clin Infect Dis 1999; 28(Suppl. 1):S29–36.
25. Bryskier A. Anti-anaerobic activity of antibacterial agents. Expert Opin Investig Drugs 2001; 10:239–67.
26. Brook I. Bacteria from solid tumours. J Med Microbiol 1990; 32:207–10.
27. Brook I, Martin WJ, Finegold SM. Neonatal pneumonia caused by members of the *Bacteroides fragilis* group. Clin Pediatr 1980; 19:541–4.
28. Brook I, Frazier EH. Microbiology of scalp abscess in newborns. Pediatr Infect Dis J 1992; 11:766–8.

29. Rechner PM, Agger WA, Mruz K, Cogbill TH. Clinical features of clostridial bacteremia: a review from a rural area. Clin Infect Dis 2001; 33:349–53.
30. Severijnen AJ, van Kleef R, Hazenberg MP, van de Merwe JP. Chronic arthritis induced in rats by cell wall fragments of *Eubacterium* species from the human intestinal flora. Infect Immun 1990; 58:523–8.
31. Leung FW, Serota AI, Mulligan ME, George WL, Finegold SM. Nontraumatic clostridial myonecrosis: an infectious disease emergency. Ann Emerg Med 1981; 10:312–4.
32. Mantadakis E, Danilatou V, Christidou A, Stiakaki E, Kalmanti M. *Capnocytophaga gingivalis* bacteremia detected only on quantitative blood cultures in a child with leukemia. Pediatr Infect Dis J 2003; 22:202–4.
33. Maderazo EC, Anton TF, Ward PA. Inhibition of leukocytes in patients with cancer. Clin Immunol Immunopathol 1978; 9:166–76.
34. Phair JP, Riesing KS, Metzger E. Bacteremic infection and malnutrition in patients with solid tumors. Investigation of host defense mechanisms. Cancer 1980; 42:2702–6.
35. Chanock SJ, Pizzo PA. Infectious complications of patients undergoing therapy for acute leukemia: current status and future prospects. Semin Oncol 1997; 24:132–40.
36. Hughes WT, Armstrong D, Bodey GP, et al. 2002 guidelines for the use of antimicrobial agents in neutropenic patients with cancer. Clin Infect Dis 2002; 15(34):730–51.
37. Dosik EM, Luna M, Valdivieso M, et al. Necrotizing colitis in patients with cancer. Am J Med 1979; 67:646–56.
38. Leach WB. Acute leukemia: a pathological study of the causes of death in 157 proved cases. Can Med Assoc J 1961; 85:345–9.
39. Viola MV. Acute leukemia and infections. JAMA 1967; 201:923–6.
40. Prella JC, Kirsner JB. The gastrointestinal lesions and complications of the leukemias. Ann Intern Med 1964; 61:1084–103.
41. Vaupel P. Oxygen transport in tumors: characteristics and clinical implications. Adv Exp Med Biol 1996; 388:341–51.
42. Nuyts S, Van Mellaert L, Theys J, et al. Clostridium spores for tumor-specific drug delivery. Anticancer Drugs 2002; 13:115–25.
43. Malmgren RA, Flanigan CC. Localization of the vegetation form of *Clostridium tetani* in mouse tumors following intravenous spore administration. Cancer Res 1955; 15:473–8.
44. Alpern RJ, Dowell VR, Jr. *Clostridium septicum* infection and malignancy. J Am Med Assoc 1969; 209:385–8.
45. Cabrera A, Tsukada Y, Pickren JW. Clostridial gas gangrene and septicemia in malignant disease. Cancer 1965; 18:800–6.
46. Caya JG, Farmer SG, Ritch PS, et al. *Clostridia septicemia* complicating the course of leukemia. Cancer 1986; 57:2045–8.
47. Brook I. Bacterial infection associated with malignancy in children. Int J Pediatr Hematol Oncol 1999; 5:379–86.
48. Larson CM, Bubrick MP, Jacobs DM, et al. Malignancy, mortality, and medicosurgical management of *Clostridium septicum* infection. Surgery 1995; 118:592–7.
49. Prinssen HM, Hoekman K, Burger CW. *Clostridium septicum* myonecrosis and ovarian cancer: a case report and review of literature. Gynecol Oncol 1999; 72:116–9.
50. Felner JM, Dowell VR, Jr. "Bacteroides" bacteremia. Am J Med 1971; 50:787–96.

5 | Virulence of Anaerobic Bacteria and the Role of Capsule

PATHOGENICITY OF ANAEROBIC BACTERIA

Most anaerobic infections are pyogenic and arise from the normal flora of the skin, oropharynx, the large intestine, or the female genital tract. Such infections typically involve multiple species of bacteria, some strict anaerobes, some strict aerobes and others that are facultative anaerobes (i.e., able to grow aerobically or anaerobically). The polymicrobial nature of infections involving anaerobic bacteria is apparent in infections of the respiratory tract, abdomen, pelvis, and soft tissue, where the number of isolates in an infectious site varies between two and five (1–3). The contributing role of anaerobes in these infections has been often questioned (4).

In the past, it was thought that treating the aerobic component of the infectious flora to cure the infection was sufficient (4). This simplistic attitude was based on the assumption that anaerobes are dependent on the aerobic and facultative components of the infection to lower the Po$_2$ of their environment (5) and to provide them with essential metabolic by-products (6). Therefore, elimination of the aerobic and facultative flora would deprive the anaerobes of that support, and hence, they would be eliminated by the host defenses. However, substantial clinical and laboratory data exist that disproves this hypothesis and demonstrates the importance of anaerobes as pathogens in single or polymicrobial infections.

Some of the uncertainty regarding the role of anaerobes was clarified following several important observations: anaerobes often may be present in infection in pure culture as the only isolate or as part of a polymicrobial infection involving only anaerobic bacteria. They have also been recovered as the sole isolate in bacteremias (7).

The factors that determine the outcome of an anaerobic infection are the balance between the bacterial and host factors. The bacterial factors include the inoculum size, the virulence, and synergistic potential of the infecting organisms, while the opposing host factors include the host defense, breaks in the anatomic barriers, and reduction in the oxidation–reduction potential.

The major virulence factors of anaerobes are: their ability to adhere and invade epithelial surfaces; the production of toxins, enzymes, or other pathogenic factors; the production of superoxide dismutase and catalase, immunoglobulin proteases; and coagulation promoting and spreading factors (such as hyaluronidase, collagenase, and fibrinolysin), and with the presence of surface constituents such as capsular polysaccharide or lipopolysaccharide. Adherence of bacterial to epithelial cells is the first essential step of colonization or infection. *Bacteroides fragilis* adherence is mitigated through a pili-like structure, their capsule, and lectin-like adhesions. *Prevotella melaninogenica* attaches to certain gram-positive organisms, with cervicular epithelium. *Fusobacterium nucleatum* also attach to that epithelium. *Porphyromonas gingivalis* possesses fimbria that assists bacterial attachment.

The immune system is active in protection against anaerobic infection. Anaerobes activate complement directly, thus attracting polymorphonuclear leukocytes. Anaerobes are susceptible to killing by macrophages and are killed by oxidative and monoxidative mechanisms intracellularly. Both humoral and cell-mediated immune mechanisms actively protect the host from anaerobes. These include circulating antibodies and complement that have been shown to protect from experimental bacteremia, and T-lymphocytes that resist abscess formation (8).

Anaerobes can adversely affect the cellular and humoral immunity. Some can deplete or bind opsonins that bind to aerobes, thus preventing their oposonization (9); they can suppress the activity of polymorphonuclear leukocytes, macrophages, and lymphocytes (8); and neutrophils killing ability can be inhibited by short chain fatty acids produced by *B. fragilis* and other anaerobic gram-negative bacilli (AGNB) (10). *B. fragilis* can also interact with peritoneal macrophages inducing procoagulant activity and fibrin deposition that impairs clearance of the infecting organisms (11).

The ability of several anaerobes to possess a capsule was found to be an important virulence factor.

Factors that enhance the virulence of anaerobes include mucosal damage, oxidation–reduction potential drop, and the presence of hemoglobin or blood in an infected site. However, this chapter will be devoted only to the role of capsule as a virulence factor.

Clinical and animal studies showed bacterial synergy between anaerobic and aerobic or other anaerobic bacteria (12,13). Data derived from therapy of mixed infection also provided support for the importance of anaerobic bacteria. Polymicrobial infection involving aerobic and anaerobic bacteria responded to therapy directed at the eradication of only the anaerobic component of the infection with either metronidazole or clindamycin (14). However, for complete eradication of the infection, animal and patient studies have demonstrated that unless therapy is directed against both aerobic and anaerobic bacteria, the untreated organisms will survive (15–18). Bartlett et al. (15) demonstrated in an intra-abdominal abscess model in rats that combined therapy of clindamycin and gentamicin was needed to prevent mortality caused by *Escherichia coli* sepsis and abscesses caused by *B. fragilis*. Thadepalli et al. (16) showed that in patients with intra-abdominal trauma, clindamycin and kanamycin were superior to cephalothin and kanamycin in preventing septic complications. This principle of double coverage against aerobes and anaerobes has since then been proven to be the golden standard of therapy in numerous studies (17,18) using combination therapy (clindamycin, metronidazole, or cefoxitin plus an aminoglycoside) and single agent therapy with agents effective against both aerobes and anaerobes such as cefoxitin (19) or imipenem (20). A similar approach was found essential in the management of pelvic inflammatory disease in adults (21), and chronic otitis media (22) and chronic sinusitis (23) in children, where mixed aerobic–anaerobic flora were recovered from the majority of cases.

SYNERGY BETWEEN ANAEROBIC AND AEROBIC OR FACULTATIVE BACTERIA

Polymicrobial infections are known to be more pathogenic for experimental animals than those involving single organisms (5).

Several studies documented the synergistic effect of mixtures of aerobic and anaerobic bacteria in experimental infection. Altemeier (13) demonstrated the pathogenicity of bacterial isolates recovered from peritoneal cultures after appendiceal rupture. Pure cultures of individual isolates were relatively innocuous when implanted subcutaneously in animals, but combinations of facultative and anaerobic strains manifested increased virulence. Similar observations were reported by Meleney et al. (24) and Hite et al. (25).

Brook et al. (26) evaluated the synergistic potentials between aerobic and anaerobic bacteria commonly recovered in clinical infections. Each bacterium was inoculated subcutaneously alone or mixed with another organism into mice, and synergistic effects were determined by observing abscess formation and animal mortality. The tested bacteria included encapsulated *Bacteroides* spp., *Prevotella*, *Fusobacterium* spp., *Clostridium* spp., and anaerobic cocci. Facultative and anaerobic bacteria included *Staphylococcus aureus*, *Pseudomonas aeruginosa*, *E. coli*, *Klebsiella pneumoniae*, and *Proteus mirabilis*. In many combinations, the anaerobes significantly enhanced the virulence of each of the five aerobes. The most virulent combinations were between *P. aeruginosa* or *S. aureus* and anaerobic cocci or AGNB.

Enhancement of growth of aerobic and facultative bacteria was also apparent when they were co-inoculated into mice and a subcutaneous abscess was formed. *Streptococcus pyogenes*, *E. coli*, *S. aureus*, *K. pneumoniae*, and *P. aeruginosa* were enhanced by *B. fragilis*, *P. melaninogenica* (27,28) *Peptostreptococcus* spp. (29,30), *Fusobacterium* spp. (31,32), and *Clostridium* spp. (33), except *Clostridium difficile*. Although mutual enhancement of growth of both aerobic and anaerobic bacteria was noticed, the number of aerobic and facultative bacteria was increased many folds more than their anaerobic counterparts. Exceptions to the mutual enhancement were noticed in combinations between organisms that are generally not recovered together in mixed infections, such as *Enterococcus faecalis* and *P. melaninogenica* (28). The above observations suggest that the aerobic and facultative bacterial benefit even more than do the anaerobes from their symbiosis.

The demonstration of the synergistic potentials of anaerobic bacteria commonly recovered in polymicrobial infections provide further support for their pathogenic role in these infections. Several hypotheses have been proposed to explain microbial synergy in mixed infections (30). When this phenomenon occurs in mixtures of aerobic and anaerobic flora, it may be due to protection from phagocytosis and intracellular killing (11,30), production of essential growth factors (6), and lowering of oxidation–reduction potentials in host tissues (5). Obligate anaerobes can interfere with the phagocytosis and killing of aerobic bacteria (35). The ability of human polymorphonuclear leukocytes to phagocytose and kill *P. mirabilis* was impaired in vitro when the human serum used to opsonize the target bacterium was pretreated with live or dead organisms of various AGNB (34). *Porphyromonas gingivalis* cells or supernatant culture fluid was shown to possess the greatest inhibitory effect among the AGNB (35). Supernatants of cultures of *B. fragilis* group, pigmented *Prevotella* and *Porphyromonas*, and *P. gingivalis* were capable of inhibiting the chemotaxis of leukocytes to the chemotactic factors of *P. mirabilis* (36).

Bacteria may also provide nutrients for each other. *Klebsiella* spp. produces succinate, which supports *P. assacharolytica* (37), and oral diphtheroids produced vitamin K which is a growth factor for *P. melaninogenica* (38).

Another possible mechanism that explains the synergistic effect of aerobic–anaerobic combinations is the lowering of local oxygen concentrations and the oxidation–reduction potential by the aerobic bacteria. The resultant physical conditions are appropriate for replication and invasion by the anaerobic component of the infection. Such environmental factors are known to be critical for anaerobic growth in vitro and may apply with equal relevance to in vivo experimental animal studies. Mergenhagen et al. noted that the infecting dose of anaerobic cocci was significantly lowered when the inoculum was supplemented with chemical reducing agents (5). A similar effect may be produced by facultative bacteria, which may provide the proper conditions for establishing an anaerobic infection at a previously well-oxygenated site.

CAPSULE FORMATION IN EXPERIMENTAL MIXED INFECTIONS

An important virulence factor of *Bacteroides* spp. is the possession of a capsule. Several studies demonstrated the pathogenicity of encapsulated anaerobes and their ability to induce abscesses when injected alone in animals. Onderdonk et al. (39) correlated the virulence of *B. fragilis* strains with the presence of capsule, and Simon et al. (40) described decreased phagocytosis of the encapsulated *B. fragilis*. Capsular material from *P. melaninogenica* also inhibits phagocytosis and phagocytic killing of other microorganisms in an in vitro system (41). Tofte et al. (42), Jones and Gemmel (34), and Ingham et al. (32) have shown that both phagocytic uptake and killing of facultative species were impaired by encapsulated *Bacteroides* spp.

The presence of capsule in *B. fragilis* was shown to provide the organism with growth advantage in vivo over unencapsulated isolates (43). Furthermore, encapsulated strains survived better in vitro than unencapsulated variants when they were grown in an aerobic environment. Thus, the presence of a capsule apparently enables a strain of *Bacteroides* to resist exposure to oxygen as well as host defenses. Another mechanism of protection is the inhibition of polymorphonuclear migration caused by the production of succinic acid by *Bacteroides* spp. (11).

The ability of the aerobic component in mixed infections to enhance the appearance of encapsulated anaerobic bacteria in these infections was studied in an abscess model in mice. The anaerobic bacteria with which they were inoculated were those commonly recovered in mixed infections.

Pigmented *Prevotella* and *Porphyromonas* spp. (44), *Prevotella bivia* (45), *B. fragilis* group (46), and anaerobic and facultative gram-positive cocci (AFGPC) (47) did not induce abscess when isolates that contained only a small number of encapsulated organisms (<1%) were inoculated. However, when these relatively nonencapsulated isolates were inoculated, mixed with abscess-forming viable or nonviable bacteria ("helpers"), the *Bacteroides, Prevotella, Porphyromonas*, and AFGPC survived in the abscess and became heavily encapsulated (> 50% of organisms had a capsule). Thereafter, these heavily encapsulated anaerobic isolates were able to induce abscesses when injected alone (Fig. 1). Of interest is the observed appearance of pili along with encapsulation in the *B. fragilis* group after co-inoculation with *K. pneumoniae* (46).

Most of the "helper" strains were encapsulated; although several of the strains were not encapsulated, and they were able to induce abscesses when inoculated alone. The "helper" organisms used in conjunction with pigmented *Prevotella* and *Porphyromonas*, and AFGPC were *S. aureus, S. pyogenes, Haemophilus influenzae, P. aeruginosa, E. coli, K. pneumoniae*, and AGNB (44,47). For the *B. fragilis* group, these organisms were *E. coli, K. pneumoniae, S. aureus, S. pyogenes*, and *Enterococcus* spp. (46). *Neisseria gonorrhoeae* was chosen as a helper for *B. fragilis*, and *Prevotella* and *Porphyromonas* spp. (45). Of interest is the observed inability of *N. gonorrhoeae* strains to survive in intra-abdominal abscesses and also their disappearance from abscesses within five days of inoculation with AGNB and *P. bivia* (45).

The virulence of *Fusobacterium* spp. was also associated with the presence of a capsule. Only encapsulated strains of *F. nucleatum, Fusobacterium necrophorum*, and *Fusobacterium varium* were able to induce abscesses when inoculated alone (31). However, following passage in animals of nonencapsulated strains, none of these organisms acquired a capsule.

The presence of a thick granular cell wall (300–360 Å) before animal passage was associated with virulence of *Clostridium* spp. (33). Such structure was observed before inoculation into animals, only in *Clostridium perfringens*, and *Clostridium butyricum*, the only organisms capable of inducing an abscess when inoculated alone. This structure was observed in other *Clostridium* species only after their co-inoculation with encapsulated AGNB or *K. pneumoniae*.

However, other undetermined factors may also contribute to the induction of an abscess, since most isolates of *C. difficile* were not able to produce an abscess even though they possessed a thick wall.

The selection of encapsulated AGNB and AFGPC with the assistance of other encapsulated or nonencapsulated but abscess-forming aerobic or anaerobic organisms may explain the conversion into pathogens of non-pathogenic organisms that are part of the normal

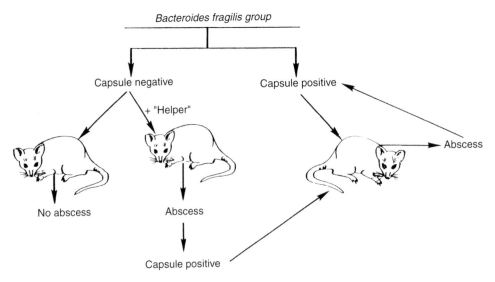

FIGURE 1 Encapsulation cycle of *B. fragilis* group after passage in mice. "Helper" is viable bacteria or formalized bacteria or capsular material.

host flora or are concomitant pathogens. Although such a phenomenon was not observed in *Fusobacterium* spp., the presence of a capsule in these organisms was a prerequisite for induction of abscesses. Some *Clostridium* spp. also manifested cell wall changes after animal passage that could be associated with increased virulence. Although the exact nature and chemical composition of the capsule or external cell wall may be different in each of the anaerobic species studied, the changes that were observed tended to follow similar patterns.

The mechanism that is responsible for the observed phenomenon is yet unknown, and may be due to either genetic transformation or a process of selection.

ROLE OF A CAPSULE OF *BACTEROIDES* SPP. AND ANAEROBIC COCCI IN BACTEREMIA

Anaerobic bacteremia account for 5% to 15% of cases of bacteremia (1,4), and are especially prevalent in polymicrobial bacteremia, associated with abscesses (7).

The role of possession of capsular material in the systemic spread of AGNB and AFGPC was investigated in mice following subcutaneous inoculation of encapsulated strains alone or in combination with aerobic or anaerobic facultative bacteria (48). Encapsulated anaerobes were isolated more frequently from infected animal blood, spleen, liver, and kidney than were nonencapsulated organisms.

After inoculation with a single encapsulated anaerobic strain, encapsulated organisms were recovered in 163 of 420 (39%) animals, whereas nonencapsulated anaerobes were recovered in only 14 of 420 (3%) animals. Following inoculation of *B. fragilis* mixed with aerobic or facultative flora, encapsulated *B. fragilis* was isolated more often and for longer periods of time than was the nonencapsulated strain. Furthermore, encapsulated *B. fragilis* was recovered more often after inoculation with other flora than it was when inoculated alone.

Therefore, encapsulated strains were found to be more virulent than their nonencapsulated strains. These data highlight the importance of encapsulated AGNB and AFGPC in increasing the mortality associated with bacteremia and the spread to different organs. A similar pathogenic quality was observed in other bacterial species, such as *Streptococcus pneumoniae* (49) and *H. influenzae* (50), where the encapsulated strains showed greater ability for systemic spread.

SIGNIFICANCE OF ANAEROBIC BACTERIA IN MIXED INFECTION WITH OTHER FLORA

Although anaerobic bacteria often are recovered mixed with other aerobic and facultative flora, their exact role in these infections and their relative contribution to the pathogenic process are unknown. The relative importance of the organisms present in the abscess caused by two bacteria (an aerobe and an anaerobe) and the effect of encapsulation on the relationship were determined by comparing the abscess sizes in (*i*) mice treated with antibiotics directed against one or both organisms and (*ii*) nontreated animals (27,31,33,34,47).

As judged by selective antimicrobial therapy, the possession of a capsule in most mixed infections involving AGNB generally made these organisms more important than their aerobic counterparts. In almost all instances, the aerobic counterparts in the infection were more important than nonencapsulated AGNB (27). Encapsulated members of the pigmented *Prevotella* and *Porphyromonas* were almost always more important in mixed infections than their aerobic counterparts (*S. pyogenes*, *S. pneumoniae*, *K. pneumoniae*, *H. influenzae*, and *S. aureus*). Encapsulated *B. fragilis* group organisms were found to be more important than or as important as *E. coli* and enterococci and less important than *S. aureus*, *S. pyogenes*, and *K. pneumoniae*.

In contrast to AGNB, encapsulated AFGPC were found more often to be less important than their aerobic counterparts (47). *Clostridium* spp. and *Fusobacterium* spp. were found to be less or equally important to enteric gram-negative rods (31–33). Although *Fusobacterium* spp., AFGPC, and *Clostridium* spp. were generally equal to or less important than their aerobic counterpart, variations in the relationship existed. However, as determined by the abscess size, most of the anaerobic organisms enhanced mixed infection.

ENCAPSULATED ANAEROBIC BACTERIA IN CLINICAL INFECTIONS

In an attempt to define the important pathogens among the isolates recovered from clinical specimens, Brook et al. studied the virulence and importance of encapsulated bacterial isolates recovered from 13 clinical abscesses (51). This was done by injecting each of the 35 isolates (30 anaerobes and 5 aerobes) subcutaneously into mice alone or in all possible combinations with the other isolates recovered from the same abscess. The ability of each isolate to induce and/or survive in a subcutaneous abscess was determined. Sixteen of the isolates were encapsulated; 15 of them were able to cause abscesses by themselves and were recovered from the abscesses even when inoculated alone. The other organisms, which were not encapsulated, were not able to induce abscesses when inoculated alone. However, some were able to survive when injected with encapsulated strains. Therefore, the possession of a capsule by an organism was associated with increased virulence, compared with the same organism's nonencapsulated counterparts, and might have allowed some of the other accompanying organisms to survive. We found this phenomenon to occur in AGNB, *Prevotella* spp. anaerobic gram-positive cocci, *Clostridium* spp., and *E. coli*. Detection of a capsule in a clinical isolate may therefore suggest a pathogenic role of the organism in the infection.

Three studies support the importance of encapsulated anaerobic organisms in respiratory infections (52–54). The presence of encapsulated and abscess-forming organisms that belong to the pigmented *Prevotella* and *Porphyromonas* spp. (previously called *B. melaninogenicus* group) was investigated in 25 children with acute tonsillitis and in 23 children without tonsillar inflammation (control) (52). Encapsulated pigmented *Prevotella* and *Porphyromonas* were found in 23 of 25 children with acute tonsillitis, compared with 5 of 23 controls ($p<0.001$). Subcutaneous inoculation into mice of the *Prevotella* and *Porphyromonas* strains that had been isolated from patients with tonsillitis produced abscesses in 17 of 25 instances, compared with 9 of 23 controls ($p< 0.05$). These findings suggest a possible pathogenic role for pigmented *Prevotella* and *Porphyromonas* spp. in acute tonsillar infection, and also suggest the importance of encapsulation in the pathogenesis of the infection.

In another study (53), the presence of encapsulated AGNB (*Prevotella* and *Porphyromonas* spp., and fragilis group) and anaerobic gram-positive cocci was investigated in 182 patients with chronic orofacial infections and in the pharynx of 26 individuals without inflammation (Table 1). Forty-nine of the patients had chronic otitis media, 45 had cervical

TABLE 1 Encapsulated Anaerobic Bacteria in Children with Abscesses and Chronic Inflammation Compared with Controls (Number of Strains Isolated)

Clinical diagnosis (number of samples)	Pigmented *Prevotella* and *Porphyromonas*	*Prevotella oralis*	*Bacteroides fragilis* group	Peptostrepto-coccus spp.	Total
Chronic otitis media (*n*= 48)	15/19	4/6	7/10	19/25	45/60 (75%)[a]
Chronic mastoiditis (*n*=24)	9/11	2/2	3/3	11/15	25/31 (81%)[a]
Chronic sinusitis (*n*=37)	10/14	3/5	—	16/20	29/39 (74%)[a]
Peritonsillar abscess (*n*= 16)	21/23	3/5	—	16/22	40/50 (80%)[a]
Periapical abscess (*n*= 12)	8/9	3/3	—	10/12	21/24 (87%)[a]
Cervical lymphadenitis (*n*=45)	4/4	—	—	6/8	10/12 (83%)[b]
Total number in all infected sites[d] (*n*=182)	67/80 (84%)[a]	15/21(71%)[c]	10/13 (77%)	78/102 (76%)[c]	170/216 (79%)[a]
Pharyngeal culture (*n*= 26) (control)	8/35 (25%)	4/13 (31%)	—	22/48 (46%)	34/96 (35%)

[a]$p<0.001$.
[b]$p<0.005$.
[c]$p<0.05$, respectively, when compared to control.
[d]Encapsulated/total (%).
Source: From Ref. 53.

lymphadenitis, 37 had chronic sinusitis, 24 had chronic mastoiditis, 10 had peritonsillar abscesses, and 12 had periodontal abscesses. One hundred seventy of the 216 (79%) isolates of *Prevotella* and *Porphyromonas*, *B. fragilis* group, and anaerobic cocci were found to be encapsulated in patients with chronic infections, compared to only 34 of 96 (35%) controls ($p < 0.001$).

The presence of encapsulated and piliated AGNB (mostly *B. fragilis* group and pigmented *Prevotella* and *Porphyromonas*) was investigated in isolates from blood, abscesses and normal flora (54). Of the strains of AGNB isolated, 45 of 54 (83%) recovered from blood and 31 of 40 (78%) found in abscesses were encapsulated. In contrast, only 7 of 71 (10%) similar strains isolated from the faeces or pharynx of healthy persons were encapsulated ($p < 0.001$). Pili were observed in 3 of 54 (6%) of strains isolated from blood, 30 of 40 (75%) of those recovered from abscesses ($p < 0.001$), and 49 of 71 (69%) of those found in normal flora ($p < 0.001$) (Fig. 2 shows only *B fragilis* group). The predominance of encapsulated forms in all strains of AGNB in blood as well as in abscesses suggests an increased virulence of these compared with nonencapsulated isolates. In contrast, the presence of pili in AGNB recovered mostly from abscesses and normal flora suggests that this structure may play a role in the ability of these organisms to adhere to mucous membranes and may interfere with their ability to spread systematically. These findings illustrate the morphologic differences that may be observed in AGNB from various anatomic sites.

The predominance of encapsulated *Bacteroides*, *Prevotella*, and *Porphyromonas* spp. recovered from blood and abscesses compared with their rate of encapsulation in the normal flora of the pharynx and faeces suggests an increased virulence of these strains as compared to nonencapsulated strains. In contrast to the emergence of encapsulated AGNB in blood and abscesses, the presence of pili was less frequent in such strains recovered from blood. The rate of piliated strains was high among those recovered from abscesses.

Since most *B. fragilis*, and *Prevotella* and *Porphyromonas* spp. recovered from infected sites probably originate from the predominantly nonencapsulated endogenous flora of mucous membranes, they may express their capsules only during the inflammatory process. The frequent recovery of encapsulated AGNB in such conditions illustrates their increased virulence as compared to their nonencapsulated counterparts.

Complete eradication of experimental AGNB infection by means of metronidazole was not achieved when these organisms were encapsulated (10). Once the organisms become encapsulated, eradication of AGNB infection becomes difficult. Therapy of infections involving nonencapsulated AGNB, however, was more efficacious. Early treatment of anaerobic infections may therefore prevent the emergence of encapsulated AGNB, and subsequent bacteraemia.

The recovery of a greater number of encapsulated anaerobic organisms in patients with orofacial infections, abscesses, and blood provides support for the potential pathogenic role of encapsulated organisms. Early and vigorous antimicrobial therapy, directed at both aerobic and anaerobic bacteria present in these mixed infections, may abort the infection before the emergence of encapsulated strains that contribute to the chronicity of the infection.

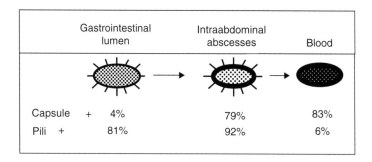

FIGURE 2 Dynamics of pili and capsule of *B. fragilis* group. *Source*: From Ref. 54.

CONCLUSION

The recovery of a greater number of encapsulated anaerobic organisms in patients with acute and chronic infections provides further support for the potential pathogenic role of these organisms. Detection of the presence of a capsule in a clinical isolate may add importance to the organisms' possible role as a pathogen in the infection. The demonstration of the importance of encapsulated organisms in mixed infection may justify directing therapy in such infections against these potential pathogens. Early and vigorous antimicrobial therapy, directed at both aerobic and anaerobic bacteria present in these mixed infections, may abort the infection before the emergence of encapsulated strains that contribute to the chronicity of the infection.

REFERENCES

1. Finegold SM. Anaerobic Bacteria in Human Disease. New York: Academic Press, 1977.
2. Brook I, Frazier EH. Aerobic and anaerobic bacteriology of wounds and cutaneous abscesses. Arch Surg 1990; 125:1445–51.
3. Brook I. A 12 year study of aerobic and anaerobic bacteria in intra-abdominal and postsurgical abdominal wound infections. Surg Gynecol Obstet 1989; 169:387–92.
4. Gorbach SL, Bartlett JG. Anaerobic infections. N Engl J Med 1974; 290:1177–84.
5. Mergenhagen SE, Thonard JC, Scherp HW. Studies on synergistic infection. I. Experimental infection with anaerobic streptococci. J Infect Dis 1958; 103:33–44.
6. Lev M, Krudell KC, Milford AF. Succinate as a growth factor for *Bacteroides melaninogenicus*. J Bacteriol 1971; 108:175–8.
7. Brook I. Anaerobic bacterial bacteremia: 12-year experience in two military hospitals. J Infect Dis 1989; 160:1071–5.
8. Tzianabos AO, Kasper DL, Cisneros RL, Smith RS, Onderdonk AB. Polysaccharide-mediated protection against abscess formation in experimental intra-abdominal sepsis. J Clin Invest 1995; 96:2727–31.
9. Klempner MS. Interactions of polymorphonuclear leukocytes with anaerobic bacteria. Rev Infect Dis 1984; 6(Suppl. 1):S40–4.
10. Brook I. Pathogenicity of encapsulated and non-encapsulated members of *Bacteroides fragilis* and *melaninogenicus* groups in mixed infection with *Escherichia coli* and *Streptococcus pyogenes*. J Med Microbiol 1988; 27:191–8.
11. Rotstein OD. Interactions between leukocytes and anaerobic bacteria in polymicrobial surgical infections. Clin Infect Dis 1993; 16(Suppl. 4):S190–4.
12. Meleney FL. Bacterial synergy in disease processes. Ann Surg 1931; 22:961–73.
13. Altemeier WA. The pathogenicity of the bacteria of appendicitis. Surgery 1942; 11:374–85.
14. Brook I, Coolbaugh JC, Walker RI. Antibiotic and clavulanic acid therapy of subcutaneous abscesses caused by *Bacteroides fragilis* alone or in combination with aerobic bacteria. J Infect Dis 1983; 148:156–9.
15. Bartlett JG, Louie TJ, Gorbach SL, Onderdonk AB. Therapeutic efficacy of 29 antimicrobial regimens in experimental intraabdominal sepsis. Rev Infect Dis 1981; 3:535–42.
16. Thadepalli H, Gorbach SL, Broido PW, Norsen J, Nyhus L. Abdominal trauma, anaerobes and antibiotics. Surg Gynecol Obstet 1973; 137:270–6.
17. Brook I. Management of anaerobic infection. Expert Rev Anti Infect Ther 2004; 2:89–94.
18. Holzheimer RG, Dralle H. Antibiotic therapy in intra-abdominal infections—a review on randomised clinical trials. Eur J Med Res 2001; 30(6):277–91.
19. Fabian TC. Infection in penetrating abdominal trauma: risk factors and preventive antibiotics. Am Surg 2002; 68:29–35.
20. Geddes AM, Stille W. Imipenem: the first thienamycin antibiotic. Rev Infect Dis 1985; 7:S353–6.
21. Barrett S, Taylor C. A review on pelvic inflammatory disease. Int J STD AIDS 2005; 16:715–20.
22. Brook I. Management of chronic suppurative otitis media: superiority of therapy effective against anaerobic bacteria. Pediatr Infect Dis J 1994; 13:188–93.
23. Brook I, Yocum P. Antimicrobial management of chronic sinusitis in children. J Laryngol Otol 1995; 109:1159–62.
24. Meleney FL. A review of antibiotic treatment for surgical infections, with special reference to the importance of local and systemic administration of specific antibiotics. J Int Coll Surg 1962; 37:260–70.
25. Hite KE, Locke M, Heseltine HC. Synergism in experimental infections with nonsporulating anaerobic bacteria. J Infect Dis 1949; 84:1.
26. Brook I, Hunter V, Walker RI. Synergistic effects of anaerobic cocci, *Bacteroides, Clostridia, Fusobacteria*, and aerobic bacteria on mouse mortality and induction of subcutaneous abscess. J Infect Dis 1984; 149:924–8.
27. Brook I, Walker RI. Significance of encapsulated *Bacteroides melaninogenicus* and *Bacteroides fragilis* groups in mixed infections. Infect Immun 1984; 44:12–5.

28. Brook I. Enhancement of growth of aerobic and facultative bacteria in mixed infections with *Bacteroides fragilis* and *melaninogenicus* groups. Infect Immun 1985; 50:929–31.

29. Brook I. Enhancement of growth of aerobic, anaerobic and facultative bacteria in mixed infections with anaerobic and facultative gram positive cocci. J Surg Res 1988; 45:222–7.

30. Hofstad T. Virulence factors in anaerobic bacteria. Eur J Clin Microbiol Infect Dis 1992; 11:1044–8.

31. Brook I, Walker RI. The relationship between *Fusobacterium* species and other flora in mixed infection. J Med Microbiol 1986; 21:93–100.

32. Ingham HR, Sisson PR, Tharagonnet D, Selkon JB, Codd AA. Inhibition of phagocytosis in vitro by obligate anaerobes. Lancet 1977; 2:1252–4.

33. Brook I, Walker RI. Pathogenicity of *Clostridium* species with other bacteria in mixed infection. J Infect 1986; 13:245–53.

34. Jones GR, Gemmel CG. Impairment by *Bacteroides* species of opsonization and phagocytosis of enterobacteria. J Med Microbiol 1982; 15:351–61.

35. Namavar F, Verweij-van Vught AMJJ, Vel WAC, Bal M, MacLaren DM. Polymorphonuclear leukocyte chemotaxis by mixed anaerobic and aerobic bacteria. J Med Microbiol 1984; 18:167–72.

36. Namavar F, Verweij AMJJ, Bal M, Martijn van Steenbergen TJ, de Graaf J, MacLaren DM. Effect of anaerobic bacteria on killing of *Proteus mirabilis* by human polymorphonuclear leukocytes. Infect Immun 1983; 40:930–5.

37. Mayrand D, McBride BG. Ecological relationships of bacteria involved in a simple mixed anaerobic infection. Infect Immun 1980; 27:44–50.

38. Cibbons RJ, MacDonald JB. Hemin and vitamin K compounds as required factors for the cultivation of certain strains of *Bacteroides melaninogenicus*. J Bacteriol 1960; 80:164–70.

39. Onderdonk AB, Cisneros DL, Bartlett JB. The capsular polysaccharide of *Bacteroides fragilis* as a virulence factor: comparison of the pathogenic potential of encapsulated strain. J Infect Dis 1977; 136:82–9.

40. Simon GL, Klempner MS, Kasper DL, Gorbach SL. Alterations in opsonophagocytic killing by neutrophils of *Bacteroides fragilis* associated with animals and laboratory passage: effect of capsular polysaccharide. J Infect Dis 1982; 145:72–7.

41. Okuda K, Takazoe I. Antiphagocytic effects of the capsular structure of a pathogenic strain of *Bacteroides melaninogenicus*. Bull Tokyo Dent Col 1973; 14:99–104.

42. Tofte RW, Peterson PK, Schmeling D, Bracke J, Kim Y, Quie PG. Opsonization of four *Bacteroides* species: role of the classical complement pathway and immunoglobulin. Infect Immun 1980; 27:78–924.

43. Patrick S, Reid JH, Larkin MJ. The growth and survival of capsulate and non-capsulate *Bacteroides fragilis* in vivo and in vitro. J Med Microbiol 1984; 17:237–46.

44. Brook I, Gillmore JD, Coolbaugh JC, Walker RI. Pathogenicity of encapsulated *Bacteroides melaninogenicus* group, *Bacteroides oralis*, and *Bacteroides ruminicola* in abscesses in mice. J Infect 1983; 7:218–26.

45. Brook I. The effect of encapsulation on the pathogenicity of mixed infection of *Neisseria gonorrhoea* and *Bacteroides* spp.. Am J Obstet Gynecol 1986; 155:421–8.

46. Brook I, Coolbaugh JC, Walker RI. Pathogenicity of piliated and encapsulated *Bacteroides fragilis*. Eur J Clin Microbiol 1984; 3:207–9.

47. Brook I, Walker RI. Pathogenicity of anaerobic gram positive cocci. Infect Immun 1984; 45:320–4.

48. Brook I. Bacteremia and seeding of encapsulated *Bacteroides* sp. and anaerobic cocci. J Med Microbiol 1987; 23:61–7.

49. Dhingra RK, Williams RC, Jr., Reed WP. Effects of pneumococcal mucopeptide and capsular polysaccharide on phagocytosis. Infect Immun 1977; 15:169–74.

50. Inzana TJ, Tosi MF, Kaplan SL, Anderson DC, Mason EO, Jr., Williams RP. Effect of *Haemophilus influenzae* type b lipopolysaccharide on complement activation and polymorphonuclear leukocyte function. Pediatr Res 1987; 22:659–66.

51. Brook I, Walker RI. Infectivity of organisms recovered from polymicrobial abscesses. Infect Immun 1983; 41:986–9.

52. Brook I, Gober AE. *Bacteroides melaninogenicus*: its recovery from tonsils of children with acute tonsillitis. Arch Otolaryngol 1984; 109:818–20.

53. Brook I. Recovery of encapsulated anaerobic bacteria from orofacial abscesses. J Med Microbiol 1986; 22:171–4.

54. Brook I, Myhal LA, Dorsey CH. Encapsulation and pilus formation of *Bacteroides* spp. in normal flora abscesses and blood. J Infect 1992; 25:251–7.

6 | Neonatal Infections

The incidence of infection in the fetus and newborn infant is high. As many as 2% of fetuses are infected in utero and up to 10% of infants are infected during delivery or in the first few months of life. The predominant microorganisms known to cause these infections are cytomegalovirus, herpes simplex virus, rubella virus, *Toxoplasma gondii*, *Treponema pallidum*, *Chlamydia*, Group B *Streptococcus*, *Enterococcus* spp., *Escherichia coli*, and anaerobic bacteria. All of these agents can colonize or infect the mother and infect the fetus or newborn either intrauterinely or during the passage through the birth canal. Although anaerobic bacteria cause a small number of these infections, the conditions predisposing to anaerobic infections in newborns are similar to those associated with aerobic microorganisms. Furthermore, the true incidence of anaerobic infections may be underestimated because techniques for the recovery and isolation of anaerobic bacteria are rarely used, or are inadequate. Several factors have been associated with acquisition of local or systemic infection in the newborn. Most of these factors are vague and difficult to define; however, most studies have described the presence of one or more risk factors in the pregnancy and delivery of these infants: premature and prolonged rupture of membranes (longer than 24 hours), maternal peripartum infection, premature delivery, low birth weight, depressed respiratory function of the infant at birth or fetal anoxia, and septic or traumatic delivery (1–3).

Maternal infection at the time of delivery, can be associated with the development of infection in the newborn. Transplacental hematogenous infection that can spread before or during delivery is another way in which the infant can be infected (4). The acquisition of infection while the newborn passes through the birth canal is, however, the most frequent mode of transfer.

During pregnancy, the fetus is shielded from the flora of the mother's genital tract. Potentially pathogenic bacteria are found in the amniotic fluid (AF) even when the membranes are intact. Prevedourakis et al. (5) documented bacterial invasion of the intact amnion in nearly 8% of the pregnant women in their sample, but this was of no consequence to the mother or the newborn infant. It was suspected that the AF may have antibacterial properties, probably owing to lack of nutritional factors (5,6). The AF actively inhibited the growth of aerobic bacteria, through a phosphate-sensitive cationic protein that is regulated by zinc (7). Its activity was independent of the muramidase and peroxidases, and spermine. The pH of the AF is the only variable predictive of bacterial growth in AF in a laboratory model (8).

The antimicrobial properties of the AF also vary with the period of gestation; it is the least inhibitory against *E. coli* and *Bacteroides fragilis* during the first trimester and most inhibitory during the third trimester (8,9). The relative scarcity of the *B. fragilis* population in the cervix at term labor and the added inhibitory effect of the AF at term may together explain the relatively low incidence of *B. fragilis* infections at full term as compared to postabortal sepsis (10–12).

Following the rupture of the membranes, the colonization of the newborn is initiated (4) by further exposure to the flora during the infant's passage through the birth canal. When premature rupture of the membranes occurs, the ascending flora can cause infection of the AF with involvement of the fetal membranes, placenta, and umbilical cord (13). Aspiration of the infected AF can cause aspiration pneumonia. Since anaerobic bacteria are the predominant organisms in the mother's genital flora (14), they become major pathogens in infections that follow early exposure of the newborn to that flora.

Genetic factors may be responsible for the predominance of sepsis in the newborn male (15). The immaturity of the immunologic system, which is manifested by decreased function of the phagocytes and decreased inflammatory reactions, may also contribute to the susceptibility of infants to microbial infection (16,17). The presence of anoxia and acidosis in the newborn may interfere also with the defense mechanisms.

The support systems and procedures used in regular nurseries and intensive care units can facilitate the acquisition of infections. Offending instruments include umbilical catheters, arterial lines, and intubation devices. Contamination of equipment such as humidifiers and supplies such as intravenous solutions and infant formulas, and poor isolation techniques can result in outbreaks of bacterial or viral infections in nurseries. Such spread is thought to contribute to clustering of cases of necrotizing enterocolitis in newborns.

CONJUNCTIVITIS AND DACRYOCYSTITIS

Conjunctivitis

Conjunctivitis in the newborn infant usually is due to chemical and mechanical irritation caused by the instillation of silver nitrate drops or ointment into the eye in order to prevent gonorrheal ophthalmia. Chemical conjunctivitis differs from infective forms in that it becomes apparent almost immediately after the instillation. The most common causes of infectious conjunctivitis in descending order of frequency are *Chlamydia trachomatis*, *Neisseria gonorrhoeae*, *Staphylococcus* spp., inclusion conjunctivitis caused by groups A and B *Streptococcus*, *Enterococcus* spp., *Streptococcus pneumoniae*, *Haemophilus influenzae*, *Pseudomonas aeruginosa*, *E. coli*, *Moraxella catarrhalis*, *Neisseria meningitidis*, *Corynebacterium diphtheriae*, herpes simplex virus, echoviruses, and *Mycoplasma hominis* (18). Clostridia and peptostreptococci were also implicated as probable causes of neonatal conjunctivitis (19).

The classical ophthalmia neonatorum caused by *N. gonorrhoeae* is an acute purulent conjunctivitis that appears from two to five days after birth. If untreated, the infection progresses rapidly until the eye becomes puffy and the conjunctiva is intensely red and swollen. The subsequent outcome would be corneal ulceration. Ophthalmia caused by organisms other than gonococcus, including *Clostridium* spp., occurs usually from 5 to 14 days following delivery, is indistinguishable clinically, and the conjunctival inflammatory reaction usually is milder than in ophthalmia caused by gonococci.

Isenberg et al. (20) who studied 106 infants, 50 delivered by cesarian section, and 56 delivered vaginally illustrated that those delivered by cesarean section had significantly fewer bacterial species and total number of organisms per subject than the infants delivered vaginally. The conjunctivae of infants delivered vaginally had significantly more bacteria characteristic of vaginal flora.

The conjunctiva of newborns acquires facultative and anaerobic bacteria during birth primarily from the mother's cervical flora during passage through the birth canal (14). The role of anaerobes in neonatal conjunctivitis was investigated by obtaining conjunctival cultures from 35 babies prior to silver nitrate application and 48 hours later (19). On initial culture, 46 facultative bacteria, and 27 anaerobes were recovered. The organisms isolated in almost all of these cases were present also in the mother's cervical cultures and in the baby's gastric aspirates, taken concomitantly. *Clostridium* spp. were recovered from two infants who developed conjunctivitis (14,19).

Clostridium perfringens was recovered from one newborn, and *Clostridium bifermentans* with *Peptostreptococcus* spp. were recovered from the other infant. Similar organisms were also recovered from the mother's cervix immediately after delivery. These infections were noted on the second and third day postdelivery. The conjunctivitis was characterized by a profuse yellow–green discharge and the eyelids were edematous in both newborns, and there were no other abnormal findings. Local therapy was initiated with 2% penicillin eye drops (two drops every two hours). The conjunctivitis subsided within three days, and repeat cultures of the eyes after 10 days were sterile. The babies were followed for three months with no residual of infection noted.

Of considerable interest is the change in the conjunctival flora after 48 hours. *Gardnerella vaginalis*, *Bacteroides* spp., and anaerobic cocci all but disappeared, whereas *Staphylococcus epidermidis*, *Micrococcus* spp., and *Propionibacterium acnes* increased in numbers. It is obvious that the conjunctiva of the newborn can be exposed to not only *N. gonorrhoeae*, but to other potentially pathogenic bacteria as well. However, most of those organisms disappeared from the conjunctiva within 48 hours.

Streptococcus mitis, a microaerophilic organisms that is part of the vaginal flora was associated with increased risk of conjunctivitis in newborns (21).

Of interest is that the silver nitrate solution of 1% currently used in newborns was efficacious in preventing in vitro growth of clostridia. However, in a concentration of 0.1% or lower, it was only bacteriostatic or ineffective (19). The common practice of rinsing the eyes with distilled water after the addition of silver nitrate to prevent chemical conjunctivitis may alter the ability of this solution to effectively inhibit certain strains of *Clostridium* spp.

Because anaerobic bacteria have been recovered from children (22) and adults (23,24) suffering from bacterial conjunctivitis, their presence in neonatal conjunctivitis is not surprising. These organisms, however, are not the most prevalent cause of inflammation of the eye in these age groups. Their presence should be suspected in children whose aerobic and chlamydial cultures are negative, in those who do not respond to conventional antimicrobial therapy, and in those at high risk of developing anaerobic infection (i.e., the presence of maternal amnionitis or premature rupture of membranes).

The experience acquired from the documented cases of anaerobic conjunctivitis indicates that local therapy with appropriate antimicrobial agents is generally adequate.

Dacryocystitis

The predominant bacteria causing acute dacryocystitis in neonates are aerobic organisms such as *S. pneumoniae* and *Staphylococcus aureus* (25,26), Anaerobic bacteria have been rarely recovered in these patients (27). We reported two newborns who developed acute dacryocystitis caused by anaerobic bacteria (28).

Peptostreptococcus micros and *Prevotella intermedia* were recovered in one newborn, and *Peptostreptococcus magnus* and *Fusobacterium nucleatum* in the other. Parenteral therapy was given to both newborns and the first patient had surgical drainage. The anaerobes isolated are likely of endogenous origin because they are members of the normal oral and skin flora (29) and normal conjunctival flora (30,31).

The actual prevalence of these organisms in dacryocystitis in infants has yet to be investigated by prospective studies. This is of particular importance because these organisms are often resistant to the antimicrobials used for therapy of dacryocystitis. We elected to treat the patients for at least 21 days to achieve complete eradication of the infection. It is recommended that specimens of dacryocystitis be cultured for both aerobic and anaerobic bacteria so that proper antimicrobial therapy can be directed against the pathogens.

PNEUMONIA

Pneumonia in the newborn can be classified according to the mode of acquiring the infection and the time when the infection takes place. The infection can be acquired in utero by transplacental route or following intrauterine infection. The pneumonia could be acquired during delivery by aspiration of bacteria that colonize the birth canal. The type of infection contracted after birth is acquired by contact with environmental objects (e.g., a tracheostomy tube) or by human contact. Aspiration can occur in up to 80% of intubated premature infants (32) and is common in newborns with gastroesophageal reflux (33) or those who require general anesthesia (34), or have swallowing dysfunction (35).

Congenital and intrauterine pneumonia usually is caused by viruses such as herpes simplex, cytomegalovirus, or rubella, and can be caused also by intrauterine exposure to *T. pallidum*, *Mycobacterium tuberculosis*, or *Listeria monocytogenes*. Aspiration during delivery or after intubation can be caused by the mother's vaginal flora, and the patient's oral flora once that had developed. Early neonatal pneumonia is mainly caused by bacteria, Group B *Streptococcus*, *E. coli* and *Listeria* being the most frequently involved (36); Herpes simplex is the main viral agent. These agents may also be responsible for late forms, as do *C. trachomatis* and the pathogen agents of community acquired pneumonia.

During vaginal delivery, the neonate is exposed to the cervical birth canal flora, which includes both aerobic and anaerobic bacteria. Almost every normal baby born by vaginal delivery swallows potentially pathogenic aerobic and anaerobic bacteria (14). These bacteria can be cultured in the infant's gastric contents. In a few instances, especially in high-risk infants, aspiration of, or exposure to, these organisms can lead to the development of infections. The diagnosis of bacterial pneumonia can be done by cultures of tracheal aspirate, pleural fluids, needle aspirate of the lungs, and blood cultures.

In approximately, 40% of the previously reported cases of neonatal pneumonia, no organisms were recovered at necropsy. Although the role of anaerobes as a cause of pulmonary infection in adults is well established (37) only two reports (38) described the isolation of *B. fragilis* from children with perinatal pneumonia.

Harrod and Stevens (38) described two newborns who presented with neonatal aspiration pneumonia that developed following maternal amnionitis. *B. fragilis* was recovered from the blood of these children.

Brook, et al. (39) reported three newborns with neonatal pneumonia caused by *B. fragilis* group. The mothers of all three infants had premature rupture of their membranes and subsequent amnionitis. The maternal membranes ruptured more than 24 hours before delivery, and the AF was foul smelling. Organisms identical to those recovered from the newborns were recovered from the AF of two of the mothers. In all three instances, the organisms were recovered from tracheal aspirates and in two from blood cultures as well. Two of the newborns were treated with ampicillin and gentamicin but succumbed to their infections; one of these infants also had meningitis. The third baby, treated with clindamycin, recovered.

Anaerobic gram-negative bacilli (e.g., *Prevotella*, *Porphyromonas*, and *Bacteroides* spp.) are part of the normal flora of the female genital tract (29). These organisms are involved frequently in ascending infections of the uterus and have been recognized as pathogens in septic complications of pregnancy, such as amnionitis, endometritis, and septic abortion, and from infection in other clinical settings (40). Amnionitis may develop prior to delivery resulting in an early exposure of the infant to the offending organism(s). Furthermore, the relative immaturity of the cellular and humoral immune systems of the newborn may permit localized infections to invade the blood stream.

Tracheal aspirates of infants who have recently had an endotracheal tube placed may be useful for diagnosing pneumonia and for identifying the causative agent (41). Repeated aspirates can reveal the presence of newly acquired organisms that may cause the pneumonia (42).

Pulmonary anaerobic infections tend to occur in association with aspiration, tissue anoxia, and trauma. Such circumstances usually are present in high-risk newborns, which make them more vulnerable to anaerobic pneumonia, especially in the presence of maternal amnionitis.

In most instances, a beta-lactam antibiotic and one of the aminoglycosides are administered for treatment of infection or pneumonia in newborns. While most anaerobic organisms are susceptible to penicillins, members of the *B. fragilis* group and growing numbers of other anaerobic gram-negative bacilli (e.g., pigmented *Prevotella* and *Porphyromonas*) can be resistant to these agents (43). The first two described newborns (39), who died of their infections, received the conventional antimicrobial therapy of a combination of ampicillin and gentamicin that was inappropriate for their infection. The third newborn, however, received a broader coverage that included therapy with clindamycin, a drug shown to be effective in the treatment of anaerobic infections in adults (44) and children (45) with aspiration pneumonia. Because clindamycin does not penetrate the blood–brain barrier in sufficient quantities, it is not recommended for treatment of meningitis. Other antimicrobial agents with better penetration to the central nervous system, such as chloramphenicol, a carbapenem (i.e., meropenem), a combination of a penicillin plus a beta-lactamase inhibitor or metronidazole, should be administered in the presence of meningitis.

ASCENDING CHOLANGITIS FOLLOWING PORTOENTEROSTOMY

Extrahepatic biliary atresia is an obliterative cholangiopathy that involves all or part of the extrahepatic biliary tree and, in many instances, the intrahepatic bile ducts. In the U.S.A., from 400 to 600 new cases of biliary atresia are encountered annually (46). The diagnosis is usually suggested by the persistence of jaundice for six weeks or more after birth. Several factors have been considered for the pathogenesis of extrahepatic biliary atresia, including viral infection (e.g., cytomegalovirus) (47), metabolic insults, and abnormalities in bile duct morphogenesis. Although selected patients benefit from prompt diagnosis and Kasai portoenterostomy surgical intervention (48,49) within the first 60 days of life, many ultimately require liver transplantation because of portal hypertension, recurrent cholangitis, and cirrhosis (50).

Infection of the biliary tract and rarely liver abscess are a known complication following Kasai's procedure. About half of the patients who undergo the Kasai procedure developed postsurgical cholangitis (51). Most episodes occurred within three months of the operation. Factors associated with cholangitis included the degree of restoration of bile flow, abnormal intrahepatic bile ducts or cavities at the porta hepatis, and the postoperative use of antibiotics. External jejunostomy is not effective in preventing cholangitis. Fever decreased bile flow, increased erythrocyte sedimentation rate and signs of shock are frequently observed.

Early bacterial studies of cholangitis following Kasai's procedure revealed coliform bacilli, *Proteus* spp., and enterococci to be the predominant isolates recovered from these patients (52). However, adequate culture methods for anaerobic bacteria were not performed in most of these studies.

The largest study reporting the bacterial growth within the biliary tract following the Kasai operation was done by Hitch and Lilly (52), who studied 19 patients over 23 months, obtaining 283 cultures. These investigators used methods for recovery of aerobic as well as anaerobic bacteria and reported the colonization of all the bilioenteric conduits with colonic flora within the first postoperative month. *E. coli*, and *Klebsiella*, *Enterococcus Pseudomonas*, *Proteus*, and *Enterobacter* spp. were the predominant aerobic isolates. *Bacteroides* spp., including *B. fragilis*, were recovered in 11% of the cultures. These authors report the recovery of similar organisms during episodes of cholangitis.

Brook and Altman studied the aerobic and anaerobic microbiology of the bile duct system in six children with cholangitis following Kasai's procedure (53). Fourteen aerobic bacteria were recovered from all six specimens, and three anaerobic organisms were recovered from three specimens. The predominant aerobes were *Klebsiella pneumoniae* (4 isolates), *Enterococcus* spp. (3), and *E. coli* (2). The anaerobes recovered were *B. fragilis* (2) and *C. perfringens* (1). Since that report, we have isolated anaerobes in three more patients, which were two strains of *C. perfringens* and one *B. fragilis*. These findings demonstrate the role of anaerobic organisms in cholangitis following hepatic portoenterostomy.

Studies in adults demonstrated that *E. coli*, and *Klebsiella*, *Enterobacter*, and *Enterococcus* spp., and anaerobes (*B. fragilis* group and *Clostridium* spp.) are the main isolates recovered from patients with biliary tract infection (54–58).

The mechanism by which both aerobic and anaerobic bacteria reach the bile ducts in patients who had undergone Kasai's procedure is probably by an ascending mode from the gastrointestinal tract. This mode of spread is favored by the surgical procedure that approximates a part of the jejunum to the bile system, by the lack of the normal choledochal sphincter action, and by the stasis that can develop after the surgery. Other mechanisms of development of cholangitis are transhepatic filtration of bacteria from the portal venous blood into the cholangiole and periportal lymphatic infection.

The anaerobes recovered in children with ascending cholangitis (52,53) are part of the normal gastrointestinal flora in infants. The initial sterile meconium becomes colonized within 24 hours with aerobic and anaerobic bacteria, predominantly *E. coli*, *Clostridium* spp., *B. fragilis*, and streptococci (59). The isolation rate of *B. fragilis* and other anaerobic bacteria in the gastrointestinal tract of term babies approaches that of adults within one week (59).

Although the number of infants studied so far is small, the data suggest that anaerobes play a major role in cholangitis following Kasai's procedure, and that specimens obtained from these patients should be cultured routinely for anaerobic as well as aerobic bacteria. It is conceivable that some of the reported failures of conventional antimicrobial therapy to cure patients with postsurgical cholangitis (60) could be due to the lack of use antimicrobial agents effective against anaerobic bacteria, especially those belonging to the *B. fragilis* group.

While most anaerobic organisms are susceptible to penicillins, members of the *B. fragilis* group are known to be resistant to these agents (55). In administering therapy to infected patients, consideration should be given to the possible presence of anaerobic organisms. It is reasonable, therefore, to treat children with this infection with antimicrobial agents effective also against *B. fragilis* and *Clostridium* spp., at least until results of cultures are known. This includes agents such as clindamycin, metronidazole, the combination of penicillin and a beta-lactamase inhibitor, or a carbapenem.

REFERENCES

1. Oray-Schrom P, Phoenix C, St Martin D, Amoateng-Adjepong Y. Sepsis workup in febrile infants 0–90 days of age with respiratory syncytial virus infection. Pediatr Emerg Care 2003; 19:314–9.
2. Waheed M, Laeeq A, Maqbool S. The etiology of neonatal sepsis and patterns of antibiotic resistance. J Coll Physicians Surg Pak 2003; 13:449–52.
3. Lott JW. Neonatal bacterial sepsis. Crit Care Nurs Clin North Am 2003; 15:35–46.
4. Benson KD, Luchansky JB, Elliott JA, et al. Pulsed-field fingerprinting of vaginal group B *Streptococcus* in pregnancy. Obstet Gynecol 2002; 100:545–51.
5. Prevedourakis C, Papadimitriou G, Ioannidou A. Isolation of pathogenic bacteria in the amniotic fluid during pregnancy and labor. Am J Obstet Gynecol 1970; 106:400–2.
6. Yoshio H, Tollin M, Gudmundsson GH, et al. Antimicrobial polypeptides of human vernix caseosa and amniotic fluid: implications for newborn innate defense. Pediatr Res 2003; 53:211–6.
7. Larson B, Snyder IS, Galask RP. Bacterial growth inhibition by amniotic fluid. Am J Obstet Gynecol 1974; 119:492–7.
8. Silver HM, Siler-Khodr T, Prihoda TJ, Gibbs RS. The effects of pH and osmolality on bacterial growth in amniotic fluid in a laboratory model. Am J Perinatol 1992; 9:69–74.
9. Talmi YP, Sigler L, Inge E, Finkelstein Y, Zohar Y. Antibacterial properties of human amniotic membranes. Placenta 1991; 12:285–8.
10. Ledger WJ, Sucet RL, Headington JT. *Bacteroides* species as a cause of severe infections in obstetrics and gynaecologic patients. Surg Gynecol Obstet 1971; 133:837–42.
11. Pearson HE, Anderson GV. Perinatal deaths associated with *Bacteroides* infections. Obstet Gynecol 1967; 30:486–92.
12. Ismail MA, Salti GI, Moawad AH. Effect of amniotic fluid on bacterial recovery and growth: clinical implications. Obstet Gynecol Surv 1989; 44:571–7.
13. Benirschke K. Routes and types of infection in the fetus and newborn. Am J Dis Child 1960; 99:714–21.
14. Brook I, Barrett CT, Brinkman CR, III, Martin WJ, Finegold SM. Aerobic and anaerobic flora of maternal cervix and newborn gastric fluid and conjunctiva: a prospective study. Pediatrics 1979; 63:451–5.
15. Washburn TC, Medearis DN, Jr., Childs B. Sex differences in susceptibility to infection. Pediatrics 1965; 35:57–64.
16. Levy O, Immunity of the newborn: basic mechanisms and clinical correlates. Net. Rev. Immunol. 2007;7:379–90.
17. Fleer A, Gerards LJ, Verhoef J. Host defence to bacterial infection in the neonate. J Hosp Infect 1988; 11(Suppl. A):320–7.
18. Teoh DL, Reynolds S. Diagnosis and management of pediatric conjunctivitis. Pediatr Emerg Care 2003; 19:48–55.
19. Brook I, Martin WJ, Finegold SM. Effect of silver nitrate application on the conjunctival flora of the newborn, and the occurrence of clostridial conjunctivitis. J Pediatr Ophthalmol Strabismus 1978; 15:179–9.
20. Isenberg SJ, Apt L, Yoshimori R, McCarty JW, Alvarez SR. Source of the conjunctival bacterial flora at birth and implications for ophthalmia neonatorum prophylaxis. Am J Ophthalmol 1988; 106:458–62.
21. Krohn MA, Hillier SL, Bell TA, Kronmal RA, Grayston JT. The bacterial etiology of conjunctivitis in early infancy. Am J Epidemiol 1993; 138:326–32.
22. Brook I. Anaerobic and aerobic bacterial flora of acute conjunctivitis in children. Arch Ophthalmol 1980; 98:833–5.
23. Perkins RE, Kundsin RB, Pratt MV, Abrahamsen I, Leibowitz HM. Bacteriology of normal and infected conjunctiva. J Clin Microbiol 1975; 1:147–9.
24. Brook I, Pettit TH, Martin WJ, Finegold SM. Anaerobic and aerobic bacteriology of acute conjunctivitis. Ann Ophthalmol 1979; 11:389–93.

25. Pollard ZF. Treatment of acute dacryocystitis in neonates. J Pediatr Ophthalmol Strabismus 1991; 28:351–3.
26. Huber-Spitzy V, Steinkogler FJ, Huber E, Arocker-Mettinger E, Schiffbanker M. Acquired dacryocystitis: microbiology and conservative therapy. Acta Ophthalmol (Copenh) 1992; 70:745–9.
27. Evans AR, Strong JD, Buck AC. Combined anaerobic and coliform infection in acute dacryocystitis. J Pediatr Ophthalmol Strabismus 1991; 28:292–4.
28. Brook I. Dacryocystitis caused by anaerobic bacteria in the newborn. Pediatr Infect Dis J 1998; 17:172–3.
29. Rosebury T. Microorganisms Indigenous to Man. New York: McGraw-Hill, 1996.
30. Matsura H. Anaerobes in the bacterial flora of the conjunctival sac. Jpn J Ophthalmol 1971; 15:116–24.
31. Perkins RE, Abrahamson I, Leibowitz HM. Bacteriology of normal and infected conjunctiva. J Clin Microbiol 1975; 1:147–9.
32. Goodwin SR, Graves SA, Haberkern CM. Aspiration in intubated premature infants. Pediatrics 1985; 75:85–8.
33. Mukhopadhyay K, Narang A, Kumar P, Chakraborty S, Mittal BR. Gastroesophageal reflux and pulmonary complication in a neonate. Indian Pediatr 1998; 35:665–8.
34. Borland LM, Sereika SM, Woelfel SK, et al. Pulmonary aspiration in pediatric patients during general anesthesia: incidence and outcome. J Clin Anesth 1998; 10:95–102.
35. Kohda E, Hisazumi H, Hiramatsu K. Swallowing dysfunction and aspiration in neonates and infants. Acta Otolaryngol Suppl (Stockh) 1994; 517:11–6.
36. Albertini M. Neonatal pneumonia. Arch Pediatr 1998; 5(Suppl. 1):57s–61.
37. Bartlett JC, Finegold SM. Anaerobic infections of the lung and pleural space. Am Rev Respir Dis 1974; 110:56–77.
38. Harrod JR, Stevens DA. Anaerobic infections in the newborn infant. J Pediatr 1974; 85:399–402.
39. Brook I, Martin WJ, Finegold SM. Neonatal pneumonia caused by members of the *Bacteroides fragilis* group. Clin Pediatr 1980; 19:541–5.
40. Price B, Martens M. Outpatient management of pelvic inflammatory disease. Curr Womens Health Rep 2001; 1:36–40.
41. Ruderman JW, Srugo I, Morgan MA, Vinstein AL, Brunell PA. Pneumonia in the neonatal intensive care unit. Diagnosis by quantitative bacterial tracheal aspirate cultures. J Perinatol 1994; 14:182–6.
42. Akhtar N, Stromberg D, Rosenthal GL, Bowles NE, Towbin JA. Tracheal aspirate as a substrate for polymerase chain reaction detection of viral genome in childhood pneumonia and myocarditis. Circulation 1999; 99:2011–8.
43. Rasmussen BA, Bush K, Tally FP. Antimicrobial resistance in anaerobes. Clin Infect Dis 1997; 24(Suppl. 1):S110–20.
44. Gorbach SL, Thadepalli H. Clindamycin in the treatment of pure and mixed anaerobic infections. Arch Intern Med 1974; 134:87–92.
45. Brook I. Clindamycin in the treatment of aspiration pneumonia in children. Antimicrob Agents Chemother 1979; 15:342–5.
46. Lefkowitch JH. Biliary atresia. Mayo Clin Proc 1998; 73:90–5.
47. Tarr PI, Haas JE, Christie DL. Biliary atresia, cytomegalovirus, and age at referral. Pediatrics 1996; 97:828–31.
48. Kasai M, Mochizuki I, Ohkohchi N, Chiba T, Ohi R. Surgical limitation for biliary atresia: indication for liver transplantation. J Pediatr Surg 1989; 24:851–4.
49. Bezerra JA. Potential etiologies of biliary atresia. Pediatr Transplant 2005; 9:646–51.
50. Kobayashi H, Stringer MD. Biliary atresia. Semin Neonatol 2003; 8:383–91.
51. Krishna M, Keaveny AP, Genco PV, et al. Clinicopathological review of 18 cases of liver allografts lost due to bile duct necrosis. Transplant Proc 2005; 37:2221–3.
52. Hitch DC, Lilly JR. Identification, quantification and significance of bacterial growth within the biliary tract after Kasai's operation. J Pediatr Surg 1978; 13:563–9.
53. Brook I, Altman P. The significance of anaerobic bacteria in biliary tract infection after hepatic portoenterostomy for biliary. Surgery 1984; 95:281–3.
54. Brook I. Aerobic and anaerobic microbiology of biliary tract disease. J Clin Microbiol 1989; 27:2373–5.
55. Finegold SM. Anaerobic Bacteria in Human Disease. New York: Academic Press, 1977.
56. England DM, Rosenblatt JE. Anaerobes in human biliary tracts. J Clin Microbiol 1977; 6:494–8.
57. Shimada K, Inamatsu T, Yamashiro M. Anaerobic bacteria in biliary disease in elderly patients. J Infect Dis 1977; 135:850–4.
58. Qureshi WA. Approach to the patient who has suspected acute bacterial cholangitis. Gastroenterol Clin North Am 2006; 35:409–23.
59. Long SS, Swenson RM. Development of anaerobic fecal flora in healthy newborn infants. J Pediatr 1977; 91:298–301.
60. Chaudhary S, Turner RB. Trimethoprim-sulfamethoxazole for cholangitis following hepatic portoenterostomy for biliary atresia. J Pediatr 1981; 99:656–8.

7 | Bacteremia and Septicemia in Newborns

Because the newborn generally is less able to overcome infections than an older child, localized infection may enter the infant's blood stream. The septic infant manifests generally clinical signs and symptoms that distinguish him from infants with transient bacteremia. Factors such as prematurity or obstetric complications can change these rates.

The awareness of the role of anaerobic bacteria in neonatal bacteremia has increased in recent years, following improvement and simplification in the methods of growing and identification of these organisms.

INCIDENCE AND BACTERIAL ETIOLOGY

Within the past 70 years, changes have occurred in the bacterial etiology of neonatal bacterial septicemia. In the preantibiotic era before 1940, the predominant organism was Group A beta-hemolytic streptococci. In the 1950s, *Staphylococcus aureus* became the major pathogen, to be replaced by *Escherichia coli* and Group B streptococci. Since the beginning of the 1960s, the latter two pathogens have accounted for up to 70% of bacteremia in the newborn (1). Early-onset sepsis (that occurring within 72 hours after birth) is currently caused by predominantly aerobic gram-positive organisms and late onset is due to predominantly aerobic gram-negative bacteria (1). The role of anaerobic bacteria in neonatal bacteremia has not been studied adequately. Most of the reports of bacteremia due to anaerobes were through case report (2,3,6–38). The true incidence of neonatal anaerobic bacteremia is difficult to ascertain since anaerobic blood cultures were not employed in the reported major series of neonatal sepsis and still are not routinely performed in some medical centers. Furthermore, many medical centers do not employ appropriate culture media for recovery of anaerobes.

Several studies attempted to recover anaerobic bacteria in newborns. However, proper techniques for isolation and identification were not always used. Tyler and Albers (2) obtained cultures from 319 newborns. These authors reported the recovery of anaerobes in four instances, which allowed them to predict an incidence of 12.5 cases per 1000 live births and 13% of all cases of neonatal bacteremia.

Another report described anaerobic bacteremia in 23 newborns. The yield of anaerobic bacteria in 23 newborns seen over a period of 3.5 years represented 1.8 cases per 1000 live births and accounted for 26% of all instances of neonatal bacteremia at that hospital (3).

In the study of Salem and Thadepalli (4), 180 per 1000 live births had self-limiting transplacental bacteremia. Thirumoorthi et al. (5) conducted a prospective survey of all neonate blood cultures that were specially processed for anaerobes and isolated anaerobes from only 1% of the 1599 blood cultures processed. It is difficult to generalize about the population of anaerobic bacteria in newborns in these studies, since cultures were obtained through the umbilical artery in many of the infants. The possibility of umbilical artery contamination occurring in some of these patients cannot be discounted. Noel et al. (17) retrospectively reviewed the presence of anaerobic bacteremia in the neonatal intensive care unit over 18 years. Blood was not collected from the umbilical cord of these patients. During that period, 1290 newborns had bacteria cultured from blood, of which 29 (2.2%) had anaerobic bacteria.

The majority of cases for neonatal bacteremia reported in the literature were obtained, from selected case reports. Table 1 summarizes 179 cases of anaerobic neonatal bacteremia

TABLE 1   Literature Summary: Neonatal Bacteremia Due to Anaerobic Bacteria

Organisms	No. of patients (deaths)	Predisposing conditions	Ref.
***Bacteroides* spp.**	14 (14)		(6)
	5 (0)	Omphalitis	(7)
	2 (1)		(8)
	1 (0)		(2)
	1 (0)		(9)
	1 (0)		(10)
	15 (1)		(3)
	1 (0)	Adrenal abscess	(11)
	1 (0)	Neonatal scalp monitoring	(12)
	1 (0)	Meningitis	(13)
	1 (0)	Meningitis	(14)
	5 (2)	Pneumonia and meningitis	(15,18)
		Necrotizing enterocolitis	
	2 (0)		(16)
	3 (0)		(19)
	1 (0)	Necrotizing enterocolitis	(20)
	1 (1)	Pneumonia	(21)
	15 (6)	Necrotizing enterocolitis and pneumonia	(17)
	1 (0)	Meningitis and amnionitis	(22)
	2 (0)	Maternal amnionitis	(23)
Subtotal	73 (25)	34% mortality	
Anaerobic gram-positive cocci	19 (0)		(7)
	3 (0)		(2)
	2 (1)		(24)
	7 (0)		(3)
	1 (0)		(25)
	3 (1)		(17)
Subtotal	35 (2)	6% mortality	
***Veillonella* spp.**	2 (0)		(25)
	1 (0)	Amnionitis and pneumonia	(3)
Subtotal	3 (0)		
***Fusobacterium* spp.**	1 (0)		(7)
	1 (0)		(26)
	1 (0)		(27)
Subtotal	3 (0)		(28)
***Clostridium* spp.**	1 (1)		(28)
	1 (1)		(29)
	1 (1)		(30)
	1 (0)		(31)
	1 (0)		(3)
	18 (0)		(32)
	2 (1)	Necrotizing enterocolitis	(20)
	9 (0)	Necrotizing enterocolitis	(33)
	1 (0)	Necrotizing enterocolitis	(34)
	1 (0)	Necrotizing enterecolitis	(35)
	13 (8)	Omphalitis	(36)
	7 (4)	Necrotizing enterocolitis amnionitis	(17)
	1 (1)	Meningitis	(38)
Subtotal	57 (17)	24% mortality	
***Eubacteria* spp.**	2 (1)	Necrotizing enterocolitis	(20)
***Bifidobacterium* spp.**	1 (1)		(17)
Propionibacterium acnes	1 (0)		(37)
	1 (0)	Periorbital cellulites	(18)
	2 (0)		(25)
	1 (1)	Necrotizing enterocolitis	(17)
Subtotal	5 (1)	20% mortality	
Total	179 (47)	26% mortality	

reported in the literature. The predominant organisms are *Bacteroides* (73 cases). Of these, the *Bacteroides fragilis* group is predominant. The other organisms, in descending order of frequency, are clostridia (57 instances), anaerobic gram-positive cocci (35), *Propionibacterium acnes* (5), veillonellae (3), fusobacteria (3), and *Eubacterium* spp. (2).

Multiple organisms, aerobic and anaerobic, were isolated from eight patients reported in one study (3): anaerobic coisolates from six patients (*Peptostreptococcus* spp., five and *Veillonella parvula*, one) and aerobic coisolates from only two patients (*E. coli* and alpha-hemolytic streptococcus). In one patient, reported by Noel et al. (17), *Bacteroides vulgatus* was isolated from a single blood culture along with four aerobic bacteria (*Enterococcus faecalis*, *E. coli*, *Enterococcus faecium*, and *Klebsiella pneumoniae*).

Simultaneous isolation of the anaerobes from other sites was reported by several authors (Table 2) (3,11–14,34,38). This was especially common with *B. fragilis* and *Clostridium* spp.

Chow and co-workers (3) reported the simultaneous isolation of *Bacteroides* organisms from gastric aspirate in four instances, from the amniotic fluid or uterus at cesarean section in two cases, and from the maternal and fetal placental surfaces and the external auditory canal in one instance each.

Brook et al. (15) reported the concomitant recovery of *B. fragilis* group from lung aspirates of two patients with pneumonitis; Harrod and Sevens (21) recovered *B. fragilis* from the inflamed placenta; Dysant and associates (14), Brook et al. (15), Kasik et al. (13), and Webber and Tuohy (22) recovered *B. fragilis* from the cerebrospinal fluid of a total of four patients with meningitis.

Brook (12) recovered *B. fragilis* from an occipital abscess that developed following neonatal monitoring with scalp electrodes. Ahonkhai and colleagues (31) reported the concomitant isolation of *Clostridium perfringens* in the placenta of a newborn.

Kosloske et al. (20) isolated *Clostridium* spp., *B. fragilis*, and *Eubacterium* spp. from the peritoneal cavity of four patients with necrotizing enterocolitis (NEC). Brook et al. (34) isolated *Clostridium difficile* from the peritoneal cavity of a newborn with NEC. Spark and Wike (36) summarized four cases of isolation of *Clostridium* spp. from omphalitis, and Heidemann et al. (38) isolated a gas-forming *C. perfringens* in the cerebrospinal fluid of a newborn with meningitis.

DIAGNOSIS

The diagnosis of septicemia can be made only by recovery of the organism from blood cultures. Blood should be obtained from a peripheral vein rather than from the umbilical vessels, which frequently are colonized by aerobic and anaerobic bacteria. Femoral vein aspiration may result in cultures contaminated with organisms from the perineum such as *Bacteroides* and coliforms. It is helpful to obtain cultures of sites other than the last two prior to initiating antimicrobial therapy.

This is of particular importance in relation to maternal amnionitis or septicemia. In many cases, organisms identical to those found in the newborn's blood can be recovered from the mother's blood or amniotic fluid (15). The rate of growth of most anaerobic bacteria, including the *B. fragilis* group, is relatively slow, and it may take several days to identify them with culture. The development of rapid methods of identification may facilitate the identification of

TABLE 2 Studies Where Anaerobic Bacteria Causing Bacteremia Were also Simultaneously Isolated (reference number in parenthesis)

Bacteroides spp.	*Clostridium* spp.
Gastric aspirates (3)	Placenta (31)
Amniotic fluid (3)	Omphalitis (36)
Placenta (3,21)	Cerebrospinal fluid (38)
Lung (15)	Peritoneal cavity (in NEC) (20)
Cerebrospinal fluid (13–16,21,24)	
Scalp abscess (12)	
Peritoneal cavity (in NEC) (20)	

Abbreviation: NEC, necrotizing enterocolitis.

these anaerobes. Examination of gastric aspirates generally is not helpful in the prediction of anaerobic sepsis, since the gastric fluid of the normal infants can contain many aerobic and anaerobic bacteria that were ingested during delivery (39). However, examination of the gastric aspirate for white blood cells may suggest the presence of maternal amnionitis.

None of the other blood tests can be helpful in the diagnosis of bacterial septicemia. The white blood count can be elevated above 20,000 cells/mL^3, but in some cases, it may be below 10,000 cells/mL^3. Clinical findings associated with sepsis are generally nonspecific. Premature infants present with apnea and jaundice more often than term infants (40).

PREDISPOSING CONDITIONS

A number of factors have been shown to dispose to aerobic neonatal septicemia, including maternal age, quality of prenatal care, sex of the infant, gestational age, and associated congenital anomalies. Perinatal maternal complications, such as abruptio placentae, placenta previa, maternal toxemia, premature rupture of the membranes, and chorioamnionitis all increase the incidence of neonatal septicemia. Congenital anomalies that cause a breakdown of anatomic barriers or of the immunologic system and the presence of central venous catheter also predispose to infection.

The factors predisposing for anaerobic bacteremia were found to be similar to predisposing factors for aerobic bacteremia. The frequency of various perinatal factors associated with anaerobic bacteremia in newborns was reported by Chow and associates (3). Prolonged time after premature rupture of membranes and maternal amnionitis were the most commonly associated obstetric factors. The median duration of time after membrane rupture until delivery in the 15 mothers studied by these authors was 57 hours. Seven out of 12 mothers who had evidence of intrapartum amnionitis were noted to have foul-smelling vaginal discharge, suggestive of an anaerobic infection. Other investigators (40–42) had also demonstrated a relationship between premature rupture of fetal membranes and neonatal bacteremia. Prolonged rupture of fetal membranes often is associated with amnionitis, and it is generally accepted that an important pathway for fetal infection is by an ascending route through the membranes from the cervix (43,44). Tyler and Albers (2) also found an increasing frequency of neonatal bacteremia directly related to the duration after membrane rupture; they further demonstrated a highly significant association of neonatal bacteremia with the presence of foul-smelling amniotic fluid.

Prematurity was reported in about a third of the newborns with anaerobic bacteremia, and a male-to-female ratio of 1.6:1, which is similar to the finding of increased male susceptibility to neonatal aerobic bacteremia (45), was also reported in anaerobic bacteremia (3). Of interest is the correlation between certain predisposing conditions and some bacterial isolates. Neonatal pneumonia, NEC, omphalitis amnionitis and, abscesses were reported in association with the recovery of *B. fragilis* group and clostridia (Table 1) (20). *Clostridium butyricum* was isolated from blood cultures obtained from 13 newborns with that disease (33). Although most reports describe the recovery of *Clostridium* spp. in newborns with NEC, the recent study by Noel et al. (17) demonstrated the high-recovery rate of *B. fragilis* as well.

Noel et al. (17) observed the association of certain clinical settings with specific anaerobic isolates. Although gram-positive and gram-negative anaerobes were isolated with similar frequency, 8 out of 12 infants bacteremic within the first 48 hours of life were infected with gram-positive, penicillin-susceptible organisms (*Peptostreptococcus* spp., *P. acnes*, and *C. perfringens*); whereas 11 out of 17 infants, two days of age and older were bacteremic with gram-negative, penicillin resistant anaerobes (*B. fragilis* and *Bacteroides* spp.). Eleven out of 17 infants with anaerobic bacteremia associated with NEC were bacteremic with gram-negative anaerobes (10 *Bacteroides* spp. and 1 *Fusobacterium* spp.). Five out of six infants with anaerobic bacteremia associated with chorioamnionitis were bacteremia with gram-positive anaerobes (anaerobic cocci and *Clostridium* spp.).

Ten of the episodes of anaerobic bacteremia occurred within the first three days of life and were associated with intrauterine infection (17). Although *Peptostreptococcus* spp. were recovered twice as often from these infants, gram-positive and gram-negative anaerobes were equally represented in those episodes. All four infants with *Bacteroides* spp., bacteremia not associated with gastrointestinal disease had congenital pneumonia. Three were born to mothers who did not have chorioaminoitis, but had premature rupture of membranes for less than 24 hours before birth. These infants may have aspirated organisms colonizing the birth canal or acquired infection in utero from mothers with subclinical infection (7). In contrast, three infants with congenital pneumonia born to mothers with apparent intrauterine infection had gram-positive anaerobic bacteremia.

PATHOGENESIS

Studdiford and Douglas (46) demonstrated placental bacteremia caused by gram-negative bacteria, with the fetal blood vessels distended. They considered this to be peculiar to neonatal deaths with vascular collapse. Mandsley and colleagues (47) examined at random the fetal adnexa in 494 patients and found evidence of inflammation in 34%. They found chorionitis in 21% and inflammation of the cord in 17%. They also have studied the bacteriology of the surface of the placenta and failed to correlate these findings with the histologic findings. They found deciduitis in 89.5%, suggesting that normal labor may not be that normal after all. Salem and Thadepalli (4) have examined the histology of the cord, placenta, and membranes and tried to correlate the cord blood cultures with the neonatal outcome in 50 consecutive births. Thirty percent of the cord blood cultures were positive for aerobic–anaerobic bacteria soon after birth. Anaerobes were found in cord cultures in nine samples (18%), anaerobic cocci dominating. Excellent correlation was found between the cord blood culture results and the morphotypes of the bacteria seen in the Gram-stained sections of the placenta, cord, and membranes. Inflammation as evidenced by leukocyte infiltration was rare, found in only one instance. It appears, therefore, that transplacental transmission of aerobic and anaerobic bacteria is a common, but fortunately benign, feature of normal labor. In most instances, it results from the contamination of the amniotic fluid with the cervical flora, followed by the transplacental influx of microorganisms created by the intrauterine pressure changes during active labor. Because amnionitis is generally a polymicrobial aerobic–anaerobic infection (48), newborns who are exposed to maternal amnionitis at term are at greater risk for anaerobic bacteremia.

CLINICAL MANIFESTATIONS

The early signs and symptoms of septicemia are caused by facultative or aerobic bacteria, are nonspecific, and frequently are recognized by the mother or nurse. Temperature imbalance, tachypnea, apnea, tachycardia, lethargy, vomiting, or diarrhea may be noted. Jaundice, petechiae, seizures, and hepatosplenomegaly are late signs and usually denote a poor prognosis.

The relative frequency of various clinical manifestations of neonatal anaerobic bacteremia in newborns is not different from those seen in aerobic bacteremia (3). Over half of the infants had evidence of fetal distress, and three-fourths had a low Apgar score. A positive correlation between the presence of foul-smelling discharge at birth and bacteremia caused by *Bacteroides* organisms was also noted (3). About two-thirds of the infants may manifest respiratory distress, with tachypnea and/or cyanosis shortly after birth. Chest films may reveal pneumonitis, confirming a correlation between prenatal aspiration of infected amniotic fluid and subsequent development of pneumonia or sepsis in the newborn infant.

Other clinical manifestations of these infants were nonspecific, and included poor sucking and feeding activity, lethargy, hypotonia, irritability, and tonic–clonic seizures. In general, the clinical manifestations of neonatal anaerobic bacteremia are indistinguishable from other causes of neonatal sepsis.

PROGNOSIS

The mortality following anaerobic bacteremia depends on such factors as age of the patient, underlying disease, nature of the organism, speed with which the diagnosis is made, and surgical or medical therapy instituted (49). The overall mortality from anaerobic bacteria in the 179 patients reported in the literature (Table 1) is 26%. The highest mortality is observed in the *Bacteroides* group (34%), while the mortality from other organisms is generally below 17%.

In the series of Chow and colleagues (3), the patients with neonatal anaerobic bacteremia had better prognosis than did newborns with bacteremia caused by facultative bacteria. Only 1 out of the 23 patients (4%) died; however, the mortality from the cases of anaerobic bacteremia reviewed from the literature was about 25%.

Several authors reported spontaneous recovery from anaerobic bacteremia (3,19). However, most of the reports in the literature describe the need to treat patients with such infection adequately (18) and describe infants who were inappropriately treated and died (15). Noel et al. (17) described one patient and Brook et al. (15) presented two patients who died after inappropriate therapy of *B. fragilis* bacteremia. Following appropriate therapy and in the absence of complicating factors such as other sites of infections (meningitis and abscesses), generally, there is complete recovery.

THERAPY

Antimicrobial therapy must be initiated as early as possible in infants suspected of bacteremia. This should be done in most cases prior to the recovery of organisms and before information about their susceptibility is available. The clinician cannot wait in most cases for this information because of the vulnerability of newborns to bacterial infection. The time needed for the recovery and performance of blood cultures for susceptibility of anaerobes generally is longer than the time needed for culture of aerobes, and delay in therapy may be deleterious.

In most instances, a beta-lactam antibiotic (ampicillin or cefotaxime) and an aminoglycoside are administered for treatment of newborns. While most anaerobic organisms are susceptible to penicillin G, members of the *B. fragilis* group, and increasing numbers of other *Bacteroides* spp. (50) are known to be resistant to that agent mostly through the production of the enzyme beta-lactamase. In one series, two newborns died after receiving the conventional antimicrobial therapy of combination ampicillin and gentamicin, treatment inappropriate for their infection by *B. fragilis* (15). The third newborn in that study, however, recovered following therapy with a broader treatment that included therapy with clindamycin, a drug known to be effective in the treatment of anaerobic infections in adults and children (51). Clindamycin was used in the treatment of anaerobic bacteremia by other authors also (21).

Because clindamycin does not penetrate the blood–brain barrier in sufficient quantities, it is not recommended for treatment of meningitis. Other antimicrobial agents such as chloramphenicol metronidazole, a carbapenem (i.e. imipenem, meropenem) and the combination of a penicillin (ticarcillin or amoxacillin) and a beta-lactamase inhibitor (clavulanic acid or sulbactam), offer the advantage of penetration to the central nervous system, should be administered in the presence of meningitis. Although the experience in newborns is limited, metronidazole has been used successfully in the treatment of neonatal bacteremia (52).

The length of treatment time for anaerobic infections is not established. It is apparent from data derived from older children (18), however, that prolonged therapy of at least 14 days is adequate in eliminating the infection.

Surgical drainage is essential when pus has collected. Organisms identical to those causing anaerobic bacteremia were recovered from other infected sites in many patients. These extravascular sites may serve as a source of persistent bacteremia in some cases; however, the majority of patients will recover completely when prompt treatment with appropriate antimicrobial agents is instituted before any complications develop. The early recognition of anaerobic bacteremia and administration of appropriate antimicrobial and surgical therapy play a significant role in preventing mortality and morbidity in newborns.

REFERENCES

1. Stoll BJ, Hansen N, Fanaroff AA, et al. Changes in pathogens causing early-onset sepsis in very-low-birth-weight infants. N Engl J Med 2002; 347:240–7.
2. Tyler CW, Albers WH. Obstetric factors related to bacteremia in the newborn infants. Am J Obstet Gynecol 1996; 94:970–6.
3. Chow AW, Leake RD, Yamauchi T, Anthony BF, Guze LB. The significance of anaerobes in neonatal bacteremia: analysis of 23 cases and review of the literature. Pediatrics 1974; 54:736–45.
4. Salem FA, Thadepalli H. Microbial invasion of the placenta, cord and membranes during normal labor. Clin Pediatr 1978; 18:50–2.
5. Thirumoorthi MC, Keen BM, Dajani AS. Anaerobic infections in children: a prospective survey. J Clin Microbiol 1976; 3:318–23.
6. Pearson HE, Anderson GV. Perinatal deaths associated with *Bacteroides* infections. Obstet Gynecol 1967; 30:486–91.
7. Kelsall GRH, Barter RA, Manessis C. Prospective bacteriological studies in inflammation of the placenta, cord and membranes. Obstet Gynaecol Brit Comm 1967; 74:401–11.
8. DuPont HL, Spink WW. Infections due to gram-negative organisms: an analysis of 860 patients with bacteremia at the University of Minnesota Medical Center, 1958–1966. Medicine 1969; 48:307–32.
9. Tynes BS, Frommeyer WB, Jr. *Bacteroides* septicemia: culture, clinical and therapeutic features in a series of twenty-five patients. Ann Intern Med 1962; 56:12–26.
10. Lee Y, Berg RB. Cephalhematoma infected with *Bacteroides*. Am J Dis Child 1971; 121:77–8.
11. Ohta S, Shimizu S, Fujisawa S, Tsurusawa M. Neonatal adrenal abscess due to *Bacteroides*. J Pediatr 1978; 93:1063–4.
12. Brook I. Osteomyelitis and bacteremia caused by *Bacteroides fragilis*. Clin Pediatr 1980; 19:639–40.
13. Kasik JW, Bolam DL, Nelson RM. Sepsis and meningitis associated with anal dilation in newborn infant. Clin Pediatr 1984; 9:509–10.
14. Dysart NK, Griswold WR, Schanberger JE, Goscienki PJ, Chow AW. Meningitis due to *Bacteroides fragilis* in a newborn. J Pediatr 1976; 89:509–10.
15. Brook I, Martin WJ, Finegold SM. Neonatal pneumonia caused by members of the *Bacteroides fragilis* group. Clin Pediatr 1980; 19:541–3.
16. Maguire GC, Nordin J, Myers MG, Koontz FP, Hierholzer W, Nassif E. Infections acquired by young infants. Am J Dis Child 1981; 135:693–8.
17. Noel J, Laufer DA, Edelson PJ. Anaerobic bacteremia in a neonatal intensive care unit: an eighteen-year experience. Pediatr Infect Dis J 1988; 7:858–62.
18. Brook I, Controni G, Rodriguez WJ, Martin WJ. Anaerobic bacteremia in children. Am J Dis Child 1980; 134:1052–6.
19. Echeverria P, Smith AL. Anaerobic bacteremia observed in a children's hospital. Clin Pediatr 1978; 17:688–95.
20. Kosloske AM, Ulrich JA. A bacteriologic basis for clinical presentation of necrotizing enterocolitis. J Pediatr Surg 1980; 15:558–64.
21. Harrod JR, Stevens DA. Anaerobic infections in the newborn infant. J Pediatr 1974; 85:399–402.
22. Webber SA, Tuohy P. *Bacteroides fragilis* meningitis in a premature infant successfully treated with metronidazole. Pediatr Infect Dis J 1988; 7:886–7.
23. Keffer GL, Monif GR. Perianal septicemia due to the *Bacteroides*. Obstet Gynecol 1988; 71:463–5.
24. Robinson SC, Krause VW, Johnson J, Zwicker B. Significance of maternal bacterial infection with respect to infection and disease in the newborn. Obstet Gynecol 1965; 25:664–70.
25. Spector S, Tickner W, Grossman M. Studies of the usefulness of clinical and hematological findings in the diagnosis of neonatal bacteremia. Clin Pediatr 1981; 20:385–92.
26. Tynes BS, Utz JP. *Fusobacterium* septicemia. Am J Med 1960; 29:879–87.
27. Robinow M, Simonelli FA. *Fusobacterium* bacteremia in the newborn. Am J Dis Child 1965; 110:92–4.
28. Wilson WR, Martin WJ, Wilkowske CJ, Washington JA, II. Anaerobic bacteremia. Mayo Clin Proc 1972; 47:639–46.
29. Freedman S, Hollander M. *Clostridium perfringens* septicemia as a postoperative complication of the newborn infant. J Pediatr 1967; 71:576–8.
30. Isenberg AN. *Clostridium welchii* infection: a clinical evaluation. Arch Surg 1966; 92:727–31.
31. Ahonkhai VI, Kim MH, Raziuddin K, Goldstein EJ. Perinatal *Clostridium perfringens* infection. Clin Pediatr 1981; 20:532–3.
32. Alpern RJ, Dowell VR, Jr. Nonhistotoxic clostridial bacteremia. Am J Clin Pathol 1971; 55:717–22.
33. Howard FM, Flynn DM, Bradley JM, Noone P, Szawatkowski M. Outbreak of necrotizing enterocolitis caused by *Clostridium butyricum*. Lancet 1977; 2:1099–192.
34. Brook I, Avery G, Glasgow A. *Clostridium difficile* in pediatric infections. J Infect 1982; 4:253–7.
35. Kliegman RM, Fanaroff AA, Izant R, Speck WT. Clostridia as pathogens in neonatal necrotizing enterocolitis. J Pediatr 1979; 95:287–9.
36. Spark RP, Wike DA. Nontetanus clostridial neonatal fatality after home delivery. Ariz Med 1983; 10:697–700.

37. Dunkle LM, Brotherton MS, Feigin RD. Anaerobic infections in children: a prospective study. Pediatrics 1976; 57:311–20.

38. Heidemann SM, Meest KL, Perrin E, Sarnaik AP. Primary meningitis in infancy. Pediatr Infect Dis J 1989; 8:126–8.

39. Brook I, Barrett CT, Brinkman CR, III, Martin WJ, Finegold SM. Aerobic and anaerobic bacterial flora of the maternal cervix and newborn gastric fluid and conjunctiva: a prospective study. Pediatrics 1979; 63:45–51.

40. Zamora-Castorena S, Murguia-de-Sierra MT. Five year experience with neonatal sepsis in a pediatric center. Rev Invest Clin 1998; 50:463–70.

41. Kobak AJ. Fetal bacteremia: a contribution to mechanism of intrauterine infection and to the pathogenesis of placentitis. Am J Obstet Gynecol 1930; 19:299–304.

42. Wilson MG, Armstrong DH, Nelson RC, Boak RA. Prolonged rupture of fetal membranes: effect on the newborn infant. Am J Dis Child 1964; 107:138–46.

43. Benirschke K. Routes and types of infection in the fetus and the newborn. Am J Dis Child 1960; 99:714–20.

44. Blanc WA. Pathways of fetal and early neonatal infection. J Pediatr 1961; 59:473–6.

45. Doyle LW, Gultom E, Chuang SL, James M, Davis P, Bowman E. Changing mortality and causes of death in infants 23–27 weeks' gestational age. J Paediatr Child Health 1999; 35:255–9.

46. Studdiford WE, Douglas GW. Placental bacteremia: a significant finding in septic abortion accompanied by vascular collapse. Am J Obstet Gynecol 1956; 71:842–58.

47. Mandsley RF, Brix GA, Hinton NA, Robertson EM, Bryans AM, Haust MD. Placental inflammation and infection. Am J Obstet Gynecol 1966; 95:648–59.

48. Hagberg H, Wennerholm UB, Savman K. Sequelae of chorioamnionitis. Curr Opin Infect Dis 2002; 15:301–6.

49. Naeye RL, Blanc WA. Relation of poverty and race to antenatal infection. N Engl J Med 1970; 283:555–9.

50. Wexler HM, Finegold SM. Current susceptibility patterns of anaerobic bacteria. Yonsei Med J 1998; 39:495–501.

51. Brook I. Clindamycin in the treatment of aspiration pneumonia in children. Antimicrob Agents Chemother 1979; 15:342–6.

52. Rom S, Flynn D, Noone P. Anaerobic infection in a neonate: early detection by gas liquid chromatography and response to metronidazole. Arch Dis Child 1977; 52:740–1.

8 | Necrotizing Enterocolitis

Necrotizing enterocolitis (NEC) is the most common gastrointestinal medical and/or surgical emergency afflicting neonates with mortality rate of about 50% in infants weighing less than 1500 g. NEC represents a significant clinical problem. Although, it is more common in premature infants, it can also be observed in term babies. It is a clinical syndrome of ischemic necrosis of the bowel of multiple etiological factors. However, not all features of NEC are explicable by this process. It is the most common gastrointestinal emergency in the neonate (1,2). The role of aerobic and anaerobic bacteria and viruses in epidemic NEC has also been suggested; however, a single causative organism has not been identified.

EPIDEMIOLOGY

NEC occurs in a sporadic and epidemic form (3). Frequency varies from nursery to nursery without correlation with season or geographic location. Outbreaks of NEC seem to follow an epidemic pattern within nurseries, suggesting an infectious etiology even though a specific causative organism has not been isolated. It is estimated to account for 1% to 5% of all admissions to newborn intensive care units. In the U.S.A., there is a relatively stable incidence, ranging from 0.3 to 2.4 cases per 1000 live births. The disease is more prevalent among the smallest preterm infants, and it is reported among term infants with perinatal asphyxia or congenital heart disease (4). Average age at onset in premature infants seems to be related to postconceptional age, with babies born earlier developing NEC at a later chronologic age. The mortality rate ranges from 10% to 44% in infants weighing less than 1500 g, compared with 0% to 20% mortality rate for babies weighing more than 2500 g. Extremely premature infants (<1000 g) are particularly vulnerable, with reported mortality rates of 40% to 100% (4,5).

The improved neonatal and obstetric care shifted the incidence of NEC away from acutely ill newborns toward smaller, less mature ones who survived the perinatal period.

PATHOGENESIS

Even though the pathogenesis of NEC remains uncertain, evidence suggests a multifactorial etiology, including the presence of abnormal intestinal ischemia, abnormal bacterial flora, and intestinal mucosal immaturity (1,2).

Ischemia induces a local inflammatory response resulting in activation of a proinflammatory cascade with mediators such as platelet-activating factor (PAF), tumor necrosis factor alpha, complement, prostaglandins, and leukotriene C4. Subsequent norepinephrine release and vasoconstriction result in splanchnic ischemia, followed by reperfusion injury. Activated leukocytes and intestinal epithelial xanthine oxidase may then produce reactive oxygen species, leading to further tissue injury and cell death (6,7).

Intestinal necrosis results in breach of the mucosal barrier, allowing for bacterial translocation and spread of bacterial endotoxin into the damaged tissue. The endotoxin then interacts synergistically with PAF and amplifies the inflammatory response (6,7).

In the preterm infant, lack of mucosal cellular maturity and antioxidative mechanisms may make the mucosal barrier more susceptible to injury. Feeding with human milk is protective because it contains secretory immunoglobulin A (IgA), and prohibits bacterial transmural translocation by binding to the intestinal luminal cells. Human milk may also mediate the inflammatory response (8).

Bifidobacteria predominate in the intestinal mucusa in healthy individuals. This is enhanced by the presence of oligofructose, a component of human milk, which also inhibits lactose-fermenting organisms. Clostridia predominate in infants not fed with oligofructose. The exposure of preterm infants to broad-spectrum antimicrobials further alters their intestinal bacterial environment. The administration of exogenous bifidobacteria and lactobacilli may moderate the risk and severity of NEC in preterm infants (9,10).

The intestinal bacteria exploit the break in the integrity of the mucosa. Adynamic ileus and stasis develop, and in the fed infant whose immunologic defenses are deficient, bacteria colonize and multiply. Strains of *Escherichia coli*, *Klebsiella pneumoniae*, and *Staphylococcus aureus* can produce enterotoxins that cause further fluid loss (1,2). The predominantly gas-forming organisms that generate pneumatosis may accumulate and rupture the intestinal wall, producing pneumoperitoneum and peritonitis. Further invasion into the lumen occurs, and bacterial proliferation extends into the lymphatics and the portal circulation and reaches the liver. Finally, there is overwhelming sepsis and death (7).

PREDISPOSING CONDITIONS

Two sequential conditions are significant in the development of NEC. In the first stage, there is an insult to the intestinal mucosa caused by ischemia, which is followed by the detrimental activity of intestinal bacteria or viruses, enhancing bacterial growth, or inducing mucosal damage, and altering the host defense. This is promoted by the availability of intraluminal substances.

The damage to the intestinal mucosa can be due to synergistic factors. In response to systemic shock and hypoxia, blood is a shunted from the intestinal tract and kidneys to the heart and brain (the "diving reflex") (7). Prolonged intestinal ischemia can cause permanent mucosal damage, including vascular thrombosis and local bowel infarction.

Some supportive procedures that may cause ischemia have been associated with NEC. It includes umbilical and venous catheterization and exchange transfusion (2,6). Perinatal factors that cause hypoxia include respiratory distress syndrome, apnea, asphyxia, hypotension, congestive heart failure, patent ductus arteriosus, hypothermia, sepsis, hypoglycemia, and polycythemia. However, some infants with no risk factors develop NEC. Maternal complications associated with fetal distress and shock, such as prolonged rupture of membranes and maternal infection, frequently are observed in these infants (11).

Diet can also be associated with mucosal damage. NEC rarely occurs before feeding, and it is especially prevalent in infants fed with hyperosmolar formulas. Many of the infants had been fed before developing NEC, and of those fed, most have not had breast milk. The few that had been fed breast milk received it from a breast milk bank and were not nursed. It was hypothesized that premature infants are relatively unable to handle large water and electrolyte loads.

ETIOLOGY

Numerous reports have implied that the fecal microflora may contribute to the pathogenesis of NEC. A broad range of organisms generally found in the distal gastrointestinal tract have been recovered from the peritoneal cavity and blood of infants with NEC. Infectious agents recovered from newborns with endemic NEC are similar to those associated with epidemic NEC. Organisms cultured from the blood usually matched with those found in the stool (1,2,12). Most reports describe the predominance of members of the neonatal gut normal flora [including Enterobacteriaceae such as *E. coli* (12,13) and *K. pneumoniae* (1,2), and clostridia (14–23)], enteric pathogens (salmonellae, Coxsackie B_2 virus, and coronavirus rotavirus), and potential pathogens (*Bacteroides fragilis*) (24–26).

The epidemic nature of NEC and the concomitant isolates of similar pathogens suggest the spread of organisms within a nursery. During the epidemic, these organisms may cause other disease manifestations, such as sepsis or diarrhea (1,2). Thus, host factors may determine the disease status. Alternatively, NEC may be a host response to multiple adverse intestinal conditions. The immature bowel may have a limited response pattern to injury, one of which is NEC.

Clostridia have been implicated as pathogens in some infants with NEC. Pedersen and colleagues (23) cultured *Clostridium perfringens* from the peritoneal fluids of babies who died of NEC and observed gram-positive bacilli resembling clostridia in nectrotic portions of the gut in six out of seven infants. Howard et al. (21) reported an outbreak of nonfatal NEC from *Clostridium butyricum*. Strum and co-workers (22) recovered *C. butyricum* from the peritoneal fluid and cerebrospinal fluid of a neonate with NEC. Brook et al. (27) recovered *Clostridium difficile* mixed with *K. pneumoniae* from the peritoneal fluid and blood of a patient with NEC. Warren et al. (16) recovered *C. perfringens* from the inflamed peritoneal cavity of two newborns with NEC with severe hemolytic anemia. Novak (18) described red blood cell alteration in four patients with NEC. *Clostridium* spp. were recovered in the blood or peritoneal cavity of three out of four patients. These strains elaborated red blood cells altering enzymes also in vitro. Alfa et al. (15) described an outbreak of NEC occurred in six neonates within a two-month period. Blood cultures from three of these neonates grew the same strain of what appears to be a novel *Clostridium* spp.

The virulence of clostridia strains in NEC could result from multiple mechanisms. Kosloske and Ulrich (28) obtained cultures of blood and peritoneal fluid with NEC. Of the 17 operated infants, 16 had bacteria in their blood and/or peritoneal fluid. The majority of resected bowel specimens from these infants contained a confirmatory morphologic type of bacterium within the wall. The clinical course of eight infants with clostridia was compared with that of eight infants with gram-negative aerobic and anaerobic bacteria (*Klebsiella, E. coli,* or *B. fragilis*). The infants with clostridia were sicker; they had more extensive pneumatosis intestinalis, a higher incidence of portal venous gas, more rapid progression to gangrene, and more extensive gangrene. These authors concluded that among infants who develop intestinal gangrene, clostridia appear to be more virulent than gram-negative bacteria. Kosloske et al. (20) recovered *Clostridium* spp. in 16 out of 50 infants with NEC. Of the 16, 9 had *C. perfringens* and 7 had other species. These nine had a fulminate form of NEC analogous to gas gangrene of the intestine, and mortality was 78%. The seven infants with other *Clostridium* spp. had mortality comparable with that of infants with nonclostridial NEC (32%). However, Kliegman et al. (29) who isolated clostridia from seven infants with NEC, reported a similar mortality among clostridial and nonclostridial infections.

The toxin of *C. difficile* has not been implicated in the pathogenesis of NEC, although it has been identified in the stools of healthy infants. Kliegman and colleagues found that 17 out of 121 stools (14%) from infants up to five months of age caused cytotoxicity in tissue culture that was consistent with the effect of *C. difficile* toxin (29). No toxin was identified in stools from 24 patients with NEC examined by Bartlett and associates (30) or from 18 patients with NEC studied by Chang and Areson (31).

Cashore and co-workers (32) found *C. difficile* toxin in 5 samples from 15 patients with confirmed or suspected NEC. In addition, they recovered clostridia in 8 out of 11 confirmed NEC cases, in 7 out of 9 suspected cases, and in 4 out of 13 asymptomatic cases.

Clostridia are implicated as a possible source of NEC by almost all studies, however, their definite role in NEC awaits further confirmation. The hypoxia and circulatory disturbances in small premature infants at risk for NEC may lead to ischemia of bowel, where multiplication of clostridia and toxin production may result in bowel ulceration, infarction, pneumatosis, and the clinical picture of NEC.

Earlier investigations failed to identify clostridia in NEC probably because peritoneal fluid was seldom cultured for anaerobes. Clostridia in the gastrointestinal tract do not cause illness unless they invade tissues and/or produce exotoxins. A low oxidation–reduction potential, which occurs in the presence of devitalized tissue, is essential for toxin production. Those infants colonized by clostridia and who have an episode of intestinal ischemia prior to the onset of NEC may, therefore, be at risk of clostridial invasion of their devitalized intestinal portions.

The gas-forming ability of some clostridia may explain the more extensive pneumatosis intestinalis and the higher incidence of portal venous gas among the infants with clostridia. The production of clostridial exotoxins, which cause cell lysis and tissue necrosis, may explain the more rapid progression to gangrene and more extensive gangrene among infants with clostridia (28). The lower platelet counts in infants with *Clostridium* may be due to their endotoxin production. The hemolysis seen in some patients with clostridial infections in NEC patients (16) may be caused by elaboration of hemolysins. Endotoxin, which has been detected both in blood and in peritoneal fluid of infants with severe NEC (33), produces thrombocytopenia by direct destruction of platelets.

Anaerobes, including clostridia, are considered to be members of the normal flora of infants of this age (34). The majority of infants are colonized by 10 days of age with aerobic gram-negative rods (most frequently *E. coli* and *Klebsiella*), as well as by anaerobic flora, including *B. fragilis* (35,36) and clostridia species are found in a third of infants. Although clostridia are normal inhabitants of the human intestinal tract, colonization rates among neonates vary from 7% to 70% (37). The source of the neonatal intestinal flora is the environment encountered by the infant after birth. The normal flora of the cervix and vagina contains many anaerobes, including clostridia (38). Differences among neonates in gestational age, route of delivery, and type of feeding are associated with different colonization patterns of aerobic and anaerobic bacteria (36).

Waligora-Dupriet et al. (39) who fed gnotobiotic quails a lactose diet with *K. pneumoniae*, *C. perfringens*, *C. difficile*, *Clostridium paraputrificum*, or *C. butyricum* (two strains) found that neither *K. pneumoniae* nor *C. difficile* induced any cecal lesions. In contrast, the four other clostridial strains led to cecal NEC-like lesions with a variable occurrence. Gross aspects of the lesions was linked to the short-chain fatty acid profiles and/or concentrations: thickening of the cecal wall (*C. butyricum* and *C. perfringens*) with high proportion of butyric acid, hemorrhages (*C. paraputrificum*) with high proportion of *iso*-butyric acid, and presence of other iso-acids. In addition, *C. butyricum* was characterized by pneumatosis, linked to a high-gas production. The authors concluded that Clostridia species seem to be implicated in NEC through excessive production of butyric acid as a result of colonic lactose fermentation.

The similarities to clostridial enterotoxemias in adults (antibiotic-associated pseudomembranous colitis) and animals (pig-bell disease) and the similarity to the histology noted in pseudomembranous colitis strengthen the epidemiological data and highlight the role of *Clostridium* spp. in NEC (1,2,32).

Epidemics of necrotizing enteritis caused by a *C. perfringens* type C exotoxin have been noted. These are preventable through administration of specific antitoxin or specific immunization of mothers. *C. perfringens* type B produces diseases in newborn fowl, calves, piglets, and lambs (40). Pig-bell is caused by *C. perfringens* type C enterotoxin (41). The disease is comparable to NEC in histology and clinical features. Treatment is possible with an antitoxin to type C alpha and beta Clostridial toxins, and prevention can be achieved by immunization with *C. perfringens* beta toxoid (42). Pseudomembranous colitis that usually follows antimicrobial therapy where *C. difficile* toxin appear to be the primary agent has histological features similar to NEC, except for the lack of pneumatosis intestinalis (43).

CLINICAL MANIFESTATION

The classic triad of symptoms includes abdominal distention, bilious vomiting, and bloody stools. Most patients, however, present with less specific symptoms. The onset of acute NEC has a bimodal pattern. It generally occurs in the first week of life (in newborns more than 34 weeks of gestational age), but in some it may be delayed to the second to the fourth week (mostly in those less than 30 weeks of gestational age). The affected term neonate is usually systemically ill with other predisposing maternal and individual conditions (see above). Premature babies are at risk for several weeks after birth, with the age of onset inversely related to their gestational age. The typical infant with NEC is premature and recovering from some form of stress, but is well enough to begin gavage feedings. Initial symptoms may include progressive subtle signs of feeding intolerance, and subtle systemic signs. In advanced disease, a fulminant systemic collapse and consumption coagulopathy occurs. Feeding intolerance can be manifested by abdominal distention/tenderness, delayed gastric emptying and vomiting. General symptoms can progress insidiously and include increased apnea and bradycardia, lethargy, and temperature instability. Fulminant NEC presents with acidosis, disseminated intravascular coagulation, peritonitis, profound apnea, rapid cardiovascular and hemodynamic collapse, and shock. Stools-reducing substance are elevated, the stools will show traces of occult blood, and diarrhea may be present. As abdominal distention progresses, the gastric residuals rise, and within a short period the urine volume decreases and osmolarity rises. Abdominal erythema can appear and gastric aspirate becomes bile stained. At this stage, the child may have hypotension and may have gross blood in diarrheal stools.

Infants with sudden onset have those symptoms more abruptly. NEC was staged by Bell et al. (44), but should also be further defined as either endemic or epidemic. Stage I (suspected NEC) of NEC is defined as the presence of abdominal distention poor feeding, and vomiting, and radiologically, there is ileus. Stage II (definite NEC) has also gastrointestinal bleeding, and radiologically is defined by pneumatosis intestinals and portal vein gas. Stage III is advanced NEC, has also septic shock, and radiologically there is pneumopentoneum. All stages are treated medically, and Stage III also surgically.

Differential diagnosis includes sepsis in the early stages, and at later stages, metabolic disorders, congenital heart diseases, intraventriculus hemorrhage, and infections. Other diagnoses included omphalitis, intestinal malabsorption or volvulus, infection enterocolitis, neonatal appendicitis, spontaneous perforation, urinary infection, and Hirschsprung disease.

DIAGNOSIS

Radiological and Other Studies

The earliest radiographic findings in NEC may be dilation of the small bowel. The pattern suggests mechanical or aganglionic obstruction, most frequently in the form of multiple dilated loops of small bowel, but sometimes as isolated loops. Air fluid levels often are observed in the erect position. Commonly, intestinal loops will appear separated and then progresses to pneumatosis intestinalis in about 30% of infants studied, and about one-third of those with pneumatosis intestinalis will also have gas within the portal venous system of the liver (1,2).

A common finding is thickened bowel wall, bubbly appearance of the intestinal contents, and loops of unequal size. Free air ultimately may be identified within the peritoneal cavity of many infants with NEC who are not successfully treated. The site of perforation often is walled off, and in some infants with gas under the diaphragm the intestinal wall may be intact. Ultrasonography is helpful for distinguishing fluid from air. Doppler study of the splanchnic arteries early in the course of NEC can help distinguish developing NEC from benign feeding intolerance in a mildly symptomatic baby (45).

Laboratory Findings

Blood and peritoneal fluid cultures will yield organisms of enteric origin in about one-fourth of patients. Yeast may be isolated from peritoneal fluid, especially in infants who had been treated with antimicrobials. In the event of an outbreak in a nursery, it is important to evaluate both cases and matched concurrent controls. Viruses can be detected antigenically or through genetic methods. In some infants, the white blood count may be very low or very high and the platelet count usually will be diminished and falling rapidly. At least 50% of infants with NEC have platelet counts of 50,000 per millimeter or less (45). Prothrombin and partial thromboplastin times are elevated. Hyponatremia is common at the outset of NEC.

MANAGEMENT

Medical Management

The goals of the initial management are preventing ongoing damage, restoring hemostasis, and minimizing complications. The management consists of withholding oral feeding, placement of nasogastric tube for suction, abdominal decompression, paracenthesis, vigorous intravenous hydration containing electrolytes and calories, support of the circulation with plasma blood or dextran, and administration of antibiotics (46). The antibiotics should be of broad spectrum appropriate for covering of *E. coli*, *K. pneumoniae*, and other enterobacteria. The antibiotic coverage should be based on the sensitivities or the expected susceptibility of those pathogens prevalent in the nursery at the time of treatment.

Broad-spectrum parenteral therapy is initiated at the onset of symptoms providing coverage for gram-positive and gram-negative organisms, with the addition of anaerobic coverage for infants less than one week with progression of radiologic disease. Antifungal therapy should be considered for premature infants with a history of recent or prolonged antibacterial therapy or for babies who continue to deteriorate clinically and/or hematologically despite adequate antibacterial coverage. Ampicillin and an aminoglycoside (i.e., gentamicin) or cefotaxime should be given parenterally. Bell and colleagues (47) found improved survival after administration of gentamicin or kanamycin by nasogastric tube in a dose of two to three times the systemic dose. Caution should be used, however, in administration of aminoglycosides through the oral route, since rapid absorption of these drugs from the intestinal tract can occur in newborns with impaired mucosa. Topical nonabsorbable antibiotics (e.g., colistin, gentamicin) can suppress the gastrointestinal flora. However, it is not currently recommended because of the development of resistant bacteria.

Antibiotic coverage for anaerobes is controversial (5,48). Clindamycin use was associated with increased strictures (49), and the resistance of *C. difficile* to this drug. Penicillin is most active against *Clostridium* spp. Vancomycin is active against *C. difficile* as well as Staphylococcal spp. In instances of bowel perforation, antimicrobial coverage should include agents effective also against *B. fragilis* group, *Clostridium* spp., as well as Enterobacteriaceae, which can cause peritonitis. These include the combination of metronidazole, clindamycin, cefoxitin, and aminoglycosides, or single agent therapy with a carbapenem. Antimicrobials should be administered for 10 to 14 days. Infants should not be fed by mouth for a minimum of three to five days after they show normal gastrointestinal function and normal abdominal radiographic picture.

Surgical Treatment

Indications for surgery include clinical deterioration, perforation, peritonitis, obstruction, and abdominal mass. When NEC has been detected early and appropriate therapy instituted promptly, only a small percentage of infants will require surgical intervention (50,51). Since perforation is an ominous complication, however, a close watch by a surgeon is essential. Infants with spontaneous perforation of the bowel are often more mature. Signs such as rapid clinical deterioration, manifested by persistent acidosis, consumption coagulopathy, a fall in the platelets, bradycardia, hyponatheremia, and urinary output deterioration in the face of adequate therapy, or if there is free air within the abdomen and if the child shows sudden onset of abdominal tenderness, the child must be promptly explored surgically. The goal of surgery is to stabilize gross peritoneal infection without sacrificing bowel length. The organisms recovered after perforation of the bowel represent the bowel flora and include Enterobacteriaceae as well as anaerobes (17). Antimicrobial coverage should therefore provide coverage against these organisms in a manner similar to the one used after any spontaneous rupture of the viscus (see chap. 22).

COMPLICATIONS

Complications include bacteremia, intestinal perforation follow by sepsis, hemolysis following transfusion, disseminated fungal infection following intestinal perforation and postsurgical wounds.

Survival improved with improvement in care. Survival is currently 98% for those treated medically and 75% for those treated also surgically. Strictures occur in about a third treated surgically, and also in many treated medically. Short-gut syndrome develops in about a third treated surgically, and dysfunction of the gastrointestinal tract occurs in 10% of infants (51).

Up to a third of infants have neurodevelopmental sequelae, which can occur in three-fourth with severe NEC.

PREVENTION

Since early presentation of NEC can be subtle, high-clinical suspicion is important when evaluating any infant with signs of feeding intolerance or other abdominal pathology (52). Generally, continuing feeding a patient with developing NEC worsens the disease. Prophylaxis with oral aminoglycosides has been shown either to reduce the incidence of NEC especially in low birth infants or to have no appreciable effect (5,53). The use of prophylactic oral aminoglycoside antibiotics carries the risk of emergence of resistant bacteria, including clostridia (52). This argument is bolstered by the description of colitis caused by *C. difficile* in a newborn (54). This is also important because clostridia have been implicated in the etiology of NEC (5) or NEC-like illnesses (14–23,28–34), and these organisms are resistant to the aminoglycosides and polymyxins. Direct gastrointestinal injury by aminoglycosides and their systemic absorption may also have an adverse effect. Because endemic NEC occurs too infrequently and unpredictably, the routine administration of oral antibiotics is not warranted. However, during epidemics, especially those associated with specific organisms, appropriate prophylaxis may be indicated.

Breastfeeding may reduce the risk of NEC. Antenatal corticosteroids can reduce the incidence of NEC (55,56). Based on the available trials, the evidence does not support that the administration of oral immunoglobulin prevents NEC. There are no randomized controlled trials of oral IgA alone for the prevention of NEC (57). Avoidance of hypertonic formulas, medications, diagnostic agents, phlebotomy, placement of venous umbilical catheters in the portal vein, and performing exchange transfusion with plasma when polycythemia is critical or helpful (52).

Two studies (9,10) demonstrated a significant benefit for the use of oral probiotics [one using *Lactobacillus acidophilus* and *Bifidobacterium infantis* (10) and the other *Bifidobacterium infantis*, *Streptococcus thermophilus*, and *Bifidobacteria bifidus* (9)] in the prevention of NEC. They confirm previous observations in experimental animal models (58,59) and findings in studies involving premature infants (60).

The mechanisms by which probiotics may protect from NEC include: shifting the intestinal balance from a microflora, which is potentially harmful to the host, to one, which is predominantly beneficial (61); strengthening the intestinal mucosal barrier function, thereby impeding translocation of bacteria or their products; and modification of host responses to microbial products (62).

Probiotics appear to be safe in neonates. However, the rare complication of sepsis is of concern. In a recent report (63) two patients, a six-week-old and a six-year-old, who received probiotic lactobacilli, developed bacteremia and sepsis attributable to *Lactobacillus* spp. Molecular DNA fingerprinting analysis showed that the Lactobacillus strain isolated from blood samples was indistinguishable from the probiotic strain ingested by these patients.

Even though two studies (9,10) support a role for probiotics in the protection from NEC, the use of probiotics in neonates must be better understood and its advantages and potential risks need further confirmation before it becomes a general practice.

Routine infection-control measures, such as glove–gown-cohort-isolation and good handwashing are of utmost importance especially in preventing and controlling outbreaks. Cohorting of infants and personnel are important. Caregivers with concurrent illnesses should not work in the nursery.

REFERENCES

1. Neu J. Neonatal necrotizing enterocolitis: an update. Acta Paediatr Suppl 2005; 94:100–5.
2. Torma MJ, Kafetzis DA, Skevaki C, Costalos C. Neonatal necrotizing enterocolitis: an overview. Curr Opin Infect Dis 2003; 16:349–55.
3. Stoll BJ. Epidemiology of necrotizing enterocolitis. Clin Perinatol 1994; 21:205–18.

4. Llanos AR, Moss ME, Pinzon MC, Dye T, Sinkin RA, Kendig JW. Epidemiology of neonatal necrotising enterocolitis: a population-based study. Paediatr Perinat Epidemiol 2002; 16:342–9.
5. Panigrahi P. Necrotizing enterocolitis: a practical guide to its prevention and management. Paediatr Drugs 2006; 8:151–65.
6. Nowicki PT. Ischemia and necrotizing enterocolitis: where, when, and how. Semin Pediatr Surg 2005; 14:152–8.
7. Horton KK. Pathophysiology and current management of necrotizing enterocolitis. Neonatal Netw 2005; 24:37–46.
8. Updegrove K. Necrotizing enterocolitis: the evidence for use of human milk in prevention and treatment. J Hum Lact 2004; 20:335–9.
9. Bin-Nun A, Bromiker R, Wilschanski M. Oral probiotics prevent necrotizing enterocolitis in very low birth weight neonates. J Pediatr 2005; 147:192–6.
10. Lin HC, Su BH, Lin TW. Oral probiotics reduce the incidence and severity of necrotizing enterocolitis in very low birth weight infants. Pediatrics 2005; 115:1–4.
11. Martinez-Tallo E, Claure N, Bancalari E. Necrotizing enterocolitis in full-term or near-term infants: risk factors. Biol Neonate 1997; 71:292–8.
12. Hsueh W, Caplan MS, Qu XW, Tan XD, De Plaen IG, Gonzalez-Crussi F. Neonatal necrotizing enterocolitis: clinical considerations and pathogenetic concepts. Pediatr Dev Pathol 2003; 6:6–23.
13. Krediet TG, van Lelyveld N, Vijlbrief DC, et al. Microbiological factors associated with neonatal necrotizing enterocolitis: protective effect of early antibiotic treatment. Acta Paediatr 2003; 92:1180–2.
14. Chan KL, Ng SP, Chan KW, Wo YH, Tam PK. Pathogenesis of neonatal necrotizing enterocolitis: a study of the role of intraluminal pressure, age and bacterial concentration. Pediatr Surg Int 2003; 19:573–7.
15. Alfa MJ, Robson D, Davi M, Bernard K, Van Caeseele P, Harding GK. An outbreak of necrotizing enterocolitis associated with a novel *Clostridium* species in a neonatal intensive care unit. Clin Infect Dis 2002; 35:S101–5.
16. Warren S, Schreiber JR, Epstein MF. Necrotizing enterocolitis and hemolysis associated with *Clostridium perfringens*. Am J Dis Child 1984; 138:686–8.
17. Kosloske AM, Ball WS, Jr., Umland E, Skipper B. Clostridial necrotizing enterocolitis. J Pediatr Surg 1985; 20:155–9.
18. Novak RW, Klein RL, Novak PE. Necrotizing enterocolitis, hemolysis, and *Clostridium perfringens*. Am J Dis Child 1985; 139:114–5.
19. Novak RW. Bacterial-induced RBC alterations complicating necrotizing enterocolitis. Am J Dis Child 1984; 138:183–5.
20. Kosloske AM, Ulrich JA, Hoffman H. Fulminant necrotising enterocolitis associated with clostridia. Lancet 1978; 2:1014–6.
21. Howard FM, Flynn DM, Bradley JM, Noone P, Szawatkowski M. Outbreak of necrotising enterocolitis caused by *Clostridium butyricum*. Lancet 1977; 2:1099–102.
22. Sturm R, Staneck JL, Stauffer LR, Neblett WW, III. Neonatal necrotizing enterocolitis associated with penicillin-resistant, toxigenic *Clostridium butyricum*. Pediatrics 1980; 66:928–31.
23. Pedersen PV, Hansen FH, Halveg AB, Christiansen ED. Necrotizing enterocolitis of the newborn—is it gas-gangrene of the bowel? Lancet 1976; 2:715–6.
24. Rousset S, Moscovici O, Lebon P, et al. Intestinal lesions containing coronavirus-like particles in neonatal necrotizing enterocolitis: an ultrastructure analysis. Pediatrics 1984; 73:218–24.
25. Rotbart HA, Levin MJ, Yolken RH, Manchester DK, Jantzen J. An outbreak of rotavirus-associated neonatal necrotizing enterocolitis. J Pediatr 1983; 103:454–9.
26. Noel GJ, Laufer DA, Edelson PJ. Anaerobic bacteremia in a neonatal intensive care unit: an eighteen-year experience. Pediatr Infect Dis J 1988; 7:858–62.
27. Brook I, Avery G, Glasgow A. *Clostridium difficile* in pediatric infection. J Infect 1982; 4:253–7.
28. Kosloske AM, Ulrich JA. A bacteriologic basis for the clinical presentations of necrotizing enterocolitis. J Pediatr Surg 1980; 15:558–64.
29. Kliegman RM, Fanaroff AA, Izant R, Speck WT. Clostridia as pathogens in neonatal necrotizing enterocolitis. J Pediatr 1979; 95:287–9.
30. Bartlett JG, Moon N, Chang TW, Taylor N, Onderdonk AB. Role of *Clostridium difficile* in antibiotic-associated pseudomembranous colitis. Gastroenterology 1978; 75:778–82.
31. Chang TW, Areson P. Neonatal necrotizing enterocolitis: absence of enteric bacterial toxins. N Engl J Med 1978; 299:424.
32. Cashore WJ, Peter G, Lauermann M, Stonestreet BS, Oh W. Clostridia colonization and clostridial toxin in neonatal necrotizing enterocolitis. J Pediatr 1981; 98:308–11.
33. Fumarola D. Endotoxemia and neonatal necrotizing enterocolitis. Am J Clin Pathol 1985; 84:409.
34. Edwards CA, Parrett AM. Intestinal flora during the first months of life: new perspectives. Br J Nutr 2002; 88(Suppl. 1):S11–8.
35. Rotimi VO, Duerden BI. The development of the bacterial flora in normal neonates. J Med Microbiol 1981; 14:51–62.

36. Long SS, Swenson RM. Development of anaerobic fecal flora in healthy newborn infants. J Pediatr 1977; 91:298–301.

37. Kindley AD, Rboerts PJ, Tulloch WH. Neonatal necrotising enterocolitis. Lancet 1977; 1:649.

38. Brook I, Barrett CT, Brinkman CR, III, Martin WJ, Finegold SM. Aerobic and anaerobic flora of maternal cervix and newborn's conjunctiva and gastric fluid: a prospective study. Pediatrics 1979; 63:451–5.

39. Waligora-Dupriet AJ, Dugay A, Auzeil N, Huerre M, Butel MJ. Evidence for clostridial implication in necrotizing enterocolitis through bacterial fermentation in a gnotobiotic quail model. Pediatr Res 2005; 58:629–35.

40. Finegold SM. Anaerobic Infections in Human Disease. New York: Academic Press, 1977.

41. Murrell TG. Pigbel in Papua New Guinea: an ancient disease rediscovered. Int J Epidemiol 1976 1983; 12:211–4.

42. Lawrence G, Shann F, Freestone DS, Walker PD. Prevention of necrotizing enteritis in Papua New Guinea by active immunization. Lancet 1979; 1:227–30.

43. Kliegman RM, Fanaroff AA. Necrotizing enterocolitis. N Engl J Med 1984; 310:1093–103.

44. Bell MJ, Ternberg JL, Feigin RD, et al. Neonatal necrotizing enterocolitis: therapeutic decisions based upon clinical staging. Ann Surg 1978; 187:1–7.

45. Faingold R, Daneman A, Tomlinson G, et al. Necrotizing enterocolitis: assessment of bowel viability with color doppler US. Radiology 2005; 235:587–94.

46. Henry MC, Moss RL. Current issues in the management of necrotizing enterocolitis. Semin Perinatol 2004; 28:221–33.

47. Bell MJ, Kosloske AM, Benton C, Martin LW. Neonatal necrotizing enterocolitis: prevention of perforation. J Pediatr Surg 1973; 8:601–5.

48. Bell MJ, Shackelford PG, Feigin RD, Ternberg JL, Brotherton T. Alterations in gastrointestinal microflora during antimicrobial therapy for necrotizing enterocolitis. Pediatrics 1979; 63:425–8.

49. Faix RG, Polley TZ, Grasela TH. A randomized, controlled trial of parenteral clindamycin in neonatal necrotizing enterocolitis. J Pediatr 1988; 112:271–7.

50. Pierro A. The surgical management of necrotising enterocolitis. Early Hum Dev 2005; 81:79–85.

51. Horwitz JR, Lally KP, Cheu HW, Vazquez WD, Grosfeld JL, Ziegler MM. Complications after surgical intervention for necrotizing enterocolitis: a multicenter review. J Pediatr Surg 1995; 30:994–8.

52. Reber KM, Nankervis CA. Necrotizing enterocolitis: preventative strategies. Clin Perinatol 2004; 31:157–67.

53. Bury RG, Tudehope D. Enteral antibiotics for preventing necrotizing enterocolitis in low birthweight or preterm infants. Cochrane Database Syst Rev 2001:CD000405.

54. Adler SP, Chandrika T, Berman WF. *Clostridium difficle* associated with pseudomembranous colitis: occurrence in a 12-week-old infant without prior antibiotic therapy. Am J Dis Child 1981; 135:820–2.

55. Nanthakumar NN, Young C, Ko JS, et al. Glucocorticoid responsiveness in developing human intestine: possible role in prevention of necrotizing enterocolitis. Am J Physiol Gastrointest Liver Physiol 2005; 288:G85–92.

56. Lee JS, Polin RA. Treatment and prevention of necrotizing enterocolitis. Semin Neonatol 2003; 8:449–59.

57. Foster J, Cole M. Oral immunoglobulin for preventing necrotizing enterocolitis in preterm and low birth-weight neonates. Cochrane Database Syst Rev 2004:CD001816.

58. Caplan MS, Miller-Catchpole R, Kaup S, et al. Bifidobacterial supplementation reduces the incidence of necrotizing enterocolitis in a neonatal rat model. Gastroenterology 1999; 117:577–83.

59. Butel MJ, Waligora-Dupriet AJ, Szylit O. Oligofructose and experimental model of neonatal necrotizing enterocolitis. Br J Nutr 2002; 87:S213–9.

60. Hoyos AB. Reduced incidence of necrotizing enterocolitis associated with enteral administration of *Lactobacillus acidophilus* and *Bifidobacterium infantis* to neonates in an intensive care unit. Int J Infect Dis 1999; 3:197–202.

61. Fuller R. Probiotics in man and animals. J Appl Bacteriol 1989; 66:365–78.

62. Neu J, Caicedo R. Probiotics: protecting the intestinal ecosystem? J Pediatr 2005; 147:143–6.

63. Land MH, Rouster-Stevens K, Woods CR, Cannon ML, Cnota J, Shetty AK. *Lactobacillus* sepsis associated with probiotic therapy. Pediatrics 2005; 115:178–81.

9 | Infant Botulism

Infant botulism (IB) results from absorption of heat-labile neurotoxin produced in situ by *Clostridium botulinum* that can colonize the intestines of infants younger than one year (1). It is an age-limited neuromuscular disease that is distinct from classic botulism in that the toxin is elaborated by the organism in the infant's intestinal lumen and is then absorbed.

MICROBIOLOGY

C. botulinum is a gram-positive spore-forming obligate anaerobe that is present in the soil worldwide and may spread by dust. It is composed of four groups of clostridia (groups I–IV), linked by their ability to produce potent neurotoxins which have identical pharmacologic modes of action. Botulinal toxin is the most potent neurotoxin known (2). The toxin does not appear to cross the blood–brain barrier and it exerts its toxicity through affecting the transmission at all peripheral cholinergic junctions. It interferes with the normal release of acetylcholine from nerve terminals in response to depolarization (3). The toxin binds irreversibly, and recovery of function depends on ultra-terminal sprouting of the nerve to form new motor end plates.

EPIDEMIOLOGY

IB is a restricted age-range disease. Ninety-five percent of all recognized cases have occurred in patients between six weeks and six months of age. The disease affects equally all major racial and ethnic groups and both sexes. More than 1500 cases of IB have been confirmed in the U.S.A. since it was recognized in 1976. IB is the most common form of botulism, with about 80 to 100 (median of 71) cases reported annually in the United States (4–7). Almost all cases of IB are caused by proteolytic *C. botulinum* group I strains that produce either type A or B (or Bf) neurotoxin. Type E neurotoxin-producing *Clostridium butyricum* was recovered from infants (7). *Clostridium baratii* strains can also produce type F botulinal toxin, and has also been recovered from infants with botulism (8–10).

IB has been reported from all inhabited continents except Africa. In the U.S.A., differences in the regional soil distribution of *C. botulinum* exist. *C. botulinum* spores that produce toxin B are mainly found east of the Mississippi River, while neurotoxin type A spores predominate in the soils west of it (11). Similar distribution in the case of IB was found. Geographic clustering of the cases had also been noted (12–14).

PREDISPOSING CONDITIONS AND PATHOPHYSIOLOGY

IB results from the ingestion of *C. botulinum* spores. Even though honey is a known source, in about 85% of patients the source is unknown. BI cases occur from six days to 12 months of age and not later. Information derived from a mouse model and clinical cases suggest that transient absence of competitive microbial intestinal flora and/or alteration in motility or pH enables outgrowth of vegetative forms from ingested spores. Recently, weaned infants that have been exclusively breast-fed and, when changes of intestinal flora occurs, are at risk for IB.

Replicating *C. botulinum*, and occasionally *C. baratii* and *C. butyricum*, produce distinctive botulinal neurotoxins (types A–G) of high potency. After systemic absorption, toxin binds to receptors on presynaptic nerve endings of cranial and peripheral nerves and blocks acetyl-choline release (15).

Excretion of the organism has persisted for as long as 158 days after the onset of constipation, well after clinical recovery had occurred. The syndrome has occurred in both breast-fed and bottle-fed infants, and the role of type of feeding is yet unsettled (16).

Colonization is believed to occur because normal bowel flora that could compete with *C. botulinum* have not been fully established.

Risk factors for IB are multifactorial and include breastfeeding, and the introduction of first-formula feeding, consumption of honey, and residence in a region of high spore density and soil disruption (13). Constipation appears to be a risk factor but also is an early manifestation of intoxication (17).

Breastfeeding is a risk factor for IB in all studies (13,16–21). This may be the case because it truly predispose to illness (13,17,20), or that it slows the illness to permit hospitalization (16). However, among hospitalized infants the formula-fed reported from California (16), had a mean age of onset (7.6±8.4 weeks) that was significantly less than that of their breast-fed counterparts (13.7±8.4 weeks). The younger age at onset for formula-fed infants may reflect their earlier availability of suitable ecologic niches for *C. botulinum* in the intestinal flora of the formula-fed infants (13,18), as well as the lack of immune factors that are contained in human milk. Long et al. (13), who reported 44 patients with IB from Southeastern Pennsylvania, found that the majority of their patients had just formula feedings or other food introduced within four weeks of onset. The resident gut microflora is capable of blocking the outgrowth and multiplication of *C. botulinum* spores. The difference in the fecal flora of breast- and formula-fed infants may account for the increased earlier susceptibility of formula-fed infants to IB. Infants fed human milk have more acidic feces (pH 5.1–5.4) that contain a large number of *Bifidobacterium* ($\sim 10^{10}$/g). *Clostridium* (as spores) are virtually absent (22).

In contrast, formula-fed infants have less acidic feces (pH 5.4–8.0), that also contain *Clostridium* spp. as well as other anaerobes and facultative bacteria (18). The difference in pH may be important, because multiplication of *C. botulinum* and toxin production declines with reduced pH.

Preformed toxin has not been identified in food ingested by the infants, but the organism has been identified in honey, vacuum cleaner, dust, and soil. *C. botulinum* organisms, but no preformed toxin, were identified in six different honey specimens fed to three California patients with IB, as well as from 10% (9/90) of honey specimens studied (23). By food exposure history, honey was significantly associated with type B IB. In California, 20% (56 of 272) of hospitalized patients had been fed honey prior to onset of constipation (24), in Utah 83% (10 of 12) (19), and in Southeastern Pennsylvania 14% (6 of 44) (13). Worldwide, honey exposure occurred in 35% (28/75) of hospitalized cases. Of all food items tested, only honey contained *C. botulinum* organisms.

The organism and its toxin have rarely been identified in the feces of normal infants (25). *C. botulinum* was isolated from the stools of three normal control infants and nine control infants who had neurologic diseases that clearly were not IB (19). These infants were termed as "asymptomatic carriers" of the organism. The occurrence of the asymptomatic carrier state suggests that a diagnosis of IB cannot be made on a basis of culture results alone, but must rest on historical and physical confirmation of progressive bulbar and extremity weakness with ultimate complete resolution of symptoms and findings over a period of several months.

A distinct seasonal incidence to IB was observed in one study done in Utah (19). All the cases were reported between March and October with no reported cases during the winter months. The seasonal incidence suggests that the temperature and moisture factors that favor proliferation of *C. botulinum* in the soil could be of major importance. No apparent temporal relationship existed between cases and season, temperature, or rainfall in the 44 cases reported from Southeastern Pennsylvania (13).

A common set of environmental features was found to be characteristic of the home environment of children with IB and asymptomatic carriers, and includes nearby constructional or agricultural soil disruption, dusty, and windy conditions, a high water table, and alkaline soil conditions (19). The conditions of high soil water and alkaline content, which are favorable for the growth of *C. botulinum* (11), were found near the homes of all affected infants.

The dissemination of the organism appeared to be further enhanced by construction and agricultural soil disruption as well as windy conditions near the homes of most affected infants and asymptomatic carriers.

About half of patients' fathers in the cases reported in Pennsylvania (13) had occupations that brought them into daily contact with soil. Spores were recovered from yard soil, window sills, cribs, or fathers' shoes in seven of nine instances in which environmental sampling was done. Forty three of the 44 cases occurred in infants who resided around the city of Philadelphia, and only 1 infant was from the city. A possible explanation for this discrepancy is the differences in the disruption of soil between the city and surrounding areas and little occupational contact with soil in the city compared to the surrounding areas.

The ubiquitous distribution of *C. botulinum* spores in nature allows for their ingestion by many infants (5). The fact that ingested spores can germinate in some, but not all, infants generally between one and six months old indicates that host factors unique to this age play a central role in pathogenesis. Host factors are of great importance, a point emphasized by the broad spectrum in the severity of disease.

CLINICAL MANIFESTATION

The onset ranges from insidious to abrupt. The syndrome is characterized by a history of constipation (defined as three or more days without bowel movement) followed by a subacute progression of bulbar and extremity weakness (within four to five days) manifest in inability to suck and swallow, weakened voice, ptosis, hypotonia, that may progress to generalized flaccidity and respiratory compromise. There is, however, a broad clinical spectrum of IB. The mild end of the spectrum appears to be represented by infants who never require hospitalization but who have feeding difficulties, mild hypotonia, and floppy neck, and failure to thrive, while the severe end of the spectrum may be characterized by a presentation resembling sudden infant death syndrome (SIDS) (26), and these patients require hospitalization for treatment of their respiratory and feeding difficulties.

The main clinical feature of the syndrome is constipation which occurs in about 95% of patients (16,27). Botulism is expressed clinically as a symmetric, descending paralysis. Early in the progression, weakness, and hypotonia are typical, and the first sign of illness is in the cranial nerves, in the form of bulbar palsies. Less vigorous crying or sucking or subdued facial expression generally is the first sign. Weakness progresses in a symmetric descending fashion over hours to a few days, from muscle innervated by cranial nerves to those of trunk and limbs. A marked dichotomy between the normal physical and abnormal neurologic findings usually occurs.

The time between the onset of constipation and onset of weakness ranges from 0 to 24 days (mean 11 days). Progression is more severe is infants younger than two months (14,28). Obstructive apnea due to the hypotonia leading to collapse of the hypopharynx support can occur rapidly in this age group. The infants also may manifest tachycardia, difficulty in sucking and swallowing, listlessness, weakening, hypotonia, general muscular weakness with a loss of head control, and pooling of oral secretion. These babies appear "floppy," and may manifest various neurologic signs such as ptosis, ophthalmoplegia, sluggish reaction of the pupils, dysphagia, weak gag reflex, and poor anal sphincter tone (29). In seriously ill babies respiratory arrest may occur.

The first signs noted in IB are classically those of autonomic blockade. The parasympathetic nervous system is more vulnerable to cholinergic blockade by botulinum toxin than the sympathetic nervous system because the parasympathetic pre- and postsynaptic transmissions are affected. In infants with botulism, recognition of the signs and symptoms associated with parasympathetic blockade is important, since these findings precede generalized motor weakness and respiratory decompensation (17,30). The autonomic nervous system dysfunction may include decreased salivation, distention of abdomen and bladder, decreased bowel sounds, fluctuation in blood pressure, heart rate, and skin color.

The orderly sequence of presentation and recovery of disease signs and symptoms in IB generally follows the order of constipation and tachycardia, followed by loss of head control, difficulty in feeding, weakening, and depressed gag reflex, followed by peripheral motor weakness and subsequent diaphragmatic weakness (30,31).

The nadir of paresis and paralysis generally occur within one or two weeks. The resolution of disease signs and symptoms occurs in the inverse order of presentation, with autonomic finding the last to regress (31). Once strength and tone begin to return, the improvement continues over the following weeks in the absence of complications. It is important to minimize interventions that increase complications.

It is important to remember that at this stage of the disease, return of peripheral motor activity does not signify complete reversed cholinergic synapse. The infant is highly susceptible to events that will additionally stress or impair neuromuscular transmission. Such events may lead to sudden respiratory arrest or gradual respiratory failure. Two specific factors have been associated with respiratory decompensation in IB: administration of aminoglycoside antibiotics and neck flexion during positioning for lumbar puncture or computerized axial tomography scan (32,33). Aminoglycoside antibiotics decrease acetylcholine release from nerve terminals innervating the diaphragm, leading to diaphragmatic weakness and respiratory failure.

DIFFERENTIAL DIAGNOSIS

The most frequent admission diagnoses of infants later found to have IB include sepsis, viral syndrome, dehydration, cerebrovascular accident, failure to thrive, myasthenia gravis, polio-myelitis, Guillain–Barré syndrome, encephalitis, and meningitis. Several hereditary-endocrine or metabolic disorders considered are amino acid metabolism disorder, Werdnig–Hoffmann disease, and drug or toxin ingestion. Diagnoses less frequently considered include subdural effusion, infectious mononucleosis, brain stem encephalitis, animal bite or sting, organopho-sphate poisoning, carbon monoxide intoxication, methemoglobinemia, myoglobinuria, glycogen or lipid storage diseases, benign congenital hypotonia, congenital muscular dystrophy, myotonic dystrophy, congenital myopathy, anterior horn cell syndrome, atonic cerebral palsy, and diffuse cerebral degenerative disease.

Even though sepsis may be considered in the differential diagnosis, infants with botulism are afebrile, alert, have robust skin color, but are hypotonic or paralyzed.

DIAGNOSIS

The diagnosis is made on clinical grounds. Routine laboratory tests such as blood chemistry, blood count, and urinalysis generally are normal. Mild dehydration and fat mobilization because of decreased oral intake may be present at admission. A few cases have shown slight elevation in the cerebrospinal fluid protein because of dehydration (30).

The only procedure that consistently corroborate the clinical diagnosis of IB is electro-myography (EMG). The EMG shows a characteristic pattern of: (*i*) brief, small amplitude, abundant, motor-unit action potential (BSAP) (34); (*ii*) enhancement of compound action potential in response to rapid repetitive nerve stimulation; (*iii*) normal nerve conduction velocity; and (*iv*) no response to edrophonium chloride or neostigmine injection (35). As clinical recovery occurs, normal motor-unit activity reappears.

EMG can provide rapid bedside substantiation of the clinical diagnosis of IB. If the BSAP pattern is present (34,36), then many of the other diagnostic tests and procedures to which patients are subjected may be deferred while laboratory examination of fecal specimens for *C. botulinum* toxin and organisms proceeds.

Unfortunately, EMG is not in itself diagnostic. Furthermore, failure to detect the BSAP pattern does not exclude the diagnosis of IB. The EMG pattern of post-tetanic facilitation, observed often in food-borne botulism, may be found in a variety of other disorders besides botulism such as diseases of the terminal motor nerve axons, the neuromuscular junction, or of muscle itself (37–39). Controversy exists regarding the sensitivity and specificity of EMG depending on the point in course of the illness and the timing and amount of nerve stimulation (39). Due to the unique clinical findings, and the availability of toxin assay, the painful EMG testing is not usually performed.

The diagnosis of IB is established unequivocally only when *C. botulinum* organisms are identified in a patient's feces, as *C. botulinum* is not part of the normal resident intestinal microflora of infants or adults (34,40,41). Confirmation of the clinical diagnosis requires the demonstration of botulinus toxin or *C. botulinum* in feces of the infant. The mouse neutralization assay is used to test for the presence of toxin in feces or the serum. Therefore, serum, and fecal specimens should be collected as soon as the diagnosis of botulism is suspected. It is sometimes possible to identify small amount of the toxin in serum if the specimen is collected early in the illness (42).

An enzyme-linked immunosorbent assay has recently been developed for rapid detection of toxins A and B in IB (43). This test allows detection within 24 hours as compared with four days that are required for the mouse assay. The toxin can be identified in stool of affected infants as long as four months after onset of symptoms, well into recovery.

Other specimens that are important for the epidemiologic investigation should be collected also, including suspected food, drug, and environmental samples. All specimens should be transported in insulated containers with cold packs and remain at temperatures of at least 4°C. Specimens for botulism investigation can be submitted to State Health Department or the Centers for Disease Control in Atlanta, Georgia.

MANAGEMENT

Children with IB presenting with mild symptoms require minimal care and can be managed as outpatients if careful follow-up is arranged. Infants with severe IB constitute a select group who are at risk for respiratory failure. These infants can be identified by their progressive sequential loss of neurologic functions.

Seriously ill patients require hospitalization for up to two months. Careful maintenance of adequate ventilation and caloric intake is of particular importance. The need for respiratory assistance, if any, generally occurs during the first week of hospitalization. Parenteral antibiotic therapy in an attempt to eradicate *C. botulinum* toxin and organisms from the intestinal tract usually is unsuccessful and should be reserved for cases with proved or suspected sepsis caused by other organisms.

Antibiotics are not recommended for IB and will not affect the course of illness or recovery. When penicillin or its derivatives have been used, neither oral nor parenteral administration succeeded in producing discernible clinical benefit or in eradicating either *C. botulinum* organisms or botulinus toxin from the intestine (17,34).

Effective antibiotics may increase the pool of toxin in the bowel available for absorption as it is liberated following bacterial cell death. Another argument against the use of antimicrobial agents is that these agents may alter the intestinal microecology in an unpredictable manner and might actually permit intestinal overgrowth by *C. botulinum* by eliminating the normal flora.

Aminoglycosides may potentiate neuromuscular weakness caused by *C. botulinum* toxin. It is, therefore, suggested that these antibiotics should be used with caution in suspected cases of IB. In large doses, gentamicin, along with other aminoglycosides, has been demonstrated to produce a non-depolarizing type of neuromuscular block (32). As *C. botulinum* toxin is known to block the release of acetylcholine from cholinergic nerve endings (2,3), gentamicin may potentiate sublethal concentrations of the toxin and result in complete neuromuscular blockade and resultant paralysis. L'Hommedieu and co-workers (32) provide clinical data and Santos et al. (44) provide animal data to support this hypothesis.

The present treatment of IB consists of meticulous supportive care, with particular attention to nutrition, pulmonary hygiene and good nursing care. Immediate access to an intensive care unit and to mechanical ventilation is especially important because aspiration or apnea may occur. Associated conditions such as dehydration, aspiration pneumonia, and anemia should be treated also. The respiratory aspects of the patient should be addressed by performing frequent suctioning and stimulation, mechanical ventilation, transcutaneous monitoring of oxygen, and administration of oxygen. When IB is suspected, monitoring for both apnea and bradycardia should be instituted; endotrachael intubation or tracheostomy may be required in some cases. Monitoring should continue until sufficient breathing, coughing, and swallowing ability have returned so that apnea and aspiration are unlikely to occur. The need for nutritional support can require gavage feeding, intravenous glucose and electrolytes, and sometimes hyperalimentation. Because bladder atony is often present, the bladder should be emptied frequently by Credé method. Tube feeding may stimulate peristalsis and has been used successfully in most patients. Patients should not be fed by mouth until they are able to gag and swallow. The patients should receive mother's milk, if available. Otherwise, formula without added iron is the next choice. Intravenous feeding has been used as a last resort. To reduce the quantity of *C. botulinum* organisms and toxin in the intestine, cathartic agents or bulk laxatives may be judiciously administered if adynamic ileus is absent, but rarely have these proved efficacious.

Since patients excrete *C. botulinum* toxin and organisms in their feces for weeks to months after they have returned home, it is important to adhere to careful hand washing and diaper disposal. Enemas and purgatives, clostridiocidal antibiotics, cholinomimetic drugs (i.e., guanidine, 4-aminopyridine) (45), and the equine botulinum antitoxin had no beneficial effects.

The intravenous botulinum immune globulin (BIG) trials in California that were completed in early 1997 demonstrated the safety and efficacy of human-derived BIG and a reduced mean hospital stay from 5.5 to 2.5 weeks. BIG is now Food and Drug administration approved and is only available from the California Department of Health Services (24-hour telephone: 510-540-2646) (46). BIG should be administered as early as possible to infants with suspected botulism to interrupt neuromuscular blockade. Equine botulinal antitoxin should not be used for IB, and human BIG is not available for use in any form of botulism other than IB.

The prognosis of IB is generally excellent. The main goal is to prevent complications while allowing neuromuscular recovery through the timely recognition and administration of antitoxin.

COMPLICATIONS

Secondary infections are common. These include acute otitis media (that is related to eustachian tube dysfunction or due to the presence of nasogastric tube), aspiration pneumonia, hypoxic encephalopathy, hyponatremia due to excretion of antidiuretic hormone in response to decreased atrial filling because of venous pooling in the paralyzed infant, urinary tract infection due to indwelling bladder catheter, *Clostridium difficile* collitis due to colonic stasis with manifestations of toxic megacolon and necrotizing enterocolitis (47), and septicemia associated with intravascular catheters.

PREVENTION

Since *C. botulinum* spores are heat resistant and may survive boiling for several hours, home cooking of foods may not destroy *C. botulinum* spores. Washing and peeling raw foods before cooking may substantially reduce the number of spores, if present.

The single food fed to patients that has been identified as a source of *C. botulinum* spores, but not of preformed botulinum toxin, is honey (34,40,48). Furthermore, honey exposure has been implicated as a significant risk factor for type B IB (48). A survey of honey samples not associated with cases of IB found that 7.5% contained *C. botulinum*, toxin-producing type A or type B or both. The honeys that contained *C. botulinum* originated in various parts of the U.S.A. (40). Since honey is not essential for infant nutrition, it is recommended that honey not be fed to infants less than one-year old. Previously corn syrup contained botulinum spores, but changes in corn syrup production have apparently eliminated this problem.

The full extent of infant morbidity and mortality that results from the intestinal production of botulinum toxin has not been determined. Although an association between infant with botulism and SIDS was suspected (26), a prospective study failed to confirm the presence of *C. botulinum* in 248 cases of SIDS (49). As the disease may mimic many other disorders, it is possible that more cases of IB may be recognized.

REFERENCES

1. Long SS. Infant botulism. Pediatr Infect Dis J 2001; 20:707–9.
2. Horowitz BZ. Botulinum toxin. Crit Care Clin 2005; 21:825–39.
3. Goonetilleke A, Harris JB. Clostridial neurotoxins. J Neurol Neurosurg Psychiatry 2004; 75 (Suppl. 3):iii35–9.
4. Jajosky RA, Hall PA, Adams DA, et al. Summary of notifiable diseases—United States, 2004. MMWR 2006; 53:1–79.
5. Shapiro R, Hatheway CL, Swerdlow D. Botulism in the United States: a clinical and epidemiologic review. Ann Intern Med 1998; 129:221–8.
6. Sobel J. Botulism. Clin Infect Dis 2005; 41:1167–73.
7. Aureli P, Fenicia L, Pasolini B, Gianfranceschi M, McCroskey LM, Hatheway CL. Two cases of type E infant botulism in Italy caused by neurotoxigenia *Clostridium butyricum*. J Infect Dis 1986; 54:207–11.
8. Suen JC, Hatheway CL, Steigerwalt AG, et al. Genetic confirmation of identities of neurotoxigenic *Clostridium barati* and *Clostridium butyricum* implicated as agents of infant botulism. J Clin Microbiol 1988; 26:2191–2.
9. Hall JD, McCroskey LM, Pincomb BJ, et al. Isolation of an organism resembling *Clostridium barati* which produces type F botulinal toxin from an infant with botulism. J Clin Microbiol 1985; 21:654–5.
10. Paisley JW, Lauer BA, Arnon SS. A second case of infant botulism type F caused by *Clostridium baratii*. Pediatr Infect Dis J 1995; 14:912–4.
11. Smith LD. The occurrence of *Clostridium botulinum* and *Clostridium tetani* in the soil of the United States. Health Lab Sci 1978; 15:74–80.
12. Centers for Disease Control and Prevention. Type B botulism associated with roasted eggplant in Oil—Italy, 1993. MMWR 1995; 44:33–6.
13. Long SS, Gajewski JL, Brown LW, Gilligan PH. Clinical, laboratory, and environmental features of infant botulism in Southeastern Pennsylvania. Pediatrics 1985; 75:935–41.
14. Istre GR, Compton R, Novotny T, et al. Infant botulism: three cases in a small town. Am J Dis Child 1986; 140:1013–4.
15. Schiavo G, Rossetto O, Tonello F, Montecucco C. Intracellular targets and metalloprotease activity of tetanus and botulism neurotoxins. Curr Top Microbiol Immunol 1995; 195:257–74.
16. Arnon SS, Damus K, Thompson B, Midura TF, Chin J. Protective role of human milk against sudden death from infant botulism. J Pediatr 1982; 100:568–73.
17. Spika JS, Shafer N, Hargrett-Bean N, et al. Risk factors for infant botulism in the United States. Am J Dis Child 1989; 143:828–32.
18. Stark PH, Lee A. The microbial ecology of the large bowel of breast-fed and formula-fed infants during the first year of life. J Med Microbiol 1982; 15:189–203.
19. Thompson JA, Glasgow LA, Warpinski JR, Olson C. Infant botulism: clinical spectrum and epidemiology. Pediatrics 1980; 66:936–42.
20. Long SS. Epidemiologic study of infant botulism in Pennsylvania: report of the infant botulism study group. J Pediatr 1985; 75:928–34.
21. Morris JG, Jr., Snyder JD, Wilson R, et al. Infant botulism in the United States: an epidemiologic study of cases occurring outside of California. Am J Public Health 1983; 73:1385–8.
22. Hentges DJ. The intestinal flora and infant botulism. Rev Infect Dis 1979; 1:668–73.
23. Johnson RO, Clay SA, Arnon SS. Diagnosis and management of infant botulism. Am J Dis Child 1979; 133:586–93.
24. Arnon SS. Infant botulism: anticipating the second decade. J Infect Dis 1986; 154:201–6.
25. Chin J, Arnon SS, Midura TF. Food and environmental aspects of infant botulism in California. Rev Infect Dis 1979; 1:693–7.
26. Arnon SS, Midura TF, Damus K, Wood RM, Chin J. Intestinal infection and toxin production by *Clostridium botulinum* as one cause of sudden infant death syndrome. Lancet 1978; 1:1273–7.
27. Long SS. Botulism in infancy. Pediatr Infect Dis 1984; 3:266–71.
28. Gunn RA, Dowell VR, Jr., Hatheway CL. Infant Botulism: Clinical and Laboratory Aspects. Atlanta: Center for Disease Control, 1978.
29. Woodruff BA, Griffin PM, McCroskey LM, et al. Clinical and laboratory comparison of botulism from toxin types A, B, and E in the United States, 1975–1988. J Infect Dis 1992; 166:1281–6.
30. Hurst DL, Marsh WW. Early severe infantile botulism. J Pediatr 1993; 122:909–11.
31. L'Hommedieu C, Polin RA. Progression of clinical signs in severe infant botulism. J Pediatr 1981; 20:90–5.
32. L'Hommedieu CS, Stough R, Brown L, Kettrick R, Polin R. Potentiation of neuromuscular weakness in infant botulism with aminoglycosides. J Pediatr 1979; 95:1065–70.
33. Paton WDM, Waud DR. The margin of safety of neuromuscular transmission. J Physiol 1967; 191:59–90.
34. Arnon SS, Midura TF, Clay SA, Wood RM, Chin J. Infant botulism. Epidemiological, clinical, and laboratory aspects. JAMA 1977; 237:1946–51.
35. Brown LW. Differential diagnosis of infant botulism. Rev Infect Dis 1979; 1:625–9.

36. Clay SA, Ramseyer JC, Fishman LS, Sedgwick RP. Acute infantile motor unit disorder: infantile botulism? Arch Neurol 1977; 34:236–43.
37. Jones HR, Jr., Darras BT. Acute care pediatric electromyography. Muscle Nerve 2000; 9(Suppl.):S53–62.
38. Graf WD, Hays RM, Astley SJ, et al. Electrodiagnosis reliability in diagnosis of infant botulism. J Pediatr 1992; 120:747–9.
39. Gutmann L, Bodensteiner J, Gutierrez A. Electrodiagnosis of botulism. J Pediatr 1992; 121:835 (Letter).
40. Tanzi MG, Gabay MP. Association between honey consumption and infant botulism. Pharmacotherapy 2002; 22:1479–83.
41. Arnon SS, Midura TF, Damus K, Wood RM, Chin J. Intestinal infection and toxin production by *Clostridium botulinum* as one cause of sudden infant death syndrome. Lancet 1978; 1:1273–7.
42. Takahashi M, Noda H, Takeshita S, et al. Attempts to quantify *Clostridium botulinum* type A toxin and antitoxin in serum of two cases of infant botulism in Japan. Jpn J Med Sci Biol 1990; 43:233–7.
43. Lindstrom M, Korkeala H. Laboratory diagnostics of botulism. Clin Microbiol Rev 2006; 19:298–314.
44. Santos JI, Swensen P, Glasgow LA. Potentiation of *Clostridium botulinum* toxin by aminoglycoside antibiotics: clinical and laboratory observations. Pediatrics 1981; 68:50–4.
45. Cherington M, Ryan DW. Treatment of botulism with guanidine: early neurophysiologic studies. N Engl J Med 1970; 282:195–7.
46. Centers for Disease Control and Prevention (CDC). Infant botulism—New York City, 2001–2002. MMWR Morb Mortal Wkly Rep 2003; 52:21–4.
47. Fenicia L, Da Dalt L, Anniballi F, Franciosa G, Zanconato S, Aureli P. A case if infant due to neurotoxigenic *Clostridium butyricum* type E associated with *Clostridium difficile* colitis. Eur. J. Clin. Microbiol. Infect. Dis. 2002; 21:736–8.
48. Arnon SS, Midura TF, Damus K, Thompson B, Wood RM, Chin J. Honey and other environmental risk factors for infant botulism. J Pediatr 1979; 94:331–6.
49. Byard RW, Moore L, Bourne AJ, et al. *Clostridium botulinum* and sudden infant death syndrome: a 10 year prospective study. J Pediatr Child Health 1992; 28:156–7.

10 | Central Nervous System Infections

The main mode of spread of anaerobes to the central nervous system (CNS) was postulated to be contiguous by dissemination from chronic otitis media, mastoiditis, or sinusitis. Although anaerobic bacteria are found rarely in acute meningeal infection, they are the major cause of intracranial abscess.

MENINGITIS

Incidence

Anaerobic bacteria are rarely the cause of acute bacterial meningitis (1,2). Because cultures of cerebrospinal fluid (CSF) for anaerobes are rarely done, the rate of anaerobic meningitis could be higher.

Microbiology and Pathogenesis

The predominant anaerobes causing meningitis are gram-negative bacilli (including *Bacteroides fragilis* group), *Fusobacterium* spp. (mostly *F. necrophorum*), and *Clostridium* spp. (mostly *Clostridium perfringens*) (1,2). *Peptostreptococcus* spp., *Veillonella*, *Actinomyces*, *Propionibacterium acnes*, and *Eubacterium* are less commonly isolated. The main predisposing conditions to anaerobic meningitis are ear, nose, and throat infections, gastrointestinal disease, and skull fractures. Less common causes are skull trauma, following lumbar puncture (LP), head and neck neoplasm, congenital dermal sinuses, myelomeningocele, meningorectal fistulae, ventricular shunts, pulmonary disease, peritonitis, and pilonidal cyst abscesses (1–3).

Meningitis caused by *F. necrophorum* has been associated with chronic otitis media and an episode of upper respiratory infection (4,5). *C. perfringens* is a cause of meningitis following head injuries or surgery (2,6), that is fatal in about a third of patients despite therapy. Contamination of these wounds with environmental or endogenous flora would explain the entry of *C. perfringens* into the CNS.

Shunt infection with *Propionibacterium* spp. was reported, especially in association with ventriculo-auricular and ventriculo-peritoneal shunts. Anaerobic meningitis is generally monomicrobial and is less likely to be a mixed anaerobic–aerobic infection. Multiple organisms mostly *B. fragilis* and Enterobacteriaceae were reported in meningitis complicating dermal sinus tract infection (5) and ventriculo-peritoneal shunt infections following perforation of the gut by the shunt's distal tube (7).

Anaerobic meningitis often is part of a more extensive intracranial infection that includes concurrent brain abscess or extradural or subdural abscesses.

Diagnosis

The symptoms, signs, and laboratory findings associated with meningitis caused by anaerobic bacteria do not generally differ from those associated with other bacteria. Patients can present with headache, vomiting, stiff neck, lethargy or irritability, seizures, and fever.

The CSF is generally cloudy and contains more than 1000 neutrophils per cubic millimeter, the protein concentration generally is above 100 mg%, the glucose content is generally low (below 30 mg%), and the lactic acid concentration is elevated (above 35 mg%). Clues to the presence of meningitis caused by anaerobic bacteria are the absence of bacterial growth in a routine CSF culture in the face of clinical findings suggesting bacterial infection. These include the presence of bacteria on Gram stain, elevated neutrophil count, and protein and a reduced glucose concentration. The presence of more than one bacterial strain in Gram stain and the ability to grow only one isolate is another clue. Patients who fail to respond to appropriate antimicrobial therapy should be examined for the presence of anaerobes because of the possibility of mixed aerobic and anaerobic infections.

Meningitis caused by anaerobes should be suspected especially in clinical predisposing situations, such as chronic otitis media and sinusitis, mastoiditis, dental abscess, ventricular-peritoneal shunt, anaerobic bacteremia, following perforation of an abdominal viscus, following surgery, and head trauma. Special consideration should be given to newborns at high risk to develop anaerobic infection, especially those who were born to mothers with amnionitis or in meningitis in a compromised neonate.

Because of the association between subdural or epidural empyema and brain abscesses with meningitis, the presence of such abscesses warrants excluding possible concurrent meningitis.

Management

Most gram-positive anaerobes are susceptible to penicillins. However, many gram-negative anaerobes resist these antibiotics, and therefore susceptibility testing is necessary to ensure proper therapy (8). These organisms are generally susceptible to several antimicrobials that penetrate the CSF, including metronidazole, chloramphenicol, ticarcillin, and carbapenems (i.e., meropenem imipenem) (9). Imipenem has been associated with an increase rate of seizures in those with CNS disorders or renal dysfunction. Clindamycin and cefoxitin are not recommended in CNS infections because of their poor penetration into the CSF (9).

Some of the newer quinolones (i.e., trovafloxacin) that are effective against anaerobes may be effective in the therapy of anaerobic meningitis (9). Metronidazole is very active in vitro against gram-negative anaerobes and achieves high levels in CSF (9). However, *P. acnes* and other gram-positive anaerobes are generally resistant to metronidazole (9).

The length of antimicrobial therapy depends on the patient's response and underlying illness. It should be given for at least 14 days.

In patients with mixed aerobic and anaerobic CNS infections, antimicrobial coverage against all organisms present is necessary. Because metronidazole is effective only against anaerobic organisms, additional coverage for the other organisms should be added in instances of mixed infection. Complete eradication of the organisms in the CSF may be difficult when insufficient antimicrobial agents penetrate into the CSF. Repeated spinal tap would ensure eradication of the organisms and allows measurement of concentration of the antimicrobial agents in the CSF. Elimination of associated foci of infection is crucial. Failure to drain inflamed foci adjacent to the CSF can prevent complete cure.

P. acnes shunt infection is treated with antimicrobials and when needed shunt removal. In cases of ventriculo-peritoneal shunt infections after perforation of the colon, surgical repair of the perforation as well as removal of the shunt is necessary (7).

Prognosis

The prognosis of anaerobic meningitis is usually grave, and the mortality rate may reach 50%. Early recognition and adequate therapy may allow survival and recovery.

INTRACRANIAL ABSCESSES

Intracranial abscesses can be classified as brain abscesses or subdural or extradural empyema. Brain abscess is an uncommon but serious life-threatening infection. It can originate from infection of contiguous structures, such as chronic otitis media and sinusitis, dental infections, mastoiditis, as the result of hematogenous spread from a remote site, after skull trauma or surgery, or following meningitis.

Microbiology

The predominant organisms causing brain abscesses are aerobic and anaerobic *Streptococcus* spp. (*Peptostreptococcus* spp. and microaerophilic streptococci, isolation frequency of 60–70%), gram-negative anaerobic bacilli [*B. fragilis* group, *Prevotella* spp., *Porphyromonas* spp., and *Fusobacterium* spp. (20–50%)], *Actinomyces* spp. (3–5%), Enterobacteriaceae (20–30%), *Staphylococcus aureus* (10–15%), and fungi (10–15%) (10). Most brain abscesses evolving anaerobic bacteria are polymicrobial, often containing aerobic bacteria.

Many of the studies of the bacteriology of intracranial abscess may be misleading for a number of reasons, including lack of appropriate sampling techniques to prevent contamination of specimens by normal flora and the failure to culture adequately for strict anaerobes (1,10).

Yeast and fungi predominate in immunocompromised patients and those with cancer. These include *Aspergillus* spp., *Candida* spp., *Cryptococcus neoformans*, *Coccidioides immitis*, and the mucormycosis agents (10–13). Protozoa and helminths may also cause brain abscess. These include *Entamoeba histolytica*, *Cysticerosis*, *Schistosoma japonicum*, and *Parogonimus* spp. (14) Patients with T-lymphocyte defects and those with acquired immune deficiency syndrome (AIDS) are susceptible to *Toxoplasma gondii*, *Nocardia asteroides*, *Mycobacterium* spp., *Listeria monocytogenes*, Enterobacteriaceae, and *Pseudomonas aeruginosa* (15).

An association generally exists between the predisposing conditions and the organisms recovered from the abscess (Table 1).

Pathogenesis

Anaerobes can spread from contiguous sites of existing infections resulting in epidural or cerebral abscesses, subdural empyema, or septic thrombophlebitis of the cortical veins or venous sinuses (16).

Infection may enter the intracranial compartment by: (*i*) Direct extension through necrotic areas of osteomyelitis, after trauma that caused open fracture or following neurosurgery. Contiguous spread could extend to various sites in the CNS, causing cavernous sinus thrombosis, retrograde meningitis, and epidural, subdural, and brain abscess (16). (*ii*) Spread through the valveless venous systems that connects the intracranial and the sinus mucosal veins (common in sinusitis). (*iii*) Hematogenic spread from a distant focus.

The site of the primary infection or the underlying condition can determine the etiology of the brain abscess (Table 1). Anaerobic gram-negative bacilli are commonly recovered in association with ear and sinus infections (17). Spread by blood usually originates in the lung. Anaerobic and microaerophilic streptococci, as well as alpha-hemolytic streptococci, are common in abscesses associated with congenital heart disease (12,18,19). Enterobacteriaceae and anaerobes may spread from intraabdominal or genitourinary sites (1). *S. aureus* is commonly isolate following trauma and neurosurgical procedures (12,18,19). Dental infections can spread into the CNS via the sinuses (20).

TABLE 1 Organisms Associated with Certain Predisposing Conditions

Sinus and dental infections—aerobic and anaerobic streptococci, anaerobic gram-negative bacilli (e.g., *Prevotella*, *Porphyromonas*, *Bacteroides*), *Fusobacterium*, *Staphylococcus aureus*, and Enterobacteriaceae
Pulmonary infections—aerobic and anaerobic streptococci, anaerobic gram-negative bacilli (e.g., *Prevotella*, *Porphyromonas*, *Bacteroides*), *Fusobacterium*, *Actinomyces*, and *Nocardia*
Congenital heart disease—aerobic and microaerophilic streptococci and *S. aureus*
Penetrating trauma—*S. aureus*, aerobic streptococci, Enterobacteriaceae, and *Clostridium*
Transplantation—*Aspergillus*, *Candida*, *Cryptococcus*, *Mucorales*, *Nocardia*, and *Toxoplasma gondii*
Neutropenia—Aerobic gram-negative bacilli, *Aspergillus*, *Candida*, and *Mucorales*
HIV infection—*T. gondii*, *Mycobacterium*, *Cryptococcus*, *Nocardia*, and *Listeria monocytogenes*

Clinical Manifestations

Brain abscess is usually manifested by low-grade fever and symptoms of a space-occupying lesion. These include persistent localized headache, drowsiness, confusion, stupor, general or focal seizures, ataxia, nausea and vomiting, and focal motor or sensory impairments. Papilledema is present in the older child and adults, and bulging fontanels may be present in the younger infant. In the initial stages, the infection is in a form of encephalitis accompanied by signs of increased intracranial pressure such as papilledema. A ruptured brain abscess may produce purulent meningitis.

Localized neurologic signs are eventually found in most patients. The signs and/or symptoms are a direct function of the intracranial location of the abscess (Table 2).

Diagnosis

Moderate leukocytosis is present, and the erythrocyte sedimentation rate and C-reactive protein (CRP) are generally elevated. Serum sodium levels may be lowered as a result of inappropriate antidiuretic hormone production. Platelet counts may be high or low. Initial tests include CBC count with differential and platelet count, serum CRP or Westergren sedimentation rate, serological tests (e.g., serum immunoglobulin G antibodies, CSF polymerase chain reaction for *Toxoplasma*), blood cultures (at least 2; preferably before antibiotic usage).

Cultures for aerobes, anaerobes, acid-fast organisms, and fungi should be obtained whenever possible from the abscess, with the assistance of CT-guided needle if necessary. The following staining should be performed: Gram stain, acid-fast stain (for *Mycobacterium*), modified acid-fast stain (for *Nocardia*), and special fungal stains (e.g., methenamine silver, mucicarmine).

The opening pressure of the CSF generally is elevated. If the diagnosis of intracranial suppuration is suspected, a LP should be deferred to avoid brain herniation. Magnetic resonance imaging (MRI) or computed tomography (CT) can evaluate the presence of brain abscess prior to LP. The usual CSF findings associated with subdural or parenchymal abscesses consist of an elevated protein, pleocytosis with a variable neutrophil count, a normal glucose, and sterile cultures. The number of white blood cells and red blood cells is elevated when the abscess ruptures.

Skull films can be important in the diagnosis of sinusitis or in the detection of free gas in the abscess cavity.

CT scanning has made other tests, such as angiography, ventriculography, pneumoencephalography, and radionuclide brain scanning, almost obsolete. CT scanning, preferably with contrast administration, provides a rapid means of detecting the size, the number, and the location of abscesses, and it has become the mainstay of diagnosis and follow-up care. This method is used to confirm the diagnosis, to localize the lesion, and to monitor the progression after treatment (21,22). However, CT scan results can lag behind clinical findings. After the injection of a contrast material, CT scans characteristically show the brain abscess as a hypodense center with a peripheral uniform enhancement ring. In the earlier cerebritis stages, CT scans show nodular enhancement with areas of low attenuation without enhancement. As the abscess forms, contrast enhancement is observed. After encapsulation, the contrast material cannot help differentiate the clear center and the CT scan is similar in appearance to those obtained during the early cerebritis stage.

Many authorities consider MRI to be the first diagnostic method to be used for the diagnosis of brain abscess (21,22). It can permit accurate diagnosis and excellent follow-up of the lesions because of its superior sensitivity and specificity. Compared with CT scanning,

TABLE 2 Association of Neurological Signs with Location of the Brain Abscess

Cerebellar abscess—nystagmus, ataxia, vomiting, and dysmetria
Brainstem abscess—facial weakness, headache, fever, vomiting, dysphagia, and hemiparesis
Frontal abscess—headache, inattention, drowsiness, mental status deterioration, motor speech disorder, and hemiparesis with unilateral motor signs
Temporal lobe abscess—headache, ipsilateral aphasia (if in the dominant hemisphere), and visual defects

it offers better ability to detect cerebritis, greater contrast between cerebral edema and the brain, and early detection of satellite lesions and the spread of inflammation into the ventricles and subarachnoid space.

Contrast enhancement with gadolinium diethylenetriaminepentaacetic acid (a paramagnetic agent) helps differentiate the abscess, the enhancement ring, and the cerebral edema around the abscess. T1-weighted images enhance the abscess capsule and T2-weighted images can demonstrate the edema zone around the abscess (21,22).

Since the advent of CT and MRI scanning, the case fatality rate has fallen by 90% (21).

Electroencephalogram occasionally can reveal a focus of high voltage with slow activity; however, this is the least accurate procedure in the diagnostic evaluation.

Management

Medical Care

Before the abscess has become encapsulated and localized, antimicrobial therapy, accompanied by measures to control increasing intracranial pressure, is essential. Once an abscess has formed, surgical excision or drainage combined with prolonged antibiotics (usually four to eight weeks) remains the treatment of choice. Some neurosurgeons advocate complete evacuation of the abscess, while others advocate repeated aspirations as indicated (23).

The first step is to verify the presence, size, and number of abscesses using contrast CT scanning or MRI. Emergency surgery should be performed if a single abscess is present. Abscesses larger than 2.5 cm are excised or aspirated, while those smaller than 2.5 cm or which are at the cerebritis stage are aspirated for diagnostic purposes only. In cases of multiple abscesses or in abscesses in essential brain areas, repeated aspirations are preferred to complete excision. High-dose antibiotics for an extended period may be an alternative approach in this group of patients.

An early effort at making a microbiologic diagnosis is important in planning appropriate antimicrobial therapy. The use of CT-guided needle aspiration may provide this important information. Frequent scanning, at least once a week, is essential in monitoring treatment response. Although surgical intervention remains an essential treatment, selected patients may respond to antibiotics alone (23).

Corticosteroid use is controversial. Steroids can retard the encapsulation process, increase necrosis, reduce antibiotic penetration into the abscess, and alter CT scans. Steroid therapy can also produce a rebound effect when discontinued. If used to reduce cerebral edema, therapy should be of short duration. The appropriate dosage, the proper timing, and any effect of steroid therapy on the course of the disease are unknown.

A number of factors should be considered when trying to decide the appropriate approach to therapy. Abscesses smaller than 2.5 cm generally respond to antimicrobial therapy, while abscesses larger than 2.5 cm have failed to respond to such treatment (24). Knowledge of the etiologic agent or agents by recovery from blood, CSF, abscess, or other normally sterile sites is essential because it allows for the most appropriate selection of antimicrobial agents.

Bacterial abscess in the brain is preceded by infarction and cerebritis. Antibiotic therapy during the early stage, when no evidence of an expanding mass lesion exists, may prevent the progress from cerebritis to abscess.

The duration of the symptoms before diagnosis is an important factor. Patients who have symptoms for less than a week have a more favorable response to medical therapy than patients with symptoms persisting longer than one week. Patients treated with medical therapy alone usually demonstrate clinical improvement before significant changes in the CT scan are observed.

CT scanning and MRI should eventually show a decrease in the size of the lesion, a decrease in accompanying edema, and a lessening of the enhancement ring. Improvement on CT scans is generally observed within one to four weeks (average, 2.5 weeks) and complete resolution in one to 11 months (average, 3.5 months) (24).

The antimicrobial treatment of the brain abscess is generally long (six to eight weeks) because of the prolonged time needed for brain tissue to repair and close abscess space.

The initial course is through an intravenous route, often followed by additional two to six months of appropriate oral therapy. A shorter course (three to four weeks) may be adequate in patients who had surgical drainage.

Because of the difficulty involved in the penetration of various antimicrobial agents through the blood–brain barrier, the choice of antibiotics is restricted, and maximal doses are often necessary.

Initial empiric antimicrobial therapy should be based on the expected etiologic agents according to the likely predisposing conditions, the primary infection source, and the presumed pathogenesis of abscess formation. When abscess specimens are available, staining of the material can help guide selection of therapy. Whenever proper cultures are taken and organisms are isolated, the initial empiric therapy can be adjusted to specifically treat the isolated bacteria (25–27).

Coverage for streptococci can be attained by a high dose of penicillin G or a third-generation cephalosporin (e.g., cefotaxime, ceftriaxone). Metronidazole is included to cover penicillin-resistant anaerobes (i.e., gram-negative bacilli).

When *S. aureus* is suspected (following neurosurgery or trauma), nafcillin or vancomycin (when methicillin resistance or penicillin allergy is present) is administered. Cefepime or ceftazidime is administered to treat *P. aeruginosa* infection.

Patients with HIV infection may require therapy for toxoplasmosis.

Specific Antibiotics

Penicillin penetrates well into the abscess cavity and is active against non-beta-lactamase–producing anaerobes and some aerobic organisms. Chloramphenicol penetrates well into the intracranial space and is also active against *Haemophilus* spp., and most obligate anaerobes. Its use has been curtailed dramatically in most U.S.A. centers because of the availability of other equally efficacious and less toxic antimicrobial combinations (i.e., cefotaxime plus metronidazole).

Metronidazole penetrates well into the CNS and is not affected by concomitant corticosteroid therapy. However, it is only active against strict anaerobic bacteria, and its activity against anaerobic gram-positive cocci and bacilli may be suboptimal.

Third-generation cephalosporins (e.g., cefotaxime, ceftriaxone) generally provide adequate therapy for aerobic gram-negative organisms. If *Pseudomonas* spp. are isolated or anticipated, the parenteral cephalosporin of choice is either ceftazidime or cefepime.

Aminoglycosides do not penetrate well into the CNS and are relatively less active because of the anaerobic conditions and the acidic contents of the abscess.

Beta-lactamase–resistant penicillins (e.g., oxacillin, methicillin, nafcillin) provide good coverage against methicillin-sensitive *S. aureus*. However, their penetration into the CNS is less than penicillin, and the addition of rifampin has been shown to be of benefit in staphylococcal meningitis.

Vancomycin is most effective against methicillin-resistant *S. aureus* and *Staphylococcus epidermidis* as well as aerobic and anaerobic streptococci and *Clostridium* species.

With the exception of the *B. fragilis* group and growing numbers of strains of *Prevotella*, *Porphyromonas*, and *Fusobacterium* spp., most of the anaerobic pathogens isolated are sensitive to penicillin. Because these penicillin-resistant anaerobic organisms predominate in brain abscesses, empiric therapy should include agents effective against them that can also penetrate the blood–brain barrier. These include metronidazole, chloramphenicol, ticarcillin plus clavulanic acid, imipenem, or meropenem (9).

Caution should be used in administering carbapenems and beta-lactamases in general, because high doses of these agents may be associated with seizure activity. Imipenem has been associated with increased risk of seizures in patients with brain abscess. Although fluoroquinolones have good penetration into the CNS, data are limited regarding their use in treating brain abscesses.

Therapy with penicillin should be added to metronidazole to cover aerobic and microaerophilic streptococci. The administration of beta-lactamase–resistant penicillin or vancomycin (if methicillin-resistant staphylococci are isolated) for the treatment of *S. aureus* is generally recommended.

Amphotericin B is administered for *Candida*, *Cryptococcus*, and *Mucorales* infections; voriconazole for *Aspergillus* and *Pseudallescheria boydii* infections (13,28).

T. gondii infection is treated with pyrimethamine and sulfadiazine.

Injection of antibiotics into the abscess cavity was advocated in the past in an effort to sterilize the area before operation. However, many antimicrobials penetrate brain abscess cavities fairly well, and instillation of antibiotics into the abscess after drainage is not needed.

Surgical Care

Patients who do not meet the criteria for medical therapy alone require surgery. Surgical drainage provides the most optimal therapy. The procedures used are stereotactic guides aspiration through a bur hole and complete excision after craniotomy. Aspiration is the most common procedure and is often performed using a stereotactic procedure with the guidance of CT scanning or MRI. Craniotomy is generally performed in patients with multiloculated abscesses and for those whose conditions failed to resolve (26–28). The risk of repeating aspiration is that the procedure may cause bleeding. Excision is clearly indicated in posterior fossa or multiloculated abscesses, those caused by fungi or helminths, and those that reaccumulate following repeated aspirations.

Ventricular drainage combined with administration of intravenous or intrathecal antimicrobials or both are used to treat brain abscesses that rupture into the ventricles.

If not recognized early, both subdural empyema and brain abscess can be fatal. Emergency surgery is needed if neurologic signs related to a mass lesion progress. Although antibiotics have improved the outlook, the management of subdural empyema requires prompt surgical evacuation of the infected site and antimicrobial therapy. Failure to perform surgical drainage can lead to a higher mortality rate.

Although proper selection of antimicrobial therapy is most important in the management of intracranial infections, surgical drainage may be required. Optimal therapy of fungal brain abscess generally requires both medical and surgical approach. A delay in surgical drainage and decompression can be associated with high morbidity and mortality.

Recent studies illustrate that brain abscess in the early phase of cerebritis may respond to antimicrobial therapy without surgical drainage. Surgical drainage may be necessary in many patients to ensure adequate therapy and a complete resolution of the infection (27).

Prognosis

Characteristics associated with an excellent prognosis include the following: young age, absence of severe neurologic defect on initial presentation, lack of neurologic deterioration, and absence of comorbid disease.

Mortality from brain abscess is approximately 10%. However, in patients with signs of herniation on initial presentation, mortality rate exceeds 50%.

Morbidity in survivors is generally due to residual focal defects, increased incidence of seizures due to scar tissue foci, or neuropsychiatric changes.

REFERENCES

1. Finegold SM. Anaerobic Bacteria in Human Diseases. New York: Academic Press, 1977.
2. Law DA, Aronoff SC. Anaerobic meningitis in children; case report and review of the literature. Pediatr Infect Dis J 1992; 11:968–71.
3. Aucher P, Saunier JP, Grollier G, et al. Meningitis due to enterotoxigenic *Bacteroides fragilis*. Eur J Clin Microbiol Infect Dis 1996; 15:820–3.
4. Jacobs JA, Hendriks JJE, Verschure PDMM, et al. Meningitis due to *Fusobacterium necrophorum* subspecies *necrophorum*: case report and review of the literature. Infection 1993; 21:57–60.
5. Brook I. Anaerobic meningitis in an infant associated with pilonidal cyst abscess. Clin Neurol Neurosurg 1985; 87:131.
6. Debast SB, van Rijswijk E, Jira PE, Meis JF. Fatal *Clostridium perfringens* meningitis associated with insertion of a ventriculo-peritoneal shunt. Eur J Clin Microbiol Infect Dis 1993; 12:720–1.
7. Brook I, Johnson N, Overturf GD, Wilkins J. Mixed bacterial meningitis: a complication of ventriculo and lumboperitoneal shunts. Report of two cases. J Neurosurg 1977; 47:961–4.

8. Rasmussen BA, Bush K, Tally FP. Antimicrobial resistance in anaerobes. Clin Infect Dis 1997; 24(Suppl. 1):S110–20.
9. Lutsar I, McCracken GH, Jr., Friedland IR. Antibiotic pharmacodynamics in cerebrospinal fluid. Clin Infect Dis 1998; 27:1117–27.
10. Brook I. Anaerobic and anaerobic microbiology of intracranial abscess. Pediatr Neurol 1992; 8:210–4.
11. Le Moal G, Landron C, Grollier G, et al. Characteristics of brain abscess with isolation of anaerobic bacteria. Scand J Infect Dis 2003; 35:318–21.
12. Tattevin P, Bruneel F, Lellouche F, et al. Bacterial brain abscesses: a retrospective study of 94 patients admitted to an intensive care unit (1980 to 1999). Am J Med 2003; 115(2):143–6.
13. Sanchez-Portocarrero J, Perez-Cecilia E, Corral O, Romero-Vivas J, Picazo JJ. The central nervous system and infection by candida species. Diagn Microbiol Infect Dis 2000; 37:169–79.
14. Hagensee ME, Bauwens JE, Kjos B, Bowden RA. Brain abscess following marrow transplantation: experience at the Fred Hutchinson Cancer Research Center, 1984–1992. Clin Infect Dis 1994; 19:402–8.
15. Bensalem MK, Berger JR. HIV and the central nervous system. Compr Ther 2002; 28:23–33.
16. Lerner DN, Choi SS, Zalzal GH, Johnson DL. Intracranial complications of sinusitis in childhood. Ann Otol Rhinol Laryngol 1995; 104(4 Pt 1):288–93.
17. Brook I. Anaerobic bacteria in upper respiratory tract and other head and neck infections. Ann Otol Rhinol Laryngol 2002; 111(5 Pt 1):430–40.
18. Jadavji T, Humpherys RP, Proper CG. Brain abscess in infants and children. Pediatr Infect Dis 1985; 4:394–8.
19. Sofianou D, Selviarides P, Sofianos E, Tsakris A, Foroglou G. Etiological agents and predisposing factors of intracranial abscesses in a Greek university hospital. Infection 1996; 24:144–6.
20. Brook I. Microbiology of intracranial abscesses associated with sinusitis of odotogenic origin. Ann Otol Rhinol Laryngol 2006; 115:917–20.
21. Wong J, Quint DJ. Imaging of central nervous system infections. Semin Roentgenol 1999; 34:123–43.
22. Karampekios S, Hesselink J. Cerebral infections. Eur Radiol 2005; 15:485–93.
23. Townsend GC, Scheld WM. Infections of the central nervous system. Adv Intern Med 1998; 43:403–47.
24. Nguyen JB, Black BR, Leimkuehler MM, Halder V, Nguyen JV, Ahktar N. Intracranial pyogenic abscess: imaging diagnosis utilizing recent advances in computed tomography and magnetic resonance imaging. Crit Rev Comput Tomogr 2004; 45:181–224.
25. Yogev R, Bar-Meir M. Management of brain abscesses in children. Pediatr Infect Dis J 2004; 23:157–9.
26. Livraghi S, Melancia JP, Antunes JL. The management of brain abscesses. Adv Tech Stand Neurosurg 2003; 28:285–313.
27. Bernardini GL. Diagnosis and management of brain abscess and subdural empyema. Curr Neurol Neurosci Rep 2004; 4:448–56.
28. Schwartz S, Thiel E. Update on the treatment of cerebral aspergillosis. Ann Hematol 2004; 83(Suppl. 1):S42–4.

11 | Ocular Infections

The increased recovery of anaerobic bacteria in clinical infection has led to greater appreciation of these organisms in ocular infections. Anaerobes play a role in several types of ocular infections: conjunctivitis, keratitis, dacryocystitis, and orbital and periorbital cellulitis.

CONJUNCTIVITIS

Conjunctivitis is defined as redness of the conjunctivae associated with hyperemia and congestion of the blood vessels, with varying severity of ocular exudate. Preauricular adenopathy may be present.

Bacteria, viruses, chlamydia, rickettsiae, fungi, parasites, and numerous noninfectious agents and metabolic diseases may induce conjunctivitis. Early etiological diagnosis of acute bacterial conjunctivitis is of utmost importance because of the potential of rapid development that may cause irreversible ocular damage. Arriving at a specific diagnosis is important for the selection of appropriate therapy.

Microbiology

The most common aerobic bacteria causing conjunctivitis are *Staphylococcus aureus*, *Staphylococcus epidermidis*, *Haemophilus influenzae* (mostly nontypable), *Streptococcus pneumoniae*, *Streptococcus* spp. including *Streptoccocus pyogenes*, and *Moraxella* spp. Others include *Neisseria gonorrhoeae* and *Neisseria meningitidis*, gram-negative rods such as *Pseudomonas* and *Proteus*, and *Corynebacterium* spp. (1). The main viral causes are adenovirus, herpes simplex, and Picornavirus.

Chlamydia trachomatis, *N. gonorrhoeae*, and *Neisseria cinerea* are commonly recovered in newborns. Others organisms recovered in neonates and children include *N. meningitidis*, gram-negative rods such as *Pseudomonas* and *Proteus*, and *Corynebacterium* spp.

The most common anaerobes in all age groups are *Peptostreptococcus* spp., isolated alone or mixed with other bacteria (2). These organisms have a high tendency for corneal ulceration. Other anaerobes are *Bacteroides fragilis*, pigmented *Prevotella* and *Porphyromonas*, Fusobacteria, Bifidobacteria, Clostridia (3–6), non-spore-forming anaerobic organisms, and *Actinomyces* spp. Anaerobic bacteria were also recovered from patients who wore contact lenses and developed conjunctivitis (7).

Pathogenesis

Spread of organisms to the ocular surface can occur through a variety of modes, however, direct contamination by the fingers is the most common one. Most of the isolates are part of the normal nasopharyngeal bacterial flora. Organisms can also be spread as airborne droplets, initiated by sneezing and coughing, or by contact with fomites.

Propionibacterium acnes and *Peptostreptococcus* spp. are present in the conjunctival sac of uninflamed eyes (8). The presence of anaerobes in the normal conjunctival sac does not exclude their ability to become pathogenic under the right circumstances. This can occur when injuries, foreign bodies, and underlying noninfectious diseases favor the establishment of conjunctival infections, thus allowing for the resident organisms to become pathogenic.

Oral flora anaerobes can be introduced to the conjunctivae by wetting contact lens with saliva.

Diagnosis

Typically, the palpebral conjunctiva is more inflamed than the bulbar, and the area around the cornea is spared. A bacterial etiology is suspected when severe conjunctivitis is present, and many polymorphonuclear leukocytes are found in conjunctival swab specimens. Severe infection, copious exudate, and matting of the eyelids are more likely to occur with bacterial or chlamydial infection than with viral infection. Preauricular lymphadenitis is generally associated with viral infections.

Conjunctivitis associated with anaerobes is indistinguishable from inflammation caused by other bacteria, although patients wearing contact lenses may be at higher risk of developing infections caused by these organisms. The presence of lymphocytes suggests viral infection, eosinophils and basophils suggest an allergic etiology, and intranuclear inclusions implicate herpes or adenoviruses. Conjunctival scraping can be helpful when they contain conjunctival epithelial cells that may harbor intracellular pathogens. Gram and giemsa stains and aerobic and anaerobic cultures are necessary for correct diagnosis.

Management

Most cases of conjunctivitis are self-limited. Treatment of bacterial conjunctivitis enhances the resolution of the infection and includes administration of proper topical antibiotics selected according to the antimicrobial susceptibility of the infecting organism. Conjunctivitis caused by anaerobes should be treated by antimicrobial agents effective against these organisms. Bacitracin is very active against *Peptostreptococcus* spp. but is generally inactive against *B. fragilis* and *Fusobacterium nucleatum* (9). Erythromycin shows good activity against pigmented *Prevotella* and *Porphyromonas*, microaerophilic and anaerobic streptococci, and gram-positive non-spore-forming anaerobic bacilli. Erythromycin has relatively good activity against *Clostridium* spp. but poor and inconsistent activity against gram-negative anaerobic bacilli. Chloramphenicol has the greatest in vitro activity against anaerobes, but should be used cautiously because it is absorbed from the conjunctivae. Anaerobic gram-positive cocci, the anaerobes most frequently recovered from inflamed conjunctivae, are susceptible to penicillins, macrolides, and chloramphenicol. Anaerobic bacteria may be relatively resistant to sulfonamide, the older quinolones, polymixin B, and aminoglyloside preparations that are commonly applied to inflamed conjunctiva. Since anaerobes may be involved in severe cases of conjunctivitis and especially with the most serious complications of bacterial conjunctivitis, such as a penetrating corneal ulcer or orbital cellulitis, specific coverage for these organisms should be considered. In such instances, administration of parenteral antimicrobial agents should supplement the topical application of medications.

KERATITIS

Microbial keratitis is a serious ocular infection that can cause corneal scarring and opacification.

Microbiology

Infective keratitis can be viral, bacterial, fungal and due to *Acanthamoeba*. The main viruses are herpes simplex, varicella-zoster, measles, mumps, rubella, adenovirus, coxsackievirus A24, and enterovirus 70. Fungal causes are rare and include *Aspergillus*, *Fusarium solani*, and *Candida albicans*. Bacterial causes include *S. pneumoniae*, *S. aureus*, and *S. epidermidis*. *Pseudomonas aeruginosa* is common in contact lens wearers; *H. influenzae* and *M. catarrhalis* cause ulcerative veratitis and enteric organisms (i.e., *Shigella*, *Serratia marcescens*) can be transferred by contaminated hands (10).

Anaerobic bacteria can also cause keratitis. The most common one associated with ocular trauma is *Clostridium perfringens*. *Clostridium tetani* was also rarely described. Other organisms include *Peptostreptococcus* spp., *P. acnes*, *Propionibacterium avidum*, *Prevotella* spp., *Fusobacterium* spp., and microaerophilic streptococci (11).

We conducted a retrospective review of the microbiological records of samples collected for aerobic and anaerobic bacteria, as well as fungi from 148 patients including 22 children with keratits (11). A total of 173 organisms (1.2/specimen)—98 aerobic or facultative aerobic, 68 anaerobic, and 7 fungi—were recovered.

The predominant aerobic and facultative were *S. aureus* (35 isolates), *S. epidermidis* (26), *Pseudomonas* spp. (9), *S. marcescens* (6), and *S. pneumoniae* (5). The most frequently recovered anaerobes were *Propionibacterium* spp. (31 isolates), *Peptostreptococcus* spp. (15), *Clostridium* spp. (11), *Prevotella* spp. (6), and *Fusobacterium* spp. (3). The predominant fungi was *C. albicans* (4 isolates).

Use of contact lenses was associated with the recovery of *Pseudomonas* spp., *Peptostreptococcus* spp., *Fusobacterium*, and *P. acnes*.

Pathogenesis

Predisposing conditions include trauma (e.g., foreign body, corneal laceration, and contact lens), corneal exposure (facial palsy, sedated or moribund state, globe prostosis, congenital abnormalities of the eyelids), immune deficiency (immunodeficiency syndrome, immunosuppressive therapy, topical steroids), and abnormalities of ocular surface (dryness, mucin deficiency, vitamin A deficiency, malnutrition, and corneal anesthesia).

Anaerobic bacteria can reach the cornea from the mucous membranes in similar manner to the one discussed in the section on conjunctivitis. However, in cases of trauma or foreign body associated infection they can be directly inoculated.

Diagnosis

The patient presents with severe pain, reflex tearing, eye redness, decreased vision, and photophobia. Gray corneal opacification is characteristic, the light reflex is dulled, and the cornea can be stained with fluorescein. An hypopyon can be observed in the anterior chamber. Corneal scraping of the leading edge and base of ulcer for smears and culture for aerobic and anaerobic and viruses are necessary. Staining with Gram and Giemsa is obtained and methenamine-silver, acridine orange, and calcoflur white staining are used for detecting fungi and *Acanthamoeba*. Chlamydia, viruses, and some fungi can be detected using recombinant DNA methods, enzyme-linked immunofluorescent assays, and fluorescein-labeled monoclonal antibodies.

Management

Topical anti-infective agents chosen based upon the results of the staining and culture of diagnostic corneal scraping, are the major therapy. These include a combination of a cephalosporin plus an aminoglycoside, or a quinolone (norfloxacin, ciprofloxacin, or ofloxacin) (12,13). Frequent administration of topical therapy is important, as they are cleared rapidly. For coverage for anaerobes, see the conjunctivitis section. After an initial application of five consecutive single drops every minute, and then every 15 minutes for four doses, the drops are given every 30 to 60 minutes for at least two days. Treatment is continued for 7 to 14 days.

Fungi are treated with frequently administered topical fluocytosine, natamycin, amphotericin B, or miconazole for 6 to 12 weeks. Parenteral therapy and excisional keratoplasty is considered to prevent deep fungal keratitis and endopthalmitis. Viral infections, excluding herpes, are self-limited and there is currently no effective therapy. Herpes virus infection can be treated with frequently administered (every hour first week, every two hours second week) topical antivirals, such as a vidarabine or trifluorothymidine. Debridement is also an option. Herpes zoster is managed with topical steroids. *Acanthamoeba* keratitis is treated with the combination of imidazole, propamide isethiocyanate, neomycin, and polyhexamethylamine biguanide.

Complication

The corneal transparency may be lost and refractive changes and central corneal scars (leukomas) may occur. Corneal grafting may be necessary.

DACRYOCYSTITIS

Dacryocystitis is a bacterial infection of the lacrimal sac. It can occur at any age as a bacterial complication of a viral upper respiratory tract infection (URTI).

Microbiology

S. pneumoniae, H. influenzae, Streptococcus agalactiae, and anaerobes are common in neonates. The most common pathogens in acute dacryocystitis in children are *S. aureus, Streptococcus* spp., and *H. influenzae.* The most frequently recovered organisms in chronic dacryocystitis are *S. aureus, S. epidermidis, P. aeruginosa, Escherichia coli,* and *C. trachomatis. S. aureus, S. epidermidis,* and rarely *P. aeruginosa* and *E. coli* have been reported in adults (14). Anaerobic bacteria alone can be recovered in about a third of cases, mixed aerobic and anaerobic bacteria in 11% of cases (14). The most frequently recovered anaerobes are *Peptostreptococcus, Propionibacterium, Prevotella,* and *Fusobacterium* spp. Polymicrobial infection was present in about half of cases.

Pathophysiology

The infection can occur as a result of tear stagnation in the lacrimal sac secondary to obstruction to the normal drainage of the tears through the nasolacrimal duct due to trauma, infection or inflammation, tumor infiltration and after surgery. Delayed opening, inspissated secretion, or anatomical abnormality are a common etiologies in infants. The organisms causing the infection can originate from the hosts oropharyngeal flora or from external causes.

Diagnosis

The infection often follows viral URTI, and the patients present with fever, erythema, edema, and tenderness over the triangular area below the medial canthus. Purulent material can be expressed from the lacrimal puncta.

Obstruction to drainage can be documented by the dye disappearance test done by instilling 2% sodium fluorescein in the lower conjunctival sac and observing its disappearance after five minutes. An alternative method is to irrigate the lacrimal excretory system. However, probing and irrigation should not be done until the inflammation has resolved. Other tests include dacryocystography, computed tomography (CT) and magnetic resonance imaging (MRI) (3). Specimen of the pus obtained from the puncta or intraoperatively should be Gram stained and cultured for aerobic and anaerobic bacteria.

Management

Admission to the hospital and parenteral antimicrobial therapy is indicated in acute cases because of the potential for extension of the infection (e.g., cavernous sinus thrombosis). The choice of therapy depends on the identification of the causative organisms. A first generation cephalosporin or a beta-lactamase-resistant penicillin (e.g., nafcillin) is adequate for *S. aureus.* Vancomycin or clindamycin are appropriate in penicillin allergic individuals, and the former for *S. aureus* resistant to methicillin. Clindamycin, a combination of penicillin plus a beta-lactamase inhibitor (e.g., amoxicillin–clavulanate), chloramphenicol, metronidazole (plus a penicillin), tigecycline or a carbapenem are adequate for anaerobes. When the infection has improved, oral therapy can be substituted for a total of 10 to 14 days.

Incision and draining plus direct application of antibiotics into the sac is indicated to drain a pointed lacrimal sac abscess (3), where surgical drainage is not necessary for most patients; however, probing is helpful in neonates. Probing of the lacrimal excretory system is often sufficient to open the localized membranous obstruction. Definite surgery is done in adults upon resolution of the infection.

Complications

Chronic ipsilateral conjunctivitis and corneal ulcers can develop and spread into the orbit causing orbital abscess. Intraorbital complication should be promptly treated surgically. Delay can lead to visual compromise and life-threatening complications.

ORBITAL AND PERIORBITAL CELLULITIS (see also Chapter 14)

Cellulitis of the orbital and periorbital tissues includes a spectrum of disorders that ranges from simple periorbital inflammation to cavernous sinus thrombosis. Orbital cellulitis can be due to hematogenous dissemination of organisms, traumatic inoculation of bacteria, and as a complication of sinusitis.

Microbiology

Bacteremic periorbital cellulitis generally occurs in children between 6 and 30 months. *S. pneumoniae* and *H. influenzae* type b are the most common causes. The introduction of *H. influenzae* and *S. pneumoniae* vaccinations in children reduced the rate of this infection (4). In cellulitis related to trauma (including insect bite) or to extension from a neighboring soft tissue area, group A beta-hemolytic streptococci, and *S. aureus* are the most likely pathogens (4).

Anaerobes could be associated with cellulitis that develops following chronic sinusitis or following sinusitis associated with dental infection. *C. perfringens* infection can follow a penetrating wound involving a foreign body.

The most common pathogens in cellulitis and orbital abscesses associated with sinusitis are those seen in acute and chronic sinusitis, depending on the length and etiology of the primary sinusitis. These include *S. pneumoniae, H. influenzae, S. aureus*, gram-negative anaerobic bacilli (*Prevotella, Porphyromonas,* and *Fusobacterium*), *Peptostreptococcus*, and microaerophilic streptococci spp. (5). The infection associated with periorbital cellulitis and maxillary sinuses of odontogenic origin is often polymicrobial and the organisms most often isolated are anaerobic gram-negative bacilli, *Peptostreptococcus* spp., *Fusobacterium* spp., and *Streptococcus* spp. The organisms isolated in cavernous sinus thrombosis (CST) are *S. aureus* (50–70% of instances), *Streptococcus* spp. (20%), and gram-negative anaerobic bacilli. Similar organisms can be recovered from subperiosteal and orbital abscesses and their corresponding maxillary sinusitis (6).

Pathogenesis

The origin of bacteremic *H. influenzae* and *S. pneumoniae* periorbital cellulitis is the nasopharynx. The orbit is separated from the ethmoid cells and maxillary sinus by a thin bony plates (lamina papyracea). Infections can spread directly by penetration of the thin bones or through the small bony dehiscences. Children are at a greater risk because of their thinner bony septa and sinus wall, greater porous bones, open suture lines, and larger vascular foramina. It can also extend directly through the anterior and posterior ethmoid foraminas. Since the ophthalmic venous system has no valves, retrograde thrombophlebitis, and spread of the infection can also occur.

Periorbital cellulitis may represent only reactive inflammatory edema in sinusitis. Orbital cellulitis is less common than periorbital cellulitis and involves the globe or orbit. It is the most frequent serious complication of sinusitis and despite antimicrobial therapy, is a potentially life-threatening infection. There is diffuse edema of the orbital contents and infiltration of the adipose tissue with inflammatory cells and bacteria. The upper molar or premolar teeth may be the primary site in cases of maxillary sinusitis. Orbital infection may also arise as a metastatic spread of a systemic infection, extension through the orbital septum or through facial veins from a neighboring inflamed soft tissue area, or from a penetrating wound.

Diagnosis

Differential diagnosis include sinus infection, infected periorbital laceration, bacteremic preseptal cellulitis, conjunctivitis, dacryocystitis, systemic or contact allergy, insect bite, seborrheic or eczematoid dermatitis, and nasal vestibular infection.

TABLE 1 Orbital Complications of Sinusitis

Class I	Inflammatory edema and preseptal cellulitis
Class II	Orbital cellulitis
Class III	Subperiosteal abscess
Class IV	Orbital abscess
Class V	Cavernous sinus thrombosis

Infection in and around the eye must initially be differentiated from trauma, malignancy, dysthyroid exophthalmos, orbital pseudotumor, or CST.

The severity of the orbital cellulitis is determined by the staging systems of I to V (Table 1) (15).

Distinguishing between infections of the superficial layers and the orbit is critical. The tissue plane separating the two types of infections is a fascial layer termed the orbital septum. Infection anterior to the orbital septum is most properly described as preseptal cellulitis (periorbital cellulitis). It is characterized by edema, erythema, tenderness, and warmth of the lid (stage I). The eye itself is not involved in preseptal cellulitis and, therefore, the conjunctivae and orbital tissues are not involved. Preauricular lymphadenopathy may be present. Vision, mobility of the globe, and intraocular pressure are normal.

Orbital cellulitis, an infection deep to the orbital septum, is characterized by marked lid edema and erythema, proptosis, chemosis, reduction of vision, restriction of mobility of the eye globe in proportion to orbital edema, pain on movement of the globe, fever, and leukocytosis (stage II). The distinctions between preseptal and orbital cellulitis may be difficult to make. If the infection is allowed to progress, subperiosteal (stage III) or orbital (stage IV) abscess and CST (stage V) may develop.

Radiographic studies are abnormal if sinusitis is involved. Generally, the ethmoid and maxillary sinuses are involved, but pansinusitis may be present. As clinical examination cannot reliably differentiate between abscess and cellulitis, CT is especially useful in defining and localizing the extent of the abscesses and for monitoring of therapy. It should be carried out when an abscess is suspected or when orbital cellulitis has not responded to medical therapy. The MRI is reserved for cases where intracranial progression is suspected. Often the swelling of the lid precludes monitoring of the visual acuity and extraocular muscular motility.

When CST involvement is suspected, CT with intravenous contrast material should be done. In cases where improvement is delayed or absent, serial clinical examinations are needed, accompanied by repeated CT, to allow early intervention and drainage. A low threshold needs to be maintained for repeating CT scans after surgical intervention.

Gram stains and cultures for aerobic and anaerobic bacteria should be obtained of any adequately collected purulent material, and blood cultures are imperative. Aspiration and culture of the advancing border of cellulitis may be helpful. In patients with purulent sinusitis, direct aspiration of the sinus can provide bacterial diagnosis.

Management

Medical treatment should be vigorous and aggressive from the early stages of periorbital cellulitis to prevent progression to orbital cellulitis and abscess. If orbital cellulitis or abscess is suspected, an ophthalmologist should be consulted. If rapidly advancing infection is suspected, time is crucial and imaging studies and therapeutic measures should be instituted without delay.

Patients with mild inflammatory eyelid edema or preseptal cellulitis (class I) can be treated with oral antibiotics and decongestants. The most effective available oral agents are the second generation cephalosporins or amoxicillin–clavulanate. However, close supervision and follow-up is mandatory, and the initiation of parenteral antimicrobial agents in the hospital should be undertaken if postseptal involvement (classes II to V) is suspected or has developed. The parenteral agents include ceftriaxone or cefotaxime plus coverage for anaerobic bacteria (addition of metronidazole or clindamycin). Drugs that have good brain–blood barrier penetration are preferred.

Anaerobic bacteria should be suspected in periorbital cellulitis associated with dental infections and chronic sinusitis. Antimicrobial agents that generally provide coverage for methicillin-susceptible *S. aureus* as well as aerobic and anaerobic bacteria include cefoxitin, tigecycline carbapenems, and the combination of a penicillin (e.g., piperacillin) and a beta-lactamase inhibitor (e.g., tazobactam). Metronidazole is administered in combination with an agent effective against aerobic or facultative streptococci and *S. aureus*. A glycopeptide (e.g., vancomycin) or linezolid should be administered in cases where methicillin-resistant *S. aureus* is present or suspected.

Treatment of CST includes high doses of parenteral wide spectrum antimicrobial agents. The use of anticoagulants and corticosteroids is controversial. Anticoagulants are used to prevent further thrombosis, and the fibrinolytic activity of urokinase helps dissolve the clot. Early diagnosis and vigorous treatment can yield a survival rate of 70% to 75%. However, permanent sequelae such as blindness and other cranial nerve palsies are common in survivors.

The medical therapy of orbital complications of sinusitis also includes topical and systemic decongestants, humidification, warm compresses, elevation of the head of the bed, analgesics, and hydration with intravenous fluids. The patient's visual acuity and extraocular muscular motility are closely monitored. Sequential CT may be needed for follow-up. Cellulitis without an abscess is treated medically. However, if symptoms progress after 24 hours of antibiotics and no improvement occurs after 72 hours, surgical intervention is indicated.

Surgical treatment is mandated by the presence of an abscess on CT, deterioration of visual acuity, signs of deterioration and progression in the orbital involvement despite adequate medical therapy, relapse of symptoms or their progression to the contralateral eye. Surgery involves drainage of the abscess and the involved sinus(es). Indicators of a deterioration are radiological or clinical, or both. Drainage should not be delayed, and should be carried out as an emergency treatment. Intranasal endoscopic ethmoidectomy is often utilized to treat subperiosteal abscess. Orbital abscess is still approached with an external incision (16). External ethmoidectomy can be reserved for instances in which the orbital signs fail to resolve completely following endoscopic ethmoidectomy, or when visualization of the ethmoid walls is not possible.

Complications

Periorbital and orbital infections pose the risk of serious complications (17). These include loss of vision owing to involvement of the optic nerve, progression to CST, meningitis, subdural or cerebral abscess, and death.

REFERENCES

1. Weiss A, Brinser JH, Nazar-Stewart V. Acute conjunctivitis in childhood. J Pediatr 1993; 122:10–4.
2. Brook I, Pettit TH, Martin WJ, Finegold SM. Anaerobic and aerobic bacteriology of acute conjunctivitis. Ann Ophthalmol 1979; 11:389–93.
3. Cahill KV, Burns JA. Management of acute dacryocystitis in adults. Ophthalm Plast Reconstr Surg 1993; 9:38–41.
4. Donahue SP, Schwartz G. Preseptal and orbital cellulitis in childhood. A changing microbiologic spectrum. Ophthalmology 1998; 105:1902–5.
5. Brook I, Friedman EM, Rodriguez WJ, Controni G. Complications of sinusitis in children. Pediatrics 1980; 66:568–72.
6. Brook I, Frazier EH. Microbiology of subperiosteal orbital abscess and associated maxillary sinusitis. Laryngoscope 1996; 106:1010–3.
7. Brook I. Presence of anaerobic bacteria in conjunctivitis associated with wearing contact lens. Ann Ophthalmol 1988; 20:397–9.
8. Perkins RE, Kundsin RB, Pratt MV, Abrahamsen I, Leibowitz HM. Bacteriology of normal and infected conjunctivitis. J Clin Microbiol 1975; 1:147–9.
9. Finegold SM. Anaerobic Bacteria in Human Disease. New York: Academic Press, 1977.
10. Clinch TE, Palmon FE, Robinson MJ, et al. Microbial keratitis in children. Am J Ophthalmol 1994; 117:65–71.
11. Brook I, Frazier EH. Aerobic and anaerobic microbiology of keratitis. Ann Ophthalmol 1999; 31:21–6.
12. Groden LR, Brinser JH. Outpatient treatment of microbial corneal ulcers. Arch Ophthalmol 1986; 104:84–6.

13. Parks DJ, Abrams DA, Sarforazi FA, Katz H. Comparison of topical ciprofloxacin to conventional antibiotic therapy in the treatment of ulcerative keratitis. Am J Ophthalmol 1993; 115:471–7.

14. Brook I, Frazier EH. Aerobic and anaerobic microbiology of dacryocystitis. Am J Ophthalmol 1998; 125:552–4.

15. Chandler JR, Laagenbrunner DJ, Stevens ER. The pathogenesis of orbital complications in acute sinusitis. Laryngoscope 1970; 80:1414–28.

16. Manning SC. Endoscopic management of medial subperiosteal orbital abscess. Arch Otolaryngol Head Neck Surg 1993; 119:789–91.

17. Wald ER. Periorbital and orbital infections. Pediatr Rev 2004; 25:312–20.

12 | Odontogenic Infections

The complexity of the oral and gingival flora has prevented the clear elucidation of specific etiologic agents in most forms of oral and dental infections. In the gingival crevice, there are approximately 1.8×10^{11} anaerobes per gram (1). Because anaerobic bacteria are part of the normal oral flora and outnumber aerobic organisms by a ratio of 1:10 to 1:100 at this site, it is not surprising that they predominant in dental infections. There are at least 350 morphological and biochemically distinct bacterial groups or species that colonize the oral and dental ecologic sites (1). Most odontogenic infections result initially from the formation of dental plaque (2). Once pathogenic bacteria become established within the plaque, they can cause local and disseminated complications including bacterial endocarditis, infection of orthopedic or other prosthesis, pleuropulmonary infection, cavernous sinus infection, septicemia, maxillary sinusitis, mediastinal infection, and brain abscess (3).

The microorganisms recovered from odontogenic infections generally reflect the host's indigenous oral flora (Table 1) (4). The organisms most commonly isolated are anaerobic streptococci, *Capnocytophaga*, *Actinobacillus*, *Fusobacterium*, *Prevotella* and *Porphyromonas* spp. Among the potential pathogens associated with oral and dental infection, the anaerobic black-pigmented gram-negative bacilli received the most attention (5). *Porphyromonas gingivalis* and *Prevotella intermedia* appear to be the most frequently isolated from periodontal lesions. Other groups of bacteria are consistently recovered from odontogenic and orofacial infections, suggesting that many pathogens may be capable of producing clinical signs and symptoms of disease (6). *Fusobacterium nucleatum* has been recovered more often from patients with severe odontogenic infections (7). The difference in recovery of these organisms is influenced by age, underlying systemic disease, and local factors (8). Most pathogens are indigenous to the oral cavity but in the immunocompromised host, bacteria such as *Escherichia coli* and *Bacteroides fragilis* can also colonize and cause infection.

DENTAL CARIES

The first step in the origination of caries is the formation of a dental plaque (2). An increase in the amount of plaque is responsible for the ultimate development of gingivitis. A variety of factors interact in the generation of dental plaque and subsequent emergence of caries. These include the presence of a susceptible tooth surface, the proper microflora, and a suitable nutritional substrate for that flora. Several oral acid producing aerobic and anaerobic bacteria, including *Streptococcus mutans*, *Lactobacillus acidophilus*, and *Actinomyces viscosus*, are capable of initiating the carious lesion. However, *S. mutans* is consistently the only organism recovered from decaying dental fissures and is isolated in greater quantities from carious teeth than in non-carious ones (9). The overwhelming majority of microorganisms isolated from carious dentin are obligate anaerobes (10). The predominant organisms are *Propionibacterium*, *Eubacteria*, *Arachnia*, *Lactobacillus*, *Bifidobacteria*, and *Actinomyces*. Some microorganisms also contribute to caries generation through synthesis of extracellular polysaccharides that adhere to the tooth surface (11). Fermentable carbohydrates are substrates for the microbial enzyme systems that produce organic acids (primarily lactic acid); sucrose is the optimum substrate for extracellular polysaccharide synthesis. In addition to providing a source of fermentable carbohydrate for conversion to acid, these extracellular polysaccharides greatly increase the bulk of the dental plaque and heighten its capacity as an area of bacterial proliferation.

TABLE 1 Microorganisms Associated with Periodontal Infections

Aerobic and facultative anaerobic	Anaerobic

I. Gram-positive cocci
   Streptococcus spp.
   Beta-hemolytic streptococci
   Streptococcus milleri group (viridans)
   Streptococcus mutans group
II. Gram-positive bacilli
   Rothia dentcocariosa
   Lactobacillus spp.
III. Gram-negative coccobacilli
   Actinobacillus spp.
   Actinobacillus actinomycentemcomitans[a]
   Campylobacter spp.
   Campylobacter rectus
   Capnocytophaga spp.
   Eikenella spp.
IV. Gram-negative rods
   Pseudomonas spp.[b]
   Enterobactericeae[b]
	I. Gram-positive cocci
	   Peptostreptococcus spp.
	   Peptostreptococcus micros
	II. Gram-negative cocci
	   Veillonella spp.
	III. Gram-positive bacilli
	   Actinomyces spp.
	   Eubacterium spp.
	   Propionibacterium spp.
	   Lactobacillus spp.
	IV. Spirochetes
	   Treponema denticola
	   Treponema sokranskii
	V. Gram-negative rods
	   Prevotella spp.
	   Prevotella intermedia
	   Prevotella nigrescens
	   Porphyromonus spp.
	   Porphyromonus gingivalis
	   Bacteriodes spp.
	   Bacteriodes forsythus
	   Fusobacterium spp.
	   Fusobacterium nucleatum
	   Selemenomas sputigena

[a] Common in juvenile periodontitis.
[b] Rare.

Ingestion of dietary carbohydrates plays a major role in caries initiation. The types of carbohydrates and the frequency of their ingestion are more important than the total quantity that is consumed. Frequent between-meal snacks, especially of sucrose-containing foods, enhance the carious process; sticky foods linger in the mouth and are potentially more harmful than non-sticky foods. Mechanisms that can shield the teeth include the cleaning action of the tongue, the buffering and protective activity of the saliva and its secretory immunoglobulin (IgA) (11).

Although caries can be arrested, none of the destroyed tooth structure will regenerate. Treatment involves removal of all affected tooth structure and proper replacement with a restorative material. Prophylaxis of caries includes ingestion of proper amounts of fluoride (about 1 mg/day) or local application of fluoride compounds. The fluoride forms a complex with the apetite crystals in enamel, as it replaces the hydroxyl group. It strengthens and increases acid resistance and promotes remineralization of carious lesions, and has also mild bacteriostatic properties. Daily brushing and mechanical removal of plaque, and adhering to proper diet that contains fewer carbohydrates are also important.

PULPITIS

Pulpitis is an inflammation of the dental pulp that can result from thermal, chemical, traumatic, or bacterial irritation. The most frequent inducer of pulpitis is dental caries that leads to destruction of enamel and dentin resulting in bacterial invasion. Secondary infection of the pulp by supragingival anaerobes occurs frequently in teeth with longstanding caries. Invasion of the pulp and spread of infection to the periapical areas can promote spreading of infection to other anatomical areas.

Microbiology

The bacteria isolated from an inflamed pulp and root canal are aerobic and facultative anaerobic organisms. *Streptococcus salivarius* generally constitutes less than 8% of the microorganisms of the infected root canal. *Enterococcus faecalis* has been reported in 10% to 30% of inflamed root canals (12). Other recovered microorganisms are yeasts and gram-negative bacteria, mostly neisseriae and gram-negative rods, such as *Proteus vulgaris* and *E. coli*. These bacteria may be difficult to eliminate from contaminated root canals.

Studies of the bacteriology of root canals have detected anaerobic bacteria. The quality of these studies varies considerably, however, and the anaerobic techniques generally are not always optimal. Most of these studies do not avoid contamination of the root canal specimen by oral flora. A variety of anaerobes have been recovered, accounting for 25% to 30% of the root canal isolates. These include anaerobic streptococci, anaerobic gram-negative bacilli (AGNB), actinomyces, propionibacteria, veillonellae, and others (13).

Using polymerase chain reaction (PCR), Rolph et al. (12) detected clones related to the genera *Capnocytophaga*, *Cytophaga*, *Dialister*, *Enterococcus*, *Eubacterium*, *Fusobacterium*, *Gemella*, *Lactobacillus*, *Mogibacterium*, *Peptostreptococcus*, *Prevotella*, *Propionibacterium*, *Selenomonas*, *Solobacterium*, *Streptococcus*, and *Veillonella*.

Several PCR studies have revealed new endodontic pathogens (14). These organisms include *Tannerella forsythensis* (formerly *Bacteroides forsythus*), *Prevotella tannerae*, *Porphyromonas endodontalis*, *P. gingivalis*, *F. nucleatum*, *Treponema* spp. (*Treponema denticola*, *Treponema socranskii*, and *Treponema vincentii*), *Dialister pneumosintes*, *Slackia exigua* (formerly *Eubacterium exiguum*), *Mogibacterium timidum* (formerly *Eubacterium timidum*) and *Eubacterium saphenum*.

The bacterial complex composed of *T. forsythensis*, *P. gingivalis*, and *T. denticola*, termed the "red complex," has been implicated in severe forms of periodontal disease (15).

Pathogenesis

The dental pulp is normally protected from infection by oral microorganisms by the enamel and dentin. This barrier may be breached allowing entrance of bacteria into the pulp or periapical areas. This can occur through a cavity caused by dental caries, trauma, or dental procedures; through the tubules of cut or carious dentin; in periodontal disease by way of the gingival crevice and by invasion along the periodontal membrane; by extension of periapical infection from adjacent teeth that are infected; or through the bloodstream during bacteremia.

Potentially virulent bacteria can migrate from the root canal into the apical regions. Toxic products from the pulp also may have a pathogenic role in the response to the inflammation. As the abscess progresses, more tissue may become involved, as well as adjacent teeth; the pressure of the accumulated pus can generate a sinus tract to the surface of the skin or to the oral or nasal cavity.

The most important route of pulp invasion is through the tubules of carious dentin. This may take place even before the pulp is exposed directly to the oral environment by cavitation. The bacteria that penetrate the dentin prior to cavitation are mostly facultative anaerobes and include streptococci, staphylococci, lactobacilli, and filamentous microorganisms (16).

After the pulp becomes necrotic, bacteria can proceed through the necrotic root canal tissue, and inflammation (apical periodontitis) develops in the periapical area.

The organisms that predominate in this stage of the infection are *Prevotella*, *Porphyromonas*, *Fusobacterium*, and *Peptostreptococcus* spp. However, the primary microorganism (5) causing pulpitis is difficult to determine because of the technical difficulties associated with obtaining samples for culturing, and because the exact time of the initial infection is difficult to ascertain.

Diagnosis

The symptoms of acute suppurative pulpitis include low-grade fever, pain, soreness of the tooth, and facial swelling. Pain is usual induced by hot liquids, a reaction believed to be caused by expansion of gases produced by gas-forming bacteria trapped inside the root canal. Sampling from the root canal for recovery of organisms, before treatment, during treatment and at the end of therapy to ensure eradication of the infection is useful, and can differentiate between infectious and non-infectious pulpitis.

The patient may experience intense pain that may be difficult to localize. It may be referred to the opposite mandible or maxilla or to areas supplied by common branches of the fifth cranial nerve. X-rays, pulp testers, percussion, and palpation are helpful aids in confirming the diagnosis.

Treatment

Cleansing of the cavity to remove debris and packing the cavity with zinc oxide–eugenol cement usually will afford relief in early pulpitis. Once pulpitis developed the infected pulpal tissue should be removed and root canal therapy instituted, or the tooth should be extracted.

Antimicrobial therapy supplementing the dental care should be considered, especially when local or systemic spread of the infection is suspected. Penicillin or amoxicillin are generally effective against most of the aerobic and anaerobic bacteria recovered. However, a growing number of patients harbor penicillin-resistant organisms and should be considered for treatment with drugs effective against these organisms. These agents include amoxicillin–clavulanate, clindamycin or the combination of metronidazole plus amoxicillin or a macolide (17).

DENTOALVEOLAR ABSCESS

An alveolar or apical abscess may be either acute or chronic. The acute alveolar abscess is an extension of necrotic or putrescent pulp into the periapical area, which induces bone and tissue necrosis and accumulation of pus. It may also occur after trauma to the teeth or from periapical localization of organisms. As the abscess growth, more tissue may be involved, including adjacent teeth, and the pressure within the abscess may produce a fistula to the gingival surface or to the oral or nasal cavities (18).

Microbiology

Anaerobic bacteria were recovered from most cases of dentoalveolar abscesses that were cultured using proper methods for their isolation (19–23). Studies done at the turn of the century of acute and chronic alveolar abscesses described the recovery of predominantly aerobic streptococci; however, fusiform bacilli and *Bacteroides* spp. were found in some abscesses, sometimes in pure culture (4). More recent studies report the isolation of a variety of anaerobes in periodontal abscesses, including anaerobic cocci, AGNB, and anaerobic gram-positive bacilli (19–23). The microflora associated with dentoalveolar abscesses was also recently determined and characterized by molecular methods (19). A quantitative and qualitative study of 50 dentoalveolar abscesses reported the presence of 3.3 isolates per abscess (20). Twenty (40%) abscesses harbored anaerobes only, and 27 (54%) abscesses had a mixture of both aerobes and anaerobes. Three-fourths of the isolates were strict anaerobes, the most common *Peptostreptococcus* spp., *Prevotella oralis*, and *Prevotella melaninogenica*.

Anaerobes were the predominant isolates, outnumbering aerobes eight to one in periodontal abscesses in 12 children (21). Anaerobes were recovered in all patients; in two thirds of the patients, they were the only organism isolated, and in the rest they were mixed with aerobes. There were 53 anaerobic isolates (4.4/specimen), 20 AGNB (including nine *P. melaninogenica*, three *P. oralis*), 17 anaerobic gram-positive cocci, 5 *Fusobacterium* spp., and 3 *Actinomyces* spp. There were six aerobic isolates (0.5/specimen), three *S. salivarius*, two alpha-hemolytic streptococci, and one gamma-hemolytic *Streptococcus*. Beta-lactamase production was noticed in four isolates three *P. melaninogenica*, and one *P. oralis*.

Brook et al. (22), who studied 39 periapical abscesses detected bacterial growth in 32 specimens. A total of 78 bacterial isolates (55 anaerobic and 23 aerobic and facultative) were recovered (2.4 isolates/specimen). Anaerobic bacteria only were present in 16 (50%) patients, aerobic and facultatives in two (6%), and mixed aerobic and anaerobic flora in 14 (44%). The predominant anaerobic isolates were AGNB (23 isolates, including 13 pigmented *Prevotella* and *Porphyromonas* spp.), *Streptococcus* spp. (20), anaerobic cocci (18), and *Fusobacterium* spp. (9). Beta-lactamase-producing organisms were recovered from seven of the 21 (33%) tested specimens.

Similar organisms were isolated from aspirate of pus from five periapical abscesses of the upper jaw and their corresponding maxillary sinusitis (23). Polymicrobial flora was found in all instances, where the number of isolates varied from two to five. Anaerobes were recovered from all specimens. The predominant isolates were *Prevotella* spp., *Porphyromonas* spp., *F. nucleatum*, and *Peptostreptococcus* spp. Concordance in the microbiological findings between periapical abscess and the maxillary sinus flora was found in all instances. However, certain organisms were only present at one site and not the other.

Diagnosis

An abscess can be focal or diffuse and present as red tender fluctuant gingival swelling. Pain from an acute abscess usually is intense and continuous. The involved tooth is painful when percussed. Hot or cold foods may increase the pain.

A chronic periapical abscess presents few clinical signs, since it is essentially a circumscribed area of mild infection that spreads slowly. In time, the infection may become granulomatous. Radiographic studies of the involved tooth can be helpful, and free air eventually can be observed in the tissues.

Complications

Complications can occur by direct extension or hemotogenous spread. If treatment is delayed, the infection may spread directly through adjacent tissues, causing cellulitis (phlegmona), varying degrees of facial edema, and fever. The infection may extend into osseous tissues or into the soft tissues of the floor of the mouth. Local swelling and gingival fistulas may develop opposite the apex of the tooth, especially with deciduous teeth.

Serious complications from periapical infections are relatively rare. The infection can spread to tissues in other portions of the oral cavity, causing submandibular or superficial sublingual abscesses; abscesses may be produced also in the submaxillary triangle or in the parapharyngeal or submasseteric space (24).

In the maxilla, periapical infection may affect only the soft tissues of the face, where it is less serious. It may extend, however, to the intratemporal space including the sinuses and then to the central nervous system, where it can cause serious complications such as subdural empyema, brain abscess, or meningitis (4,25).

Other potential complications include mediastinitis, suppurative jugular thrombophlebitis (Lemierre syndrome), maxillary sinusitis, carotid artery erosion, and osteomyelitis of the mandible and maxilla (4,26).

The finding of anaerobic bacteria in periodontal abscesses is of importance because of the association of anaerobes with many serious infections arising from dental foci, such as bacteremia, endocarditis, sinusitis, meningitis, subdural empyema, brain abscess, and pulmonary empyema (4). The spread of dental infections into the central nervous system via the sinuses has been documented (4,26).

Intracranial suppuration following tooth extraction or dental infection is an uncommon but extremely serious complication. Intracranial infections of buccodental origin may evolve cavernous sinus thrombosis, at times associated with brain abscess or subdural empyema (4,27). Isolated brain abscesses occur much less frequently, and subdural empyema of odontogenic origin is quite rare. Infections of the molar teeth are more likely to cause intracranial complications because pus arising in the back of the jaw tends to collect between the muscles of mastication and spread upward in the fascial planes, whereas infection arising in the front of the jaw has free access to the oral cavity (28).

Management

Extraction or root canal therapy and drainage of pus usually are indicated. Antibiotic prophylaxis is recommended if extraction or drainage is contemplated in patients at risk of developing endocarditis. Penicillin and erythromycin have been used. However, although the incidence of bacteremia caused by aerobic and anaerobic oral flora is reduced by such therapy, antimicrobial therapy does not prevent it (29). If high fever persists, antibiotics should be administered. Antibiotic should also be given if drainage is not adequate or when the infection perforates the cortex and spread into surrounding soft tissue. Most of the aerobic and anaerobic pathogens isolated from the abscesses are sensitive to penicillin. Some strains of *Fusobacterum* and pigmented *Prevotella* and *Porphyromonas* recovered from patients with periodontal abscesses may be resistant to penicillin, however (30). In patients who require therapy, the recovery of these penicillin-resistant organisms may mandate the administration of antimicrobial agents also effective against these organisms. These include clindamycin, chloramphenicol, cefoxitin, a combination of a penicillin and a beta-lactamase inhibitor or a carbapenem (31). Metronidazole should be administered with an agent effective against the aerobic or facultative streptococci (i.e. a macrolide). Although the need for judicious selection of antimicrobial agents must be emphasized, it is essential to note that the treatment of periapical abscess generally require surgical intervention and that surgical drainage of these cases is, therefore, an integral part of the management.

GINGIVITIS AND PERIODONTITIS

Pathogenesis and Complications

The healthy gingiva is a pink, keratinized mucosa, attached to the teeth and alveolar bone that forms the interdental papilla between the teeth. A 1–2 mm deep crevice of free gingiva surrounds each tooth. The gingival crevice is heavily colonized by anaerobic gram-negative bacilli and spirochetes.

Periodontal disease is a term referring to all diseases involving the supportive structures of the teeth (periodontium). It most commonly begins as gingivitis and progresses to periodontitis. How rapidly these infections progress depends on the type of bacteria present and the resistance and self-care of the patient. Although children are more resistant to gingivitis as compared to adults, it is the most common periodontal disease during childhood and peaks in adolescence (32).

The host response to the inflammation varies and depends on many factors including the type of the bacterial insult and its duration, the local and environmental contributing factors, immunological and inflammatory responses, predisposing genetic factors, and association with systemic diseases (33).

Purulent gingival pockets or gingival abscesses may complicate periodontal disease. Gingivitis results from accumulation of plaque and bacteria in the gingival crevice. Gingivitis is an inflammation of the gingivae, characterized by swelling, redness, change of normal contours, and bleeding. Swelling deepens the crevice between the gingivae and the teeth, forming gingival pockets. Although the patient usually experiences no pain, a mild foul smell may be noticed (32,34,35). Gingivitis may be acute or may be chronic with remissions and exacerbations.

Subgingival plaque is associated with periodontal diseases. The bacteria that colonize the area are primarily anaerobic. Both gram-negative and gram-positive species are regularly isolated. Most of these bacteria utilize protein and other nutrients provided in the subgingival environment by the gingival fluid. Once established in the subgingival areas, periodontal infections usually drain into the oral cavity via a periodontal pocket. If the drainage of the periodontal pocket is obstructed, an acute process results.

Abscess formation is usually limited to the alveolar process. In some cases, spread to adjacent spaces may be noted. Focal or diffuse periodontal abscesses can develop. They appear as red fluctuant swelling of the gingiva or mucosa, which are tender. As the underlying tissues are affected, a complete destruction of the periodontium occurs, with subsequent loss of teeth.

Aspiration pneumonia and lung abscess can develop as a complication of gingival disease, especially in individuals with poor dental hygiene. This has been noted especially following aspiration of the contents of a spontaneously drained periodontal abscess, in the neurologically impaired, who constantly aspirate their oral secretions and in those with gingivitis associated with dilantin therapy (36).

Epidemiological studies have indicated that untreated periodontal disease could be a risk factor to preterm delivery of low birth infants, coronary heart disease, and cerebral vascular accidents. This is explained by the production of lipopolysaccharides, heat-shock proteins, and proinflammatory cytokines by the AGNB that cause periodontal disease (37).

Classification and Manifestations of Periodontal Diseases

Until recently, the accepted standard for the classification of periodontal diseases was the one agreed upon at the 1989 World Workshop in Clinical Periodontics. This classification system, however, had its weaknesses as some of the criteria for diagnosis were unclear, disease categories overlapped, and patients did not always fit into any one category. Additionally, over emphasis was placed on the age of disease onset and the rate of progression, which are commonly difficult to determine. In 1999, an International Workshop for a Classification of Periodontal Diseases and Conditions was created by the American Academy of Periodontology to revise the classification system (Table 2) (38).

Gingivitis

The most fulminate form of gingivitis is necrotizing ulcerative gingivitis (NUG) (previously called acute NUG, "trench mouth" or "Vincent's infection"). It is a very painful, fetid, ulcerative disease that occurs most often in persons under severe stress with no or very poor oral hygiene. It is manifested by acutely tender, inflamed, bleeding gums associated with the interdental papillae necrosis and loss. Halitosis and fever are often present. Microbiological examinations of the bacterial biofilms found in NUG revealed high numbers of spirochetes and fusobacteria (39–41).

Another form of fulminate gingivitis is acute streptococcal gingivitis. It is caused by Group A beta-hemolytic streptococci (*Streptococcus pyogenes*) and is generally associated with acute streptococcal tonsillitis.

Periodontitis

Periodontitis often develops as a progression of gingivitis to the point that loss of supporting bone has begun because of destruction of alveolar bone. Tooth mobility, bleeding gingivae, and increased spaces between the teeth are common but are not necessarily signs of advanced disease. In some cases purulent exudate is present. Periodontal infection tends to localize to intraoral soft tissue but can spread to adjacent sites. The two main forms of periodontitis are *chronic* and *aggressive periodontitis* (Table 2).

Chronic periodontitis (replaced adult periodontitis) occurs mostly in adults, but can be also seen in younger individuals. Destruction is consistent with the amount of plaque present

TABLE 2 Outline of the 1999 Classification of Periodontal Disease

1. Gingival disease
     Dental plaque-induced
     Non-plaque-induced
2. Chronic periodontitis[a,b]
     Localized
     Generalized (>30% of sites involved)
3. Aggressive periodontitis[c]
     Localized
     Generalized (>30% of sites involved)
4. Periodontitis associated with systemic diseases (hematological, genetic and other)
5. Necrotizing periodontal diseases (necrotizing ulcerative gingivitis or periodontitis)
6. Abscesses of the periodontium (gingival, periodontal and pericoronal)
7. Periodontal diseases associated with endodontic lesions (combined)
8. Developmental or acquired deformities and conditions (including Trauma)

[a] Can be further classified on basis of extent and severity.
[b] Chronic periodontitis replaced adult periodontitis.
[c] Aggressive periodontitis replaced early onset, destructive and juvenile periodontitis.
Source: From Ref. 38.

and other local factors (i.e., anatomic and other factors that retain plaque next to a tooth such as overhanging restorations, open contacts and palato-radicular grooves); subgingival calculus is also commonly found. The disease progresses slowly but there may be bursts of destruction. Local factors, systemic diseases and extrinsic factors such as smoking can modify the rate of disease progression. Chronic periodontitis has been further classified as localized or generalized depending on whether <30% or >30% of sites are involved. Severity is based on the amount of clinical attachment loss (CAL) and is designated as slight (1–2 mm CAL), moderate (3–4 mm CAL), or severe (>5 mm CAL).

Aggressive Periodontitis

Aggressive periodontitis (replaced early onset, destructive and juvenile periodontitis) is diagnosed based on clinical, radiographic, and historical findings which show rapid attachment loss and bone destruction, and possible familial aggregation of disease. Except for periodontal disease, patients are healthy. Other features that may be present are periodontal tissue destruction that is greater than would be expected given the level of local factors.

Microbiology

Gingivitis

The healthy gingival sulcus contains relatively few organisms, usually Streptococci and *Actinomyces* (Table 1). The development of gingivitis is associated with a significant increase in AGNB (*F. nucleatum, P. intermedia* and *Bacteroides* spp.), spirochetes and motile rods.

NUG is known to be caused by synergistic infection between unusually large spirochetes and fusobacteria (39–41), which are part of the normal oropharyngeal flora. Loesche et al. (40) found that the bacteria associated with the infection are fairly constant and include oral *Treponemes* and *Selenomonas* spp., which represent these *Spirochete* and *Spirochete*-like organisms, and *P. intermidia* and *Fusobacterium* spp.

Periodontitis

All forms of periodontitis are polymicrobial aerobic–anaerobic bacterial infection. Periodontal disease develops usually because of two events in the oral cavity: an increase in bacterial quantity of AGNB and a change in the balance of bacterial types from harmless to disease-causing bacteria. Among the bacteria most implicated in periodontal disease and bone loss are *Actinobacillus actinomycetemcomitans* and *P. gingivalis*. Other bacteria associated with periodontal disease are *B. forsythus, T. denticola, Treponema sokranskii* and *P. intermedia* (32,42).

Bacteria listed in Table 1 have been implicated in chronic periodontitis. Those most prevalent can be identified with cultures and DNA probes. These include *P. intermedia, B. forsythus, Actinomyces* spp., *Capnocytophaga*, and *Peptostreptococcus micros*.

Examinations of subgingival biofilms with a phase contrast microscope can be helpful with patient education and motivation and with follow-up. Following the prevalence of spirochetes provides insight into patient compliance and the adequacy of their self-care. The microorganisms involved are generally acquired from another person's saliva, possibly over a period of years, and the self-care the patients have used has not controlled them.

Aggressive periodontitis is now recognized as a contagious infection that can be passed between family members. *A. actinomycetemcomitans* and *P. gingivalis*, are believed to play a major role in this infection.

The role of anaerobic organisms in this infection is strengthened by the finding of elevated levels of serum IgG antibodies specific for these organisms in patients with periodontitis (43). This immunoserologic observation is strongly supportive of several bacteriologic studies (44,45) that have indicated that *P. gingivalis* is a predominant isolate from advancing chronic periodontitis lesions. Several oral anaerobes and streptococci including *P. gingivalis, P. intermedia, P. melaninogenica, Capnocytophaga* spp; *S. sanguis* and *Streptococcus mitis*, produce IgA proteases (46), that may impair local immunity.

Management

Gingivitis

Treatment of gingivitis involves removing dental plaques and maintaining good oral hygiene. Personal plaque/calculus control and professional debridement, oral hygiene care, correction of plaque retentive sites, and if these are unhelpful, chlorhexidine gluconate 0.12% mouthwash or baking soda plus hydrogen peroxide rinses should be used.

Antibiotics are generally not recommended for gingivitis. The types of gingivitis that require systemic antimicrobial therapy include streptococcal gingivitis and NUG.

Local and systemic antimicrobials are used in the therapy of NUG. Some of the agents that can be used topically in the dental office include a 3% solution of hydrogen peroxide mixed with sodium bicarbonate, and a 0.12% solution of chlorhexidine gluconate. Systemic antibiotic therapy is very beneficial because it provides continuous bacterial control (Table 3).

Periodontitis

Therapy of chronic periodontitis should include debridement and thorough scaling and root planing to remove the subgingival and supragingival deposits of calculus and plaque (bacterial biofilm) (32,47). When pockets are more than 5 mm deep, local therapy rarely suppresses the involved pathogens adequately. Therefore, subgingival irrigation to disinfect the gingival crevices can be accomplished with the use of either ultrasonic scalers or individual irrigating syringes. Effective antiseptic solutions are povidone iodine, chlorhexidine, chloramine-T, or salt water. Helpful measures may include twice-daily rinsing with chlorhexidine–gluconate 0.12% mouthwash, brushing with a mixture of baking soda plus hydrogen peroxide, and/or frequent salt-water rinses. Local therapy with antimicrobial delivery systems is to be considered as adjunctive therapy and not as an alternative to instrumentation. Since there is negligible calculus and firm plaque in aggressive periodontitis, traditional scaling and root planing is not needed. Pockets may be irrigated with an antibacterial solution and the patient receives systemic antibiotics (Table 3).

The use of systemic antimicrobials is especially indicated in aggressive periodontitis and is sometimes needed in chronic periodontitis (Table 3). Appropriate systemic antibiotic regimens should be based on culture and susceptibility testing of the subgingival flora whenever possible. Cultures should also be taken after therapy to ensure eradication of pathogens.

TABLE 3 Oral Antimicrobial Therapy of Periodontal Infections

Antimicrobial	Adult dose/duration	Children dose/duration
Narrow spectrum agents		
Penicillin VK	250–500 mg q6 h×7–10 day	50 mg/kg q8 h×7–10 day
Amoxicillin	500 mg q8 h×7–10 day	15 mg/kg q8 h×7–10 day
Erythromycin[a]	250 mg q6 h×7–10 day	10 mg/kg 16 h×7–10 day
Azithromycin[a,b]	500 mg first day, then 250 or 500 mg q24 h×4 day	10 mg/kg/d first day, then 5 mg/kg/d q24 h×4 day
Broad spectrum agents		
Clindamycin[a]	150–300 mg q8 h×7 day	10 mg/kg q8 h×7 day
Amoxicillin/clavulanate	875 mg q12 h×7 day	45 mg/kg q12 h×7 day
Metronidazole plus[a]	250 mg q6 h or 500 mg q12 h×7 day	7.5 mg/kg q6 h or 15 mg/kg q12 h×7 day
Penicillin VK or	250–500 mg q6 h×7 day	50 mg/kg q6 h×7 day
Amoxicillin or	500 mg q8 h×7 day	15 mg/kg q8 h×7 day
Erythromycin[a]	250 mg q6 h×7 day	10 mg/kg q6 h×7 day
Doxycycline[a,c]	100 mg q12 h×7 day	1–2 mg/kg q12 h×1d, then 1–2 mg/kg q24 h×6 day
Tetracycline[a,c]	250 mg q6 h×7 day	12.5–25 mg/kg q12 h×7 day

[a] Also in penicillin-allergic patients.
[b] First dose is a loading dose and should have double the regular amount.
[c] In children more than seven years.

Periodontal Abscess

Treatment includes drainage of puss and debridement. Antimircobial therapy is necessary whenever local or systemic spread is present (Table 3). Extraction of the involved tooth may be necessary if antibiotic therapy fails.

General Guidelines for Use of Antimicrobial Agents

Since periodontal infections are generally mixed anaerobic and facultative anaerobic infection, identifying the causative organisms in the subgingival flora and determining their antimicrobial susceptibility is helpful in selecting the proper antimicrobial therapy. Identification can be done by culture or DNA probing methods (45). Cultures should also be taken after therapy to ensure eradication of pathogens.

Antimicrobials utilized in odontogenic infections can be divided into broad and narrow spectrum. Many patients can be treated with narrow spectrum antimicrobials. However, three categories of patients need to be treated with broad spectrum antimicrobials to prevent failure and complications: patients infected by resistant bacteria (48,49), and those with underlying serious medical conditions or are suffering from a severe dental infection. The risk factors prompting use of broad spectrum agents are listed in Table 4.

Narrow spectrum antimicrobials include penicillin, amoxicillin, cephalexin, the macrolides (erythromycin, clarithromycin, and azithromycin), and the tetracyclines (including doxycycline). These agents have a limited antimicrobial efficacy as they are not effective against aerobic and anaerobic beta-lactamase producers as well as other specific organisms.

Broad spectrum antimicrobials or antimicrobial combinations include clindamycin, the combination of a penicillin (i.e., amoxicillin) plus a beta-lactamase inhibitor (i.e., clavulanate), tigecycline and carbapenems and the combination of metronidazole plus penicillin, amoxicillin or a macrolide (31). These possess a broad spectrum of activity against most odontogenic pathogens including aerobic and anaerobic beta-lactamase producers. Furthermore, some of these agents (clindamycin and amoxicillin–clavulante) provide better pharmacokinetic and pharmacodynamic indexes against the odontogenic pathogens compared to the other agents (48,49). Pharmacokinetic and pharmacodynamic indexes of each antimicrobial can predict their clinical efficacy by considering their concentrations at the site of the infection and the susceptibility of the pathogens.

The choice between broad and narrow spectrum antimicrobials should be individualized in each patient. Utilization of broad spectrum antimicrobial can ensure efficacy against all potential pathogens especially those resistant to antimicrobials.

Anti-infectives should be given a chance to work. Improvement may take time and therefore therapy should not be changed until it is given for at least 48 to 72 hours. The short-term

---

TABLE 4 Risk Factor Prompting Use of Broad Spectrum Agents

Conditions that may increase the risk of infection with antimicrobial resistant organisms
  Recent antimicrobial therapy or prophylaxis (within the past six weeks)
  Close contact with individual(s) recently treated with an antimicrobial. (i.e., household, school, daycare center)
  Failure of first line antimicrobial
  Direct or indirect exposure to smoking
  Antimicrobial resistance high in the community
  Winter season
Increased risk of infection due to medical history or condition
  The young (<2 years) and the old (>55 years)
  Serious, complicated, or spreading infection
  Malignancy (i.e., leukemia, Hodgkin's disease, other hematological malignancies)
  Metabolic disorder (i.e., out-of-control diabetes mellitus, hemodialysis patients)
  Immunosupression (congenital or acquired)
  Drug-related immunosuppression (i.e., corticosteroids, immunosuppressants, cytotoxic agents, cancer chemotherapy)
  Other conditions that are associated with immunosuppression (i.e., Radiotherapy/osteoradionecrosis of head and neck, transplant patients, neutropenia, granulocytopenia, patients with an indwelling intravascular catheter, those with immunocompromising procedures)

use of an anti-infective, effective as it may be, may not produce long-term results because the patient may become re-infected.

PERICORONITIS

Pericoronitis is an infection of the pericoronal soft tissue associated with gum flaps (opercula) that partially overlie the crown of the tooth. The teeth most often involved are the third mandibular molars. The infection is caused by microorganisms and debris that become entrapped in the gingival pocket between the tooth and the overlying soft tissue. If the overlying soft tissue becomes swollen, the drainage is obstructed and inflammatory exudate is entrapped and will spread to other anatomical sites. Pericoronitis is usually accompanied by swelling of the soft tissues and marked trismus. However, the underlying alveolar bone is not usually involved. In most cases, antibiotic treatment is necessary to avoid spread of the infection. The microorganisms most often isolated from acute pericoronitis are anaerobic cocci, *Fusobacteria* spp. and AGNB (50). Treatment of pericoronitis also includes gentle debridement and irrigation under the tissue flap. Excision of the gum flap may be considered. Antibiotics and incision and drainage may be needed if fascial plains cellulitis develops.

DEEP FACIAL INFECTIONS AND LEMIERRE SYNDROME

The source of most deep neck infections before the era of the antibiotics were pharyngeal and tonsillar infections in about 75% of instances and dental in about 25%. With the common use of antimicrobials, this ratio has been reversed and dental infections account for the majority of cases and pharyngo-tonsillar are less commonly encountered. Other sources include nasal, otologic, salivary gland, dermatologic infections, hematogenic spread, cervical adenitis, and trauma.

Odontogenic infections that generally originate from infected or necrotic pulp may spread to fascial spaces of the lower head and upper neck. These space infections can be divided into those around the face (masticator, buccal, cannine, and parotid), the suprahyoid area (submandibular, sublingual, and lateral pharyngeal), and those in the infrahyoid region or lateral neck (retropharyngeal and pretracheal spaces) (51). If penetration of the infection occurs above the attachment of the buccinator muscle on the mandible or below the attachment in the maxilla, the pus will drain intraorally. However, penetration above or below these attachments will result in extraoral drainage.

Management of deep facial infections and Lemierre syndrome evolves surgical drainage as well as directing appropriate antimicrobial therapy against potential bacterial pathogens. The recent increased recovery of anaerobic bacteria from these infections has led to greater appreciation of their role in these conditions and to revaluation of their proper management.

Microbiology

The predominant organisms recovered from deep facial infections are *Staphylococcus aureus* and Group A streptococci and anaerobic bacteria of oral origion. These include pigmented *Prevotella* and *Porphyromonas* as well as *Fusobacterium* spp. (4). These organisms are mostly recovered in polymicrobial infections mixed with aerobic bacteria. The recovery of anaerobic bacteria from these infections is not surprising because these bacteria outnumber aerobic bacteria in the oralsc cavity by a ratio of 10 to 100:1 (1). Furthermore, these organisms were also isolated from chronic upper respiratory infections, such as otitis and sinusitis, and from periodontal infections (52).

DEEP FACIAL INFECTIONS

Masticator Spaces

Masticator spaces include the masseteric, pterygoid, and temporal spaces, which communicate with each other as well as with the buccal submandibular and lateral pharyngeal spaces, allowing extension of the infection. The molar teeth, particularly the third molar, are often the source of infection. Patients generally present with trismus and mandibular pain. Swelling is not always present. The infection can spread internally, pressing the lateral pharyngeal wall and causing dysphagia. Deep temporal space infections often originate from posterior maxillary molars. As the infection progresses, the swelling increases, and involves the cheeks, eyelids, and the side of the face.

Management includes surgical drainage and antimicrobial therapy. The principles of antimicrobial therapy are outlined in a separate section (see below).

Buccal, Canine, and Parotid Spaces

Buccal space infections often originate from an intraoral extension of infection of the bicuspid or molar teeth. This infection is characterized by significant cheek swelling with minimal trismus and systemic symptoms. Often, antimicrobial therapy alone is sufficient. However, extraoral superficial drainage may be required.

Canine space infections often follow maxillary incisor involvement. The typical swelling involves the upper lip, canine fossa, and periorbital tissues. Extension into the maxillary sinuses can occur. Intraoral surgical drainage and antibiotic therapy are often advocated.

Parotid space infections are generally a sequela of masseteric space infection and are characterized by swelling of the angle of the jaw, and pain, fever, and chills. These types of infections can extend directly into the posterior mediastinum and visceral spaces.

Submandibular and Sublingual Spaces

Infection of the submandibular and sublingual spaces usually arises from the second and third mandibular teeth. Swelling and minimal trismus are generally present. Sublingual space infection generally originates from the mandibular incisors and is characterized by a brawny, erythematous, tender swelling of the floor of the mouth. In the later stages, tongue elevation may also be noted.

The classic Ludwig's angina involves a bilateral infection of both the submandibular and sublingual spaces (53). A dental source of the infection usually can be found, and the second and third mandibular molars are often involved. The infection begins in the mouth floor and spread rapidly, causing indurating cellulitis that often induces lymphatic involvement or abscess formation. The clinical presentation includes a brawny, boardlike non pitting swelling of the mandibular spaces and general toxicity. The mouth is generally held open, and the floor is elevated, which pushes the tongue upward. Eating, swallowing, and breathing may be impaired. Rapid progression can induce neck and glottis edema, which precipitates asphyxiation (54).

A variety of microorganisms has been isolated from cases of Ludwig's angina. In recent years, anaerobic bacteria have predominated, including *Fusobacterium* spp., AGNB, and *Peptostreptococcus* spp. Often, one or more of the following also have been found: staphylococci, streptococci, pneumococci, *E. coli*, Vincent's spirochetes, *Haemophilus influenzae*, and *Candida albicans* (4). Management includes high doses of parenteral antibiotics, airway monitoring, early intubation or tracheostomy, soft tissue decompression, and surgical drainage (55).

Lateral Pharyngeal Space

The lateral pharyngeal space is continuous with the carotid sheath. Involvement of this space may follow pharyngitis, tonsillitis, otitis, parotitis, and odontogenic infections. Anterior compartment involvement is characterized by fever, chills, pain, tremors, and swelling below the angle of the jaw. Posterior compartment infection is characterized by septicemia, often with few local signs. Other complications include edema of the larynx, asphyxiation, internal carotid artery, and erosion internal jugular vein thrombosis. Close observation is mandatory and tracheostomy may be required. Surgical drainage and parenteral antibiotic therapy are needed.

Retropharyngeal and pretracheal spaces

The retropharyngeal space includes the posterior part of the visceral compartment in which the esophagus, trachea, and thyroid gland are enclosed by the middle layers of deep cervical fasci, which extend into the superior mediastinum. This space may become infected as a result from direct extension of a pharyngeal space infection or through lymphatics from the nasopharynx. The onset of the infection is insidious, although dyspnea, dysphagia, nuchal rigidity, fever, and chills may be present. Bulging of the posterior pharyngeal wall may be present. Soft tissue radiography or computed tomography (CT) scan disclose widening of the retropharyngeal space. Hemorrhage, rupture into the airway, laryngeal spasm, bronchial erosion, and jugular vein thrombosis are the main complications. The pretracheal space that surrounds the trachea generally becomes involved following perforation of the anterior esophageal wall or from an extension of a retropharyngeal infection. Patients usually present with hoarseness, dyspnea, and difficulty in swallowing. Prompt surgical drainage is needed to prevent mediastinal extension.

LEMIERRE SYNDROME

Lemierre syndrome (or suppurative thrombophlebitis of the internal jugular vein) was originally described as a complication of postanginal sepsis (56–60). Lemierre, in 1936, wrote a comprehensive article on the subject and called this syndrome "postanginal septicemia" (59).

This syndrome is a rare but severe life-threatening complication of oral infections, particularly those resulting in lateral pharyngeal space infection. It is characterized as thrombosis and suppurative thrombophlebitis of the internal jugular vein that is associated with spread of septic emboli to the lungs and other sites. Before the availability of antimicrobial agents, death was the common result, unless patients were treated with surgical ligation of the vein (57,58).

Fusobacterium is the predominant genus and *Fusobacterium necrophorum* is the most prevalent species. Other Fusobacteria include *F. nucleatum*, *Fusobacterium gonidiaforum* and *Fusobacterium varium*. Other isolates recovered alone or in combination include pigmented *Prevotella*, *Bacteroides* and *Peptostreptococcus* spp. (61–63).

The source of the infection is pharyngitis, exudative tonsillitis, peritonsillar abscess or oral procedure (i.e., tonsillectomy), which precedes the onset of septicemia. The initiating event is generally a localized infection in an area drained by the large cervical veins. Thereafter, the infection quickly progresses to cause a pathognomic triad of findings: (*i*) local symptoms of neck pain, torticollis, trismus, dysphagia or dysarthria ascribable to involvement of the hypoglossal, glossopharyngeal, vagus or accessory nerves; (*ii*) development of thrombophlebitis; (*iii*) embolic infection of the lungs, viscera, joints or brain, or direct extension of the infection to the internal ear, middle ear or mastoid. Death can occur as a result of the erosion of a blood vessel wall with rupture into the mediastinum, ear, or crania vault (60).

Most patients with Lemierre's syndrome are older than 10 years (62). The patients look toxic and manifest fever, sore throat, cough neck, pain, dyspnea, and arthralgia. Palpable jugular arch can be detected in about 20% of patients. Swelling and tenderness at the angle of the jaw and along the sternocleidomastoid muscle with signs of severe sepsis along with evidence of pleuropulmonary emboli, is very suggestive of thrombophlebitis of the internal jugular vein (61).

Pulmonary emboli are found in most untreated patients, as most present with pleuritic pain. Empyema is however rare. Seeding of other body sites occurs, mostly to the joints. Other potential sites that are involved are the liver causing "bacteremic jaundice" (64). Chest x-ray is indicated.

High resolution ultrasonography can confirm the diagnosis of suppurative thrombophlebitis (65). CT can also demonstrate intravascular thrombus; however, it is more expensive, produces higher morbidity because of intravascular contrast agents and is probably less sensitive than high resolution ultrasonography for identifying small mural thrombi (65–67). Radionuclide gallium scans can localize the source of the original infection in the internal jugular vein (68). However, inability to document a thrombus should not delay initiation of appropriate antibiotic therapy for anaerobic sepsis.

Treatment

Prolonged high dose antimicrobial therapy is important in ensuring cure and preventing local and systemic extension of these infections. These agents should be directed at the eradication of the predominant organisms causing these infections. To assure that therapy is individualized, appropriate specimens should be collected from the infected site and processed for aerobic and anaerobic bacteria. The choice of the proper antibiotics depends on the antimicrobial susceptibility of the etiologic agent. Most patients respond adequately to proper antimicrobial therapy; however, once an abscess has formed surgical drainage is required. Ultrasonography or CT scan can be used to detect suppuration. Progressive induration, edema, and toxicity are also an indication for drainage.

Broad antimicrobial therapy is indicated to cover all possible aerobic and anaerobic pathogens, including adequate coverage for *S. aureus*, hemolytic streptococci, and beta-lactamase producing AGNB. Many of the AGNB causing these infections can produce beta-lactamase (30,69). These include pigmented *Prevotella* and *Porphyromonas* as well as *Fusobacterium* spp.

Clindamycin, cefoxitin, chloramphenicol, a carbapenem (i.e., imipenem, meropenem), tigecycline, the combination of a penicillin (i.e., amoxicillin) plus beta-lactamase inhibitor (i.e., clavulanate) or metronidazole plus a macrolide, will provide adequate coverage for anaerobic as well as aerobic bacteria. A penicillinase-resistant penicillin (i.e., nafcillin) or first-generation cephalosporin is generally adequate when the infection is caused only by staphyloccoci. However, the presence of methicillin-resistant staphylococci may mandate the use of vancomycin, linezolid or tigecycline.

Prevention of suppuration can be achieved by early and proper therapy of odontogenic infections. A poor response in the treatment of Lemierre syndrome may require the need for anticoagulation, rather than for a change in antibiotics. However, the use of these agents is controversial (70). Because this syndrome is due to an endovascular infection, surgical draining of purulent collection (empyema, septic arthritis, soft-tissue abscess) is needed. Ligation and resection of the internal jugular vein is unnecessary in the majority of the cases (61).

REFERENCES

1. Moore WEC, Holdeman LV, Cato EP, et al. Variation in periodontal floras. Infect Immun 1984; 46:720–6.
2. Dahlen G. Microbiology and treatment of dental abscesses and periodontal-endodontic lesions. Periodontol 2000 2002; 28:206–39.
3. Deroux E. Complications of dental infections. Rev Med Brux 2001; 22:A289–95.
4. Finegold SM. Anaerobic Bacteria in Human Disease. New York: Academic Press, 1977.
5. White D, Maynand D. Association of oral *Bacteroides* with gingivitis and adult periodontitis. J Periodontal Res 1981; 16:259–65.
6. Socransky SS. Microbiology of periodontal disease: present status and future consideration. J Periodontol 1977; 48:497–504.
7. Heimdhal A, von Konow L, Satoh T, Nord CE. Clinical appearance of orofacial infections of odontogenic origin in relationship to findings. J Clin Microbiol 1985; 22:299–302.
8. Zambon JJ. Periodontal diseases: microbialfactors. Ann Periodontol 1996; 1:879–925.
9. Hanada N. Current understanding of the cause of dental caries. Jpn J Infect Dis 2000; 53:1–5.
10. Hoshino E. Predominant obligate anaerobes in human carious dentin. J Dent Res 1985; 64:1195–8.
11. Bowden GH, Hamilton IR. Survival of oral bacteria. Crit Rev Oral Biol Med 1998; 9:54–85.
12. Rolph HJ, Lennon A, Riggio MP, et al. Molecular identification of microorganisms from endodontic infections. J Clin Microbiol 2001; 39:3282–9.
13. Liljemark WF, Bloomquist C. Human oral microbial ecology and dental caries and periodontal diseases. Crit Rev Oral Biol Med 1996; 7:180–98.
14. Siqueira JF, Jr., Rocas IN. PCR methodology as a valuable tool for identification of endodontic pathogens. J Dent 2003; 31:333–9.
15. Socransky SS, Haffajee AD, Cugini MA, Smith C, Kent RL, Jr. Microbial complexes in subgingival plaque. J Clin Periodontol 1998; 25:134–44.

16. Siqueira JF, Jr. Aetiology of root canal treatment failure: why well-treated teeth can fail. Int Endod J 2001; 34:1–10.

17. Kinder SA, Holt SC, Korman KS. Penicillin resistance in the subgingival microbiota associated with adult periodontitis. J Clin Microbiol 1986; 23:1127–33.

18. Johnson BR, Remeikis NA, Van Cura JE. Diagnosis and treatment of cutaneous facial sinus tracts of dental origin. J Am Dent Assoc 1999; 130:832–6.

19. Dymock D, Weightman AJ, Scully C, Wade WG. Molecular analysis of microflora associated with dentoalveolar abscesses. J Clin Microbiol 1996; 34:537–42.

20. Lewis MAO, MacFarlane TW, McGowan OA. Quantitative bacteriology of acute dentoalveolar abscesses. J Med Microbiol 1986; 21:101–4.

21. Brook I, Grimm S, Kielich RB. Bacteriology of acute periapical abscess in children. J Endod 1981; 7:378–80.

22. Brook I, Frazier EH, Gher ME. Aerobic and anaerobic microbiology of periapical abscess. Oral Microbiol Immunol 1991; 6:123–5.

23. Brook I, Frazier EH, Gher ME, Jr. Microbiology of periapical abscesses and associated maxillary sinusitis. J Periodontol 1996; 67:608–10.

24. Brook I, Friedman EM, Rodriguez WJ, Controni G. Complications of sinusitis in children. Pediatrics 1980; 66:568–72.

25. Brook I, Friedman E. Intracranial complications of sinusitis in children—a sequela of periapical abscess. Ann Otol Rhinol Laryngol 1982; 91:41–3.

26. Brook I. Brain abscess in children: microbiology and management. J Child Neurol 1995; 10:283–8.

27. Corson MA, Postlethwaite KP, Seymour RA. Are dental infections a cause of brain abscess? Case report and review of the literature. Oral Dis 2001; 7:61–5.

28. Colville A, Davies W, Heneghan M, Goodwin A, Griffiths T. A rare complication of dental treatment: *Streptococcus oralis* meningitis. Br Dent J 1993; 175:133–4.

29. Josefsson K, Heimdahl A, von Konow L, Nord CE. Effect of phenoxymethyl-penicillin and erythromycin prophylaxis on anaerobic bacteremia after oral surgery. J Antimicrob Chemother 1985; 16:243–51.

30. Brook I, Calhoun L, Yocum P. Beta lactamase producing isolates of *Bacteroides* species for children. Antimicrob Agents Chemother 1980; 18:164–6.

31. Brook I, Douma M. Antimicrobials Therapy Guide for the Dentist. Newtown, PA: Handbooks in Health Care Co., 2004.

32. Oh TJ, Eber R, Wang HL. Periodontal diseases in the child and adolescent. J Clin Periodontol 2002; 29:400–10.

33. Van Dyke TE, Tohme ZN. Periodontal diagnosis: evaluation of current concepts and future needs. J Int Acad Periodontol 2000; 2:71–8.

34. Loesche WJ. Bacterial mediators in periodontal disease. Clin Infect Dis 1993; 16:S203–10.

35. Kureishi K, Chow AW. The tender tooth-dentoalveolar, pericoronal, and periodontal infections. Infect Dis Clin North Am 1988; 2:163–82.

36. Brook I, Finegold SM. Bacteriology of aspiration pneumonia in children. Pediatrics 1980; 65:1115–20.

37. Loesche WJ. Association of the oral flora with important medical diseases. Curr Opin Periodontol 1997; 4:21–8.

38. International workshop for classification of periodontal diseases and conditions. Ann Periodontol 1999; 4:1–112.

39. Stammers AF. Vincent's infection: observations and conclusions regarding the aetiology and treatment of 1017 civilian cases. Br Dent J 1944; 76:147–53.

40. Loesche WJ, Syed SA, Laughon BE, Stoll J. The bacteriology of acute necrotizing ulcerative gingivitis. J Periodontol 1982; 53:223–30.

41. Socransky SS, Haffajee AD. Evidence of bacterial etiology: a historical perspective. Periodontol 2000 1994; 5:7–25.

42. Darby I, Curtis M. Microbiology of periodontal disease in children and young adults. Periodontol 2000 2001; 26:33–53.

43. Kinane DF, Mooney J, Ebersole JL. Humoral immune response to *Actinobacillus actinomycetemcomitans* and *Porphyromonas gingivalis* in periodontal disease. Periodontol 2000 1999; 20:289–340.

44. Slots J. Microbial analysis in supportive periodontal treatment. Periodontol 2000 1996; 12:56–9.

45. Conrads G. DNA probes and primers in dental practice. Clin Infect Dis 2002; 35(Suppl. 1):S72–7.

46. Gronbaek Frandsen EV. Bacterial degradation of immunoglobulin A1 in relation to periodontal diseases. APMIS Suppl 1999; 87:1–54.

47. Slots J, Ting M. Systemic antibiotics in the treatment of periodontal disease. Periodontol 2000 2002; 28:106–76.

48. Heimdhal A, Von-Konow L, Nord CE. Isolation of beta-lactamase producing *Bacteroides* strains associated with clinical failures with penicillin treatment of human orofacial infections. Arch Oral Biol 1980; 25:689–92.

49. Brook I. Beta-lactamase-producing bacteria recovered after clinical failure with various penicillin therapy. Arch Otolaryngol 1984; 110:228–31.
50. Rajasuo A, Jousimies-Somer H, Savolainen S, Leppanen J, Murtomaa H, Meurman JH. Bacteriologic findings in tonsillitis and pericoronitis. Clin Infect Dis 1996; 23:51–60.
51. Baker AS, Montgomery WW. Oropharyngeal space infections. Curr Clin Top Infect Dis 1987; 8:227–65.
52. Brook I. Anaerobic bacteria in upper respiratory tract and other head and neck infections. Ann Otol Rhinol Laryngol 2002; 111:430–40.
53. Finch RG, Snider GE, Sprinkle PM. Ludwig's angina. JAMA 1980; 243:1171–3.
54. El-Sayed Y, Al Dousary S. Deep-neck space abscesses. J Otolaryngol 1996; 25:227–33.
55. Hartmann RW, Jr. Ludwig's angina in children. Am Fam Physician 1999; 60:109–12.
56. Beck AL. A study of 24 cases of neck infections. Trans Am Acad Ophthalmol 1932; 37:342–81.
57. Reuben M. Postanginal sepsis: report of 9 cases. Arch Pediatr 1935; 52:152–86.
58. Boharas S. Postanginal sepsis. Arch Intern Med 1943; 71:844–53.
59. Lemierre A. On certain septicemias due to anaerobic organisms. Lancet 1936; 2:701–3.
60. Chase S. Infective thrombophlebitis secondary to neck infections. J Iowa Med Soc 1935; 25:252–9.
61. Sinave CP, Hardy GJ, Fardy PW. The Lemierre syndrome: suppurative thrombophlebitis of the internal jugular vein secondary to oropharyngeal infection. Medicine (Baltimore) 1989; 68:85–94.
62. Goldhagen J, Alford BA, Prewitt LH, Thompson L, Hostetter MK. Suppurative thrombophlebitis of the internal jugular vein: report of three cases and review of the pediatric literature. Pediatr Infect Dis J 1988; 7:410–4.
63. Moreno S, Garcia Altozano J, Pinilla B, et al. Lemierre's disease: postanginal bacteremia and pulmonary involvement caused by *Fusobacterium necrophorum*. Rev Infect Dis 1989; 11:319–24.
64. Zimmerman HJ, Fane M, Utili R, Seeff LB, Hoofnagle J. Jaundice due to bacterial infection. Gastroenterology 1979; 77:363–74.
65. Gudinchet F, Maeder P, Neveceral P, Schnyder P. Lemierre's syndrome in children: high-resolution CT and color Doppler sonography patterns. Chest 1997; 112:271–3.
66. deWitte BR, Lameris JS. Real-time ultrasound diagnosis of internal jugular vein thrombosis. J Clin Ultrasound 1986; 14:712–7.
67. Sanders RV, Kirkpatrick MB, Dasco CC, Bass JB, Jr. Suppurative thrombophlebitis of the internal jugular vein. Ala J Med Sci 1986; 23:92–5.
68. Yau PC, Norante JD. Thrombophlebitis of the internal jugular vein secondary to pharyngitis. Arch Otolaryngol 1980; 106:507–8.
69. Brook I. Infections caused by beta-lactamase-producing *Fusobacterium* spp. in children. Pediatr Infect Dis J 1993; 12:532–3.
70. Mitre RJ, Rotheram EB, Jr. Anaerobic septicemia from thrombophlebitis of the internal jugular vein: successful treatment with metronidazole. JAMA 1974; 230:1168–9.

13 | Ear Infections

Otitis media is one of the most common diseases of early childhood. The incidence is highest between 6 and 18 months. There are four defined types of otitis media (1): (*i*) acute otitis media (AOM) is characterized by a rapid onset of signs and symptoms of middle-ear inflammation. Earache, bulging of the tympanic membrane, and purulent exudate characterize the early phase of infection. Even though clinical signs and symptoms resolve rapidly, the effusion can persist; (*ii*) otitis media with effusion (OME) refers to the presence of asymptomatic effusion. It may follow acute otitis media with effusion (AOME) or appear as silent or secretory otitis media; (*iii*) chronic otitis media with effusion (COME) denotes a persistence of fluid for three months or longer. The fluid is more mucoid, so-called *glue ear*; and (*iv*) chronic suppurative otitis media (CSOM) signifies chronic drainage through a perforation of the tympanic membrane.

ACUTE OTITIS MEDIA

Microbiology

Streptococcus pneumoniae, *Haemophilus influenzae*, and *Moraxella catarrhalis* are the principal etiologic agents in bacterial AOM accounting for about 80% of the bacterial isolates (2,3). *S. pneumoniae* has constantly been found more commonly, irrespective of age group, but its predominance has tended to decrease following the introduction of the pneumococcal conjugate vaccine in 2000 (4), where the frequency of isolation of *H. influenzae* increased. Of special concern is the increased rate of isolation of penicillin-resistant strains of *S. pneumoniae* (5) and amoxicillin-resistant *H. influenzae* (5,6) from infected ears. The incidence of such strains may reach 50% in some areas.

Other organisms that less frequently cause AOM include group A beta-hemolytic streptococci (GABHS), *Staphylococcus aureus*, *Turicella otitidis*, *Alloiococcus otitis* *Chlamydia* spp., and *Staphylococcus epidermidis*, and various aerobic and faculatative gram-negative bacilli (7) including *Escherichia coli*, *Klebsiella pneumoniae*, *Pseudomonas aeruginosa*, and *Proteus* spp. Gram-negative bacilli and staphylococci are implicated as dominant etiologic agents in otitis media of the neonate. However, even among very young infants, *S. pneumoniae* and *H. influenzae* constitute the most common etiologic agents. Viruses were recovered in the middle-ear fluid of 14.3% of children (8).

The role of anaerobic bacteria was evaluated in four studies (9–13). In a study of 186 children (9,10), aerobic bacteria alone, predominantly pneumococci and *H. influenzae*, were isolated from 118 (63.4%) patients (Table 1). Anaerobes alone, most often *Peptostreptococcus* spp., were isolated from 24 (12.9%) patients. Mixed flora including aerobes and anaerobes were present in 26 (14%) patients. No bacterial growth was noted in 18 (9.7%) patients. Thus, the addition of anaerobic methodology to the processing of specimens enabled the isolation of bacteria from 90% of the patients studied. This rate is higher than that obtained in studies in which anaerobic techniques were not used (2). Even though the ear canal was not sterilized prior to the procedure, it is unlikely that the *Peptostreptococcus* spp. isolates were of ear canal origin as that site is mainly colonized by *Propionibacterium acnes* (14).

In the second study (11), where the tympanic membrane was disinfected, three anaerobes were recovered from 28 infants: two *Clostridium* spp. and one *Peptostreptococcus magnus*.

TABLE 1 Bacteria Isolated from 186 Cases of Acute Otitis Media

Isolates	Number of isolates	Percentage of patients with positive cultures
Aerobic bacteria		
Streptococcus pneumoniae	62	37
Haemophilus influenzae	52	30
Staphylococcus aureus	15	9
Group A beta-hemolytic streptococci	9	5
Pseudomonas aeruginosa	3	2
Group D Enterococcus	3	2
Others	12	7
Total number of aerobic bacteria	156	
Anaerobic bacteria		
Peptostreptococcus spp.	39	21
Propionibacterium spp.	12	7
Others[a]	5	3
Total number of anaerobic bacteria	56	
Total number of aerobic and anaerobic bacteria	212	

[a] One each of *Veillonella* spp., *Bifidobacterium* spp., *Eubacterium* spp., *Clostridium ramosum*, and microaerophilic streptococci.
Source: From Ref. 10.

In the third study, two anaerobes (*Bacteroides fragilis* and *Porphyromonas gingivalis*) were recovered from 2 of 80 children (13).

The fourth study was of middle-ear aspirates and external auditory canals of 50 children with spontaneous perforation (12). Bacterial growth was present in 51 of 61 ear aspirates obtained from 46 (92%) patients. The organisms isolated mainly from the external ear canal were *S. epidermidis* isolates, *P. acnes*, and alpha-hemolytic streptococci. Aerobic bacteria alone were found in the ear aspirates of 47 patients (92%), anaerobes alone in 1 (2%), and both aerobes and anaerobes in three (6%). The predominant middle-ear isolates were *S. pneumoniae*, *H. influenzae*, GABHS, and *M. catarrhalis*. The anaerobes recovered in the middle ear were *Peptostreptococcus* spp. (2) and *P. acnes* (2).

The study demonstrate that specimens of otorrhea collected from the external auditory canals can be misleading as only 44 of the 61 (72%) isolates recovered from the middle ear were also present in the ear canal. Peptostreptococci were recovered from 17% of inner ear aspirates but were recovered from only 3% of external ear canal specimens obtained in this study (12). This difference further supports their possible role in AOM. On the other hand, the rate of isolation of *P. acnes* from the external ear canal was 18%, which is higher than its recovery rate from inner ear aspirates (7%) (14).

Pathogenesis

The pathogenesis of AOM is multifactorial. Viral respiratory tract infection precedes AOM in 41% of children (8,15). The most common viruses were respiratory syncytial virus, influenza A and B, and adenoviruses. Viruses might facilitate bacterial infection due to their ability to increase nasopharyngeal colonization by potential bacterial pathogens, alter host defenses, and impair cellular and humoral immunity, through production of inflammation that obstructs the Eustachian tube which can lead to introduction of nasopharyngeal flora to the middle ear (16). These virus-induced effects may be partially responsible for the high rate of unresponsiveness of AOM to antimicrobials and probably contribute to the frequency of relapse, recurrence, or chronicity (8,15).

The horizontally placed Eustachian tube, which opens at a lower level in the infant's nasopharynx than in that of the child or adult, may allow easy access to infection through regurgitated milk or vomitus. The infant has a poorly developed immunity to upper respiratory infections of viral origin or bacterial sequela.

Obstruction of the tube can result in the formation of negative pressure in the middle ear and subsequent formation of a transudate in that space. This space can become contaminated with bacteria through reflux of mucus from the nasopharynx, causing middle-ear infection. This mode of infection can explain the route by which aerobic and anaerobic bacteria, which are part of the oral flora, gain access to the middle ear.

The anaerobic organisms that were recovered from the middle ear of infected children are part of the normal oropharyngeal flora. The isolation of anaerobes, all known pathogens of the upper and lower respiratory tracts, suggests a primary or ancillary role for these bacteria in the etiology of AOM.

Some anaerobic (*Prevotella* and *Peptostreptococcus* spp.) and aerobic (alpha- and gamma-hemolytic streptococci) bacteria that are part of the normal oropharyngeal flora can possess in vitro interference capability against oropharyngeal pathogens. These interfering organisms were found in greater numbers in the oropharynx and adenoids of children who are not otitis media prone, compared with otitis media-prone individuals (17,18). The utilization of antimicrobials that spare the normal flora can assist in preserving the interfering flora and reduce colonization by potential pathogens. Two recent study compared the effect of antimicrobials used to treat AOM in children on the nasopharyngeal flora (19,20). Both of these studies compared treatment with amoxicillin–clavulanate in one study to a second generation cephalosporin (cefprozil) (19), and the other to an extended-spectrum third generation cephalosporin (cefdinir) (20). Amoxicillin–clavulanate has a broad spectrum of antimicrobial efficacy-including activity against potentially interfering organisms, while the cephalosporins are less inhibitory of these organisms. The oropharyngeal flora at the end of treatment of AOM with amoxicillin–clavulanate therapy was more depleted of organisms with protective potential than the oral flora following cefprozil or cefdinir therapies (19,20). The patients in one of the studies were followed for three months and these changes were still apparent (20). Recolonization with pathogens occurred more rapidly in those treated with amoxicillin–clavulanate even after three months.

Diagnosis

The child may present with crying, irritability, and restless sleep. These may be the only signs in an infant, or the infant may rub or pull at the ear. Older children will complain of pain, dizziness, and headache. Fever in infants may be very high, or it may be absent. Symptoms of an upper respiratory tract infection are usually present. Vomiting or diarrhea, or both, may be prominent. The symptoms of AOM involving anaerobes are similar to those found in infections caused by aerobes and facultatives. Examination of the ear may reveal distortion or absence of clear landmarks and light reflex, impaired drum mobility, opaqueness, thickening, flaming and diffusely red drum rather than the normal pearl-gray, and the drum may bulge. If the tympanic membrane has ruptured, an opening may be seen as discharging pus or serous fluid. A foul-smelling exudate or pus is associated with the presence of anaerobic bacteria.

A conductive-type hearing loss is always present. It should be noted that mild redness of the drum in the presence of high fever is often entirely nonspecific and is related only to the fever. Hyperemia of the drum may occur with crying.

Under certain circumstances, tympanocentesis or myringotomy should be performed (21). Indications for tympanocentesis include failure to respond to antimicrobial therapy, neonatal age, the presence of severe symptoms including severe otalgia or high fever, and suppurative complications. This procedure could be beneficial for some patients for whom the determination of the etiology of the AOM and the antimicrobial sensitivity of the organism(s), drainage of pus, and relief of pain and acute symptoms is important. Bacterial cultures for aerobic and anaerobic bacteria should be obtained. A simplified technique, using a modified Medicut*, can prevent gross contamination of the specimen (22).

Management

Supportive therapy, including analgesics, antipyretics, and local heat, can be helpful. Although an oral decongestant may relieve some nasal congestion and antihistamines may help patients with known or suspected nasal allergy, their efficacy has not been proved.

The goal of antimicrobial therapy is to eradiate the pathogen(s), prevent recurrences and complications, and facilitate recovery. Although spontaneous resolution of AOM is common and may occur in about two-thirds of patients, it is impossible to predict which child will require antimicrobials to improve (23).

The recently published American Academy of Pediatrics Guidelines for the treatment of AOM suggest the observation option and use of antimicrobials only for those younger than six months or those with a certain diagnosis between six months and two years and with a certain diagnosis and severe symptoms in older age (24). However, concern about the implementations of these guidelines exists as antibiotics provide more rapid and enhanced resolution of symptoms, better outcomes as compared with no treatment, fewer suppurative complications (e.g., acute mastoiditis), corrective surgeries, and recurrences.

The duration of therapy is also controversial. Although most physician use 10 days of therapy, a shorter course of five to seven days can be given to children older than two years, those who have no history of recurrences or other serious medical problem (25), and those who do not attend a day care center (26). The selection of the antimicrobial agents for treatment of the infection should depend on the bacterial cause of the infection. Since the common offending microbiological agents are *S. pneumoniae* and *H. influenzae,* most of the patients respond favorably to amoxicillin. However, the growing resistance of *H. influenzae* and *M. catarrhalis* to amoxcillin through the production of beta-lactamase, and *S. pneumoniae* through changes in the protein-binding site increased the risk of antimicrobials failing to clear the infection. The addition of clavulanic acid (a beta-lactamase inhibitor) to amoxicillin, however, and the increase in the dose of amoxicillin to 90 mg/kg per day has made this agent effective against resistant organisms. The second (cefuroxime axetil) and third generation cephalosporins (cefdinir and cefpedoxime proxetil) are also effective because of their activity against *H. influenzae* and *M. catarrhalis* and, intermediately, penicillin-resistant *S. pneumoniae*. One third of *S. pneumoniae* resist all macrolides and azithromycin has poor in vivo efficacy against *H. influenzae.*

Amoxicillin (90 mg/kg per day) is recommended as first-line agent. For patients with clinically defined treatment failure after two to three days of therapy, alternative agents include oral amoxicillin–clavulanate, cefdinir, cefuroxime, and intramuscular ceftriaxone. Clindamycin is recommended as therapy for AOM due to intermediately resistant *S. pneumoniae* infection. In patients who are allergic to penicillin, a macrolide (i.e., azithromycin, clarithromycin) or trimethoprim-sulfamethoxazole (TMP-SMX) may be given (24).

The anaerobes recovered in AOM are susceptible to penicillins and the other antibiotics that are commonly used to treat AOM. However, TMP-SMX is effective against only 50% of *Peptostreptococcus* spp., the major anaerobe isolated in AOM.

Complications

Complications are relatively uncommon and include perforation of drum resulting in CSOM, hearing loss, chronic serous otitis (glue ear), acquired cholesteatoma, mastoiditis, petrositis, meningitis, brain epidural and subdural abscesses. Fortunately, the intracranial suppurative complications are uncommon in recent years. These complications usually occur following CSOM or mastoiditis through direct extension or by vascular channels.

Facial paralysis secondary to involvement of facial nerves may occur during an episode of AOM. Suppurative labyrinthitis may occur during an episode of AOM from the direct invasion of bacteria through the round or oval windows.

OTITIS MEDIA WITH EFFUSION

OME is a common cause of mild hearing loss in children, most often between the ages of two and seven years. The middle ear contains fluid that varies from a thin transudate to a very thick consistency (glue ear). Eustachian tube obstruction is usually caused by primary congenital tube dysfunction. Other possible contributing factors are allergic rhinitis, adenoidal hyperplasia, supine feeding position, or a submucous cleft. Middle-ear effusion was found to persist for at least one month in up to 40% of children who had suffered from AOM, and for at least three months in 10% of afflicted children (27).

Microbiology

Organisms similar to those isolated in AOM (*S. pneumoniae*, *H. influenzae*, *M. catarrhalis*, and GABHS) were recovered from 22% to 45%(28) of aspirates of COME. Bacteria were more often recovered in those below two years (41%) as compared to older children (17%) (29). Polymerase chain reaction (PCR) methodology revealed the presence of bacterial DNA for *M. catarrhalis*, *H. influenzae*, or *S. pneumoniae* in up to 94.5% of the ear aspirates (30,31).

None of these studies, however, employed techniques for transportation and cultivation of anaerobes, and the external canal was not sterilized. In a study that employed methodology adequate for isolation of anaerobes, Brook et al. (32) recovered bacteria from 23 of 57 (41%) patients (Table 2) including anaerobes. Anaerobic bacteria were the only isolates in 17% of the culture-positive aspirates, and in an additional 26%, they were present mixed with aerobes. Aerobic organisms alone were recovered in 13 aspirates (57%). A total of 45 bacterial isolates, 31 aerobes (*H. influenzae*, *S. aureus*, and *S. pneumoniae*) and 14 anaerobes (*Peptostreptococcus* spp., pigmented *Prevotella* and *Porphyromonas*, and *P. acnes*) were recovered. Interestingly, similar anaerobes were recovered from patients with acute (10) and chronic (33) otitis media. Nine beta-lactamase-producing bacteria (BLPB) were recovered from 8 patients (35%). These included all five isolates of *S. aureus*, three of the five pigmented *Prevotella* and *Porphyromonas*, and one of eight *H. influenzae*.

Using PCR, Beswick et al. (34) detected *P. acnes* in 4 of 12 serous effusion, and *Peptostreptococcus* and *Clostridium* spp. in one patient each, along with *A. otitis* in 6.

The microbiology of CSOM in children was found to correlate with the duration of the condition and the patient's age (35). Bacterial growth was noted in 47 of 114 (41%) children with CSOM. Aerobes alone were recovered in 27 aspirates (57% of the culture-positive aspirates), anaerobes alone in 7 (15%), and mixed aerobic and anaerobic bacteria in 13 (28%). Thus, 57 aerobes (15 *H. influenzae*, 13 *S. pneumoniae*, and 12 *Staphylococcus* spp.) and 26 anaerobes (10 *Peptostreptococcus* spp., 8 *Prevotella* spp., and 4 *P. acnes*) were isolated. The rate of positive cultures (20 of 36; 56%) was higher in patients below two years of age than in those above two years of age (27 of 78; 35%). *S. pneumoniae* and *H. influenzae* were more often isolated in children below two years of age and those with effusion for three to five months, whereas anaerobes were recovered more often in those above two years of age and those with effusion for 6 to 13

TABLE 2 Bacteria Isolated from 23 Culture-Positive Serous Effusions

Isolates	Number of isolates[a]
Aerobic bacteria	
Streptococcus pneumoniae	5
Group D streptococci	1
Alpha-hemolytic streptococci	4
Gamma-hemolytic streptococci	1
Staphylococcus aureus	5(5)
Staphylococcus epidermidis	4
Diphtheroids	2
Haemophilus influenzae	8(1)
Escherichia coli	1
Subtotal aerobes	31
Anaerobic bacteria	
Porphyromonas asaccharolyticus	3
Peptostreptococcus micros	1
Streptococcus constellatus	1
Veillonella alcalescens	1
Propionibacterium acnes	3
Prevotella melaninogenica	3(2)
Prevotella intermedius	2(1)
Subtotal anaerobes	14
Total bacteria	45

[a] Values in parentheses denote the number of beta-lactamase-producing strains.
Source: Modified from Ref. 32.

months. These data illustrate the effects of the length of effusion and age on the recovery of aerobic and anaerobic bacteria in COME.

Brook et al. (36) correlated the past use of antimicrobials with the recovered organism's antimicrobial susceptibility in 129 children with COME. Resistance to the antimicrobial used was found in 60 (65%) isolates, recovered from 41 (71%) of the patients, 37 (90%) of those had been treated within three months of culture and 4 (10%) had completed treatment more than three months ($p<0.01$).

Concordance in recovery of organisms was observed in 69% of 30 children with concomitant COME and chronic sinusitis, illustrating the common bacterial etiology between these conditions (37). A total of 42 isolates, 24 aerobic and 18 anaerobic, were recovered; 27 were isolated from both sites, four from the ear alone, and 11 from the sinus alone. The most common isolates were 9 *H. influenzae*, 7 *S. pneumoniae*, 8 *Prevotella* spp., and 6 *Peptostreptococcus* spp.

Pathogenesis

Eustachian tube dysfunction is the primary cause of OME. All such patients have poor tubal function. There are two types of Eustachian tube obstruction that can result in middle-ear effusion: mechanical and functional (38). Mechanical obstruction results from inflammation by bacteria or viruses, allergy, hypertrophic adenoids, or tumors of the nasopharynx. Functional obstruction results from persistent collapse of the cartilaginous tube. This collapse may be due to increased tubal compliance or an inadequate opening mechanism, or both. Currently, the continued presence of fluid is believed to be due to chronic stimulation of inflammatory mediators (39). Symptoms appear quickly in OME, but resolved gradually over several months.

Evidence regarding the role of bacteria, viruses, and mycoplasmae in the etiology and pathogenesis of acute inflammatory disease in the middle ear is conflicting. The bacteria associated with OME in young children are *S. pneumoniae*, *H. influenzae*, and GABHS (2). Although there is a general agreement that otitis media with a purulent effusion is usually a bacterial infection, there is no uniformity of opinion on the role of bacteria in the serous, seromucinous, and mucoid OME. However, their persistence in the middle-ear fluid may stimulate inflammatory mediators.

The presence of aerobic and anaerobic bacteria in some nonsuppurative effusions suggests that both are involved in the pathogenesis of OME.

Diagnosis

Diagnosis is often delayed because of vague or absent symptoms. Symptoms may include slight earache, a feeling of watery bubbles in the ear, or a sensation that the head is full. If the middle ear is not completely filled with fluid, there may be air bubbles or a meniscus visible through the tympanic membrane. The eardrum is thin, shows a loss of translucency, may be retracted, have diminished movement, and exhibit a change in color from the normal gray to a pale or even bluish hue.

Management

The role of bacteria in the pathogenesis of this ear disease is not yet clear; however, antimicrobial agents often are used in an attempt to clear the ear effusion of bacteria. The benefit of antimicrobial therapy is controversial, although a meta-analysis of 10 studies showed a 22% benefit of their use (40). A recent study showed that antibiotic treatment improves the middle-ear status in patients with OME and amoxicillin–clavulanate is superior to penicillin V (41).

However, the recent Guidelines by the American Academies of Family Physicians, Otolaryngology—Head and Neck Surgery, and Pediatrics concluded that (*i*) because anti-histamines and decongestants are ineffective for OME, they should not be used for treatment and (*ii*) antimicrobials and corticosteroids do not have long-term efficacy and should not be used for routine management (42).

It is important to distinguish the child with OME who is at risk for speech, language, or learning problems from other children with OME and more promptly evaluate hearing, speech, language, and need for intervention in children at risk. The child with OME who is not at risk is managed with watchful waiting for three months from the date of effusion onset or diagnosis. It is also recommended that hearing testing be conducted when OME persists for three months or longer or at any time that language delay, learning problems, or a significant hearing loss is suspected. Children with persistent OME not at risk should be reexamined at three-to-six-month intervals until the effusion is no longer present, significant hearing loss is identified, or structural abnormalities of the eardrum or middle ear are suspected, and when a child becomes a surgical candidate for tympanostomy tube insertion. Adenoidectomy is not recommended unless a distinct indication such as nasal obstruction or chronic adenoiditis exists. Repeat surgery consists of adenoidectomy plus myringotomy with or without tube insertion. Tonsillectomy alone or myringotomy alone is not used to treat OME (42).

The presence of anaerobic as well as aerobic bacteria in the serous ear aspirate raises the question of whether the antimicrobial agents currently used are adequate and whether antibiotics effective also against some of the BLPB should be used. The high recovery rate of organisms in COME that are resistant to the antibiotics used to treat AOM suggests that failure of these antibiotics to completely eradicate these organisms may contribute to their persistence (36). Additional controlled studies are needed to define the value of antimicrobial treatment in children with AOM and OME and to clarify the role of bacteria in the pathogenesis of this form of otitis media.

CHRONIC SUPPURATIVE OTITIS MEDIA AND CHOLESTEATOMA

CSOM can be insidious, persistent, and very often destructive, with sometimes irreversible sequelae, such as hearing deficit and subsequent learning disabilities in children. In many patients with CSOM, a cholesteatoma may develop; a cholesteatoma is a pocket of skin that invades the middle ear and mastoid spaces from the edge of a perforation (43).

CSOM and cholesteatoma tend to be persistent and progressive and very often cause destructive irreversible changes in the bony structure of the ear. In many cases, the perforation of the tympanic membrane that occurs during AOM persists into the chronic stage.

Microbiology

Although past studies reported the recovery of anaerobic organisms from many cases of CSOM, aerobic organisms, mainly *S. aureus* and gram-negative enteric bacilli, were considered to be the major pathogens. Several studies reaffirmed the role of anaerobes in CSOM (33,44–55) and reported the recovery of anaerobes from 8% to 59% of patients (Table 3) (45–55). The variability in the rate of recovery of anaerobes in these studies may be a result of differences in geographic locations and laboratory techniques. In several of these studies, the delays in cultivation were extensive and the length of incubation was inadequate for anaerobic bacteria. The predominant anaerobic organisms recovered in these studies were anaerobic gram-positive cocci and pigmented *Prevotella* and *Porphyromonas* spp.

In a study of pediatric patients suffering from CSOM (33), anaerobic bacteria were isolated from 56% of ear aspirates (Table 3). The majority of the anaerobic organisms isolated were gram-positive anaerobic cocci, gram-negative bacilli (including the *B. fragilis* group), and *Fusobacterium nucleatum*. The predominant aerobic bacteria isolated were enteric gram-negative rods (mostly *P. aeruginosa*) and *S. aureus*. Anaerobic isolates usually were mixed with other anaerobic or aerobic bacteria and the number of isolates ranged between two and four per specimen, thereby demonstrating the polymicrobial etiology of CSOM.

Another study demonstrated that only half of the bacteria recovered from the middle ear were also present in the external auditory canal (48). Furthermore, external ear canal culture in many cases yielded bacteria that were not present in the middle ear. These findings demonstrate that cultures collected from the external auditory canal prior to its sterilization can be misleading. This is particularly important in the case of *P. aeruginosa*, which is more frequently recovered from the external auditory canal than from the middle ear. Although this

TABLE 3 Frequency of Recovery of Anaerobic and Aerobic Organisms Recovered in Chronic Suppurative Otitis Media

Author (reference)	Number of cases where anaerobes were recovered/total number cases (%)	Anaerobic cocci	Anaerobic gram-negative bacilli	Fusobacterium spp.	Clostridium spp.	Staphylococcus aureus	Pseudomonas spp.	Other aerobic gram-negative rods
Karma et al. (45)	38/114 (33)	15	29	2	2	32	16	37
Sugita et al. (46)	62/760 (8)	38	18	6	2	8	12	31
Aygagari et al. (47)	68/115 (59)	33	43	7	6	22	29	32
Brook (48)	35/68 (51)	31	21	4	3	15	33	31
Sweeney et al. (49)	52/130 (44)	7	54	9	1	33	25	86
Constable and Butler (50)	20/100 (20)	9	7	—	—	29	15	34
Papastavros et al. (51)	19/44 (43)	10	12	—	—	2	20	
Rotimi et al. (52)	59/140 (42)		59	—	—	—	67	84
Erkan et al. (53)	111/183 (61)	20	63				68	
Ito et al. (54)	9/31 (29)	9	3	1	—	16	7	10
Brook and Santosa (55)	27/38 (71)	14	21	8	4	8	11	14

organism is a common inhabitant of the external auditory canal, it can also be recovered from the middle ear where the organism may participate in the inflammatory process. Direct middle-ear aspirations through the perforation in the eardrum are therefore more reliable in establishing the bacteriology of CSOM and can assist in the selection of proper antimicrobial therapy.

The role of anaerobic bacteria in this infection is suggested also by their higher recovery rate from the middle ear alone, compared with their recovery from the external canal (48). This is more apparent when *P. acnes* isolates are deleted from the total number of isolates. Thirty-eight anaerobic strains were recovered from the middle ear alone, compared with seven from the external canal.

We evaluated the bacteriology of 48 middle-ear aspirates from children with CSOM (56). Aerobic bacteria alone were involved in 22 cases (46%), anaerobic organisms alone in five cases (12%), and mixed aerobic and anaerobic isolates were recovered in 21 cases (44%). Anaerobes and aerobes BLPB were recovered in two-third of patients. These included *S. aureus*, *B. fragilis* groups, pigmented *Prevotella* and *Porphyromonas* group, *H. influenzae*, *M. catarrhalis*, and *Staphylococcus* spp. (56) Furthermore, the enzyme beta-lactamase detected in 79% of the ear aspirates contained BLPB in excess of 10^4 colony forming units (CFU)/mL (Table 4) (57).

The bacteriology of cholesteatomas present in chronically infected ears provides further support for the role of anaerobes in chronic ear infection. Cholesteatoma specimens were obtained from 28 patients undergoing surgery for CSOM and cholesteatoma (58). A total of 74 bacterial isolates were present in 24 (40 aerobes and 34 anaerobes) specimens (Table 5). Aerobes alone were isolated from 8 (33.3%) patients, 4 (26.7%) yielded only anaerobes, and 12 (50%) had both aerobic and anaerobic bacteria. Fifty isolates (27 aerobes and 23 anaerobes) were present in a concentration $>10^6$ CFU/g. The most commonly isolated aerobes were *P. aeruginosa* (9), *Proteus* spp. (7), *K. pneumoniae* (5), *S. aureus* (5), and *E. coli* (4). The most common anaerobes were gram-positive anaerobic cocci (12), anaerobic gram-negative bacilli (AGNB; 12 including five *B. fragilis* group), *Clostridium* spp. (3), and *Bifidobacterium* spp. (3). These findings indicate the polymicrobial aerobic and anaerobic bacteriology of CSOM with cholesteatoma and concur with data obtained in other studies of the bacteriology of CSOM (45–55). Similar data were also found by Iino et al. (59), who also detected organic volatile acids (a product of the anaerobic bacteria metabolism) in the cholesteatoma.

Pathogenesis

Cholesteatoma that accompanies CSOM induces absorption of the underlying bone, but the mechanism by which this occurs is not well understood. Various theories attempt to explain the possible role of different factors in the process of expansion of the cholesteatoma and the collagen degradation that occurs in its vicinity. The volatile acids produced by anaerobic bacteria may play a role in this process (59).

TABLE 4 Recovery of BLPB and "free" Beta-Lactamase in Chronically Infected Ear Aspirates

	38 of 54 (70%)	
	Number of BLPB/total isolates	Percentage of samples with detectable free enzyme
Staphylococcus aureus	15	90
Moraxella catarrhalis	2/4	75
Haemophilus influenzae	5/11	100
Pseudomonas aeruginosa	7/10	71
Klebsiella pneumoniae	15/21	71
Gram-negative anaerobic bacilli[a]	12/15	80

[a] Pigmented *Prevotella* and *Porphyromonas* spp. and *Bacteroides* spp.
Abbreviation: BLPB, beta-lactamase-producing bacteria.
Source: From Ref. 57.

TABLE 5 Bacterial Isolates Obtained from Surgical Specimens in 24 Patients with Cholesteatoma

	Concentrations of bacteria (CFU/g)		
	$>10^6$	$<10^6$	**Total number of isolates**
Aerobes and facultatives			
Gram-positive cocci	2		2
Group A beta-hemolytic streptococci		1	1
Staphylococcus aureus	1	4	5
Staphylococcus epidermidis	2	1	3
Gram-negative bacilli	3	4	7
Proteus mirabilis			
Proteus rettgeri		2	2
Pseudomonas aeruginosa	2	7	9
Klebsiella pneumoniae		5	5
Escherichia coli	1	3	4
Serratia marcescens	2		2
Total number of aerobes	13	27	40
Anaerobes			
Peptostreptococcus spp.	3	9	12
Anaerobic gram-positive bacilli	5	3	8
Gram-negative bacilli			
Fusobacterium nucleatum		2	2
Pigmented *Prevotella* and *Porphyromonas*		3	3
Bacteroides fragilis group	1	4	5
Bacteroides spp.	2	2	4
Total number of anaerobes	11	23	34
Total number of bacteria	24	50	74

Abbreviation: CFU, colony forming units.
Source: From Ref. 58.

A possible role of anaerobic and aerobic bacteria in the destructive process is suggested, and further study to ascertain their effects on the surrounding bone and collagen is warranted.

Clearly, cholesteatoma contains bacteria similar to that recovered from aspirates of chronically infected ears. It seems reasonable that the cholesteatoma present in a chronically infected ear serves as a nidus of chronic infection.

Bacterial synergy was demonstrated between the aerobic organisms commonly found in CSOM and AGNB and anaerobic cocci and was especially apparent between *P. aeruginosa* and *S. aureus* and the anaerobes (60). These findings are of particular relevance to the pathologic role of these organisms in CSOM in that the combination of *P. aeruginosa* and anaerobic cocci was isolated from 40% of patients with CSOM, and *S. aureus* and anaerobic cocci were recovered in 9% of these patients (33,55,56).

The demonstration of synergy between the anaerobic and aerobic bacteria commonly recovered in ear infections further suggests their pathogenic role in these infections.

The microbial dynamics of persistent otitis media that eventually became chronic was also investigated (61). The study was done over a period of 36 to 55 days when the aerobic–anaerobic microbiology of ear aspirate was established for children who presented with AOM with spontaneous perforation, did not respond to initial empiric therapy, and developed a persistent infection. Repeated aspirates of middle-ear fluid revealed the dynamic of emergence of new microbial pathogens and the response of the patients to antimicrobials.

Failure to respond to antimicrobial therapy was associated with the emergence of resistant anaerobic and aerobic bacteria in the following third and fourth cultures. These organisms were pigmented *Prevotella* and *Porphyromonas* spp, *F. nucleatum*, and *P. aeruginosa*. The infection was cured in all instances following administration of antimicrobials effective against these bacteria (Fig. 1).

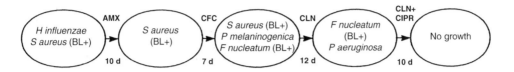

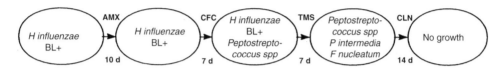

FIGURE 1 Dynamics of the microbiology and therapy of persistent otitis media. *Abbreviations*: AMX, amoxicillin; BL+, beta-lactamase producer; CFC, cefaclor; CIPR, ciprofloxacin; CLN, clindamycin; TMS, trimethoprim. *Source*: From Ref. 61.

Diagnosis

The common symptom is the presence of recurrent or persistent ear drainage. CSOM may be painless and free of fever in the intervals between acute exacerbations.

The eardrum can be perforated and foul-smelling pus may be present which suggests the presence of anaerobic bacteria. Peripheral perforations provide a greater risk of cholesteatoma formation. Mastoid tenderness may be present.

Radiographic studies for evidence of mastoid involvement may reveal pathologic findings. Aerobic and anaerobic bacteriologic cultures obtained using tympanocentesis or through the perforation are imperative. Pus collected from the ear canal can be misleading as it can contain isolates that are part of the ear canal flora and are absent from the middle ear. This is of particular importance in the case of *P. aeruginosa*, which is a known colonizer of the ear canal (14). Secondary invaders following perforations are frequent causes of chronic drainage and are much more resistant to therapy.

Management

Attempts to treat CSOM using antimicrobial therapy alone generally are not successful. The organisms usually treated are the aerobic isolates, mainly *S. aureus* and the gram-negative enteric bacilli. In an open study, Brook (62) used parenteral carbenicillin or clindamycin to treat CSOM. Combined therapy with gentamicin was used when aerobic gram-negative rods were also recovered. Although therapy was successful in only half of the patients, this study demonstrated that therapy directed against the organisms isolated from a patient's effusion could eradicate the infection in many instances. Kenna et al. (63) were able to achieve an improvement in 32 of 36 (89%) patients with CSOM with parenteral antimicrobial agents and daily aural toilet. Although the authors did not obtain cultures of anaerobic bacteria, many of the antimicrobial agents they used were effective against anaerobic bacteria.

The importance of coverage for anaerobic bacteria was demonstrated in a retrospective study that compared the efficacy of clindamycin, amoxicillin, erythromycin, and cefaclor (64). Anti-pseudomonal therapy was added to either therapy whenever *Pseudomonas* was present in the middle ear. The most rapid time for resolution of the infection was noticed with clindamycin (8.3 ± 0.6 days, $p < 0.001$), as compared with ampicillin (12.0 ± 0.8 days), erythromycin (16.5 ± 1.6 days), and cefaclor (14.6 ± 2.3 days). Resolution of the infection was achieved in 16 of 20 (80%) of those treated with clindamycin, 12 of 24 (50%) treated with ampicillin, 6 of 13 (46%) treated with erythromycin, and 4 of 12 (33%) treated with cefaclor. Organisms resistant to the antimicrobial used were recovered in 26 of 31 patients who failed to respond to therapy.

Until recently, most of the anaerobes recovered from respiratory tract and orofacial infections were susceptible to penicillin. *S. aureus* and *B. fragilis* groups are known to resist penicillin through production of beta-lactamase. However, an alarming number of AGNB, mostly pigmented *Prevotella* and *Porphyromonas* and *Fusobacterium* spp., formerly susceptible to penicillins, are currently showing increasing resistance to these drugs by virtue of production of the enzyme beta-lactamase (65).

The isolation of BLPB from over two-thirds of chronically inflamed ears (56) and the ability to actually measure the activity of the enzyme in the ear aspirate (57) have important implications for chemotherapy. Such organisms can release the enzyme and degrade penicillins or cephalosporins in the area of the infection. In this way, they can protect not only themselves but also penicillin-sensitive pathogens. Penicillin therapy directed against a susceptible pathogen might be rendered ineffective by the presence of a penicillinase-producing organism (66).

These findings raise the questions of whether the treatment of CSOM with penicillins is adequate and whether therapy should be directed at the eradication of these organisms whenever they are present.

Antimicrobials or their combinations that are effective against BLPB include clindamycin, cefoxitin, a combination of metronidazole and a macrolide, and ampicillin, amoxicillin, or a penicillin (i.e., ticarcillin, piperacillin) plus a beta-lactamase inhibitor (i.e., clavulanic acid, sulbactam). In instances where *P. aeruginosa* is considered to be a true pathogen, parenteral therapy with aminoglycosides or an anti-pseudomonal cephalosporin (i.e., ceftazidime, cefepime), or oral or parenteral treatment with a fluoroquinoline (only in postpubertal patients) should be added. Parenteral therapy with a carbapenem or tigecycline will provide adequate coverage for all potential pathogens, anaerobic as well as aerobic bacteria. Coverage for methicillin resistant *S. aureus* can be achieved with vancomycin, tigecycline, or lizezolid.

Topical instillation of appropriate antibiotic drops is also sometimes recommended, alone or in combination with systemic therapy. Topical otic agents include the combination of neomycin, polymyxin, and hydrocortisone, and polymyxin B, neomycin, and fluoroquinoline (ciprofloxacin, ofloxacin). However, their penetration into the middle-ear cavity is unpredictable. Combination of medical treatment and surgical debridement is often needed. Myringoplasty or tympanoplasty is done at about age 10 or older. Cholesteatoma should be treated surgically when diagnosed.

Complications

Mastoiditis or inflammation of the mastoid air cell system frequently accompanies CSOM. The intracranial complications of CSOM are meningitis, focal encephalitis, intracranial abscesses (brain abscess, extradural abscess, and subdural abscess), and otitic hydrocephalus.

A patient with CSOM who develops signs of intracranial complications should be treated rapidly and thoroughly. Intracranial involvement is signaled by severe earache, constant and persistent headache, nausea and vomiting, seizures, fever, or localized neurologic findings.

ACUTE OTITIS EXTERNA (SWIMMER'S EAR)

External otitis is defined as a varying degree of an inflammation of the auricle, external ear canal, or outer surface of the tympanic membrane (67). The etiology of the inflammation can be an infection, inflammatory dermatoses, trauma, or a combination of these.

The clinical infection is divided to be either localized or diffuse, and acute or chronic. Predisposing factors to infection include extraneous trauma, loss of the canal's protective water-repellent coating provided by the cerumen, maceration of the skin from water or excessive humidity, and glandular obstruction.

Sudden onset of diffuse infection involving the external auditory canal is termed acute otitis externa (68). The most predominant cause of the acute infection is *P. aeruginosa*. The diffuse infection needs to be differentiated from a localized furunculosis of the hair follicles that is caused by aerobic gram-positive bacteria. Chronic otitis externa results from persistence of the infection that causes thickening of the canal skin. Extension of the infection that encompasses the bone and cartilage is termed necrotizing otitis externa (69,70).

Microbiology

The most predominant isolates causing the infection are *P. aeruginosa*, and *S. aureus*. Other pathogens that are less often received are *E. coli*, *Proteus* spp., *K. pneumoniae*, *Enterobacter* spp., and anaerobic bacteria (68,71,72).

The role of anaerobic bacteria in external otitis was retrospectively evaluated in 46 patients including 12 children (71). A total of 42 aerobes, 22 anaerobes, and three *Candida albicans* were recovered. Aerobes alone were isolated from 31 patients (67%), anaerobes alone from 8 (17%), and mixed aerobic and anaerobic bacteria were isolated from 4 (9%). The most common isolates were *P. aeruginosa* (19 isolates), *Peptostreptococcus* spp. (11), *S. aureus* (7), and *Bacteroides* spp. (5). One isolate was recovered from 30 patients (65%), two isolates were recovered from 11 (24%), and three isolates were recovered from 5 (11%).

Another study prospectively evaluated the microbiological agents in 23 patients with otitis externa (72). A total of 33 aerobic and two anaerobic bacteria were recovered. The most common isolates were *P. aeruginosa* (14 isolates), *S. aureus* (7), *Acinetobacter calcoaceticus* (2), *Proteus mirabilis* (2), *Enterococcus faecalis* (2), *B. fragilis* (1), and *P. magnus* (1).

Diagnosis

Acute otitis externa causes different signs and symptoms depending on the severity and progression of the infection. The earlier stages are pre-inflammatory where itching, edema, and fullness sensation predominate (70). This is followed by the acute inflammatory stages divided into mild, moderate, and severe pain, where itching, auricular tenderness, purulent secretion, edema, and external auditory canal pain gradually intensify.

Management

Cultures obtained from the deeper portion of the canal can be helpful in tailoring therapy to the offending pathogen(s). The most important step in therapy is a thorough gentle-cleansing, suction, and instrumentation of the external auditory canal under direct microscopic inspection. In instances where the debris is hard, crusted, and difficult to take out, topical ophthalmic/otic drops or hydrogen peroxide can help in softening the canal's contents. In cases with advanced inflammation where the canal may be obliterated, a gentle dilatation of the canal can be done and a wick can be placed to allow solutions to reach the infected tissues. A wick or gauze strip can be placed inside the canal. The wick can be left alone for a few days or changed in conjunction with ear cleansing until the edema subsides, allowing the drops to penetrate throughout the external canal. The frequency of canal cleansing depends on the amount of debris and secretion, and may vary once every one to five days.

The administration of topical therapy is made possible by adequate cleansing of the canal. The dose of topical therapy is three to four drops given three to four times per day for 7 to 14 days. The topical agents include acidifying agents, topical antibiotics, and/or antifungals. The acidifying agents' pH varies from 3.0 to 6.0, providing antibacterial and antifungal activities. The low pH induces a burning and stinging sensation. Topical steroids can also be employed, mixed with antibacterial agents, to assist in the resolution of the local edema. Topical otic preparations are more acidic than ophthalmic preparations and may be less tolerated. Ophthalmic solutions are of lesser viscosity and can penetrate with less difficulty through a narrow canal. Topical antifungals' pH is higher and therefore more easily tolerated.

The topical antimicrobial agents include tobamycin (with or without steroids), gentamicin, chloramphenicol (with or without steroids), ciprofloxacin, ofloxacin, norfloxacin, sulfactamide (with or without steroids), and polymyxin-B (with steroids). Antifungal agents include nystatin and clotrimazole (with or without steroids). Acidic solutions include acetic acid 2% (with or without steroids), methylrosaniline chloride 1% and 2%, merthiolate 1:1000, and phenol 1.5%.

Systemic antimicrobials are indicated when the infection extends into the surrounding periauricular area inducing local cellulitis or lymphadenitis. This generally occurs in infection caused by *P. aeruginosa* or *S. aureus*. Mild infection can be treated with oral antibiotics and followed up closely. Oral anti-pseudomonas antibiotics that can be given in mild infection are the quinolones (i.e., ciprofloxacin, ofloxacin) (73,74). However, their use in children is not yet approved and should be done with caution. These patients need to be closely followed because many infections caused by *P. aeruginosa* are difficult to treat on an outpatient basis, and experience with such therapy is limited. If *S. aureus* infection is present, an anti-staphylococcal agent such as dicloxacillin or cephalexin can be used. Vancomycin or linezolid may be needed to treat methicillin-resistant *S. aureus*. When parenteral therapy is needed, especially in severe infections, in the immunocompromised host or when quinolone therapy is not effective, the combination of ticarcillin–clavulanate, an aminoglycoside, or an anti-pseudomonal cephalosporin (i.e., ceftazidime, cefepime) can be used.

In cases where anaerobes are isolated or suspected, the administration of effective agents may be warranted. These include clindamycin, chloramphenicol, metronidazole, cefoxitin, imipenem or meropenem, or the combination of penicillin and a beta-lactamase inhibitor.

The choice of systemic antimicrobial therapy should be guided whenever possible by Gram-stain preparation of the culture smear and the results of cultures and susceptibility testing.

Pain control should not be neglected. This can be achieved according to the patient's needs by either topical or systemic medication. Topical therapy can be with steroid preparation that decreases the inflammation and edema. Systemic therapy can be with nonsteroidal antiinflammatory drugs or opioids.

Patients and parents should be educated to prevent repeated infection. This can be accomplished by the use of topical acidifying and canal drying agents, and non-traumatic drying of the canal following intense exercise, swimming, or bathing. Patients should also avoid swimming in, and exposure to contaminated water (75). Wearing ear canal obstructive equipment for prolonged periods of time can induce changes in the ear canal flow and induce infection (76).

REFERENCES

1. Gates GA, Klein JO, Lim DJ, et al. Recent advances in otitis media 1. Definitions, terminology, and classification of otitis media. Ann Otol Rhinol Laryngol Suppl 2002; 188:8–18.
2. Pichichero ME, Pichichero CL. Persistent otitis media: causative pathogen. Pediatr Infect Dis J 1995; 14:178–83.
3. Brook I. Microbiology of common infections in the upper respiratory tract. Prim Care 1998; 25:633–48.
4. Casey JR, Pichichero ME. Changes in frequency and pathogens causing acute otitis media in 1995–2003. Pediatr Infect Dis J 2004; 23:824–8.
5. Leibovitz E, Raiz S, Piglansky L, et al. Resistance pattern of middle ear fluid isolates in acute otitis media recently treated with antibiotics. Pediatr Infect Dis J 1998; 17:463–9.
6. Brook I, Gober AE. Microbiologic characteristics of persistent otitis media. Arch Otolaryngol Head Neck Surg 1998; 124:1350–2.
7. Schwartz RH, Brook I. Gram-negative rod bacteria as a cause of acute otitis media in children. Ear Nose Throat J 1981; 60:9–15.
8. Heikkinen T, Thint M, Chonmaitree T. Prevalence of various respiratory viruses in the middle ear during acute otitis media. N Engl J Med 1999; 340:260–4.
9. Brook I, Anthony BF, Finegold SM. Aerobic and anaerobic bacteriology of acute otitis media in children. J Pediatr 1978; 92:13–6.
10. Brook I. Otitis media in children: a prospective study of aerobic and anaerobic bacteriology. Laryngoscope 1979; 89:992–5.
11. Brook I, Schwartz R. Anaerobic bacteria in acute otitis media. Acta Otolaryngol 1981; 91:11–4.
12. Brook I, Gober AE. Reliability of the microbiology of spontaneously draining acute otitis media in children. Pediatr Infect Dis J 2000; 19:571–3.
13. del Castillo F, Barrio Gómez MI, Garcia A. Bacteriologic study of 80 cases of acute otitis media in children. Enferm Infecc Microbiol Clin 1994; 12:82–5.
14. Brook I. Microbiological studies of the bacterial flora of the external auditory canal in children. Acta Otolaryngol 1981; 91:285–6.

15. Chonmaitree T, Owen MJ, Howie VM. Respiratory viruses interfere with bacteriological response to antibiotic in children with acute otitis media. J Infect Dis 1990; 162:546–9.
16. Nokso-Koivisto J, Hovi T, Pitkaranta A. Viral upper respiratory tract infections in young children with emphasis on acute otitis media. Int J Pediatr Otorhinolaryngol 2006; 70:1333–42.
17. Brook I, Yocum P. Bacterial interference in the adenoids of otitis media prone children. Pediatr Infect Dis J 1999; 18:835–7.
18. Brook I, Gober AE. Bacterial interference in the nasopharynx of otitis media prone and non-otitis media prone children. Arch Otolaryngol Head Neck Surg 2000; 126:1011–3.
19. Brook I, Gober AE. Bacterial interference in the nasopharynx following antimicrobial therapy of acute otitis media. J Antimicrob Chemother 1998; 41:489–92.
20. Brook I, Gober AE. Long-term effects on the nasopharyngeal flora of children following antimicrobial therapy of acute otitis media with cefdinir or amoxycillin–clavulanate. J Med Microbiol 2005; 54:553–6.
21. Brook I. Tympanocentesis in the diagnosis and treatment of otitis media. Infect Med 2001; 18:363–6.
22. Brook I. A practical technique for tympanocentesis for culture of aerobic and anaerobic bacteria. Pediatrics 1980; 65:626–7.
23. Takata GS, Chan LS, Shekelle P, Morton SC, Mason W, Marcy SM. Evidence assessment of management of acute otitis media: I. The role of antibiotics in treatment of uncomplicated acute otitis media. Pediatrics 2001; 108:239–47.
24. American Academy of Pediatrics Subcommittee on Management of Acute Otitis Media. Diagnosis and management of acute otitis media. Pediatrics 2004; 113:1451–65.
25. Pichichero ME, Cohen R. Shortened course of antibiotic therapy for acute otitis media, sinusitis, and tonsillopharyngitis. Pediatr Infect Dis J 1997; 16:680–95.
26. Raoul L, Wientzen MD, Jr., Charlotte Barbey-Morel MD. Current concepts of therapy for otitis media. Curr Infect Dis Rep 1999; 1:22–6.
27. Klein JO, Teele DW, Pelton SI. New concepts in otitis media: results of investigations of the greater boston otitis media study group. Adv Pediatr 1992; 39:127–56.
28. Fergie N, Bayston R, Pearson JP, Birchall JP. Is otitis media with effusion a biofilm infection? Clin Otolaryngol 2004; 29:38–46.
29. Jero J, Karma P. Bacteriological findings and persistence of middle ear effusion in otitis media with effusion. Acta Otolaryngol (Stockh) 1997; 529(Suppl.):22–6.
30. Post JC, Preston RA, Aul JJ, et al. Molecular analysis of bacterial pathogens in otitis media with effusion. JAMA 1995; 273:1598–604.
31. Gok U, Bulut Y, Keles E, Yalcin S, Doymaz MZ. Bacteriological and PCR analysis of clinical material aspirated from otitis media with effusions. Int J Pediatr Otorhinolaryngol 2001; 60:49–54.
32. Brook I, Yocum P, Shah K, Feldman B, Epstein S. The aerobic and anaerobic aerobic and anaerobic bacteriologic features of serous otitis media in children. Am J Otolaryngol 1983; 4:389–92.
33. Brook I, Finegold SM. Bacteriology of chronic otitis media. JAMA 1979; 241:487–9.
34. Beswick AJ, Lawley B, Fraise AP, Pahor AL, Brown NL. Detection of alloiococcus otitis in mixed bacterial populations from middle-ear effusions of patients with otitis media. Lancet 1999; 354:386–9.
35. Brook I, Yocum P, Shah K, Feldman B, Epstein S. Microbiology of serous otitis media in children: correlation with age and length of effusion. Ann Otol Rhinol Laryngol 2001; 110:87–90.
36. Brook I, Yocum P, Shah K, Feldman B, Epstein S. Increased antimicrobial resistance in organisms recovered from otitis media with effusion. J Laryngol Otol 2003; 117:449–53.
37. Brook I, Yocum P, Shah K. Aerobic and anaerobic bacteriology of concurrent chronic otitis media with effusion and chronic sinusitis in children. Arch Otolaryngol Head Neck Surg 2000; 126:174–6.
38. Takahashi H, Hayashi M, Saato H, Honjo I. Primary deficits in eustachian tube function in patients with otitis media with effusion. Arch Otolaryngol Head Neck Surg 1989; 115:581–4.
39. Sato K, Liebeler CL, Quartey MK, Le CT, Giebink GS. Middle ear fluid cytokine and inflammatory cell kinetics in the chinchilla otitis media model. Infect Immun 1999; 67:1943–6.
40. Rosenfeld RM, Post C. Meta-analysis of antibiotics for the treatment of otitis media with effusion. Otolaryngol Head Neck Surg 1992; 106:378–86.
41. Thomsen J, Sederberg-Olsen J, Balle V, Hartzen S. Antibiotic treatment of children with secretory otitis media. Amoxicillin–clavulanate is superior to penicillin V in a double-blind randomized study. Arch Otolaryngol Head Neck Surg 1997; 123:695–9.
42. American Academy of Family Physicians, American Academy of Otolaryngology—Head and Neck Surgery, American Academy of Pediatrics Subcommitee on Otitis Media with Effusion. Otitis media with effusion. Pediatrics 2004; 113:1412–29.
43. Wintermeyer SM, Nahata MC. Chronic suppurative otitis media. Ann Pharmacother 1994; 28:1089–99.
44. Fulghum RS, Daniel H, III, Yarborough JG. Anaerobic bacteria in otitis media. Ann Otol Rhinol Laryngol 1977; 86:196–203.
45. Karma P, Jokippi L, Ojala K, et al. Bacteriology of the chronically discharging middle ear. Acta Otolaryngol 1986; 86:110–6.

46. Sugita R, Kawamura S, Ichikawa G, et al. Studies of anaerobic bacteria in chronic otitis media. Laryngoscope 1981; 9:816–21.

47. Aygagari A, Pancholi VK, Pandhi SC, et al. Anaerobic bacteria in chronic suppurative otitis media. Indian J Med Res 1981; 73:860–4.

48. Brook I. Microbiology of chronic otitis media with perforation in children. Am J Dis Child 1980; 130:564–6.

49. Sweeney G, Picozzi GL, Browning GG. A quantitative study of aerobic and anaerobic bacteria in chronic suppurative otitis media. J Infect 1982; 5:47–55.

50. Constable L, Butler I. Microbial flora in chronic otitis media. J Infect 1982; 5:57–60.

51. Papastavros T, Giamarellou H, Varlejides S. Role of aerobic and anaerobic microorganisms in chronic suppurative otitis media. Laryngoscope 1986; 96:438–42.

52. Rotimi VO, Olabiyi DA, Banjo TO, Okeowo PA. Randomised comparative efficacy of clindamycin, metronidazole, and lincomycin, plus gentamicin in chronic suppurative otitis media. West Afr J Med 1990; 9:89–97.

53. Erkan M, Aslan T, Sevuk E, Guney E. Bacteriology of chronic suppurative otitis media. Ann Otol Rhinol Laryngol 1994; 103:771–4.

54. Ito K, Ito Y, Mizuta K, et al. Bacteriology of chronic otitis media, chronic sinusitis, and paranasal mucopyocele in Japan. Clin Infect Dis 1995; 20:S214–9.

55. Brook I, Santosa G. Microbiology of chronic suppurative otitis media in children in Surabaya, Indonesia. Int J Pediatr Otolaryngol 1995; 31:23–8.

56. Brook I. Prevalence of beta-lactamase-producing bacteria in chronic otitis media. Am J Dis Child 1985; 139:280–4.

57. Brook I, Yocum P. Quantitative bacterial cultures and beta-lactamase activity in chronic suppurative otitis media. Ann Otol Rhinol Laryngol 1989; 98:293–7.

58. Brook I. Aerobic and anaerobic bacteriology of cholesteatoma. Laryngoscope 1981; 91:250–3.

59. Iino Y, Hoshino E, Tomioka S, Takasaka T, Kaneko Y, Yuasa R. Organic acids and anaerobic microorganisms in the contents of the cholesteatoma sac. Ann Otol Rhinol Laryngol 1983; 92:91–6.

60. Brook I, Hunter V, Walker RI. Synergistic effects of anaerobic cocci, *Bacteroides, Clostridia, Fusobacteria,* and aerobic bacteria on mouse mortality and induction of subcutaneous abscess. J Infect Dis 1984; 149:924–8.

61. Brook I, Frazier EH. Microbial dynamics of persistent purulent otitis media in children. J Pediatr 1996; 128:237–40.

62. Brook I. Bacteriology and treatment of chronic otitis media in children. Laryngoscope 1979; 89:1129–34.

63. Kenna MA, Bluestone CD, Reilly JS, et al. Medical management of chronic suppurative otitis media without cholesteatoma in children. Laryngoscope 1986; 96:146–51.

64. Brook I. Management of chronic suppurative otitis media: superiority of therapy effective against anaerobic bacteria. Pediatr Infect Dis J 1994; 13:188–93.

65. Brook I, Calhoun L, Yocum P. Beta-lactamase-producing isolates of *Bacteroides* species of children. Antimicrob Agents Chemother 1980; 18:164–6.

66. Brook I. The role of beta-lactamase-producing bacteria in the persistence of streptococcal tonsillar infection. Rev Infect Dis 1984; 6:601–7.

67. Marcy SM. Infections of the external ear. Pediatr Infect Dis 1985; 4:192–201.

68. Bojrab DI, Bruderly TE, Abdulrazzak Y. Otitis externa. Otolaryngol Clin North Am 1996; 29:761–82.

69. Sobie S, Brodsky L, Stanievich JF. Necrotizing external otitis in children: report of two cases and review of the literature. Laryngoscope 1987; 97:598–601.

70. Senturia BH. External otitis, acute diffuse: evaluation of therapy. Ann Otol Rhinol Laryngol 1973; 82:1–23.

71. Brook I, Frazier EH, Thompson DH. Aerobic and anaerobic microbiology of external otitis. Clin Infect Dis 1992; 15:955–8.

72. Clark WB, Brook I, Bianki D, Thompson DH. Microbiology of otitis externa. Otolaryngol Head Neck Surg 1997; 116:23–5.

73. Sade J, Lang R, Goshen S, Kitzer-Cohen R. Ciprofloxacin treatment of malignant external otitis. Am J Med 1989; 87(Suppl. 5A):138S–415.

74. Zikk D, Rapoport Y, Rediana C, Salit I, Himmelfarb MZ. Oral ofloxacin therapy for invasive external otitis. Ann Otol Rhinol Laryngol 1991; 100:632–7.

75. Brook I, Coolbaugh JC, Williscroft RG. Effect of diving and diving hoods on the bacterial flora of the external ear canal and skin. J Clin Microbiol 1982; 15:855–9.

76. Brook I, Coolbaugh JC. Changes in the bacterial flora of the external ear canal from the wearing of the occlusive equipment. Laryngoscope 1984; 94:963–5.

14 | Sinusitis

Sinusitis is defined as an inflammation of the mucous membrane lining the paranasal sinuses (Fig. 1). Sinusitis can be classified chronologically into five categories (1):

- acute sinusitis;
- recurrent acute sinusitis;
- subacute sinusitis;
- chronic sinusitis;
- acute exacerbation of chronic sinusitis (AECS).

Acute sinusitis is a new infection that may last up to four weeks and can be subdivided symptomatically into severe and non-severe.

Recurrent acute sinusitis is diagnosed when four or more episodes of acute sinusitis, which all resolve completely in response to antibiotic therapy, occur within one year.

Subacute sinusitis is an infection that lasts between 4 and 12 weeks, and represents a transition between acute and chronic infection.

Chronic sinusitis is diagnosed when signs and symptoms last for more than 12 weeks.

AECS occurs when the signs and symptoms of chronic sinusitis exacerbate but return to baseline following treatment.

The infant is born with mainly the maxillary and ethmoid sinuses present. The sinuses develop gradually throughout childhood and reach full development during adolescence. The frontal sinuses rarely become infected before six years of age.

Sinuses are involved in most cases of viral upper respiratory tract infection (URTI), but sinus infection usually does not persist after the nasal infection has subsided.

MICROBIOLOGY

The pattern of many upper respiratory infections including sinusitis evolves several phases (Fig. 2). The early stage often is a viral infection that generally lasts up to 10 days where complete recovery occurs in 99% of individuals (2). However, in a small number of patients a secondary acute bacterial infection may develop. This is generally caused by aerobic bacteria (i.e., *Streptococcus pneumoniae*, *Haemophilus influenzae*, and *Moraxella catarrhalis*). If resolution does not take place, anaerobic bacteria of oral flora origin become predominant over time.

The dynamics of these bacterial changes were demonstrated in patients with maxillary sinusitis (3). Repeated endoscopic aspirations illustrated the transition from acute to chronic sinusitis in five patients who initially presented with acute maxillary sinusitis that did not respond to antimicrobials (3). Most bacteria isolated from the first culture were aerobic or facultative bacteria—*S. pneumoniae*, *H. influenzae*, and *M. catarrhalis*. Failure to respond to therapy was associated with the emergence of resistant aerobic and anaerobic bacteria. These organisms included *Fusobacterium nucleatum*, pigmented *Prevotella*, *Porphyromonas*, and *Peptostreptococcus* spp. (Fig. 3). Eradication of the infection was finally achieved following administration of effective antimicrobial agents and in three cases also by surgical drainage.

This above study illustrates that as chronicity develops, the aerobic and facultative species are replaced by anaerobes (3). This may result from the selective pressure of

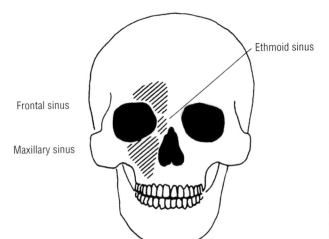

FIGURE 1 Diagram of the skull; *shaded areas* indicate frontal, ethmoid, and maxillary sinuses.

antimicrobial agents that enable resistant organisms to survive, and from the development of conditions appropriate for anaerobic growth, which include the reduction in oxygen tension and an increase in acidity within the sinus. These are caused by the persistent edema and swelling, which reduces blood supply, and by the consumption of oxygen by the aerobic bacteria (5). Another explanation for the slower emergence of anaerobes as pathogens is that expression of some of their virulence factors such as a capsule is slow (6).

Microbiology of Acute Sinusitis

Viral infection (mostly Rhino, influenza, adeno, and para-influenza viruses) is the most common predisposing factor for URTIs, including sinusitis. Viral infection can also concur with the bacterial infection. The mechanism whereby viruses predispose to sinusitis may involve viral–bacterial synergy, induction of local inflammation that blocks the sinus ostia, increase of bacterial attachment to the epithelial cells, and disruption of the local immune defense.

The bacteria recovered from pediatric and adult patients with community-acquired acute purulent sinusitis, using sinus aspiration by puncture or surgery, are the common respiratory pathogens (*S. pneumoniae*, *H. influenzae*, *M. catarrhalis*, and Group A beta-hemolytic streptococci) and *Staphylococcus aureus* (Table 1) (7–12). Following the introduction of vaccination of children with the 7-valent pneumococcal vaccine on 2000 in the U.S.A., the rate of *S. pneumoniae*

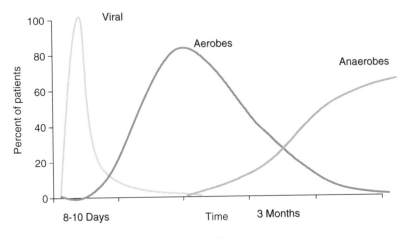

FIGURE 2 Viral and bacterial causes of sinusitis.

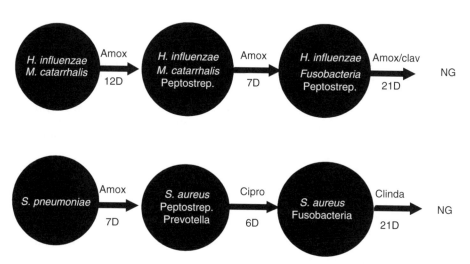

FIGURE 3 Dynamic of sinusitis: changes in bacteria recovered from the sinuses of two patients over time. *Abbreviations*: amox, amoxicillin; amox\clav, amoxicillin\clavulanic acid; cipro, ciprofloxacin; clinda, clindamycin. *Source*: From Ref. 3.

declined and *H. influenzae* increased (13). *S. aureus* is a common pathogen in sphenoid sinusitis (14), while the other organisms are common in other sinuses.

The infection is polymicrobial in about a third of the cases. Enteric bacteria are recovered less commonly, and anaerobes were recovered only from a few cases with acute sinusitis. However, appropriate methods for their recovery were rarely employed in most studies of acute sinusitis.

Anaerobic bacteria account for about 8% of isolates and are commonly recovered from acute sinusitis associated with odontogenic origin, mostly as an extension of the infection from the roots of the premolar or molar teeth (15,16).

Pseudomonas aeruginosa and other aerobic gram-negative rods are common in sinusitis of nosocomial origin (especially in patients who have nasal tubes or catheters), the immunocompromised, patients with human immunodeficiency virus (HIV) infection and cystic fibrosis (17). However, anaerobic bacteria can also be recovered in these patients.

TABLE 1 Microbiology of Sinusitis (Percentage of Patients)

	Maxillary		Ethmoid		Frontal		Splenoid	
Bacteria	Acute	Chronic $N=66$	Acute $N=26$	Chronic $N=17$	Acute $N=15$	Chronic $N=13$	Acute $N=16$	Chronic $N=7$
Aerobic								
Staphylococcus aureus	4	14	15	24	—	15	56	14
Streptococcus pyogenes	2	8	8	6	3	—	6	—
Streptococcus pneumoniae	31	6	35	6	33	—	6	—
Haemophilus infuenzae	21	5	27	6	40	15	12	14
Moraxella catarrhalis	8	6	8	—	20	—	—	
Enterobactiaceae	7	6	—	47	—	8	—	28
Pseudomonas aeruginosa	2	3	—	6	—	8	6	14
Anaerobic								
Peptostreptococcus spp.	2	56	15	59	3	38	19	57
Propionibacterium acnes		29	12	18	3	8	12	29
Fusobacterium spp.	2	17	4	47	3	31	6	54
Prevotella and *Porphyromonas* spp.	2	47	8	82	3	62	6	86
Bacteroides fragilis		6	—	—	—	15	—	—

Source: From Ref. 8–12.

Bacteriology of Chronic Sinusitis

Although the etiology of the inflammation associated with chronic sinusitis is uncertain, bacteria can be isolated in the sinus cavity in these patients (18,19). Bacteria are believed to play a major role in the etiology and pathogenesis of most cases of chronic sinusitis, and antimicrobials are often prescribed for the treatment of this infection.

Numerous studies have examined the bacterial pathogens associated with chronic sinusitis. However, most of these studies did not employ methods that are adequate for the recovery of anaerobic bacteria. Studies have described significant differences in the microbial pathogens present in chronic as compared with acute sinusitis. *S. aureus, Staphylococcus epidermidis*, and anaerobic gram-negative bacilli (AGNB) predominate in chronic sinusitis. The pathogenicity of some of the low virulence organisms, such *S. epidermidis*, a colonizer of the nasal cavity is questionable (4,20).

Gram-negative enteric rods were also reported in recent studies (21–23). These included *P. aeruginosa, Klebsiella pneumoniae, Proteus mirabilis, Enterobacter* spp. and *Escherichia coli*. Since these organisms are rarely found in cultures of the middle meatus obtained from normal individuals, their isolation from these symptomatic patients suggests their pathogenic role. These organisms may have been selected out following administration of antimicrobial therapy in patients with chronic sinusitis.

The usual pathogens in acute sinusitis (e.g., *S. pneumoniae, H. influenzae, M. catarrhalis*) are found with lower frequency (Table 1) (7–11,24–26). Polymicrobial infection is common in chronic sinusitis, which is synergistic (6) and may be more difficult to eradicate with narrow-spectrum antimicrobial agents. Chronic sinusitis caused by anaerobes is a particular concern clinically because many of the complications associated with this condition (e.g., mucocele formation, osteomyelitis, abscess) are associated with the recovery of these organisms (27).

That anaerobes play a role in chronic sinusitis is supported by the ability to induce chronic sinusitis in a rabbit by intra sinus inoculation of *Bacteroides fragilis* (28) and the rapid production of serum IgG antibodies against this organism in the infected animals (29). The pathogenic role of these organisms is also supported by the detection of antibodies (IgG) in patients with chronic sinusitis to two anaerobic organisms that were recovered from their sinus aspirates (*F. nucleatum* and *Prevotella intermedia*) (30). Antibody levels to these organisms declined in those who responded to therapy and were cured, but did not decrease in those who failed therapy (Fig. 4).

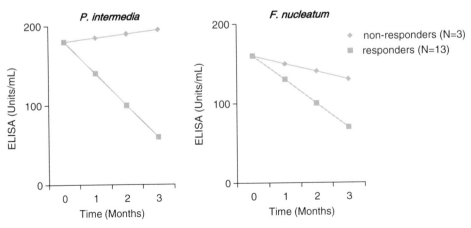

FIGURE 4 Serum antibodies of *Fusobacterium nucleatum* and *Prevotella intermedia* in 16 patients with chronic sinusitis. *Source*: From Ref. 30.

Studies in Children

Anaerobes were recovered in three studies, the only one that employed methods for their isolation (7,31,32). Brook (7) studied 40 children with chronic sinusitis. The sinuses infected were the maxillary (15 cases), ethmoid (13), and frontal (7). Pansinusitis was present in five patients. A total of 121 isolates (97 anaerobic and 24 aerobic) were recovered. Anaerobes were recovered from all 37 culture-positive specimens, and in 14 cases (38%) they were mixed with aerobes. The predominant anaerobes were AGNB (35), gram-positive cocci (27), and *Fusobacterium* spp. (13). The predominant aerobes were alpha-hemolytic streptococci (7), *S. aureus* (7), and *Haemophilus* spp. (4).

Brook et al. (31) correlated the microbiology of concurrent chronic otitis media with effusion and chronic maxillary sinusitis in 32 children. Two-third of the patients had a bacterial etiology. The most common isolates were *H. influenzae* (9 isolates), *S. pneumoniae* (7), *Prevotella* spp. (8), and *Peptostreptococcus* spp. (6). Microbiological concordance between the ear and sinus was found in 22 (69%) of culture-positive patients.

Erkan et al. (32) studied 93 chronically inflamed maxillary sinuses in children. Anaerobes were isolated in 81 of 87 (93%) culture-positive specimens and were recovered alone in 61 cases (70%) and mixed with aerobic or faculative bacteria in 20 (23%). The predominant anaerobic organisms were *Bacteroides* spp. and anaerobic cocci; the predominant aerobes or facultatives were *Streptococcus* spp. and *S. aureus*.

Studies in Adults

The presence of anaerobic bacteria in chronic sinusitis in adults is clinically significant. Finegold et al. (25) in a study of chronic maxillary sinusitis, found recurrence of signs and symptoms twice as frequent when cultures showed anaerobic bacterial counts above 10^3 colony-forming units per milliliter.

Anaerobes were identified in chronic sinusitis in adults whenever techniques for their cultivation were employed (24,33). The predominant isolates were pigmented *Prevotella*, *Fusobacterium*, and *Peptostreptococcus* spp. The predominant aerobic bacteria were *S. aureus*, *M. catarrhalis*, and *Haemophilus* spp.

A summary of 13 studies of chronic sinusitis done since 1974, including 1758 patients (133 were children) is shown in Table 2 (7,25,32,34–42). Anaerobes were recovered in 12% to 93%. The variability in recovery may result from differences in the methodologies used for transportation and cultivation, patient population, geography, and previous antimicrobial therapy.

Brook and Frazier (43) who correlated the microbiology with the history of sinus surgery in 108 patients with chronic maxillary sinusitis found a higher rate of isolation of *P. aeruginosa* and other aerobic gram-negative bacilli in patients with previous sinus surgery. Anaerobes were, however, isolated significantly more frequently in patients who had not had prior surgery.

TABLE 2 Anaerobes in Chronic Sinusitis

References		Anaerobes		
		No. of patients	Percentage points	Percentage organisms
Frederick & Braude (34)	U.S.A.	83	75	52
Van Cauwenberge et al. (42)	Belgium	66	39	39
Karma et al. (35)	Finland	40 (adult)	—	19
Brook (7)	U.S.A.	40	100	80
Berg et al. (36)	Sweden	54 (adult)	≥33	42
Tabaqchali (37)	U.K.	35	70	39
Brook (8)	U.S.A.	72	88	71
Fiscella & Chow (38)	U.S.A.	15 (adult)	38	48
Erkan et al. (39)	Turkey	126 (adult)	88	71
Erkan et al. (32)	Turkey	93 (ped.)	93	74
Ito et al. (40)	Japan	10	60	82
Klossek et al. (41)	France	394	26	25
Finegold et al. (25)	U.S.A.	150 (adult)	56	48

Brook et al. evaluated the microbiology of 13 chronically infected frontal (9), seven sphenoid (10), and 17 ethmoid sinuses (11). Anaerobic bacteria were recovered in over 2/3 of the patients. The predominant anaerobes included *Prevotella*, *Peptostreptococcus*, and *Fusobacterium* spp. The main aerobic organisms were gram-negative bacilli (*H. influenzae*, *K. pneumoniae*, *E. coli*, and *P. aeruginosa*).

Nadel et al. (22) also recovered aerobic and facultative gram-negative rods more commonly in patients who had previous surgery or those who had sinus irrigation. *P. aeruginosa* was also more common in patients who received systemic steroids. Other studies have also noted this shift toward aerobic and facultative gram-negative organisms in patients who have been extensively and repeatedly treated (21,44). The bacterial flora includes *Pseudomonas* spp., *Enterobacter* spp., methicillin-resistant *S. aureus*, *H. influenzae*, and *M. catarrhalis*.

Bacteriology of Acute Exacerbation of Chronic Sinusitis

Brook et al. evaluated the microbiology of maxillary AECS by performing repeated endoscopic aspirations in seven patients over a period of 125 to 242 days (45). Bacteria were recovered from all aspirates and the number of isolates varied between two and four. The aerobes isolated were *H. influenzae*, *S. pneumoniae*, *M. catarrhalis*, *S. aureus*, and *K. pneumoniae*. The anaerobes included pigmented *Prevotella* and *Porphyromonas*, *Peptostreptococcus*, *Fusobacterium* spp., and *Propionibacterium acnes*. A change in the types of isolates was noted in all consecutive cultures obtained from the same patients, as different organisms emerged, and previously isolated bacteria were no longer found. An increase in antimicrobial resistance was noted in six instances. These findings illustrate the microbial dynamics of AECS where anaerobic and aerobic bacteria prevail, and highlight the importance of obtaining cultures from patients with this infection for guidance in the selection of proper antimicrobial therapy.

Brook et al. (46) also compared the microbiology of maxillary AECS in 30 patients with the microbiology of chronic maxillary sinusitis in 32 individuals. The study illustrated the predominance of anaerobic bacteria and polymicrobial nature of both conditions (2.5–3 isolates/sinus). However, aerobic bacteria that are usually found in acute infections (e.g., *S. pneumoniae*, *H. influenzae*, and *M. catarrhalis*) emerged in some of the episodes of AECS.

Bacteriology of Nosocomial Sinusitis

Nosocomial sinusitis often develops in patients who require extended periods of intensive care (postoperative patients, burn victims, and patients with severe trauma) involving prolonged endotracheal or nasogastric intubation. *P. aeruginosa* and other aerobic and facultative gram-negative rods are common in sinusitis of nosocomial origin (especially in patients who have nasal tubes or catheters), the immunocompromised, patients with human immune deficiency viral infection and patients who suffer from cystic fibrosis (17,47).

Nasotracheal intubation places the patient at a substantially higher risk for nosocomial sinusitis than orotracheal intubation. Approximately 25% of patients requiring nasotracheal intubation for more than five days develop nosocomial sinusitis (48). In contrast to community-acquired sinusitis, the usual pathogens are gram-negative enterics (i.e., *P. aeruginosa*, *K. pneumoniae*, *Enterobacter* spp., *P. mirabilis*, *Serratia marcescens*) and aerobic gram-positive cocci (occasionally streptococci and staphylococci). Whether these organisms are actually pathogenic is unclear as their recovery may represent only colonization of an environment with impaired mucociliary transport and foreign body presence in the nasal cavity.

Evaluation of the microbiology of nosocomial sinusitis in nine children with neurologic impairment revealed anaerobic bacteria, always mixed with aerobic and facultative bacteria, in six (67%) sinus aspirates and aerobic bacteria only in three (33%) (49). There were 24 bacterial isolates, 12 aerobic or facultative, and 12 anaerobic. The predominant aerobic isolates were *K. pneumoniae*, *E. coli*, and *S. aureus* and *P. mirabilis*, *P. aeruginosa*, *H. influenzae*, *M. catarrhalis*, and *S. pneumoniae*. The predominant anaerobes were *Prevotella* spp., *Peptostreptococcus* spp., *F. nucleatum*, and *B. fragilis*. Organisms similar to those recovered from the sinuses were also found in the tracheostomy site and gastrostomy wound aspirates in five of seven instances. This study demonstrates the uniqueness of the microbiologic features of sinusitis in neurologically impaired children, in which, in addition to the organisms known to cause infection in children without neurologic impairment, aerobic, facultative and anaerobic gram-negative organisms that can colonize other body sites are predominant.

Bacteriology of Sinusitis in the Immunocompromised Hosts

Sinusitis occurs in a wide range of immunocompromised hosts including neutropenics, diabetics, patients in critical care units, and patients infected with HIV.

Fungal and *P. aeruginosa* are the most common forms of sinusitis in neutropenic patients. *Aspergillus* spp. is frequently the causative organism, although mucor, rhizopus, alternaria, and other molds have been implicated (50). Fungi and *S. aureus*, streptococci and gram-negative enterics are the most common isolates in diabetics (51). The organisms most commonly isolated in nosocomial sinusitis are gram-negative enteric bacteria (such as *P. aeruginosa*, *K. pneumoniae*, Enterobacteriaceae, *P. mirabilis*, and *S. marcescens*) streptococci and staphylococci (52) and anaerobic bacteria (53). The causative organisms in patients with HIV infection included *P. aeruginosa*, *S. aureus*, streptococci, anaerobes, and fungi (Aspergillus, Cryptococcus, and Rhizopus) (54). Refractory parasitic sinusitis caused by *Microsporidium*, *Cryptosporidium*, and *Acanthamoeba* has also been described in these with advanced immunosuppression. Other etiologic agents include cytomegalovirus, atypical mycobacteria, and *Mycobacterium kansasii* (47).

Bacteriology of Sinusitis of Odontogenic Origin

Odontogenic sinusitis is a well-recognized condition and accounts for approximately 10% to 12% of cases of maxillary sinusitis. Brook (16) studied the microbiology of 20 acutely and 28 chronically infected maxillary sinuses that were associated with odontogenic infection. Polymicrobial infection was very common with 3.4 isolates/specimen and 90% of the isolates were anaerobes in both acute and chronic infections. The predominant anaerobic bacteria were AGNB, *Peptostreptococcus* spp., and *Fusobacterium* spp. The predominant aerobes were alpha-hemolytic streptococci, microaerophilic streptococci, and *S. aureus*.

S. pneumoniae, *H. influenzae*, and *M. catarrhalis*, the predominate bacteria recovered from acute maxillary sinusitis not of odontogenic origin (12,18), were mostly absent in acute maxillary sinusitis that was associated with an odontogenic origin. In contrast, anaerobes predominated in both acute and chronic sinusitis.

The microorganisms recovered from odontogenic infections generally reflect the host's indigenous oral flora. The association between periapical abscesses and sinusitis was established in a study of aspirate of pus from five periapical abscesses of the upper jaw and their corresponding maxillary sinusitis (15). Polymicrobial flora was found in all instances, where the number of isolates varied from two to five. Anaerobes were recovered from all specimens. The predominant isolates were *Prevotella*, *Porphyromonas*, *Peptostreptococcus* spp., and *F. nucleatum*. Concordance in the microbiological findings between periapical abscess and the maxillary sinus flora was found in all instances. The concordance in recovery of organisms in paired infections illustrates the dental origin of the infection, with subsequent extension into the maxillary sinus. The proximity of the maxillary molar teeth to the floor of the maxillary sinus allows such a spread.

PATHOGENESIS

Because the mucous membranes lining the nasal chambers and the sinuses are alike histologically and are continuous with each other through the natural ostium, URTI commonly result in an inflammatory sinusitis. Sinusitis of nondental genesis is considered to be preceded by a viral, mechanical, or allergic stage when the nasal and paranasal mucosa are hyperemic and the permeability of the ostium is decreased. At that stage, the sealed-off sinus that fails to drain freely is prone to secondary infection.

The osteomeatal complex (OMC) is an important anatomical site at which the ostia and drainage channels of the maxillary and frontal sinuses are anatomically related to the anterior ethmoids. The complex consists of the anterior ethmoid sinuses, the ostia of the frontal and maxillary sinus and infundibulum, and the middle meatus of the nasal cavity. It is bounded by the middle turbinate medially, the basal lamella posteriorly and superiorly and the lamina papyracea lateraly. It is open for drainage enteriorly and inferiorly. Blockage or inflammation at the OMC is responsible for the development of bacterial sinusitis, as it interferes with effective mucociliary clearance (55).

Sinus ostium occlusion is the major predisposing factor causing suppurative infection and most often is the result of viral or upper respiratory infection, a common event in early childhood. Other important contributory factors are congenital and genetical factors (56) and acquired immune deficiencies (57).

Mechanical obstruction resulting in sinusitis can be related to various causative factors such as septal dislocation owing to birth trauma, unilateral choanal atresia, foreign bodies placed in the nose, or fractures of the nose following trauma. Up to 30% of cystic fibrosis patients may have polyps complicating the already abnormal sinus secretions that predispose them to sinusitis (58).

Allergy, especially asthma, is an important predisposing factor in sinusitis (59). Cyanotic congenital heart disease is frequently complicated by sinusitis. Dental infections also are a source of sinusitis (16).

The origin of organisms introduced into the sinuses that eventually cause sinusitis is the nasal cavity. The normal flora of that site comprises certain bacterial species, which include *S. aureus*, *S. epidermidis*, alpha- and gamma-streptococci, *P. acnes* and aerobic diphtheroid (60,61). Potential sinus pathogens have rarely been isolated from healthy nasal cavity.

The flora of the nasal cavity of patients with sinusitis is different from healthy flora. While the recovery of *Staphylococcus* spp. and diphtheroids is reduced, the isolation of pathogens increases (62).

The uninfected sinus contains "normal" aerobic and anaerobic bacterial flora similar to those present in the infected sinus (63). This may explain the chain of events that lead to formation of an infection following the occlusion of the ostium as well as the pathophysiology of acute and chronic sinusitis.

When sinusitis occurs, oxygen is being absorbed mostly by the sinus mucosa (5). The possible implication of the reduction of oxygen in the diseased sinus is the formation of a bacteria–host relationship in favor of certain bacteria. The mean oxygen tension in serous secretions obtained from acutely inflamed maxillary sinuses was 12.3% (compared to about 17% in the normal sinuses) (5). The bacteria recovered from these aspirates were predominantly *S. pneumoniae*. The oxygen tension in purulent secretion was zero, however, and an accumulation of carbon dioxide was found, particularly when anaerobic bacteria were recovered. It is therefore plausible that the reduced oxygen tension in the sinus during the serous phase better meets the requirements for the growth of those bacteria isolated in acute sinusitis, *S. pneumoniae* and *H. influenzae*, while the complete lack of oxygen in the purulent secretion supports the growth of the anaerobic organisms recovered in chronic sinusitis.

The frequent involvement of anaerobes in chronic sinusitis may be related to the poor drainage and increased intranasal pressure that occur during inflammation. This can reduce the oxygen tension in the inflamed sinus by decreasing the mucosal blood supply and depressing the ciliary action (64). The lowering of the oxygen content and pH of the sinus cavity supports the growth of anaerobic organisms by providing an optimal-oxidation reduction potential (5,64).

Anaerobes frequently are recovered from infectious conditions associated with complications of sinusitis (24,27,33), including periorbital cellulitis, brain abscess, subdural or epidural empyema, cavernous sinus thrombosis, and meningitis. This relationship ascertains their role in sinus infections and warrants appropriate antimicrobial therapy.

Some anaerobic and aerobic bacteria that are part of the normal oropharyngeal flora can possess in vitro interference capability with the growth of sinus pathogens. Interfering organisms were found in higher numbers in the nosopharynx of non sinusitis-prone patients, as compared to those who were sinusitis prone (65).

TABLE 3   Major and Minor Criteria of Bacterial Sinusitis[a]

Major criteria	Minor criteria
Facial pain/pressure (requires a second major criterion to constitute a suggestive history)	Headache
Facial congestion/fullness	Fever (for subacute and chronic sinusitis)
Nasal congestion/obstruction	Halitosis
Nasal discharge/purulence/discolored postnasal drainage	Fatigue
Hyposmia/anosmia	Dental pain
Fever (for acute sinusitis; requires a second major criterion to constitute a strong history)	Cough
Purulence on intranasal examination	Ear pain/pressure/fullness

[a] Diagnosis of bacterial sinusitis based on major and minor criteria. Strong history requires the presence of two major criteria or one major and two or more minor criteria. Suggestive history requires the presence of one major criterion or two or more minor criteria.
Source: From Ref. 66.

DIAGNOSIS

Practical criteria for the diagnosis of bacterial sinusitis are based on either major or minor symptoms, signs, and findings (Table 3) (66). The presence of bacterial sinusitis is suspected when at least two major or one major and two minor criteria are found.

The most common presentation is a persistent (and unimproved) nasal discharge or cough (or both) lasting longer than 10 days (18). A 10-day period separates simple viral URTI from bacterial sinusitis because most uncomplicated viral URTIs last between five and seven days—by day 10 most patients are improving.

The quality of the nasal discharge varies, and it can be thin or thick, clear, mucoid, or purulent.

The symptoms and signs of acute bacterial sinusitis can be divided into non-severe and severe forms (Table 4) (1). The severe form carries a higher risk of complications and mandates earlier use of antimicrobial therapy (67,68). The combination of high fever and purulent nasal discharge lasting for at least three to four days points to a bacterial infection of the sinuses.

In those with subacute or chronic bacterial sinusitis, the symptoms are protracted. Fever is rare, the cough and nasal congestion persist, and a sore throat (as a result of mouth breathing) is common.

The location of the facial pain can point to which of the sinuses is involved. Maxillary bacterial sinusitis is often associated with pain in the cheeks, frontal with the forehead, ethmoid with medial canthus, and sphenoid with occipital pain. Other suggestive factors are action or position that makes the sinus worse or better, and clues that suggest the presence of chronic infection.

Disease in the upper molar teeth may be the source of maxillary sinusitis.

Further workup and consideration for hospitalization include suspicion of nosocomial sinusitis (recent intubation, feeding or suction device), patients who are immunocompromised, possible meningitis or other intracranial complications, or frontal or sphenoid sinusitis.

Acute Sinusitis

The patient generally presents with edema of the mucous membranes of the nose, mucopurulent nasal discharge, and persistent postnasal drip, cough, fever, and malaise. Tenderness over

TABLE 4   Symptoms and Signs of Bacterial Sinusitis

Non-severe acute sinusitis	Severe acute sinusitis
Rhinorrhea (of any quality)	Purulent (thick, colored, opaque) rhinorrhea
Nasal congestion	Nasal congestion
Cough	Facial pain or headache
Headache, facial pain, and irritability (variable)	Periorbital edema (variable)
Low-grade or no fever	High fever (temperature $\geq 39°C$)

the involved sinus is present, and so is pain, which can be induced over the affected sinus upon percussion. Cellulitis can be observed in the area overlying the affected sinus. Other occasional findings, especially in acute ethmoiditis, are periorbital cellulitis, edema, and proptosis. Failure to transilluminate the sinus and nasal voice are also evident in many patients. Direct smear of the secretions usually reveals mostly neutrophils and may aid in the detection of associated allergy if many eosinophils are present.

Radiologically, clouding, opacity, and thickening of the mucosal interface (≥ 4 mm) of the affected sinus usually are present. Fluid level can often be observed.

Generally, plain film radiographs is difficult to use in documenting the presence of infection, and is not as specific and sensitive as computed tomography (CT) scanning for analysis of the degree of sinus abnormalities. As a result of this limitation, its use has declined and it has now been replaced by CT.

For children, CT is especially advantageous because their sinuses are smaller than those in adults and are often asymmetrical in shape and size, which makes them difficult to evaluate (69).

Chronic Sinusitis

Symptoms of chronic sinusitis vary considerably. Fever may be absent or be of low grade. Frequently symptoms are protracted and include malaise, easy fatigability, difficulty in mental concentration, anorexia, irregular nasal or postnasal discharge, frequent headaches, and pain or tenderness to palpation over the affected sinus.

Plain radiography and especially CT scanning can assist in diagnosing chronic infection and its complications. CT is useful in investigating any anatomical finding that can lead to obstruction and poor chainage.

MANAGEMENT

Role of Beta-Lactamase–Producing Bacteria

Bacterial resistance to the antibiotics used for the treatment of sinusitis has consistently increased in recent years. Production of the enzyme beta-lactamase is one of the most important mechanisms of penicillin resistance. Several potential aerobic and anaerobic BLPB occur in sinusitis.

BLPB have been recovered from over a third of patients with acute and chronic sinusitis (8–11,18). *H. influenzae* and *M. caterrhalis* are the predominate BLPB in acute sinusitis (18) and *S. aureus*, pigmented *Prevotella* and *Porphyromonas* spp. and *Fusobacterium* spp., predominate in chronic sinusitis (8–11).

Most *Prevotella* and *Fusobacterium* spp. strains were considered susceptible to penicillin. However, within the past two decades, penicillin-resistant strains have been reported with increasing frequency (70). These species are the predominant AGNB in the oral flora and are most commonly recovered in anaerobic infections in and around the oral cavity (33).

BLPB may shield penicillin-susceptible organisms from the activity of penicillin, thereby contributing to their persistence. The ability of BLPB to protect penicillin-sensitive microorganisms has been demonstrated in vitro and in vivo (71).

The actual activity of the enzyme beta-lactamase and the phenomenon of "shielding" were demonstrated in acutely and chronically inflamed sinuses fluids (72). BLPB were isolated in 4 of 10 acute sinusitis (Table 5) and in 10 of 13 chronic sinusitis aspirates. The predominate BLPB isolated in acute sinusitis were *H. influenzae* and *M. catarrhalis*, and those found in chronic sinusitis were *Prevotella* and *Fusobacterium* spp. The recovery of BLPB is not surprising, since over two-thirds of the patients with acute and all of the patients with chronic sinusitis received antimicrobial agents that might have selected for BLPB. These data suggest that therapy should be directed at the eradication of BLPB whenever present.

TABLE 5 Beta-Lactamase Detected in Chronic Sinusitis Aspirates

Organism	Patient No.			
	1	2	3	4
Staphylococcus aureus (BL +)		+		+
Streptococcus pneumoniae	+			
Peptostreptococcus spp.	+			+
Propionibacterium acnes	+			
Fusobacterium spp. (BL +)		+		+
Fusobacterium spp. (BL −)		+		+
Prevotella spp. (BL +)			+	
Prevotella spp. (BL −)	+	+	+	
Bacteroides fragilis group (BL +)	+			+
Beta-lactamase activity in pus	+	+	+	+

Abbreviations: BL +, Beta-lactamase–producing bacteria; BL −, Non-beta-lactamase–producing bacteria.
Source: From Ref. 71.

Antimicrobial Treatment of Acute Sinusitis

Treatment is aimed at establishing good drainage by using decongestants, nasal saline irrigation/spray, humidification, and mucolytic agents. Systemic decongestants or antihistamines may be helpful, especially in allergic individuals. Anatomic deformities should be corrected.

Appropriate antibiotic therapy is of paramount importance. Antimicrobial therapy has been shown to be beneficial and effective in preventing septic complications (49,73). Endoscopic examination and culture can assist in the selection of antimicrobials in the treatment of patients who fail to respond (3).

Amoxicillin can be appropriate for the initial treatment of acute uncomplicated mild sinusitis. (Table 6). However, antimicrobials that are more effective against the major bacterial pathogens (including those that are resistant to multiple antibiotics) may be indicated as initial therapy and for the re-treatment of those who have risk factors prompting a need for more effective antimicrobials (Table 7) and those who had failed amoxicillin therapy. These agents include amoxicillin and clavulanic acid, the "newer" or "respiratory" quinolones (e.g., levofloxacin, gatifloxacin, and moxifloxacin), and some of the 2nd & 3rd generation cephalosporins (cefdinir, cefuroxime-axetil, and cefpodoxime proxetil).

These agents should be administered to patients where bacterial resistance is likely (i.e., recent antibiotic therapy, winter season, increased resistance in the community), the presence of a moderate-to-severe infection, the presence of co-morbidity (diabetes, chronic renal, hepatic or cardiac pathology), and when penicillin allergy is present. Agents that may be less effective because of growing bacterial resistance may however be considered for patients with antimicrobial allergy. These include the macrolides, trimethoprim-sulfamethoxazole (TMP-SMX), tetracyclines, and clindamycin (74).

A number of antimicrobial agents have been studied in the therapy of acute sinusitis over the past 25 years, with the use of pre- and post-treatment aspirate cultures. Those studied were ampicillin, amoxicillin, amoxicillin–clavulanic acid, cefuroxime axetil, cefprozil, loracarbef, levofloxacin, gatifloxacin, moxifloxacin, and gemifloxacin. For a 10-day course of therapy, the success rate was a bacteriological cure over 80% to 90%. Appropriate antibiotic therapy is of paramount importance, even though it is estimated that spontaneous recovery occurs in about half of patients (73,74).

The recommended length of therapy for acute sinusitis is at least 14 days, or seven days beyond the resolution of symptoms, whichever is longer. However, no controlled studies have established the duration of therapy sufficient to resolve the infection.

Antimicrobial Therapy of Chronic Sinusitis

Many of the pathogens found in chronically inflamed sinuses are resistant to penicillins through the production of beta-lactamase (8–11). These include both aerobic (*S. aureus*, *H. influenzae*, and *M. catarrhalis*) and anaerobic isolates (*B. fragilis* group and over half of the

TABLE 6   Empirical Antimicrobial Therapy in Acute Bacterial Sinusitis

Amoxicillin Therapy (high-dose)
 Mild illness
 No history of recurrent acute sinusitis
 During summer months
 When no recent antimicrobial therapy has been used
 When patient has had no recent contact with patient(s) on antimicrobial therapy
 When community experience shows high success rate of amoxicillin
Risk factors prompting a need for more effective antimicrobials[a]
  Bacterial resistance is likely
   Antibiotic use in the past month, or close contact with a treated individual(s)
   Resistance common in community
   Failure of previous antimicrobial therapy
   Infection in spite of prophylactic treatment
   Child in daycare facility
   Winter season
   Smoker or smoker in family
  Presence of moderate-to-severe infection
   Presentation with protracted (more than 30 days) or moderate-to-severe symptoms
   Complicated ethmoidal sinusitis
   Frontal or sphenoidal sinusitis
   Patient history of recurrent acute sinusitis
  Presence of co-morbidity and extremes of life
   Co-morbidity (i.e., chronic cardiac, hepatic or renal disease, diabetes)
   Immunocompromised patient
   Younger than two years of age or older than 55 years
  Allergy to penicillin
   Allergy to penicillin or amoxicillin

[a] Amoxicillin and clavulanic acid, 2nd and 3rd generation cephalosporins, and the "respiratory" quinolones.

Prevotella and *Fusobacterium* spp.). Retrospective studies illustrate the superiority of therapy effective against both aerobic and anaerobic BLPB in chronic sinusitis (26,75). Antimicrobials used for treatment of chronic sinusitis should be effective against both aerobic and anaerobic BLPB, as well as those resistant through other mechanisms. These agents include the combination of a penicillin (e.g., amoxicillin) and a beta-lactamase inhibitor (e.g., clavulanic acid), clindamycin, chloramphenicol, the combination of metronidazole and a macrolide, and the "newer" or "respiratory" quinolones (e.g., moxifloxacin). All of these agents (or similar ones) are available in oral and parenteral forms. Other effective antimicrobials are available only in parenteral form (e.g., cefoxitin, cefotetan, and carbapenems). Parenteral therapy with a

TABLE 7   Recommended Antibacterial Agents for Initial Treatment of Acute Sinusitis or After No Improvement

Factors prompting more effective antibiotics[a]	At diagnosis	Clinical treatment failure at 48–72 hr after starting treatment
No	High-dose amoxicillin	High-dose–amoxicillin/clavulanate or a "new" quinolone[b] or cefuroxime or cefdinir or cefpodoxime proxetil
Yes	High-dose amoxicillin/clavulanate or a "new" quinolone[b] or cefuroxime-axetil or cefdinir or cefpodoxime proxetil	High-dose amoxicillin/clavulanate or a "new" quinolone[b] or cefuroxime-axetil or cefdinir or cefpodoxime proxetil

[a] See Table 7.
[b] Not approved for children (less than 18 yr).

carbapenem (i.e., imipenem, meropenem, ertapenem) or tigecycline is more expensive, but provides coverage for most potential pathogens, both anaerobes and aerobes. If aerobic gram-negative organisms, such as *P. aeruginosa*, are involved, parenteral therapy with an aminoglyco-sides, a fourth-generation cephalosporin (cefepime or ceftazidime) or oral or parenteral treatment with a fluoroquinolone (only in postpubertal patients) is added. A beta lactam resistant penicillin is adequate for *S. aureus*. However, for methicillin resistant *S. aureus*, vancomycin, linezolid or tigecycline is needed. Therapy is given for at least 21 days, and may be extended up to 10 weeks. Fungal sinusitis can be treated with surgical debridement of the affected sinuses and antifungal therapy (76).

In contrast to acute sinusitis, which is generally treated vigorously with antibiotics, surgical drainage is the mainstay of the treatment of chronic sinusitis, especially in patients who had not responded to medical therapy. Impaired drainage may contribute to the development of chronic sinusitis, and correction of the obstruction helps to alleviate the infection and prevent recurrence. The use of antimicrobial therapy alone without surgical drainage of collected pus may not result in clearance of the infection. The chronically inflamed sinus membranes with diminished vascularity may not allow for an adequate antibiotic level to accumulate in the infected tissue, even when the blood level is therapeutic. Furthermore, the reduction in the pH and oxygen tension within the inflamed sinus can interfere with the antimicrobial activity, which can result in bacterial survival despite a high antibiotic concentration (5).

In the past, it was often necessary to resort to surgical intervention to cure chronic sinusitis. However, with improvements in the medical care, surgery is avoided more often. Functional endoscopic sinus surgery (FESS) has become the main surgical technique used; other surgical procedures serve only as a backup and are used especially when sinusitis is complicated by orbital and/or intracranial involvement. Although endoscopic surgery can provide up to 80% to 90% success in adults and children (77,78), a substantial number of patients suffer from complications (79) that warrant medical therapy being used to its full extent before resorting to surgery.

The surgeon's goals are to prevent persistence, recurrence, progression and complications of chronic sinusitis. This is achieved by complete removal of diseased tissue, preservation of normal tissue, production of drainage (or obliteration, if this is not possible) and consideration of the cosmetic outcome. Radical procedures should only be carried out if a simple approach, such as sinus lavage and medical therapy, fails or the disease is extensive.

ADJUVANT THERAPIES

Acute Bacterial Sinusitis

Patients with a viral URTI may benefit from symptomatic therapy, aimed at improving their quality of life during the acute illness. The use of normal saline as a spray or lavage can provide symptomatic improvement by liquefying secretions to encourage drainage. The short-term (three days) use of topical alpha-adrenergic decongestants can also provide symptomatic relief, but their use should be restricted to older children and adults due to the potential for undesirable systemic effects in infants and young children. Topical glucocorticosteroids may also be useful in reducing nasal mucosal edema, mostly in those cases where a patient who has seasonal allergic rhinitis develops the complication of an acute URTI. The antipyretic and analgesic effects of nonsteroidal anti-inflammatory agents can relieve or ameliorate the associated symptoms of fever, headache, generalized malaise, and facial tenderness. Until the clinical diagnosis of acute bacterial sinusitis is established, management of an URTI should be only symptomatic. Furthermore, symptomatic care can be useful in the management of acute bacterial sinusitis as adjunctive therapy, but no adjunct, has been shown essential in improving the outcome achieved by antimicrobial therapy or effective in preventing the development of acute bacterial sinusitis in persons who have a viral URTI or allergic rhinitis.

Chronic Bacterial Sinusitis

Anti-Inflammatories

Long-term, low dose macrolide therapy represents one attempt at controlling the inflammation associated with chronic sinusitis (80). Medicines that have anti-inflammatory properties and are well tolerated are sought to help ease the reliance on systemic corticosteroids that affect both the number and function of inflammatory cells. When used in a topical form, nasal steroid sprays have been shown to be safe and effective in reducing the symptoms of alleric rhinitis (81). Their use in patients with chronic sinusitis can decrease the size of nasal polyps, and diminish sinomucosal edema (82). There are no set guidelines for the duration of use, and the expected side effects from long-term use are not yet known. Experience in using oral steroids for the treatment of chronic sinusitis is only anectodal. The extended use of oral steroid may result in serious side effects that include muscle wasting and osteoporosis. Because of the side effects, steroids are tapered and given in short courses that may span only three to four weeks.

Adjunctive Therapy

Adjunctive therapy is intended to promoted drainage of secretions and improve oxygenation to the obstructed sinus ostia. Multiple agents with different mechanisms of action are often administered. These include decongestants that are alpha-adrenergic agonists that constrict the capacitance vessels and decrease mucosal edema. Topical therapy such as oxymetazoline or neosynephrine may be used in an acute setting, but overuse can cause a rebound effect and rhinitis medicamentosa. Systemic decongestants can be used for longer periods of time, but may cause insomnia and exacerbation of underlying systemic hypertension.

Antihistamines are used in patients with underlying allergic rhinitis. They can relieve symptoms of itching, rhinorrhea, and sneezing in allergic patients, but in nonallergic patients they can cause thickening of secretions, which may prevent needed drainage of the sinus ostia.

Guaifenesin (glyceryl guaicolate) given in a daily dose of 2400 mg thins secretions, thus facilitating drainage. Nasal saline irrigations are helpful in thinning secretions and may provide a mild benefit in nasal congestion. Hypertonic saline irrigations improve patient comfort and quality of life, decrease medication use, and diminish the need for surgical therapy (83).

Leukotriene inhibitors are systemic medications that block the receptor and/or production of leukotrienes, potent lipid mediators that increase eosinophil recruitment, goblet cell production, mucosal edema, and airway remodeling. Their role in chronic sinusitis and nasal polyposis is not yet well established (84).

COMPLICATIONS

Sinus infection when not treated promptly and properly may spread via anastomosing veins or by direct extension to nearby structures (Fig. 5). Orbital complication was categorized by Chandler et al. (67) into five separate stages according to its severity (see chapter 11). Contiguous spread could reach the orbital area, resulting in periorbital cellulitis, subperiosteal abscess, orbital cellulitis, and abscess. Orbital cellulitis may complicate acute ethmoiditis if a thrombophlebitis of the anterior and posterior ethmoidal veins leads to a spread of infection to the lateral, or orbital, side of the ethmoid labyrinth. Sinusitis may extend also to the central nervous system, causing cavernous sinus thrombosis, retrograde meningitis, and epidural, subdural, and brain abscesses (67,85,86). Monitoring for possible intracranial complication is therefore warranted. Orbital symptoms frequently precede intracranial extension of the disease (27,86).

The most common pathogens in cellulitis and abscesses are those seen in acute and chronic sinusitis, depending on the length and aetiology of the primary sinusitis. These include *S. pneumoniae*, *H. influenzae*, *S. aureus*, and anaerobic bacteria (*Prevotella*, *Porphyromonas*, *Fusobacterium*, and *Peptostreptococcus* spp.) (9,24).

The organisms isolated in cavernous sinus thrombosis are *S.aureus* (50–70% of instances), *Streptococcus* spp. (20%), and AGNB (pigmented *Prevotella* and *Porphyromonas*, and *Fusobacterium* spp.) (87,88). Similar organisms can be recovered from orbital abscesses and their corresponding maxillary sinusitis (88).

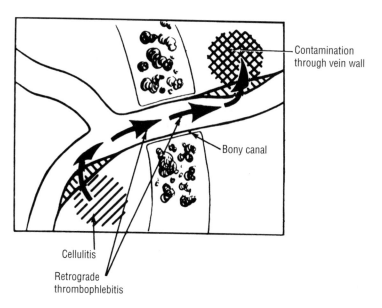

Contamination through vein wall

Bony canal

Cellulitis

Retrograde thrombophlebitis

FIGURE 5 The route of spread of infection from the site of periorbital cellulitis into the cranial cavity through retrograde thrombophlebitis.

The organisms recovered from brain abscesses that complicated sinusitis are anaerobic, aerobic, and microaerophilic bacteria. Anaerobes can be isolated in over two-thirds of the patients, and include pigmented *Prevotella* and *Porphyromonas, Fusobacterium,* and *Peptostreptococcus* spp. (27,85,86). Microaerophilic streptococci are also very common, and can be isolated from abscesses caused by maxillary sinusitis that originates from the dental infection of the upper jaw. The most common aerobe is *S. aureus,* and *H. influenzae* is rarely isolated.

Brook et al. (86) reported eight children who had complications of sinusitis. Subdural empyema occurred in four patients; in one patient it was accompanied by cerebritis and brain abscess and in another by meningitis. Periorbital abscess was present in two children who had ethmoiditis. Alveolar abscess in the upper incisors was present in two children whose infection had spread to the maxillary and ethmoid sinuses. Anaerobic bacteria were isolated from the infected sinuses in all the patients. Three of the four patients with intracranial abscess did not respond initially to appropriate antimicrobial therapy directed against the organisms recovered from their abscesses. They improved only after both the subdural empyema and infected sinus were drained. Surgical drainage and appropriate antimicrobial therapy resulted in complete eradication of the infection in all patients.

Arjmand et al. treated 22 children with subperiosteal orbital abscesses (SPOAs) (90). *S. aureus* and anaerobic bacteria were the predominant isolates. Gerald and Haris (91) evaluated 37 patients with subperostal abscess of the orbit. Polymicrobial infections including anaerobes were recovered in most cases. These included AGNB, *Peptostreptococcus, Veillonella parvulla, Eubacterium* spp., and microaerophilic streptococci.

Dill et al. (92) studied 32 patients (including 16 childen) with subdural empyema, associated with sinusitis in 56% of cases. The predominant organisms isolated from these patients were anaerobes and streptococci.

Brook & Frazier (88) studied aspirate of pus from eight SPOAs and their corresponding infected sinuses. Polymicrobial flora was found in all instances, and the number of isolates varied from two to five. Anaerobes were recovered from all specimens. The predominant isolates were *Peptostreptococcus,* AGNB, *S. aureus,* and microaerophilic streptococci. Concordance in the microbiological findings between SPOA and the infected sinus was found in all instances. However, certain organisms were only present at one site and not the other.

Even though the judicious selection of antimicrobial agents is of utmost importance, the treatment of the complications of sinusitis frequently requires surgical intervention. The morbidity and mortality are reduced when therapy includes surgical drainage, and it is an integral part of patient management.

Other complications of acute and chronic sinusitis are sinobronchitis, maxillary osteomyelitis, and osteomyelitis of the frontal bone.

We have reported three children with anaerobic osteomyelitis following chronic sinusitis (93). One child developed frontal bone infection, another had ethmoid sinusitis, and the third child had frontal and ethmoid osteomyelitis. All were associated with the infection of the corresponding sinuses.

Acute osteomyelitis of the maxilla may be produced by surgery of an inflamed antrum or by dental abscess or extractions.

Osteomyelitis of the frontal bone generally arises from a spreading thrombophlebitis. A periostitis of the frontal sinus leads to osteitis and periostitis of the outer membrane, which gives rise to a tender, puffy swelling of the forehead.

Diagnosis of osteomyelitis is made by finding local tenderness and dull pain, and is confirmed by CT and nuclear isotope scanning. The causes are anaerobic bacteria and *S. aureus*. Obtaining a culture is an important guide for therapy. Management consists of surgical drainage and antimicrobial therapy. Surgical debridement is infrequently needed after a properly extended course of parenteral antimicrobial therapy (94) Antibiotics should be given for at least six weeks. Hyperbaric oxygen therapy may be useful, but it has not been tested in controlled studies (95).

In persistent sinusitis, bronchitis may occur from the bronchial aspiration of infected material from the draining sinuses. This clinical combination is frequently associated with a chronic cough, and chronic bronchitis may develop.

REFERENCES

1. Clement PAR, Bluestone CD, Gordts F, et al. Management of rhinosinusitis in children. Consensus Meeting, Brussels, Belgium, September 13 1996. Arch Otolaryngol Head Neck Surg 1998; 124:31–4.
2. Gwaltney JM, Jr., Sydnor A, Sande MA. Etiology and antimicrobial treatment of acute sinusitis. Ann Otol Rhinol Laryngol 1981; 90(Suppl. 84):68–71.
3. Brook I, Frazier EH, Foote PA. Microbiology of the transition from acute to chronic maxillary sinusitis. J Med Microbiol 1996; 45:372–5.
4. Jiang RS, Hsu CY, Jang JW. Bacteriology of the maxillary and ethmoid sinuses in chronic sinusitis. J Laryngol Otol 1998; 112:845–8.
5. Carenfelt C, Lundberg C. Purulent and non-purulent maxillary sinus secretions with respect to Po_2, Pco_2 and pH. Acta Otolaryngol 1977; 84:138–44.
6. Brook I. Role of encapsulated anaerobic bacteria in synergistic infections. Crit Rev Microbiol 1987; 14:171–93.
7. Brook I. Bacteriologic features of chronic sinusitis in children. JAMA 1981; 246:967–9.
8. Brook I. Bacteriology of chronic maxillary sinusitis in adults. Ann Otol Rhinol Laryngol 1989; 98:426–8.
9. Brook I. Bacteriology of acute and chronic frontal sinusitis. Arch Otolaryngol Head Neck Surg 2002; 128:583–5.
10. Brook I. Bacteriology of acute and chronic sphenoid sinusitis. Ann Otol Rhinol Laryngol 2002; 111:1002–4.
11. Brook I. Bacteriology of acute and chronic ethmoid sinusitis. J Clin Microbiol 2005; 43:3479–80.
12. Gwaltney JM, Jr., Scheld WM, Sande MA, Sydnor A. The microbial etiology and antimicrobial therapy of adults with acute community-acquired sinusitis: a fifteen-year experience at the University of Virginia and review of other selected studies. J Allergy Clin Immunol 1992; 90:457–62.
13. Brook I, Foote PA, Hausfeld JN. Frequency of recovery of pathogens causing acute maxillary sinusitis in adults before and after introduction of vaccination of children with the 7-valent pneumococcal vaccine. J Med Microbiol 2006; 55:943–6.
14. Lew D, Southwick FS, Montgomery WW, Weber AL, Baker AS. Sphenoid sinusitis. A review of 30 cases. N Engl J Med 1983; 309:1149–54.
15. Brook I, Frazier EH, Gher ME, Jr. Microbiology of periapical abscesses and associated maxillary sinusitis. J Periodontal 1996; 67:608–10.
16. Brook I. Microbiology of acute and chronic maxillary sinusitis associated with an odontogenic origin. Laryngoscope 2005; 115:823–5.

17. Shapiro ED, Milmoe GJ, Wald ER, et al. Bacteriology of the maxillary sinuses in patients with cystic fibrosis. J Infect Dis 1982; 146:589–93.
18. Wald ER. Microbiology of acute and chronic sinusitis in children and adults. Am J Med Sci 1998; 316:13–20.
19. Biel MA, Brown CA, Levinson RM, et al. Evaluation of the microbiology of chronic maxillary sinusitis. Ann Otol Laryngol Rhinol 1998; 107:942–5.
20. Gordts F, Halewyck S, Pierard D, et al. Microbiology of the middle meatus: a comparison between normal adults and children. J Laryngol Otol 2000; 14:184–8.
21. Hsu J, Lanza DC, Kennedy DW. Antimicrobial resistance in bacterial chronic sinusitis. Am J Rhinol 1998; 12:243–8.
22. Nadel DM, Lanza DC, Kennedy DW. Endoscopically guided cultures in chronic sinusitis. Am J Rhinol 1998; 12:233–41.
23. Bahattacharyya N, Kepnes LJ. The microbiology of recurrent rhinosinusitis after endoscopic sinus surgery. Arch Otolaryngol Head Neck Surg 1999; 125:1117–20.
24. Nord CE. The role of anaerobic bacteria in recurrent episodes of sinusitis and tonsillitis. Clin Infect Dis 1995; 20:1512–24.
25. Finegold SM, Flynn MJ, Rose FV, et al. Bacteriologic findings associated with chronic bacterial maxillary sinusitis in adults. Clin Infect Dis 2002; 35:428–33.
26. Brook I, Thompson DH, Frazier EH. Microbiology and management of chronic maxillary sinusitis. Arch Otolaryngol Head Neck Surg 1994; 120:1317–20.
27. Brook I. Brain abscess in children: microbiology and management. Child Neurol 1995; 10:283–8.
28. Westrin KM, Stierna P, Carlsoo B, Hellstrom S. Mucosal fine structure in experimental sinusitis. Ann Otol Rhinol Laryngol 1993; 102(8 Pt 1):639–45.
29. Jyonouchi H, Sun S, Kennedy CA, et al. Localized sinus inflammation in a rabbit sinusitis model induced by *Bacteroides fragilis* is accompanied by rigorous immune responses. Otolaryngol Head Neck Surg 1999; 120:869–75.
30. Brook I, Yocum P. Immune response to *Fusobacterium nucleatum* and *Prevotella intermedia* in patients with chronic maxillary sinusitis. Ann Otol Rhinol Laryngol 1999; 108:293–5.
31. Brook I, Yocum P, Shah K. Aerobic and anaerobic bacteriology of concurrent chronic otitis media with effusion and chronic sinusitis in children. Arch Otolaryngol Head Neck Surg 2000; 126:174–6.
32. Erkan M, Ozcan M, Arslan S, Soysal V, Bozdemir K, Haghighi N. Bacteriology of antrum in children with chronic maxillary sinusitis. Scand J Infect Dis 1996; 28:283–5.
33. Finegold SM. Anaerobic Bacteria in Human Disease. Orlando, FL: Academic Press Inc., 1977.
34. Frederick J, Braude AI. Anaerobic infections of the paranasal sinuses. N Engl J Med 1974; 290:135–7.
35. Karma P, Jokipii L, Sipila P, Luotonen J, Jokipii AM. Bacteria in chronic maxillary sinusitis. Arch Otolaryngol 1979; 105:386–90.
36. Berg O, Carenfelt C, Kronvall G. Bacteriology of maxillary sinusitis in relation to character of inflammation and prior treatment. Scand J Infect Dis 1988; 20:511–6.
37. Tabaqchali S. Anaerobic infections in the head and neck region. Scand J Infect Dis Suppl. 1988; 57:24–34.
38. Fiscella RG, Chow JM. Cefixime for the teatment of maxillary sinusitis. Am J Rhinology 1991; 5:193–7.
39. Erkan M, Aslan T, Ozcan M, Koc N. Bacteriology of antrum in adults with chronic maxillary sinusitis. Laryngoscope 1994; 104(3 Pt 1):321–4.
40. Ito K, Ito Y, Mizuta K, et al. Bacteriology of chronic otitis media, chronic sinusitis, and paranasal mucopyocele in Japan. Clin Infect Dis 1995; 20(Suppl. 2):S214–9.
41. Klossek JM, Dubreuil L, Richet H, Richet B, Beutter P. Bacteriology of chronic purulent secretions in chronic rhinosinusitis. J Laryngol Otol 1998; 112:1162–6.
42. Van Cauwenberge P, Verschraegen G, Van Renterghem L. Bacteriological findings in sinusitis (1963–1975). Scand J Infect Dis Suppl. 1976; 9:72–7.
43. Brook I, Frazier EH. Correlation between microbiology and previous sinus surgery in patients with chronic maxillary sinusitis. Ann Otol Rhinol Laryngol 2001; 110:148–51.
44. Bhattacharyya N, Kepnes LJ. The microbiology of recurrent rhinosinusitis after endoscopic sinus surgery. Arch Otolaryngol Head Neck Surg 1999; 125:1117–20.
45. Brook I, Foote PA, Frazier EH. Microbiology of acute exacerbation of chronic sinusitis. Laryngoscope 2004; 114:129–31.
46. Brook I. Bacteriology of chronic sinusitis and acute exacerbation of chronic sinusitis. Arch Otolaryngol Head Neck Surg 2006; 132:1099–101.
47. Del Borgo C, Del Forno A, Ottaviani F, et al. Sinusitis in HIV-infected patients. J Chemother 1997; 9:83–8.
48. Arens JF, LeJeune FE, Jr., Webre DR. Maxillary sinusitis, a complication of nasotracheal intubation. Anesthesiology 1974; 40:415–6.
49. Brook I, Shah K. Sinusitis in neurologically impaired children. Otolaryngol Head Neck Surg 1998; 119:357–60.

50. Gillespie MB, O'Malley BW, Jr., Francis HW. An approach to fulminant invasive fungal rhinosinusitis in the immunocompromised host. Arch Otolaryngol Head Neck Surg 1998; 124:520–6.
51. Jackson RM, Rice DH. Acute bacterial sinusitis and diabetes mellitus. Otolaryngol Head Neck Surg 1987; 97:469–73.
52. Talmor M, Li P, Barie PS. Acute paranasal sinusitis in critically ill patients: guidelines for prevention, diagnosis and treatment. Clin Infect Dis 1997; 25:1441–6.
53. Brook I. Microbiology of nosocomial sinusitis in mechanically ventilated children. Arch Otolaryngol Head Neck Surg 1998; 124:35–8.
54. Godofsky EW, Zinreich J, et al. Armstrong. Sinusitis in HIV-infected patients. A clinical and radiographic review. Am J Med 1992; 93:163–70.
55. Dunham ME. New light on sinusitis. Contemp Pediatr 1994; 1:102–17.
56. Handelsman DJ, Conway AJ, Boylan LM, Turtle JR. Young's syndrome: obstructive azoospermia and chronic sinopulmonary infections. N Engl J Med 1984; 310:3–9.
57. Umetsu DT, Ambrosino DM, Quinti I, Siber GR, Geha RS. Recurrent sinopulmonary infections and impaired antibody response to bacterial capsular polysaccharide antigen in children with selective IgG subclass deficiency. N Engl J Med 1985; 313:1247–51.
58. Lyon E, Miller C. Current challenges in cystic fibrosis screening. Arch Pathol Lab Med 2003; 127:1133–9.
59. Bachert C, Patou J, Van Cauwenberge P. The role of sinus disease in asthma. Curr Opin Allergy Clin Immunol 2006; 6:29–36.
60. Brook I. Aerobic and anaerobic bacteriology of purulent nasopharyngitis in children. J Clin Microbiol 1988; 26:592–4.
61. Avolainen S, Ylikoski J, Jousimies-Somer H. The bacterial flora of the nasal cavity in healthy young men. Rhinology 1986; 24:249–55.
62. Jousimies-Somer HR, Savolainen S, Ylikoski JS. Comparison of the nasal bacterial floras in two groups of healthy subjects and in patients with acute maxillary sinusitis. J Clin Microbiol 1989; 27:2736–43.
63. Brook I. Aerobic and anaerobic bacterial flora of normal maxillary sinuses. Laryngoscope 1981; 91:372–6.
64. Aust R, Drettner B. Oxygen tension in the human maxillary sinus under normal and pathological conditions. Acta Otolaryngol (Stockh) 1974; 78:264–9.
65. Brook I, Gober AE. Bacterial interference in the nasopharynx and nasal cavity of sinusitis prone and non-sinusitis prone children. Acta Otolaryngol 1999; 119:832–6.
66. Lanza DC, Kennedy DW. Adult rhinosinusitis defined. Otolaryngol Head Neck Surg 1997; 117:51–7.
67. Chandler JR, Langenbrunner DJ, Stevens EF. The pathogenesis of orbital complications in acute sinusitis. Laryngoscope 1970; 80:1414–28.
68. Wald ER, Guerra N, Byers C. Upper respiratory tract infections in young children: duration of and frequency of complications. Pediatrics 1991; 87:129–33.
69. Aalokken TM, Hagtvedt T, Dalen I, Kolbenstvedt A. Conventional sinus radiography compared with CT in the diagnosis of acute sinusitis. Dentomaxillofac Radiol 2003; 32:60–2.
70. Brook I. Beta-lactamase producing bacteria in head and neck infection. Laryngoscope 1988; 98:428–31.
71. Brook I. The role of beta-lactamase-producing bacterial in the persistence of streptococcal tonsillar infection. Rev Infect Dis 1984; 6:601–7.
72. Brook I, Yocum P, Frazier EH. Bacteriology and beta-lactamase activity in acute and chronic maxillary sinusitis. Arch Otolaryngol Head Neck Surg 1996; 122:418–22.
73. Wald ER, Chiponis D, Leclesma-Medina J. Comparative effectiveness of amoxicillin and amoxicillin–clavulanate potassium in acute paranasal sinus infection in children: a double-blind, placebo-controlled trial. Pediatrics 1998; 77:795–800.
74. Brook I, Gooch WM, III, Jenkins SG, et al. Medical management of acute bacterial sinusitis. Recommendations of a clinical advisory committee on pediatric and adult sinusitis. Ann Otol Rhinol Laryngol 2000; 109:1–20.
75. Brook I, Yocum P. Management of chronic sinusitis in children. J Laryngol Otol 1995; 109:1159–62.
76. Decker CF. Sinusitis in the immunocompromised host. Curr Infect Dis Rep 1999; 1:27–32.
77. Gross CW, Gurucharri MJ, Lazar RH, et al. Functional endoscopic sinus surgery (FESS) in the pediatric age group. Laryngoscope 1989; 99:272–5.
78. Kennedy DW. Prognostic factors, outcomes and staging in ethmoid sinus surgery. Laryngoscope 1992; 102:1–18.
79. Stankiewicz JA. Complications of endoscopic intranasal ethmoidectomy. Laryngoscope 1987; 97:1270–3.
80. Cervin A, Wallwork B. Anti-inflammatory effects of macrolide antibiotics in the treatment of chronic rhinosinusitis. Otolaryngol Clin North Am 2005; 38:1339–50.
81. Nuutinen J, Ruoppi P, Suonpaa J. One dose beclomethasone dipropionate aerosol in the treatment of seasonal allergic rhinitis. A preliminary report. Rhinol 1987; 25:121–7.
82. Chalton R, Mackay I, Wilson R, Cole P. Double blind placebo controlled trial of betamethasone nasal drops for nasal polyposis. Br Med J Clin Res Educ 1985; 291:788.

83. Brown SL, Graham SG. Nasal irrigations: good or bad? Curr Opin Otolaryngol Head Neck Surg 2004; 12:9–13.
84. Parnes SM, Chuma AV. Acute effects on anti-leukotrienes on sinonasal polyposis and sinusitis. Ear Nose Throat J 2000; 79:18–20.
85. Brook I. Microbiology of intracranial abscesses and their associated sinusitis. Arch Otolaryngol Head Neck Surg 2005; 131:1017–9.
86. Brook I, Friedman E, Rodriguez WJ, Controni G. Complications of sinusitis in children. Pediatrics 1980; 66:568–72.
87. Baker AS. Role of anaerobic bacteria in sinusitis and its complications. Ann Otol Rhinol Laryngol Suppl. 1991; 154:17–22.
88. Brook I, Frazier EH. Microbiology of subperiosteal orbital abscess and associated maxillary sinusitis. Laryngoscope 1996; 106:1010–3.
89. Clayman GL, Adams GL, Paugh DR, et al. Intracranial complications of paranasal sinusitis: a combined institutional review. Laryngoscope 1991; 101:234–9.
90. Arjmand EM, Lusk RP, Muntz HR. Pediatric sinusitis and subperiosteal orbital abscess formation: diagnosis and treatment. Otolaryngol Head Neck Surg 1993; 109:886–94.
91. Gerald J, Harris MD. Subperiosteal abscess of the orbit age as a factor in the bacteriology and response to treatment. Ophthalmology 1994; 101:585–95.
92. Dill SRC, Cobbs G, McDonald CK. Subdural empyema: analysis of 32 cases and review. Clin Infect Dis 1995; 20:372–86.
93. Brook I. Anaerobic osteomyelitis in children. Pediatr Infect Dis 1986; 5:550–6.
94. Stankiewicz JA, Newell DJ, Park AH. Complications of inflammatory diseases of the sinuses. Otolaryngol Clin North Am 1993; 26:639–55.
95. Lentrodt S, Lentrodt J, Kübler N, Mödder U. Hyperbaric oxygen for adjuvant therapy for chronically recurrent mandibular osteomyelitis in childhood and adolescence. J Orad Maxillofac Surg 2007; 65:186–91.

15 | Mastoiditis

Acute or chronic mastoiditis are a serious intratemporal complication of otitis media. Before the use of antibiotics, acute Mastoiditis (M) was the most common complication of acute otitis media (AOM). However, antibiotic treatment of AOM has decreased the incidence of this infection.

Mastoiditis defined as an inflammation of the mastoid antrum and air cells with bone necrosis.

INCIDENCE

The incidence of M parallels that of AOM, peaking in those aged 6 to 13 months. The incidence of M has decreased since the advent of antimicrobial agents and has become quite rare. The incidence of M from AOM in the U.S.A., and other developed countries is currently 0.004% (1–3). However, developing countries have a higher incidence of M, mostly as a consequence of untreated otitis media. Although the incidence of the disease has significantly declined in the U.S.A., it is still a significant infection with the potential of life-threatening complications. Of great concern is the sharp increase noted in the last decade in the incidence of acute M in several locations (2). This increase may be due to the greater recovery rate of resistant organisms, increased virulence of the pathogens and a lower use of antibiotics for the therapy of AOM (3).

MICROBIOLOGY

Acute Mastoiditis

Streptococcus pneumoniae, Streptococcus pyogenes, Staphylococcus aureus, Haemophilus influenzae are the most common organisms recovered (4–8). Rare organisms are *Pseudomonas aeruginosa* and other gram-negative aerobic bacilli, and anaerobes (6–12). Several studies demonstrated the predominance of *P. aeruginosa* in acute M. This organism is a known pathogen in chronic otitis media and chronic M (13). Since this organism is a common colonizer of the ear canal (14) it is possible that some of these isolates recovered from pus collected from the ear canal do not represent a true infection. Mastoiditis is rarely caused by tuberculosis.

Except for a study by Maharaj et al. (11) anaerobic bacteria were rarely recovered in high numbers in acute M. Maharaj et al. (11) described 35 children with acute mastoiditis treated in South Africa. Bacteria were isolated from specimens of 32 children (91%). Aerobes alone were cultured from four children (11%); six cultures (17%) yielded only anaerobes; and 22 cultures (63%) had both aerobic and anaerobic organisms. Thus, anaerobes were cultured from a total of 28 children (80%). The anaerobes recovered were similar to those described by Brook (15) in chronic M. Possibly, the microbiology of acute infection in the lower socioeconomic groups in some parts of the world is similar to chronic infection. Also, these cases may represent chronic rather than acute infection.

Chronic Mastoiditis

P. aeruginosa, Enterobacteriaceae, and *S. aureus* are the predominant isolates that have been recovered most frequently from inflamed mastoids *S. pneumoniae* and *H. influenzae* are rarely recovered (15–22).

In a study that employed anaerobic methodology, aspirates from 24 children undergoing mastoidectomy for chronic M were cultured for aerobes and anaerobes (Table 1) (15). Bacterial growth occurred in all samples. Anaerobes alone were isolated from four specimens (17%), aerobes alone from one (4%), and mixed aerobic and anaerobic flora were obtained from 19 (79%). There were 61 anaerobic isolates (2.5/specimen). The predominant anaerobic organisms were anaerobic gram-negative bacilli, gram-positive cocci, and six *Actinomyces* spp. There were 29 aerobic isolates (1.3/specimen). The predominant ones were *S. aureus*, *P. aeruginosa*, and *E. coli*. Beta-lactamase production was noted in 20 isolates recovered from 17 patients (97%). These included isolates of *S. aureus* (8), the *Bacteroides fragilis* group (3), and *Prevotella oralis* (2), as well as six of 11 pigmented *Prevotella* and *Porphyromonas* and one of two *Bacteroides* spp. This study demonstrated the polymicrobial aerobic, facultative, and anaerobic bacteriology of chronic M and reinforces studies done at the turn of the century (23). Still more evidence for the role of anaerobes in this infection is their recovery from 33% to 55% of patients with chronic otitis media in studies in which anaerobic methodology was employed (23,24).

PATHOGENESIS

Middle ear inflammation spreads to the mastoid air cells, resulting in inflammation, infection, and destruction of the mastoid bone. The mastoid at birth consists of a single cell, the antrum, located in the petromastoid part of the temporal bone (25). The tympanic cavity of the middle ear is connected to the antrum by a small canal. Soon after birth, the mastoid air cells invade the antrum. By two years of age small mastoid processes form, giving the mastoid a honeycomb appearance. Surrounding the mastoid are the posterior cranial fossa, the middle cranial fossa, the canal of the facial nerve, the sigmoid and lateral sinuses, and the petrous tip of the temporal bone. Mastoiditis can erode through the antrum and extend to any of the above contiguous sites, causing significant morbidity and life-threatening disease (17). It is not surprising to find a correlation between the aerobic and anaerobic bacteria present in chronic otitis media and cholesteatoma and the organisms recovered from acute or chronic mastoiditis (Table 1).

The presence of anaerobes is expected in patients with chronic M as they are the predominant organisms in the oropharynx, where they outnumber aerobes at a ratio of 10:1 (26). The importance of anaerobes in chronic M is supported further by their isolation from sites associated with complications of this infection. Complications include brain abscess, subdural,

TABLE 1 Bacteria Isolated from 24 Children with Chronic Mastoiditis

Isolates	No. of isolates
Aerobic and facultative	
Gram-positive cocci (total)	15
Group A beta-hemolytic streptococci	2
Staphylococcus aureus	8
Gram-negative bacilli (total)	14
Pseudomonas aeruginosa	7
Escherichia coli	5
Total	29
Anaerobic isolates	
Anaerobic cocci	23
Gram-positive bacilli (total)	14
Actinomyces sp.	6
Clostridium spp.	3
Gram-negative bacilli	
Fusobacterium nucleatum	2
Bacteroides spp.	8
Pigmented *Prevotella* and *Porphyromonas* spp.	11
B. fragilis group	3
Total	61

Note: Only the important pathogens are listed in detail. The total number of the groups of organisms is represented.
Source: From Ref. 15.

and epidural empyema, and meningitis (1,27). The frequent involvement of anaerobes in chronic M probably is related to the poor drainage and increased pressure that occur during inflammation.

DIAGNOSIS

Specimens from the mastoid cells obtained during surgery and myringotomy fluid, when obtained, should be sent for cultures for both aerobic and anaerobic bacteria, Gram and acid-fast stains. If the tympanic membrane already is perforated, the external canal can be cleaned and a sample of the fresh drainage taken. Care must be taken to obtain fluid from the middle ear and not the external canal. Culture and susceptibility testing of the isolates can assist in modifying the initial empiric antibiotic therapy and the definite choice of therapy should be guided by the results of properly collected culture for both aerobic and anaerobic bacteria. Gram stain preparation of the specimen can provide initial guidance for the empirical choice of antimicrobial therapy.

Acute Mastoiditis

This infection should be suspected when there is pain, tenderness, edema, and erythema of the postauricular area. The pinna is displaced inferiorly and anteriorly, and swelling or sagging of the posterosuperior canal wall also may be present. The eardrum usually shows changes of AOM and the child may be irritable and febrile. Radiographical studies including computed tomography may be warranted.

Chronic Mastoiditis

The onset of this infection is insidious. Clinically, there is a persistent painless, purulent, foul-smelling, scanty discharge that is unresponsive to conventional antibiotic therapy. It is often the odor that prompts the patients to seek advice. There is conductive hearing loss that is shown audiometrically. Otomicroscopic examination of the middle ear should be done (18). Specimens should be collected for Gram and acid-fast stains and cultures for aerobic and anaerobic bacteria, mycobacteria and fungi. Biopsy of suspicious tissue should be obtained.

Radiological Studies

Radiography obtained in the acute phase show diffuse inflammatory clouding of the mastoid cells; there is no evidence of bone destruction. With accumulation of the exudate there is resorption of the calcium of the mastoid cells so that they are no longer visible. Subsequently, there is destruction of the cells and areas of radiolucency representing abscesses. Axial and coronal computed tomography scanning can detect adital obstruction, osteitis, polyps, and cholesteatom (9).

With chronic M, an increase in thickness of the mastoid cells and sclerosis of the bone usually occurs. This is associated with a reduction in size of the cells. Small abscess cavities may persist in the sclerotic bone.

MANAGEMENT

The management of either acute or chronic M requires guidance provided by recovery of the offending pathogens through appropriate bacterial cultures. This requires collecting proper specimens through tympanocenthesis or surgery, and their prompt shipment to the microbiology laboratory in media supportive for the growth of both aerobic and anaerobic bacteria.

Acute Mastoiditis

The management of uncomplicated acute M includes the administration of parenteral antimicrobial therapy and myrinyotomy with or without the placement of tympanostomy tube (28). The main goal of therapy is to prevent spread of the infection to the central nervous system and to localize the infection. The antimicrobials used are vancomycin plus either ceftriaxone, or the combination of a penicillin plus a beta-lactamase inhibitor (i.e., ampicillin plus sulbactam). Oral therapy can substitute parenteral one if improvement occurred for a total of four weeks. Successful therapy markedly reduces the abscess size, the periosteal thickening, and tenderness decreases within 48 hours.

If no improvement occurs as may be evident by the patient's skin remaining red over a fluctuating abscess, or if fever and tenderness persist and do not improve within 48 hours, or if progression of the infection occurs manifested by the presence of increasing toxicity and extension of the disease process, surgical intervention and drainage may be necessary. Mastoidectomy is often required if cholesteatoma is present, or if suppurative complications occur (29). Mastoidectomy is rarely needed when adequate antibiotic therapy is administered early in the course of the disease. A recent study reported that mastoidectomy was performed in five of 21 (24%) patients (30). The surgical procedure that is generally used is simple mastoidectomy, accompanied by tympanostomy tube placement. Radical mastoidectomy is done only if no improvement occurs after simple mastoidectomy. The presence of osteitis is also an indication for surgery to prevent further intratemporal or intracranial complications.

The experience in the treatment of 72 children admitted to Children's Hospital of Pittsburgh between 1980 and 1995 with acute M complicating AOM showed that 54 (75%) were treated conservatively with broad-spectrum intravenous antibiotics and myringotomy and 18 (25%) needed mastoidectomy for treatment of a subperiosteal or Bezold's abscess or cholesteatoma, or because of poor response to conservative treatment (13). This data illustrate that patients with acute M who had only periostitis generally respond to conservative therapy, whereas those with acute mastoid osteitis usually require mastoidectomy.

Chronic Mastoiditis

Chronic suppurative otitis media that often acompanies chronic M is treated with topical antimicrobial therapy and thorough aural toilet and system antimicrobials are given if this approach fails. The empirical choice of systemic antimicrobials for chronic M is directed at the eradication of both aerobic and anaerobic bacteria. Some of the anaerobic organisms, such as *B. fragilis*, and many pigmented *Prevotella* and *Porphyromonas* and *Fusobacterium* spp. are resistant to penicillins through the production of the enzyme beta-lactamase.

Clindamycin, cefoxitin, metronidazole, chloramphenicol, or the combination of amoxicillin or ticarcillin and clavulanic acid provides coverage for anaerobic bacteria (31). Coverage for some aerobic bacteria is achieved by several of these agents. Antimicrobials effective against *S. aureus* and the aerobic gram-negative bacilli including *P. aeruginosa*, may be also needed. Whenever methicillin-resistant *S. aureus* is present vancomycin, tigecycline or linezolid should be administered instead of beta-lactam resistant penicillin (i.e., oxacillin). An aminoglycoside, a third generation cephalosporin (i.e., ceftazidine or cefepime), or a quinolone (in adults) should be considered for coverage of aerobic gram-negative bacilli (16–21). The carbapenems (i.e., imipenem, meropenem) or tigecycline provide single agent therapy for all potential pathogens. Oral therapy can substitute parenteral agent(s) if improvement occurred, for a total of six weeks of treatment.

Surgical drainage is indicated in many cases. The drained material should be Gram-stained and cultured. The reading of the Gram's stain and the results of the cultures and sensitivities allows for adjustments in the choice of antimicrobial agents.

COMPLICATIONS

Extracranial complications include temporal bone osteomyelitis, subperiosteal abscess, bezold abscess, facial nerve paralysis, dislocation of the incus, penetration of the middle or posterior fossa, labyrinthitis, and labyrinthine transgression and destruction, persistent deafness, meatal stenosis and osteomyelitis (1,28). We have described seven children who developed anaerobic osteomyelitis associated with chronic M (32). Subdural empyema developed in one patient, and aerobic bacteria were concomitantly recovered in three.

Intracranial complications of acute and particularly chronic M include facial palsy, sinus thrombosis, meningitis, rupture of the sigmoid sinus, epidural or subdural empyema and temporal lobe or cerebellum abscess.

The experience of Children's Hospital of Pittsburgh between 1980 and 1995 in 19 patients who had facial paralysis associated with M, showed that 15 recovered normal facial function but four were left with partial paralysis (13). Three patients presented with serous labyrinthitis and recovered completely with conservative therapy. Of the two patients who presented with suppurative labyrinthitis, one was treated conservatively, but the other needed tympanomastoidectomy with cochleotomy; both patients had permanent, profound sensorineural hearing loss in the affected ear. Four patients presented with acute petrositis, and in all four it resolved with mastoidectomy. These findings illustrate that even in the antibiotic era, intratemporal complications of M still occur in otherwise healthy children, often after inadequate treatment of AOM.

REFERENCES

1. Fliss DM, Leiberman A, Dagan R. Acute and chronic mastoiditis in children. Adv Pediatr Infect Dis 1997; 13:165–85.
2. Van Zuijlen DA, Schilder AG, Van Balen FA, Hoes AW. National differences in incidence of acute mastoiditis: relationship to prescribing patterns of antibiotics for acute otitis media? Pediatr Infect Dis J 2001; 20:140–4.
3. Nussinovitch M, Yoeli R, Elishkevitz K, Varsano I. Acute mastoiditis in children: epidemiologic, clinical, microbiologic, and therapeutic aspects over past years. Clin Pediatr (Phila) 2004; 43:261–7.
4. Hawkins DB, Dru D, House JW, Clark RW. Acute mastoiditis in children: a review of 54 cases. Laryngoscope 1983; 93:568–72.
5. Nadal D, Herrmann P, Baumann A, Fanconi A. Acute mastoiditis: clinical, microbiological, and therapeutic aspects. Eur J Pediatr 1990; 149:560–4.
6. Harley EH, Sdralis T, Berkowitz RG. Acute mastoiditis in children: a 12-year retrospective study. Otolaryngol Head Neck Surg 1997; 116:26–30.
7. Petersen CG, Ovesen T, Pedersen CB. Acute mastoidectomy in a Danish county from 1977 to 1996 with focus on the bacteriology. Int J Pediatr Otorhinolaryngol 1998; 45:21–9.
8. Niv A, Nash M, Peiser J, et al. Outpatient management of acute mastoiditis with periosteitis in children. Int J Pediatr Otorhinolaryngol 1998; 46:9–13.
9. Eykin S, Philips I. Anaerobic infections in surgical patients. Surg Rev 1979; 1:82–95.
10. Swantson AR, Grace ARH, Drake-Lee AB, et al. Anaerobic infection in acute mastoiditis. J Laryngol Otol 1983; 97:633–4.
11. Maharaj D, Jadwat A, Fernandes CMC, et al. Bacteriology in acute mastoiditis. Arch Otolaryngol Head Neck Surg 1987; 113:514–5.
12. Moloy PJ. Anaerobic mastoiditis: a report of two cases with complications. Laryngoscope 1982; 92:1311–5.
13. Goldstein NA, Casselbrant ML, Bluestone CD, Kurs-Lasky M. Intratemporal complications of acute otitis media in infants and children. Otolaryngol Head Neck Surg 1998; 119:444–54.
14. Brook I. Chronic otitis media in children: microbiological studies. Am J Dis Child 1980; 134:560–3.
15. Brook I. Aerobic and anaerobic bacteriology of chronic mastoiditis in children. Am J Dis Child 1981; 135:478–9.
16. Kenna MA, Rosane BA, Bluestone CD. Medical management of chronic suppurative otitis media without cholesteatoma in children–update 1992. Am J Otolaryngol 1993; 14:469–73.
17. Fliss DM, Houri Z, Leiberman A. Medical management of chronic suppurative otitis media without cholesteatoma in children. J Pediatr 1990; 1165:991–6.
18. Dagan R, Fliss DM, Einhorn M, Kraus M, Leiberman A. Outpatient management of chronic suppurative otitis media without cholesteatoma in children. Pediatr Infect Dis J 1992; 11:542–6.
19. Lang R, Goshen S, Raas-Rothscheld A, et al. Oral cefprofloxacin in the management of chronic suppurative otitis media without cholesteatoma in children: preliminary experience in 21 children. Pediatr Infect Dis J 1992; 11:925–9.
20. Arguedas AG, Herrera JF, Faingerzicht I, Molis E. Ceftazidime for therapy of children with chronic suppurative otitis media without cholesteatoma. Pediatr Infect Dis J 1993; 12:246–7.
21. Kenna MA, Bluestone CD, Reilly JS, Lusk RP. Medical management of chronic suppurative otitis media without cholesteatoma in children. Laryngoscope 1986; 96:146–51.
22. Fliss DM, Dagan R, Meidan N, Leiberman A. Aerobic bacteriology of chronic suppurative otitis media without cholestiatoma in children. Ann Otol Rhinol Laryngol 1992; 101:866–9.
23. Finegold SM. Anaerobic Bacteria in Human Disease. New York: Academic Press, 1977.
24. Brook I, Finegold SM. Bacteriology of chronic otitis media. JAMA 1979; 241:487–9.

25. Myer CM, III. The diagnosis and management of mastoiditis in children. Pediatr Ann 1991; 20:622–6.
26. Brook I. Indigenous microbial flora of humans. In: Howard R, Simmons RL, eds. Surgical Infectious Diseases. 3rd ed. Norwalk, CT: Appleton & Lange, 1995:37–46.
27. Brook I. Aerobic and anaerobic bacteriology of intracranial abscesses. Pediatr Neurol 1992; 8:210–4.
28. Bluestone CD. Acute and chronic mastoiditis and chronic supporative otitis media. Semin Pediatr Infect Dis 1998; 9:12–26.
29. Taylor MF, Berkowitz RG. Indications for mastoidectomy in acute mastoiditis in children. Ann Otol Rhinol Laryngol 2004; 113:69–72.
30. De S, Makura ZG, Clarke RW. Paediatric acute mastoiditis: the Alder Hey experience. J Laryngol Otol 2002; 116:440–2.
31. Brook I. Management of chronic suppurative otitis media: superiority of therapy effective against anaerobic bacteria. Pediatr Infect Dis J 1994; 13:188–93.
32. Brook I. Anaerobic osteomyelitis in children. Pediatr Infect Dis 1986; 5:550–6.

16 | Tonsillitis, Adenoiditis, Purulent Nasopharyngitis, and Uvulitis

TONSILLITIS

Tonsillitis is a common disease of childhood. It is extremely infectious in that it spreads easily by droplets. The incubation period is two to four days. The diagnosis of tonsillitis generally requires the consideration of group A beta-hemolytic *Streptococcus* (GABHS) infection. However, numerous other bacteria alone or in combinations (including *Staphylococcus aureus* and *Haemophilus influenzae*), viruses, and other infectious and noninfectious causes should be considered. Recognition of the cause and choice of appropriate therapy are of utmost importance in assuring rapid recovery and preventing complications.

The role of anaerobic bacteria in this infection is hard to elucidate because anaerobes are normally prevalent on the surface of the tonsils and pharynx, so that cultures taken directly from these areas are difficult to interpret. The anaerobic species that have been implicated in tonsillitis are *Actinomyces*, *Fusobacterium*, and pigmented *Prevotella* and *Porphyromonas* spp.

Anaerobes have been isolated from the cores of tonsils of children with recurrent GABHS (1) and non-GABHS (2,3) tonsillitis and peritonsillar abscesses (4). Beta-lactamase-producing strains of *Bacteroides fragilis*, *Fusobacterium* spp., *H. influenzae*, and *S. aureus* were isolated from the tonsils of 73% to 80% of children with GABHS recurrent tonsillitis (RT) (1,5,6) and from 40% of children of non-GABHS tonsillitis (2).

The failure to make a microbiological diagnosis for a known aerobic bacteria or viral pathogen in many cases of acute and RT argues for the possible role of anaerobes in this infection. A possible explanation is that the bacteria sampled by the surface swabbing technique are not an accurate reflection of the flora of the tonsillar tissue.(7–9)

It is known that deep tonsillar cultures yielded more GABHS and *S. aureus* (7–10). Comparison of surface and core cultures in a study of 23 chronically inflamed tonsils (9) showed discrepancies between the surface and core cultures in 30% of the aerobic isolates and in 43% of the anaerobic isolates. Although it is impractical to culture the core of the tonsil in patients, these findings indicate that the routine cultures obtained from the surface of the tonsils do not always represent the nature of the bacterial flora of the core of the tonsil, where potential pathogens such as GABHS or anaerobic bacteria may persist. Several investigators have suggested that hitherto unrecognized penicillin-sensitive bacteria may be responsible for many cases of non-streptococcal tonsillitis. The etiologic role of anaerobic bacteria, however, has received little attention until recently.

Microbiology

Reilly et al. (5) isolated anaerobic bacteria from all 41 tonsils removed from children at routine tonsillectomy; 75.6% of specimens yielded moderate-to-heavy growth and 80% of tonsils contained more than one anaerobic species. This recovery rate fell to 56% after a 10-day course of metronidazole before tonsillectomy—in only 14.6% of cases were anaerobes isolated in significant numbers. Surface swabbing of the tonsils permitted recovery of a similar spectrum of anaerobic bacteria but resulted in an overall loss of both aerobes and anaerobes. A comparison was made between the flora of acutely inflamed tonsils and "healthy" tonsils: over 90% of both groups yielded anaerobes, but they were present in significant numbers in 56.2% of acutely inflamed tonsils compared with 24% of healthy children. The isolation rates for anaerobes were 37.5% and 16%, respectively. *Prevotella melaninogenica* was the most prevalent anaerobe, present in all specimens yielding anaerobic flora.

Several studies (1,5–13) were conducted to determine the aerobic and anaerobic flora present in the tonsil core of children with RT (Table 1). Beta-lactamase-producing bacteria (BLPB) were present in 74% to 100% of these tonsils.

Brook et al. (12) summarized the microbiology of tonsils removed from 50 children with recurrent GABHS tonsillitis in three periods each: 1977–1978 (period 1), 1984–1985 (period 2), and 1992–1993 (period 3). Mixed flora were present in all tonsils, with 8.1 organisms per tonsil (3.8 aerobes and 4.3 anaerobes). The predominant isolates in each period were *S. aureus*, *Moraxella catarrhalis*, and *Peptostreptococcus*; pigmented *Prevotella* and *Porphyromonas*; and *Fusobacterium* spp. The rate of recovery of *H. influenzae* type b increased from 24% in period 1 to 76% in period 2 ($p < 0.001$); a decline to 12% in period three correlated with a concomitant increase in the frequency of recovery of non-type b strains of *H. influenzae* from 4% and 10% in periods 1 and 2, respectively, to 64% in period 3 ($p < 0.001$). These changes may be due to the introduction of vaccination against *H. influenzae* type b. Both the rate of recovery of BLPB and the number of these organisms per tonsil increased over time. Specifically, BLPB were detected in 37 tonsils (74%) during period 1, in 46 tonsils (92%) during period 2, and in 47 tonsils (94%) during period 3, and the number of such strains per tonsil increased from 1.1 in period 1 to 2.9 and 3.3 in periods 2 and 3, respectively. These findings indicate the polymicrobial aerobic and anaerobic nature of deep tonsillar flora in children with recurrent GABHS tonsillitis.

The microbiology of RT is different in children when compared with adults. Tonsils removed from 25 children were compared with those removed from 23 adults (15). More bacterial isolates per tonsil were recovered in adults (10.2/tonsil) than in children (8.4/tonsil). The difference between these groups was related to a higher recovery rate in adults of pigmented *Prevotella* and *Porphyromonas* (1.6 isolates/adult, 0.8 isolates/child) and *B. fragilis* group (0.4 isolates/adult, 0.2 isolates/child) (Table 2). Conversely, GABHS were isolated in seven (28%) children and only one (4%) adult. More BLPB per tonsil were recovered in adults: 1.9/patient when compared with 1.2/patient in children ($p = 0.04$). The differences in the tonsillar flora may be the result of the many more courses of antimicrobials given to adults and the changes in tonsillar tissue, which occur in this age group.

Similar aerobic–anaerobic organisms were recovered in 22 young adults (mean age 23 years) who suffered from chronic tonsillitis (3). Mixed aerobic and anaerobic flora was obtained from core tonsillar cultures in all patients, yielding an average of 9.0 isolates (5.3 anaerobes and 3.7 aerobes) per specimen. The predominant anaerobic isolates were anaerobic gram-negative bacilli (AGNB), *Fusobacterium* spp., and gram-positive cocci. The predominant aerobic isolates were alpha-hemolytic streptococci, *S. aureus*, *M. catarrhalis*, beta-hemolytic streptococci, and *Haemophilus* spp. From 18 tonsils, 32 BLPB (82%) were isolated. These included all eight isolates of *S. aureus* and 5 *B. fragilis*, and 11 of 24 *P. melaninogenica* group (46%). Because the known

TABLE 1   Microbiology of Excised Tonsils (268 Patients)

Investigators	No. of patients	% BLPB	Predominate BLPB isolated	Reference
Brook et al., U.S.A., 1980	50	74	Pigmented *Prevotella* and *Porphyromonas* *Bacteroides fragilis* *Staphylococcus aureus*	9
Reilly et al., U.K., 1981	41	78	Pigmented *Prevotella* and *Porphyromonas*	5
Tunér and Nord, Sweden, 1983	167	73	*Prevotella oris-buccae* Pigmented *Prevotella* and *Porphyromonas* *S. aureus*	13
Chagollan et al., Mexico, 1984	10	80	*S. aureus* *Prevotella oralis* *B. fragilis*	6
Kielmovitch et al., U.S.A., 1989	25	100	Pigmented *Prevotella* and *Porphyromonas*	14
Mitchelmore et al., U.K.	50	82	Pigmented *Prevotella* and *Porphyromonas*	10
Brook et al., U.S.A., 1995	50	94	Pigmented *Prevotella* and *Porphyromonas*	12

Abbreviation: BLPB, beta-lactamase-producing bacteria.

TABLE 2 Predominate Organisms Isolated in 48 Excised Tonsils from 25 Children and 23 Adults with Recurrent Tonsillitis

	No. of isolates	
	Children	Adults
Aerobic and facultative		
Streptococcus pneumoniae	2	—
Group A, beta-hemolytic streptococci	7	1
Group B, beta-hemolytic streptococci	2	5
Group C, beta-hemolytic streptococci	2	1
Staphylococcus aureus	11 (11)[a]	10 (10)[a]
Moraxella catarrhalis	13 (2)[a]	16 (3)[a]
Haemophilus influenzae type b	6 (2)[a]	4 (2)[a]
Haemophilus parainfluenzae	3 (1)[a]	1
Total	101 (16)[a]	87 (15)[a]
Anaerobic		
Peptostreptococcus spp.	18	21
Fusobacterium spp.	20	24
Bacteroides spp.	15	13
Pigmented *Prevotella* and *Porphyromonas* spp.	21 (9)[a]	37 (16)[a]
Prevotella oralis	2 (1)[a]	5 (2)[a]
Prevotella oris-buccae	3	4
Bacteroides fragilis group	5 (5)[a]	10 (10)[a]
Bacteroides ureolyticus	4	6
Total	110 (15)[a]	148 (28)[a]

[a] The number of organisms producing beta-lactamase is given in parentheses.
Source: From Ref. 15.

pathogen of tonsillitis, the GABHS, was rarely recovered (9% of patients), it is likely that other organisms, including anaerobes, have a pathogenic role in tonsillar infection and contribute to the inflammation.

The microbiology of hypertrophic tonsils after non-GABHS tonsillitis was also studied (2). The microbial flora of tonsils removed from 20 children who suffered from recurrent GABHS tonsillitis and 20 who had tonsillar hypertrophy, following recurrent non-GABHS tonsillitis, were evaluated. Similar polymicrobial aerobic–anaerobic flora was recovered in each group: an average of 9.4 isolates/tonsil (3.75 aerobic and 5.65 anaerobic) in the recurrent GABHS tonsillitis group and 8.8 isolates/tonsil (3.4 aerobic and 5.4 anaerobic) in the non-GABHS tonsillitis group. BLPB were recovered more often in the recurrent GABHS tonsillitis group—1.6/patient when compared with 0.85/patient ($p < 0.005$). These differences were due to the lower incidence of beta-lactamase-producing strains of *M. catarrhalis* and AGNB in hypertrophic tonsils. Beta-lactamase-producing *S. aureus* were found with equal frequency in both groups. These findings demonstrate that although BLPB are recovered more often in recurrently inflamed tonsils following GABHS infection, BLPB can also be found in hypertrophic tonsils following non-GABHS tonsillitis. Because many of the aerobic and anaerobic organisms are potential pathogens, they may play a role in the inflammatory process in non-GABHS tonsillitis. Whether the presence of these bacteria in the core of hypertrophic tonsils contributes to the pathologic process in these tonsils is yet to be determined.

Kuhn et al. (16) studied the aerobic and anaerobic microbiology of tonsillar specimens from children who had undergone elective tonsillectomy: six patients with RT, nine with recurrent tonsillitis with hypertrophy (RTH), and eight with obstructive tonsillar hypertrophy (OTH). Mixed flora was present in all tonsils, yielding an average of 6.7 isolates (5.6 aerobic and 1.1 anaerobic bacteria). The highest recovery rate of organisms was in patients with OTH (7.7/tonsil), compared with 6.3/tonsil in RT and 5.9/tonsil in RTH. The predominant aerobic and facultative organisms were *H. influenzae* (22 isolates), *Neisseria* spp. (16), *S. aureus* (14), and *Eikenella corrodens* (14), and the predominant anaerobes were *Fusobacterium* spp. (8), *Bacteroides* spp. (7), and *P. melaninogenica* (5). The number of bacteria per gram of tonsillar tissue varied between 10^4 and 10^8. A higher concentration of *S. aureus* and *H. influenzae* was found in hypertrophic tonsils (RTH and OTH) when compared with RT. These findings suggest the presence of an increased bacterial load in hypertrophic tonsils with and without inflammation (RTH and OTH).

A study that evaluated the effect of selective antimicrobial therapy directed at these organisms suggested a potential option for the management of hypertrophic tonsils. In a prospective, randomized, double-blind, placebo-controlled trial of 167 children, Sclafani et al. (17) evaluated the short- and long-term effects of treatment of symptomatic chronic adenotonsillar hypertrophy with a 30-day course of 40 mg/kg amoxicillin–clavulanate (86 patients) compared with placebo (81 patients). The treatment group showed a significant reduction in the need for surgery up to two years following therapy. The effect of amoxicillin–clavulanate may be due to its efficacy against the aerobic and anaerobic BLPB recovered in higher numbers in the cores of hypertrophic tonsils.

Other anaerobes that may have a role in tonsillar infection are species of *Actinomyces*. Actinomycetes have been cultured on routine oral examination and are part of the normal oral flora. Mucosal disruption is required for these bacteria to become infective (18). The most common clinical presentation for the cervicofacial actinomycotic infection is a chronic, slowly progressive indurated mass, usually involving the submaxillary gland and frequently occurring after dental extraction or trauma (19). Several reports acknowledged the presence of actinomycetes in tonsil tissue (19).

Pathogenesis

Anaerobes are abundant among the indigenous flora of the oropharynx (20). Anaerobic bacteria capable of interfering with the in vitro growth of GABHS as well as other potential pathogens are part of the normal on pharyngeal flora and may play a role in maintaining the homeostatic balance in the flora. The frequency of recovery of aerobic and anaerobic bacteria with interfering capability for GABHS from the tonsils of 20 children with and 20 without the history of recurrent GABHS pharyngotonsillitis was investigated (11). Eleven aerobic and anaerobic isolates with interfering capability for GABHS were recovered from 6 of the 20 (30%) children with recurrent GABHS, and 40 such organisms were isolated from 17 of the 20 (85%) without recurrences ($p < 0.01$). The interfering organisms included aerobic (alpha- and nonhemolytic streptococci) and anaerobic organisms (*Prevotella* and *Peptostreptococcus* spp.). The study illustrates that the tonsils of children with the history of recurrent GABHS infection contain less aerobic and anaerobic bacteria with interfering capability of GABHS than those without that history. It also suggests that the presence of interfering bacteria may play a role in preventing GABHS infection.

The pathogenic potential of anaerobes is realized in a variety of localized infection: lung abscess, peritonsillar abscess (4), cervical adenitis, otitis media, and mastoiditis (18,21).

Using quantitative methods, Brook and Foote (22) found a similarity in the polymicrobial aerobic and anaerobic bacterial flora recovered from the cores of four normal tonsils when compared with four recurrently inflamed tonsils. The concentration of several species of organisms, however, was higher in children with recurrently inflamed tonsils (10^6–10^8/ Gram) when compared with those with normal tonsils (10^4–10^6/Gram). This was particularly true for the encapsulated pigmented *Prevotella* and *Porphyromonas* spp. isolates.

The possible role of anaerobes in the acute inflammatory process in the tonsils is supported by several clinical observations: their recovery from tonsillar (4) and retropharyngeal abscesses (23) in many cases without any aerobic bacteria, their isolation in well-established anaerobic infections of the tonsils (Vincent's angina) (24), the increased recovery rate of encapsulated pigmented *Prevotella* and *Porphyromonas* spp. in acutely inflamed tonsils when compared with noninflamed ones (25), their isolation from the cores of recurrently inflamed non-GABHS tonsils (2), and the response to antibiotics effective against them in patients with non-GABHS tonsillitis (26–31).

The pathogenicity of pigmented *Prevotella* and *Porphyromonas*, which were recovered from tonsillar tissue, was demonstrated in animal models (32). Subcutaneous and intraperitoneal abscesses were induced in mice by inoculating these organisms alone and the ability to cause an abscess correlated with the presence of a capsule.

Furthermore, immune response against *Prevotella intermedia* (33) and *Fusobacterium nucleatum* (33,34) can be detected in patients with acute non-streptococcal and GABHS tonsillitis, and those who recovered from peritonsillar cellulitis or abscesses (35) and infectious mononucleosis (36).

Several studies in which metronidazole was administered to patients with infectious mononucleosis provided support of the role of anaerobes in tonsillitis (26,27). Metronidazole alleviated the clinical symptoms of tonsillar hypertrophy and shortened the duration of fever. Metronidazole has no antimicrobial activity against aerobic bacteria and is only effective against anaerobes. A possible mechanism of its action could be the suppression of the oral anaerobic flora that might have contributed to the inflammatory process induced by the Epstein–Barr virus (26,27). This explanation is supported by the increase recovery of *P. intermedia* and *F. nucleatum* during the acute phases of infectious mononucleosis (37) and the immune response against these organisms in these patients (36).

McDonald et al. (28) demonstrated a reduction in the severity of symptoms of adults with non-GABHS tonsillitis following the administration of erythromycin. Merenstein and Rogers (29) illustrated an improvement in the symptoms of patients with acute non-GABHS tonsillitis following penicillin therapy when compared with placebo. Putto (30) showed an earlier defervescence following penicillin therapy of children with non-GABHS tonsillitis when compared with patients with viral tonsillitis. Brook (31) demonstrated the efficacy of clindamycin over penicillin in the therapy of 40 patients with recurrent non-GABHS. From the second day following therapy on, significantly fewer patients who received clindamycin showed fever, pharyngeal infection, and sore throat. In one year following RT, infection was noted in 13 of the patients who received penicillin and in two patients who were treated with clindamycin ($p<0.001$). Brook and Gober (38) found that reduction in fever, sore throat, pharyngeal injection, and tonsillar size occurred more rapidly in 20 children with non-GABHS tonsillitis, who were treated with metronidazole when compared with 20 untreated patients.

All of these studies suggest that bacteria other than GABHS, including anaerobes, may be involved in acute and recurrent tonsillitis.

Diagnosis

Distinguishing between viral and bacterial aerobic or anaerobic tonsillitis is difficult.

The patients with anaerobic infection may manifest fever, malaise, and pain on swallowing. On examination the tonsils are enlarged, and may be ulcerated. A foul-smelling discharge frequently has been observed.

Vincent (24) has described the classical findings of anaerobic tonsillitis. At the early stages of the infection, the tonsil is covered with a thin white or gray film that can be detached to leave a bleeding surface. There may be a superficial ulcer underneath the membrane. By the third or fourth day, the pseudomembrane is thick and caseous in appearance and contributes a foul smell to the breath. With anaerobic tonsillitis enlarged submandibular lymph nodes, periadenitis, edema, and even trismus can be noted.

The differential diagnosis includes diphtheria, GABHS infection, viral pharyngitis, and infectious mononucleosis. The most unique features of anaerobic tonsillitis or pharyngotonsillitis are the fetid or foul odor and the presence of fusiform bacilli, spirochetes, and other organisms that have the unique morphology of anaerobes on direct smear of the membrane. It must be remembered that anaerobic pharyngotonsillitis may coexist with other types of tonsillitis.

Management

Penicillin has been the mainstay for treatment of tonsillar infections because of its effectiveness against GABHS. However, the rate of penicillin failure in eradicating GABHS from infected tonsils has slowly increased over the past 50 years from about 7% to 38% (39,40). As a final resort, many of these patients are referred for tonsillectomy. Penicillin failure in eradicating GABHS tonsillitis has several explanations. These include noncompliance with 10-day course of therapy, carrier state, GABHS intracellular internalization, reinfection, the absence of bacterial interfering bacteria, and penicillin tolerance. One explanation is that repeated penicillin administration results in a shift in the oral microflora with selection of aerobic (*S. aureus, Haemophilus* spp., *M. catarrhalis*) and anaerobic (*Fusobacterium* spp. and pigmented *Prevotella* and *Porphyromonas* spp.) BLPB.

The emergence of anaerobic BLPB has important implications for chemotherapy (41). These bacteria can produce enzymes that degrade penicillins or cephalosporins in the tonsils protecting not only themselves but also GABHS. The presence of aerobic and anaerobic BLPB in recurrently inflamed tonsils has been extensively studied (1,5,6,12,13) (Table 2). Assays of the free enzyme in the tissues demonstrated its presence in 33 of 39 (85%) tonsils that harbored BLPB, while the enzyme was not detected in any of the 11 tonsils without BLPB (42).

The ability of BLPB to protect penicillin-sensitive microorganisms has been demonstrated in vitro. When mixed with cultures of *B. fragilis*, the resistance of GABHS to penicillin increased at least 8500-fold (43). Simon and Sakai (44) have demonstrated the ability of *S. aureus*, and Scheifele and Fussel (45) showed the ability of *Haemophilus parainfluenzae* to protect GABHS from penicillin.

These phenomena are demonstrated in Figure 1. *S. aureus* is resistant to penicillin (it grew close to the penicillin disk), while GABHS is very susceptible to it (i.e., growth on the plate was inhibited to a large extent, as is evident by the zone of the beta-hemolysis). When these two organisms were plated mixed together (middle plate), however, GABHS were able to grow in close proximity to the penicillin disk, thus showing resistance to the penicillin that was acquired by the beta-lactamase produced by *S. aureus*.

This phenomenon was demonstrated in vivo by studies of mixed infections of penicillin-resistant and penicillin-susceptible bacteria. Hackman and Wilkins (46,47) showed that penicillin-resistant strains of *B. fragilis, P. melaninogenica*, and *Prevottela oralis* protected *Fusobacterium necrophorum*, a penicillin-sensitive pathogen, from penicillin therapy in mice.

Brook et al. (48), utilizing subcutaneous abscess models in mice, demonstrated protection of GABHS from penicillin by *B. fragilis* and *P. melaninogenica*. However, clindamycin, or the combination of penicillin and clavulanic acid (a beta-lactamase inhibitor), active against both GABHS and AGNB, was effective in eradicating the infection.

Brook and Gober (49,51) and Tunér and Nord (50) have demonstrated the rapid emergence of BLPB following penicillin therapy. Brook and Gober followed 26 children treated with penicillin (51) and observed continued colonization with BLPB in 35% of children 40 to 45 days after completion of therapy and in 27% of children 85 to 90 days after therapy.

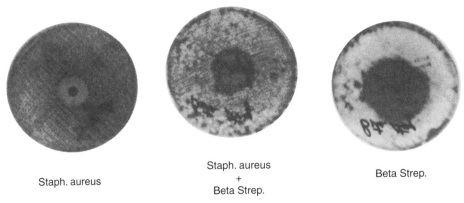

Staph. aureus

Staph. aureus
+
Beta Strep.

Beta Strep.

FIGURE 1   Effect of *Staphylococcus aureus* on the susceptibility of GABHS to penicillin. A 10-U (6 µg) penicillin G disk is placed in the center of each blood agar plate. (*Left*): *S. aureus* is resistant to penicillin. (*Right*): *GABHS* is susceptible to penicillin. (*Middle*): Mixed with *S. aureus*, GABHS is resistant to penicillin. *Abbreviation*: GABHS, group A beta-hemolytic *Streptococcus*.

A direct association was demonstrated between the presence of BLPB even before therapy and the outcome of 10-day oral penicillin therapy (52). Roos et al. (53) found that patients with recurrent GABHS tonsillitis had significantly more often detectable amounts of beta-lactamase in their saliva when compared with healthy individuals or patients who did not fail penicillin treatment.

ELIMINATION OF GABHS

Antimicrobials that are effective against BLPB as well as GABHS have been shown to be effective in the elimination of GABHS in acute and chronic infections or the eradication of GABHS carrier state. These include lincomycin, clindamycin (54–69), penicillin plus rifampin, and the combination of amoxicillin and clavulanic acid (65) (Table 3). Other drugs that may also be effective are the combination of metronidazole and a macrolide. Clindamycin was also found to be superior to penicillin in alleviating the signs and symptoms of acute non-GABHS tonsillitis and in the prevention of recurrence (31).

The superiority of these drugs may be due not only to their effectiveness against GABHS but also to their efficacy against other aerobic and anaerobic organisms that may "protect" the pathogenic streptococci by producing beta-lactamase (such as *S. aureus* and AGNB).

The combination of penicillin plus rifampin was found to be superior to penicillin in curing acute GABHS tonsillitis (65) and the eradication of GABHS carrier (64). Clindamycin was found superior to penicillin plus rifampin in the eradication of GABHS carrier state (66). Although these studies did not correlate efficacy with the presence of BLPB, the activity of rifampin and clindamycin against *S. aureus* and clindamycin against AGNB may have accounted for their success.

Brook and Leyva (67) treated with clindamycin for 7 to 10 days, 20 children who were chronic carried of GABHS and had a history of RT. All these patients responded to the therapy and a two-year follow-up showed the elimination of their carrier state for GABHS, and the lack of recurrence of streptococcal tonsillitis. In another study, Brook (68) treated 38 children who had RT and were also chronic carriers of GABHS. GABHS were completely eliminated after clindamycin therapy, and the numbers of *Bacteroides* spp. and *S. aureus* were reduced. BLPB were detected prior to therapy in 57 isolates recovered from all patients' tonsils. Only four isolates of BLPB were recovered after the conclusion of therapy. Follow-up study of 33 children for eight to 16 months showed no recurrence of GABHS in 31.

A double-blind study compared penicillin with erythromycin and clindamycin in the eradication of recurrent streptococcal tonsillitis (60). With penicillin therapy, only two of 15

TABLE 3 Studies Comparing Penicillin and Other Agents in the Therapy of Acute and Recurrent Group A Streptococcal Tonsillopharyngitis

	Failure rate		
	Penicillins	**Other drugs**	
Acute tonsillopharyngitis			
Breese et al. (54, 56)	38/131 (29%)	Lincomycin	17/131 (13%)
Randolph and DeHaan (58)	37/267 (14%)	Lincomycin	20/258 (8%)
Howie and Ploussard (61)	32/80 (40%)	Lincomycin	10/76 (13%)
Randolph et al. (59)	15/72 (21%)	Clindamycin	4/56 (7%)
Stillerman et al. (62)	9/51 (18%)	Clindamycin	5/52 (10%)
Chaudhary et al. (65)	11/39 (28%)	Penicillin and rifampin	0/60 (0%)
Massell (prophylaxis) (57)	26/102 (25%)	Clindamycin	12/100 (12%)
Recurrent tonsillopharyngitis			
Brook and Hirokawa (60)	12/15 (87%)	Erythromycin	9/15 (60%)
		Clindamycin	1/15 (7%)
Tanz et al. (carriers) (64)	10/22 (45%)[a]	Clindamycin	2/26 (8%)
Brook (63)	6/20 (30%)	Clindamycin	2/26 (8%)
Smith et al. (39)	20/24 (83%)	Amoxicillin and clavulanic acid	0/20 (0%)
Orrling et al. (55)	14/22 (64%)	Dicloxacillin	9/18 (50%)
		Clindamycin	0/26 (0%)

[a] With rifampin.

children; with erythromycin, six of 15; and with clindamycin, 14 of 15 were cured. Four children who received penicillin and two who received erythromycin required a tonsillectomy. No tonsillectomies were required in the clindamycin group.

In a randomized, prospective study of 50 patients scheduled for tonsillectomy, Foote and Brook (69) compared the relative efficacy of penicillin with clindamycin in eradicating both GABHS and BLPB in electively excised tonsillar cores. No GABHS survived treatment with clindamycin. Patients with BLPB were 94% in the nontreatment group, 82% in the penicillin-treated group, and 32% in the clindamycin-treated group. The reduction in the number of BLPB in patients who received clindamycin was especially apparent in children younger than 12 years of age.

Brook (63) compared the efficacy of penicillin with the combination of amoxicillin and clavulanic acid in the eradication of GABHS in children with a history of recurrent GABHS tonsillitis. Twenty children were studied in each group. BLPB were present in 34 of 40 (85%) of tonsillar cultures. GABHS was eradicated in 14 of 20 (70%) treated with penicillin and in all of those treated with amoxicillin and clavulanic acid ($p < 0.001$). In a year, 11 of 19 children treated with penicillin, and two of 18 children treated with amoxicillin and clavulanic acid had RT.

Tanz et al. (70) compared 10-day courses of orally administered penicillin and amoxicillin–clavulanic acid in 89 patients (43 penicillin, 46 amoxicillin–clavulanic acid). BLPB were isolated before therapy from the throats of 67% of patients treated with penicillin and 63% treated with amoxicillin–clavulanic acid. Throat cultures after completion of therapy were positive for GABHS in seven (7.9%) of 89 patients. The initial GABHS T type persisted (treatment failure) in only four (4.5%) of 89 patients, including three (6.5%) of 46 who received amoxicillin–clavulanic acid and in one (2.3%) of 43 who received penicillin. Bacteriologic treatment failure was unrelated to recovery of BLPB at the time of enrollment or after treatment.

Dykhuizen et al. (71) treated 165 patients with acute GABHS pharyngitis with amoxicillin–clavulanic acid (79 patients) or penicillin (86 patients). At follow-up after seven days, GABHS were recovered in seven patients (9.6%) in the penicillin V group; three of these patients had tonsillitis clinically. In the amoxicillin–clavulanic acid group, these figures were three (3.8%) and two, respectively ($p > 0.05$). Within the 12-month follow-up period, there were four clinical recurrences (6.1%) in the penicillin V group and seven (9.3%) in the amoxicillin–clavulanic acid group ($p > 0.1$). Beta-lactamase activity in the saliva was demonstrated in 29 patients (19.2%). Fourteen (74%) of 19 bacteriologic failures or clinical recurrences had beta-lactamase activity, versus 15 (12%) of 129 successfully treated patients ($p > 0.001$). The authors concluded that there is no evidence that amoxicillin–clavulanic acid is better than penicillin V for the first treatment of acute GABHS pharyngitis, but bacteriologic failure and clinical recurrence are strongly associated with the presence of beta-lactamase activity in commensal flora.

In meta-analysis of 35 randomized trials involving 7125 patients with acute GABHS tonsillitis that were done between 1970 and 2000, Casey and Pichichero (72) found bacterial failure three times more frequently with penicillin than cephalosporins. This was evident even in several instances when cephalosporins were given for less than 10 days (73). Their efficacy may be due to their ability to inhibit aerobic BLPB, as well as spare potential interfering organism.

Increased resistance of GABHS to the macrolides in up to 70% of the isolates has been noticed worldwide, especially in countries when these agents were used extensively (74). Only after their use was reduced, did the rate of resistance decline to less than 10% (75). The current rate of macrolide resistance in the U.S.A. is about 6% (76), but rates as high as 50% were noted in some locations (77).

Complications

Peritonsillar abscess, in which anaerobes are the dominant organisms (4), can emerge following acute tonsillitis. Uncommonly, the tonsillar and pharyngeal infections may spread to involve the prevertebral muscles, and this allows a subluxation of the atlantoaxial joint. Other complications may occur because of the increased size of the tonsils and include inability to swallow solid food, and cor pulmonale. Bacteremia and sepsis also can develop following tonsillitis. In a review of the literature from 1925 to 1974 by Finegold (78), more than 200 cases of anaerobic bacteremia and sepsis were preceded by serious tonsillar or nasopharyngeal (NP) infection (Lemierre's syndrome). (see chap. 12). The organisms most frequently recovered in these cases were *Fusobacterium* spp., AGNB, and anaerobic gram-positive cocci (79–81).

Lemierre's syndrome or postanginal septicemia (necrobacillosis) is caused by an acute oropharyngeal infection with secondary septic thrombophlebitis of the internal jugular vein and frequent metastatic infections (82). *F. necrophorum* is the most common pathogen isolated from the patients. The interval between the oropharyngeal infection and the onset of the septicemia is usually short. The most common sites of septic embolisms are the lungs and joints, and other locations can be affected. A high degree of clinical suspicion is needed to diagnose the syndrome. Computed tomography of the neck with contrast is the most useful study to detect internal jugular vein thrombosis. Treatment includes intravenous antibiotic therapy and drainage of septic foci. The role of anticoagulation is controversial. Ligation or excision of the internal jugular vein may be needed in some cases.

In the review of the literature on *Bacteroides* septicemia (83), NP infection was the most common site of the primary lesion in those cases of sepsis present in 54 of 148 reported cases (36%). The oropharynx was the source of anaerobic bacteremia in 7% of 296 cases (84).

The advent of the antimicrobials had a significant impact on this type of infection. While local tonsillar infection still occurs, it is seldom recognized as being due to anaerobes, and the use of antimicrobial therapy has resulted in the prompt response of the infection without the development of the serious complications that were very frequent in the past.

ADENOIDITIS

The adenoid tissues are part of Waldeyer's ring and form part of the body's defense mechanisms against infection. They arise from the juncture of the roof and posterior wall of the nasopharynx and are composed of vertical ridges of lymphoid tissue separated by deep clefts. This tissue differs from tonsillar tissue in that it contains no crypts, is bounded by no capsule, and is covered by ciliated epithelium. Adenoids are present at birth, survive throughout childhood, and atrophy at puberty, although persistence into adulthood is common.

Adenoids are susceptible to inflammatory changes and frequently are infected concomitantly with the tonsils. It is, therefore, difficult to differentiate isolated adenoid infection from combined infection with the tonsils. Adenoid hypertrophy is defined as an enlargement of the adenoids, which may be simple or inflammatory, and the symptoms may be due to hypertrophy, to infection, or to both. Recurrent adenotonsillitis (RAT) is often a bacterial–viral illness.

Pathogenesis and Microbiology

Microbiologically, patients suffering from adenoiditis harbor an abnormal NP and oropharyngeal microflora. Typically, this flora is characterized by the persistent presence of two to five bacterial species that are frequently associated with clinical infections of the head and neck: GABHS, *S. aureus*, *H. influenzae*, *Streptococcus pneumoniae*, *Candida albicans*, enteric gram-negative aerobes and AGNB. The viruses often present are adenoviruses and Epstein–Barr virus (85,86).

The adenoids are believed to play a role in several infectious and noninfectious upper airway illnesses. They may be implicated in the etiology of otitis media (87–91), rhinosinusitis (92,93), adenotonsillitis (94), and chronic nasal obstruction due their hypertrophy (95,96).

Establishing the unique microbiology of the adenoids in patients with a variety of pathologic conditions is of importance, as it can assist in their management. Several studies have explored the aerobic bacteria microbiology of the adenoids (87,96).

Brook (97) compared the aerobic and anaerobic bacteria recovered from the core of adenoids obtained from 18 children with chronic adenotonsillitis (group A) and those of 12 children with adenoid hypertrophy and persistent middle ear effusion (group B) (Tables 4 and 5). Mixed aerobic and anaerobic flora was obtained from all patients, yielding an average of 7.8 isolates (4.6 anaerobes and 3.2 aerobes) per specimen. There were 97 anaerobes isolated. The predominant isolates in both groups were AGNB (including *Prevotella* and *Porphyromonas* spp.),

TABLE 4 Aerobic and Facultative Organisms Isolated from Excised Adenoids from 18 Children with Chronic Adenotonsillitis (Group A) and 12 with Adenoid Hypertrophy (Group B)

Isolates	Group A (18 patients)	Group B (12 patients)	Total number (30 patients)
Gram-positive cocci			
Streptococcus pneumoniae	5	4	9
Alpha-hemolytic streptococci	14	9	23
Gamma-hemolytic streptococci	7	5	12
Group A, beta-hemolytic streptococci	6	4	10
Group B, beta-hemolytic streptococci	2	1	3
Group C, beta-hemolytic streptococci		1	1
Group F, beta-hemolytic streptococci	1	2	3
Staphylococcus aureus	9 (9[a])	2 (2[a])	11 (11[a])
Gram-negative cocci			
Neisseria spp.	15	12	27
Gram-positive bacilli			
Lactobacillus spp.	2	3	5
Diphtheroids	7	3	10
Gram-negative bacilli			
Haemophilus influenzae type b	7 (2[a])	1	8 (2[a])
Haemophilus parainfluenzae	3	1	4
Eikenella corrodens	2	1	3
Pseudomonas aeruginosa	2		2
Escherichia coli	3		3
Yeast			
Candida albicans	3	1	4
Total number of aerobes and facultatives	88 (11[a])	50 (2[a])	138 (13[a])

[a] Number of beta-lactamase-producing organisms.
Source: From Ref. 97.

Fusobacterium spp., gram-positive anaerobic cocci, and *Veillonella* spp. There were 138 aerobic isolates. The predominant isolates in both groups were alpha- and gamma-hemolytic streptococci, beta-hemolytic streptococci (groups A, B, C, and F), *S. aureus*, *S. pneumoniae*, *Haemophilus* spp. *H. influenzae* type b and *S. aureus* were more frequently isolated in group A. *B. fragilis* was

TABLE 5 Anaerobic Organisms Isolated in Excised Adenoids from 18 Children with Chronic Adenotonsillitis (Group A) and 12 with Adenoid Hypertrophy (Group B)

Isolates	Group A (18 patients)	Group B (12 patients)	Total number (30 patients)
Gram-positive cocci			
Peptostreptococcus spp.	12	7	19
Gram-negative cocci			
Veillonella parvula	3	2	5
Gram-positive bacilli			
Bifidobacterium adolescentis	1		1
Eubacterium spp.	2	2	4
Actinomyces spp.	2	1	3
Gram-negative bacilli			
Fusobacterium spp.	2	1	3
Fusobacterium nucleatum	10	6	16
Bacteroides spp.	4	1	5
Pigmented Prevotella and Porphyromonas spp.	13 (7[a])	9 (1[a])	22 (8[a])
Prevotella oralis	6 (3[a])	5 (1[a])	11 (4[a])
Prevotella oris-buccae	4	2	6
Bacteroides fragilis group	2 (2[a])		2 (2[a])
Total number of anaerobes	61 (12[a])	36 (2[a])	97 (14[a])
Total number of aerobes, facultatives, and anaerobes	149 (23[a])	86 (4[a])	235 (27[a])

[a] Number of beta-lactamase-producing organisms.
Source: From Ref. 97.

recovered only in group A. There were 27 BLPB isolated from 18 patients. Fifteen (83%) of these patients belonged to group A, while three (25%) were members of group B.

Brook et al. (98) determined the qualitative and quantitative microbiology of core adenoid tissue obtained from four groups of 15 children each: with recurrent otitis media (ROM), RAT, obstructive adenoid hypertrophy (OAH), and occlusion or speech abnormalities (controls).

Polymicrobial aerobic–anaerobic flora was present in all instances. A total of 89 organisms were isolated from controls, 146 from ROM, 142 from RAT, and 149 from OAH. The predominant aerobes in all groups were alpha- and gamma-hemolytic streptococci, *H. influenzae*, *S. aureus*, GABHS, and *M. catarrhalis*. The prominent anaerobes were *Peptostreptococcus*, *Prevotella*, and *Fusobacterium* spp. The number and distribution of types of most organisms did not vary among the three groups of diseased adenoids. However, the number of all organisms, those that are potential pathogens and BLPB, was lower in the control than the diseased adenoids ($p < 0.001$). The study highlights the importance of the bacterial load in the adenoids in contributing to the etiology of ROM, RAT, and OAH.

H. influenzae is more commonly recovered in patients with chronic adenotonsillitis when compared with those with adenoid hypertrophy (87,88,97). Another striking difference is the presence of BLPB in 83% of patients with chronic adenotonsillitis when compared with 25% in those with adenoid hypertrophy (98). Of particular interest is the higher prevalence of *B. fragilis* and the beta-lactamase-producing pigmented *Prevotella* and *Porphyromonas* and *B. oralis*. This could be due to the selective pressure of repeated antimicrobial therapy administered to these patients, which could select these BLPB.

The existence of BLPB, many of them anaerobic, within the core of the adenoids may explain the persistence of many pathogens in that area, where they may be shielded from the activity of the penicillins. The chronically infected adenoid tissue may also be a factor in the recurrence of middle ear disease by causing Eustachian tube dysfunction and serving as a source for pathogenic organisms (88).

Similarity and differences exist in individuals between the bacteriology of recurrently inflamed adenoids and tonsils. A recent study investigated the microbiology of the adenoids and tonsils electively removed from 25 children with a history of recurrent GABHS adenotonsillitis (99). Mixed flora was present in all instances with an average of 9.1 isolates/specimen. The predominant aerobes were *Streptococcus* spp., *H. influenzae*, GABHS, and the prevalent anaerobes were *Peptostreptococcus*, *Prevotella*, and *Fusobacterium* spp. BLPB were detected in 75 isolates recovered from 22 (88%) tonsils and 74 from 21 (84%) adenoids. Discrepancies in the recovery of organisms were found between the tonsils and adenoids. Of the aerobic isolates, 18% were only isolated in tonsils and 18% only in adenoids. Of the anaerobes, 20% were found only in tonsils and 26% only in adenoids. This study demonstrates the similar polymicrobial aerobic–anaerobic flora in both adenoids and tonsils, and the discrepancies in recovery of pathogens. The adenoids may serve as a potential source of tonsillitis due to this organism.

Clinical Signs and Diagnosis

Acute adenoiditis may occur alone or in association with rhinitis or tonsillitis. It produces pain behind the nose and postnasal catarrh, lack of resonance of the voice, nasal obstruction, and feeding difficulties in infants, and it is often accompanied by cervical adenitis. Chronic adenoiditis may result from repeated acute attacks or from infection in small adenoid remnants. The main symptom is postnasal drip. This secretion is seen to hang down behind the soft palate as tenacious mucopus.

Mouth breathing and persistent rhinitis are characteristic symptoms. With severe adenoid hypertrophy, the mouth is kept open during the day as well as during sleep, and the mucous membranes of the mouth and lips are dry. Chronic nasopharyngitis may be constantly present or recur frequently. The voice is altered, with a nasal, muffled quality. The breath is foul smelling and frequently offensive, and taste and smell are impaired. A harassing cough may be present, especially at night, resulting from irritation of the larynx by inspired air that has not been warmed and moistened by passage through the nose. Impaired hearing is common.

Chronic otitis media may be associated with infected, hypertrophied adenoids and blockage of the Eustachian tube orifices.

Adenoid size can be assessed in the young infant by digital palpation. Fiber-optic bronchoscopy and lateral roentgenogram can assist in evaluating the size of the adenoids.

Management

Adenoidectomy and tonsillectomy frequently are performed to relieve recurrent ear infections and chronic adenoiditis associated with persistent ear effusions in children (85). Adenoidectomy may be indicated with symptoms such as persistent mouth breathing, nasal speech, and adenoid facies.

There are no solid data to support adenoidectomy for the treatment of recurrent nasopharyngitis. However, a limited and short-term efficacy was noted on the rate of recurrent acute otitis media (100) and otitis media with effusion (90, 101) after adenoidectomy. These patients usually are treated with multiple courses of antibiotics prior to surgery; however, many continue to harbor pathogenic bacteria in the pharynx.

Various theories were suggested to explain the persistence of these pathogenic organisms in the oropharynx, including appearance of penicillin tolerant GABHS and increased numbers of BLPB such as *S. aureus* and some strains of *H. influenzae*. Removal of the tonsils and adenoids is associated, in many instances, with a reduction of pathogenic organisms such as GABHS and *S. aureus* (85,90).

The isolation of pathogenic aerobic and anaerobic BLPB from chronically inflamed adenoids raises the question of whether the currently used antimicrobial therapy of chronic adenotonsillitis is always adequate and whether therapy for this infection should be directed also at the eradication of the more prevalent of these potential pathogens.

Indirect evidence for the potential importance of microorganisms in adenoid hypertrophy was provided by Sclafani et al. (17) who demonstrated a significant reduction for the need of adenotonsillectomy following 30 days therapy with amoxicillin–clavulanate compared with placebo in children with hypertrophic adenoids and tonsils. The effect of amoxicillin–clavulanate therapy may be due to its activity against aerobic and anaerobic BLPB that are found in higher numbers in the cores of hypertrophic adenoids and tonsils with or without a history of recurrent infection.

Although no other prospective studies were done of children with adenotonsillitis, when antibiotics such as lincomycin (54,56,58,61), clindamycin (55, 59,60,62,66,67,69,102), oxacillin (39, 44), and amoxicillin and clavulanic acid (63) were administered to patients suffering from chronic RT, they were found to be more efficacious than penicillin. This may be due to the effectiveness of those drugs not only against GABHS, but also against BLPB that may protect the pathogens.

PURULENT NASOPHARYNGITIS

Purulent nasopharyngitis is commonly found in children, especially in the fall, winter, and early spring. This infection is often part of an inflammatory response of the upper respiratory tract that also involves the tonsils, adenoids, uvula, and soft palate. The role of bacteria in the infectious process is yet undetermined.

Etiology

The overwhelming majority of nasopharyngitis occurrence is caused by viral infections. Adenoviruses are the most common cause of nasopharyngitis and types 1 to 7, 7a, 9, 14, and 15, accounting for the majority of illnesses (103). Nasopharyngitis is also common with influenza and parainfluenza viral infections. Although rhinoviral and respiratory syncytial viral infections are common in children and both always have nasal manifestations (rhinitis), the occurrence of objective pharyngeal manifestations is uncommon (103).

S. pneumoniae, H. influenzae, S. aureus, and GABHS are often isolated from the purulent discharge (104–106). *Corynebacterium diphtheriae* and *Neisseria meningitidis* are rarely recovered. However, the role of anaerobic bacteria was rarely explored.

Brook reported the recovery of both aerobic and anaerobic bacteria in patients with purulent nasopharyngitis (105). Cultures of aerobic and anaerobic bacteria were obtained from the inferior nasal meatus of 25 children with purulent nasopharyngitis and from 25 controls. A total of 98 isolates (3.9/patient), 45 aerobes (1.8/patient), and 53 anaerobes (2.1/patient) were isolated in patients with purulent nasopharyngitis. Seventy-three isolates (2.9/patient) were found in the controls, 47 aerobes (1.9/patient) and 26 aerobes (1.0/patient) (Table 6). The organisms recovered in statistically significantly higher numbers in patients with nasopharyngitis were *S. pneumoniae, Haemophilus* spp., *Peptostreptococcus* spp., *Fusobacterium* spp., and *Bacteroides* spp. The organism recovered in significantly higher numbers in controls was *Propronibacterium acnes.* Beta-lactamase activity was detected in 19 isolates recovered from 15 individuals (nine patients and six controls).

The nasopharynx of healthy children is generally colonized by relatively nonpathogenic aerobic and anaerobic organisms, some of which possess the ability to interfere with the growth of potential pathogen (107–109). The organisms with interference potential include aerobic alpha-hemolytic streptococci (mostly *Streptococcus mitis* and *Streptococcus sanguis*), anaerobic streptococci (*Peptostreptococcus anaerobius*), and *P. melaninogenica* (110). Conversely, carriage of potential respiratory pathogen such as *S. pneumoniae, H. influenzae,* and *M. catarrhalis* increases

TABLE 6 Bacteria Isolated in Children with Nasopharyngitis and Controls

Isolates	Patients with nasopharyngitis		Controls ($n=25$)
	Pharyngeal culture	Nostril culture	
Aerobic and facultative			
Streptococcus pneumoniae	5	6[a]	1
Alpha-hemolytic streptococci	4	6	8
Gamma-hemolytic streptococci	6	5	6
Group A, beta-hemolytic streptococci	4	2	—
Group C, beta-hemolytic streptococci	0	1	—
Group F, beta-hemolytic streptococci	1	—	1
Staphylococcus aureus	2	3	8
Staphylococcus epidermidis	1	1	5
Moraxella catarrhalis	6	8	7
Haemophilus influenzae	7	5[a]	1
Haemophilus spp.	1	2	—
Diphtheroid spp.	2	4	7
Escherichia coli		1	2
Proteus spp.	—	1	1
Subtotal	39	45	47
Anaerobic			
Peptostreptococcus spp.		17[b]	4
Microaerophilic streptococci		4	3
Propronibacterium acnes		3	12[c]
Veillonella parvula		2	3
Fusobacterium spp.		3[b]	—
Fusobacterium nucleatum		6[b]	1
Bacteroides spp.		4[b]	1
Pigmented *Prevotella* and *Porphyromonas*		11[b]	2
Prevotella oris		3	—
Subtotal		53	26
Total number of organisms		98	73

Statistically higher number of isolates than other group (nostril vs. control).
[a] $p<0.05$.
[b] $p<0.001$.
[c] $p<0.01$.
Source: From Ref. 105.

significantly in otitis media–prone children and in the general population of young children during respiratory illness (111). Brook and Gober characterized the aerobic and anaerobic bacterial flora of nasal discharge (ND) obtained from children at different stages of uncomplicated nasopharyngitis (104). A correlation was made between the bacterial flora and the eventual course of the illness. It also investigated the relationship between colonization of the nasopharynx with organisms with interfering capability and the subsequent development of purulent nasopharyngitis.

Serial semiquantitative NP and quantitative ND cultures were taken every three to five days from 20 children who eventually developed purulent discharge (group 1), and a single culture was obtained from a group of 20 who had only clear discharge (group 2). Aerobic and anaerobic bacteria were isolated from all NP cultures. Bacterial growth was present in 8 (40%) ND of group 2. Only 7 (35%) of the clear ND of group 1 showed bacterial growth; the number increased to 14 (70%) at the mucoid stage and 20 (100%) in the purulent stage. It declined to 6 (30%) at the final clear stage. The number of species and total number of organisms increased in the ND of group 1. Group 1 patients had higher recovery rate of *S. pneumoniae* and *H. influenzae* in their NP cultures than those in group 2 ($p < 0.05$). During the purulent stage, *Peptostreptococcus* spp. was isolated in 15 (75%), *Prevotella* spp. in 9 (45%), *Fusobacterium* spp. in 8 (40%), *H. influenzae* in 8 (40%), *S. pneumoniae* in 6 (30%), and beta-hemolytic streptococci in 5 (25%) of ND of group 1. This was higher than their recovery in the clear stages of both groups and the mucoid stage of group 1. A total of eight organisms with interfering capability of the growth of potential pathogens were isolated from the NP of group 1, when compared with 35 from group 2 ($p < 0.001$).

This study illustrated that the development of purulent nasopharyngitis is associated with the preexisting presence of potential pathogens and the absence of interfering organisms. The potential oropharyngeal pathogens, *S. pneumoniae*, *H. influenzae*, and GABHS, were recovered in over three-fourths of patients with purulent ND. In contrast, these organisms were rarely recovered in patients who do not develop purulent ND. It also illustrates that the development to a purulent stage is associated with the preexisting presence of these organisms in the NP of the patients. This was associated with decrease in recovery of organisms with interfering capabilities in these patients. In contrast, patients who are not colonized with potential respiratory pathogens but are colonized with interfering bacteria, or non pathogens such as *P. acnes* and *Corynebacterum* spp. are not prone to develop purulent ND.

In addition to the higher recovery of the above aerobic organisms during the purulent stage, several anaerobic organisms were also found in over three-fourths of the patients. These included *Peptostreptococcus* spp., *Fusobacterium* spp., and pigmented *Prevotella* and *Porphyromonas* spp. all members of the oral flora. Since their increased recovery was associated with isolation of *S. pneumoniae*, *H. influenzae*, and GABHS their role in the inflammation may be secondary.

Pathogenesis

Numerous bacterial isolates can be recovered from the noses of children with purulent nasopharyngitis as well as from the noses of normal controls. Although *S. aureus* and *Propionibacterium acnes* were more frequently isolated in normal individuals, *S. pneumoniae*, *H. influenzae*, *Peptostreptococcus* spp., *Fusobacterium* spp., and pigmented *Prevotella* and *Porphyromonas* were more often isolated in the mucopurulent discharges. The isolation of anaerobes in purulent NP discharge is not surprising because these organisms can be found as part of the normal oropharyngeal flora (78), as well as in the normal nasal mucosa. The anaerobes found to normally colonize the nasal mucosa were *Peptostreptococcus* spp., *Veillonella parvula*, and *P. acnes* (20). Pigmented *Prevotella* and *Porphyromonas* and *Fusobacterium* spp. that are found as normal flora in the oropharynx were not isolated in the nose.

The recovery of several aerobic and anaerobic (104–106) bacteria that are not generally found as part of the nasal flora, from patients with purulent nasopharyngitis, may signify a potential pathogenic role for these organisms. A pathogenic role was suggested for *H. influenzae* and GABHS in nasal and perinasal infection by Cherry and Dudley (112). Further studies are indicated to investigate the pathogenic role of anaerobic bacteria in this infection.

Clinical Signs

The ND in children is generally initially clear and watery; however, in cases that progress, it becomes viscous, opaque, and discolored (white, yellow, or green). Usually the purulent discharge resolves or becomes watery again before disappearing without specific therapy (104). Nasopharyngitis is caused by many different etiologic agents and therefore has varied clinical manifestations. In nasopharyngitis with *H. influenzae* and *N. meningitidis* infections, the nasal symptomatology (coryza) usually precedes the pharyngitis and the severe systemic disease that may occur (septicemia and meningitis) by a few to several days. With diphtheria, the exudative pharyngitis and constitutional symptoms are most prominent. The presence of foul-smelling purulent discharge is often associated with the predominance of anaerobic bacteria.

Fever occurs in many of the cases of nasopharyngitis. With adenoviral and influenza viral disease, the pharyngeal findings are prominent, but with other respiratory viruses, rhinitis is more notable. In adenoviral infections, follicular pharyngitis and exudate are common. In contrast, the other respiratory viruses usually induce only pharyngeal erythema. Nasopharyngitis of a viral etiology is most often an acute, self-limited disease lasting from 4 to 10 days. Adenoviral illnesses tend to be more prolonged than other respiratory viruses. Other symptomatology in nasopharyngitis is related to the causative virus.

Management

Symptomatic relief can be achieved with antipyretics. Administration of decongestants and antihistamines may be helpful; however, they were associated with significantly more side effects (106). The use of antimicrobial agents may be justified in the therapy of severe bacterial nasopharyngitis. However, controversy exists as to whether these agents should be employed in nonbacterial infection that has become secondarily infected with bacteria.

Todd et al. (106) attempted to modify the progression of purulent nasopharyngitis using cephalexin. Although some bacterial strains susceptible to cephalexin were eradicated, the clinical outcome was not affected. However, because the antibacterial spectrum of cephalexin is limited, these authors suggested the need for further studies using antimicrobials with a wider spectrum of activity. The finding of several aerobic and anaerobic BLPB in the purulent exudate may warrant the need to use antimicrobial agents resistant to this enzyme.

UVULITIS

Infectious uvulitis is a rare infection. It is present when the uvula is the most inflamed structure in the posterior pharynx of a febrile child.

Microbiology

H. influenzae type b and GABHS are the most common etiologic agents (113,114). Although these organisms were isolated from the blood of patients with uvulitis (113,114), in other instances, they were recovered only from the surface of the uvula (114). Uvulitis caused by *H. influenzae* can occur concurrently with epiglottitis or as an isolated infection (age three months to five years) (115,116). Uvulitis caused by GABHS appears always to occur in concert with pharyngitis (age 5–15 years).

The recovery of anaerobic bacteria was reported in two children (117). *F. nucleatum* was recovered from the blood, and *H. influenzae* type b was isolated from a surface uvular culture of one patient. Beta-lactamase-producing *P. intermedia* was isolated from the blood of the other patient.

Pathogenesis

Uvulitis is characterized by significant swelling and erythema of the uvula. Infection originates most probably from direct invasion by normal NP flora organisms. Concomitant epiglottitis may also arise by direct extension, and the presence of bacteremia may be secondary to either the uvula or the epiglottis as a primary location of infection.

Diagnosis

Patients with streptococcal uvulitis and pharyngitis present with low-grade fever, sore throat, choking or gagging sensation, coughing, spitting and drooling. The uvula is edematous and red. Respiratory distress is absent.

Those with uvulitis and epiglottitis (118,119) generally present as an epiglottitis with a sudden onset of high fever, dysphagia, and respiratory distress. Those with uvulitis without epiglottitis generally present as epiglottitis (acute onset of fever, odynophagia, and drooling) or less specifically with fever, irritability, and decreased appetite (115,116). The diagnosis relies on detection of swollen and erythematous uvula.

Cultures of the uvula should be done for aerobic and facultative bacteria, and blood should be cultured for both aerobic and anaerobic bacteria. The recovery of GABHS from a surface culture of the throat or uvula or both confirms the diagnosis of streptococcal uvulitis.

H. influenzae type b is generally recovered from the surface of the uvula or the blood. A lateral neck radiograph is done to evaluate the possibility of epiglottitis unless there are obvious signs of upper airway obstruction, in which case immediate endoscopy is necessary.

The differential diagnosis includes epiglottitis, severe pharyngitis, herpetic gingivostomatitis, and peritonsillar or retropharyngeal abscess. Extreme caution is warranted in examining the pharynx in case of epiglottitis. A lateral neck radiograph should be done if no gingivostomatitis or abscesses are observed.

Management

When pharyngitis or epiglottitis are also present, treatment is directed at them. If epiglottitis is present, the airway must be secured and appropriate parenteral antimicrobials effective against *H. influenzae* (up to 50% can produce beta-lactamase) initiated with second or third generation cephalosporin, or a combination of a penicillin and beta-lactamase inhibitor. For the treatment of GABHS pharyngitis, penicillin or a cephalosporin for 10 days is adequate. Coverage for oral anaerobes, many of which produce beta-lactamase, as well as GABHS can be attained by using clindamycin, chloramphenicol, metronidazole, or the combination of a penicillin (e.g., amoxicillin) plus a beta-lactamase inhibitor (e.g., clavulanate).

REFERENCES

1. Brook I, Yocum P, Friedman EM. Aerobic and anaerobic flora recovered from tonsils of children with recurrent tonsillitis. Ann Otol Rhinol Laryngol 1981; 90:261–3.
2. Brook I, Yocum P. Comparison of the microbiology of group A streptococcal and non-group A streptococcal tonsillitis. Ann Otol Rhinol Laryngol 1988; 97:243–6.
3. Brook I, Yocum P. Bacteriology of chronic tonsillitis in young adults. Arch Otolaryngol 1984; 110:803–5.
4. Brook I. Aerobic and anaerobic bacteriology of peritonsillar abscess in children. Acta Paediatr Scand 1981; 70:831–5.
5. Reilly S, Timmis P, Beeden AG, Willis AT. Possible role of the anaerobe in tonsillitis. J Clin Pathol 1981; 34:542–7.
6. Chagollan JJ, Ramirez MJ, Gil JS. Flora indigena de las amigdalas. Invest Med Int 1984; 11:36–44.
7. Rosen G, Samuel J, Vered I. Surface tonsillar microflora versus deep tonsillar microflora in recurrent tonsillitis. J Laryngol Otol 1977; 91:911–3.
8. Brodsky L, Nagy M, Volk M, Stanievich J, Moore L. The relationship of tonsil bacterial concentration to surface and core cultures in chronic tonsillar disease in children. Int J Pediatr Otorhinolaryngol 1991; 21:33–9.
9. Brook I, Yocum P, Shah K. Surface vs. core-tonsillar aerobic and anaerobic flora in recurrent tonsillitis. JAMA 1980; 244:169–86.
10. Mitchelmore IJ, Reilly PG, Hay AJ, Tabaqchali S. Tonsil surface and core cultures in recurrent tonsillitis: prevalence of anaerobes and beta-lactamase producing organisms. Eur J Clin Microbiol Infect Dis 1994; 13:542–8.

11. Brook I, Gober AE. Interference by aerobic and anaerobic bacteria in children with recurrent group A beta-hemolytic streptococcal tonsillitis. Arch Otolaryngal Head Neck Surg 1999; 125: 225–554.
12. Brook I, Yocum P, Foote PA. Changes in the core tonsillitis bacteriology of recurrent tonsillitis: 1977–1993. Clin Infect Dis 1995; 21:171–6.
13. Tunér K, Nord CE. Beta-lactamase-producing microorganisms in recurrent tonsillitis. Scand J Infect Dis 1983; 39(Suppl.):83–5.
14. Kielmovitech IH, Keltel G, Bluestone C, et al. Microbiology of obstructive tonsillar hypertrophy and recurrent tonsillitis. Arch Otolaryngol Head Neck Surg 1989; 115:721–5.
15. Brook I, Foote PA. Comparison of the microbiology of recurrent tonsillitis between children and adults. Laryngoscope 1986; 93:1385–8.
16. Kuhn JJ, Brook I, Waters CL, Church LW, Bianchi DA, Thompson DH. Quantitative bacteriology of tonsils removed from children with tonsillitis hypertrophy and recurrent tonsillitis with and without hypertrophy. Ann Otol Rhinol Laryngol 1995; 104:646–52.
17. Sclafani AP, Ginsburg J, Shah MK, Dolisky JN. Treatment of symptomatic chronic adenotonsillar hypertrophy with amoxicillin/clavulanate potassium: short- and long-term results. Pediatrics 1998; 101:675–81.
18. Brook I. Anaerobic bacteria in upper respiratory tract and other head and neck infections. Ann Otol Rhinol Laryngol 2002; 111:430–40.
19. Pransky SM, Feldman JI, Kearns DB, Seid AB, Billman GF. Actinomycosis in abstructive tonsillar hypertrophy and recurrent tonsillitis. Arch Otolaryngol Head Neck Surg 1991; 117:883–5.
20. Socransky SS, Manganiello SD. The oral microbiota of man from birth to senility. J Periodontol 1971; 42:485–96.
21. Brook I. Anaerobic infections in children. Microbes Infect 2002; 4:1271–80.
22. Brook I, Foote PA, Jr. Microbiology of "normal" tonsils. Ann Otol Rhinol Laryngol 1990; 99:980–3.
23. Brook I. Microbiology of retropharyngeal abscesses in children. Am J Dis Child 1987; 141:202–3.
24. Folayan MO. The epidemiology, etiology, and pathophysiology of acute necrotizing ulcerative gingivitis associated with malnutrition. J Contemp Dent Pract 2004; 5:28–41.
25. Brook I, Gober AE. *Bacteroides melaninogenicus*: its recovery from tonsils of children with acute tonsillitis. Arch Otolaryngol 1984; 109:818–21.
26. Davidson S, Kaplinsky C, Frand M, Rotem J. Treatment of infectious mononucleosis with metronidazole in the pediatric age group. Scand J Infect Dis 1982; 14:103–4.
27. Helstrom SA, Mandl PA, Ripa T. Treatment of anginose mononucleosis with metronidazole. Scand J Infect Dis 1978; 10:7–9.
28. McDonald CJ, Tierney WM, Hui SL. A controlled trial of erythromycin in adults with non streptococcal pharyngitis. J Infect Dis 1985; 152:1093–4.
29. Merenstein JH, Rogers KD. Streptococcal pharyngitis: early treatment and management by nurse practitioners. JAMA 1974; 227:1278–82.
30. Putto A. Febrile exudative tonsillitis: viral or streptococcal. Pediatrics 1987; 80:6–12.
31. Brook I. Medical treatment of non-streptococcal recurrent tonsillitis. Am J Otolaryngol 1989; 10:227–33.
32. Brook I, Gillmore JD, Coolbaugh JC, Walker RI. Pathogenicity of encapsulated *Bacteroides melaninogenicus* group, *Bacteroides oralis*, and *Bacteroides ruminicola* in abscesses in mice. J Infect 1983; 7:218–26.
33. Brook I, Foote PA, Jr., Slots J, Jackson W. Immune response to *Prevotella intermedia* in patients with recurrent non-streptococcal tonsillitis. Ann Otol Rhinol Laryngol 1993; 102:113–6.
34. Brook I, Foote PA, Slots J. Immune response to *Fusobacterium nucleatum, Prevotella intermedia* and other anaerobes in children with acute tonsillitis. J Antimicrob Chemother 1997; 39:763–9.
35. Brook I, Foote PA, Slots J. Immune response to *Fusobacterium nucleatum* and *Prevotella intermedia* in patients with peritonsillar cellulitis and abscess. Clin Infect Dis 1995; 20:S220–1.
36. Brook I, de Leyva F. Immune response to *Fusobacterium nucleatum* and *Prevotella intermedia* in patients with infectious mononucleosis. J Med Microbiol 1996; 44:131–4.
37. Brook I, de Leyva F. Microbiology of tonsillar surfaces in infectious mononucleosis. Arch Pediatr Adolesc Med 1994; 148:171–3.
38. Brook I, Gober AE. Treatment of non-streptococcal tonsillitis with metronidazole. Int J Pediatr Otorhinolaryngol 2005; 69:65–8.
39. Smith TD, Huskins WC, Kim KS, Kaplan EL. Efficacy of beta-lactamase-resistant penicillin and influence of penicillin in eradicating streptococci for the pharynx after failure of penicillin therapy for Group A streptococcal pharyngitis. J Pediatr 1987; 110:777–82.
40. Pichichero ME, Green JL, Francis AB, et al. Recurrent group A streptococcal tonsillopharyngitis. Pediatr Infect Dis J 1998; 17:809–15.
41. Brook I. The role of beta-lactamase-producing bacteria in the persistence of streptococcal tonsillar infection. Rev Infect Dis 1984; 6:601–7.

42. Brook I, Yocum P. Quantitative measurement of beta-lactamase levels in tonsils of children with recurrent tonsillitis. Acta Otolaryngol 1984; 98:556–60.

43. Brook I, Yocum P. In vitro protection of group A beta-hemolytic streptococci from penicillin and cephalothin by *Bacteroides fragilis*. Chemotherapy 1983; 29:18–23.

44. Simon HJ, Sakai W. Staphylococcal antagonism to penicillin group therapy of hemolytic streptococcal pharyngeal infection effect of oxacillin. Pediatrics 1963; 31:463–9.

45. Scheifele DW, Fussell SJ. Frequency of ampicillin resistant *Haemophilus parainfluenzae* in children. J Infect Dis 1981; 143:495–8.

46. Hackman AS, Wilkins TD. In vivo protection of *Fusobacterium necrophorum* from penicillin by *Bacteroides fragilis*. Antimicrob Agents Chemother 1975; 7:698–703.

47. Hackman AS, Wilkins TD. Influence of penicillinase production by strains of *Bacteroides melaninogenicus* and *Bacteroides oralis* on penicillin therapy of an experimental mixed anaerobic infection in mice. Arch Oral Biol 1976; 21:385–9.

48. Brook I, Pazzaglia G, Coolbaugh JC, Walker RI. In vivo protection of group A beta hemolytic streptococci from penicillin by beta lactamase producing bacteroides species. J Antimicrob Chemother 1983; 12:599–606.

49. Brook I, Gober AE. Emergence of beta lactamase-producing aerobic and anaerobic bacteria in the oropharynx of children following penicillin chemotherapy. Clin Pediatr 1984; 23:338–41.

50. Tunér K, Nord CE. Emergence of beta-lactamase producing anaerobic bacteria in the tonsils during penicillin treatment. Eur J Clin Microb 1986; 5:399–404.

51. Brook I. Emergence and persistence of beta-lactamase-producing bacteria in the oropharynx following penicillin treatment. Arch Otolaryngol Head Neck Surg 1988; 114:667–70.

52. Brook I. Role of beta lactamase-producing bacteria in penicillin failure to eradicate group A streptococci. Pediatric Infect Dis 1985; 4:491–5.

53. Roos K, Grahn E, Holm SE. Evaluation of beta lactamase activity and microbial interference in treatment failures of acute streptococcal tonsillitis. Scand J Infect Dis 1986; 18:313–9.

54. Breese BB, Disney FA, Talpey WB. Beta-hemolytic streptococcal illness: comparison of lincomycin, ampicillin, and potassium penicillin in treatment. Am J Dis Child 1966; 112:21–7.

55. Orrling A, Stjernquist-Desatnik A, Schalen C, Kamme C. Clindamycin in persisting streptococcal pharyngotonsillitis after penicillin treatment. Scand J Infect Dis 1994; 26:535–41.

56. Breese BB, Disney FA, Talpey WB, Green J. Beta-hemolytic streptococcal infection: comparison of penicillin and lincomycin in the treatment of recurrent infections of the carrier state. Am J Dis Child 1969; 117:147–52.

57. Massell BF. Prophylaxis of streptococcal infection and rheumatic fever: a comparison of orally administered clindamycin and penicillin. JAMA 1979; 241:1589–94.

58. Randolph MF, DeHaan RM. A comparison of lincomycin and pencillin in the treatment of group A streptococcal infection. Del Med J 1969; 41:51–62.

59. Randolph MF, Redys JJ, Hibbard EW. Streptococcal pharyngitis: III. Streptococcal recurrence rates following therapy with penicillin or with clindamycin (7-chlorolincomycin). Del Med J 1970; 42:87–92.

60. Brook I, Hirokawa R. Treatment of patients with a history of recurret tonsillitis due to group A beta-hemolytic streptococci. Clin Pediatr 1985; 24:331–6.

61. Howie VM, Plousard JH. Treatment of group A streptococcal pharyngitis in children: comparison of lincomycin and penicillin G given orally and benzathine penicillin G given intramuscularly. Am J Dis Child 1971; 121:477–80.

62. Stillerman M, Isenberg HD, Facklam RR. Streptococcal pharyngitis therapy: comparison of clindamycin palmitate and potassium phenoxymethyl penicillin. Antimicrob Agents Chemother 1973; 4:514–20.

63. Brook I. Treatment of patients with acute recurrent tonsillitis due to group A beta-haemolytic streptococci: a prospective randomized study comparing penicillin and amoxycillin/clavulanate potassium. J Antimicrob Chemother 1989; 24:227–33.

64. Tanz RR, Shulman ST, Barthel MJ, Willert C, Yogev R. Penicillin plus rifampin eradicate pharyngeal carrier of group A streptococci. J Pediatr 1985; 106:876–80.

65. Chaudhary S, Bilinsky SA, Hennessy JL, et al. Penicillin V and rifampin for the treatment of group A streptococcal pharyngitis: a randomized trial of 10 days penicillin vs. 10 days penicillin with rifampin during the final 4 days of therapy. J Pediatr 1985; 106:481–6.

66. Tanz RR, Poncher JR, Corydon KE, Kabat K, Yogev R, Shulman ST. Clindamycin treatment of chronic pharyngeal carriage of group A streptococci. J Pediatr 1991; 119:123–8.

67. Brook I, Leyva F. The treatment of the carrier state of group A beta hemolytic streptococci with clindamycin. Chemotherapy 1981; 27:360–7.

68. Brook I. The presence of beta-lactamase-producing bacteria as a guideline in the management of children with recurrent tonsillitis. Am J Otolaryngol 1984; 5:382–6.

69. Foote PA, Jr., Brook I. Penicillin and clindamycin therapy in recurrent tonsillitis. Arch Otolaryngol Head Neck Surg 1989; 116:856–9.

70. Tanz RR, Shulman ST, Sroka PA, Marubio S, Brook I, Yogev R. Lack of influence of beta-lactamase-producing flora on recovery of group A streptococci after treatment of acute pharyngitis. J Pediatr 1990; 117:859–63.
71. Dykhuizen RS, Golder D, Reid TM, Gould IM. Phenoxymethyl penicillin versus co-amoxiclav in the treatment of acute streptococcal pharyngitis, and the role of beta-lactamase activity in saliva. J Antimicrob Chemother 1996; 37:133–8.
72. Casey JR, Pichichero ME. Meta-analysis of cephalosporin versus penicillin treatment of group A streptococcal tonsillopharyngitis in children. Pediatrics 2004; 113:866–82.
73. Pichichero ME, Cohen R. Shortened course of antibiotic therapy for acute otitis media, sinusitis and tonsillopharyngitis. Pediatr Infect Dis J 1997; 16:680–95.
74. Cizman M, Pokorn M, Seme K, Paragi M, Orazem A. Influence of increased macrolide consumption on macrolide resistance of common respiratory pathogens. Eur J Clin Microbiol Infect Dis 1999; 18:522–4.
75. Seppala H, Klaukka T, Vuopio-Varkila J, et al. The effect of changes in the consumption of macrolide antibiotics on erythromycin resistance in group A streptococci in Finland. Finnish Study Group for Antimicrobial Resistance. N Engl J Med 1997; 337:441–6.
76. Green MD, Beall B, Marcon MJ, et al. Multicentre surveillance of the prevalence and molecular epidemiology of macrolide resistance among pharyngeal isolates of group A streptococci in the U.S.A. J Antimicrob Chemother 2006; 57:1240–3.
77. Martin JM, Green M, Barbadora KA, Wald ER. Erythromycin-resistant group A streptococci in schoolchildren in Pittsburgh. N Engl J Med 2002; 346:1200–6.
78. Finegold SM. Anaerobic Bacteria in Human Diseases. New York: Academic Press, 1977.
79. Irigoyen MM, Katz M, Larsen JG. Post-anginal sepsis in adolescence. Pediatr Infect Dis 1983; 2:247–50.
80. Shank GD, Berman JD. Anaerobic pulmonary abscesses: hematogenous spread from head and neck infections. Clin Pediatr 1986; 25:520–2.
81. Goldhagen J, Alford BA, Prewitt LH, Thompson L, Hostetter MK. Suppurative thrombophlebitis of the internal jugular vein: report of three cases and review of the pediatric literature. Pediatr Infect Dis J 1988; 7:410–4.
82. Golpe R, Marin B, Alonso M. Lemierre's syndrome (necrobacillosis). Postgrad Med J 1999; 75:141–4.
83. Goldstein EJ. Anaerobic bacteremia. Clin Infect Dis 1996; 23:S97–101.
84. Brook I. Anaerobic bacterial bacteremia: 12-year experience in two military hospitals. J Infect Dis 1989; 160:1071–5.
85. Veltri RW, Sprinkle PM, Keller SA, Chicklo JM. Ecological alterations of oral microflora subsequent to tonsillectomy and adenoidectomy. J Laryngol Otol 1972; 86:893–903.
86. Huminer D, Pitlik S, Levy R, Samra Z. Mycoplasma and Chlamydia in adenoids and tonsils of children undergoing adenoidectomy or tonsillectomy. Ann Otol Rhinol Laryngol 1994; 103:135–8.
87. Tomonaga K, Kurono Y, Chaen T, Mogi G. Adenoids and otitis media with effusion: nasopharyngeal flora. Am J Otolaryngol 1989; 10:204–7.
88. Bernstein JM, Reddy MS, Scannapieco FA, Faden HS, Ballow M. The microbial ecology and immunology of the adenoid: implications for otitis media. Ann N Y Acad Sci 1997; 830:19–31.
89. Gates GA, Avery CA, Prihoda TJ, Cooper JC. Effectiveness of adenoidectomy and tympanostomy tubes in the treatment of chronic otitis media with effusion. N Engl J Med 1987; 317:1444–51.
90. Gates GA, Avery CA, Prihoda TJ. Effect of adenoidectomy upon children with chronic otitis media with effusion. Laryngoscope 1988; 98:58–63.
91. Fujita A, Takahashi H, Honjo I. Etiological role of adenoids upon otitis media with effusion. Acta Otolaryngol Stockh 1988; 454:210–3.
92. Fukuda K, Matsune S, Ushikai M, Imaura Y, Ohyama M. A study of the relationship between adenoid vegetation and rhinosinusitis. Am J Otolaryngol 1989; 10:214–6.
93. Wilson TG. The aetiology of chronic rhinitis and sinusitis in children. Laryngol Otol 1965; 79:365–83.
94. Fearon M, Bannatyne RM, Fearon BW, Turner A, Cheung R. Differential bacteriology in adenoid disease. J Otolaryngol 1992; 21:434–6.
95. Klein GL, Timms R, Ziering RW. Obstructive sleep apnea presenting as mouth breathing in a five year old. Immunol Allergy Pract 1984; 6:59–61.
96. Schiffman R, Faber J, Eidelman AL. Obstructive hypertrophic adenoids and tonsils as a cause of infantile failure to thrive: reversed by tonsillectomy and adenoidectomy. Int J Pediatr Otorhinolaryngol 1985; 9:183–7.
97. Brook I. Aerobic and anaerobic bacteriology of adenoids in children: a comparison between patients with chronic adenotonsillitis and adenoid hypertrophy. Laryngoscope 1980; 91:377–82.
98. Brook I, Shah K, Jackson W. Microbiology of healthy and diseased adenoids. Laryngoscope 2000; 110:994–9.
99. Brook I, Shah K. Bacteriology of adenoids and tonsils in children with recurrent adeno-tonsillitis. Ann Otol Rdinol Laryngol 2001; 110:844–8.

100. Paradise JL, Bluestone CD, Colborn DK, et al. Adenoidectomy and adenotonsillectomy for recurrent acute otitis media: parallel randomized clinical trials in children not previously treated with tympanostomy tubes. JAMA 1999; 282:945–53.
101. Marchant CD, Collison LM. Serous and recurrent otitis media. Pharmacological or surgical management? Drugs 1987; 34:695–701.
102. Levine MK, Beman JD. A comparison of clindamycin and erythromycin in beta-hemolytic streptococcal infections. J Med Assoc Ga 1972; 6:108–11.
103. Mackie PL. The classification of viruses infecting the respiratory tract. Paediatr Respir Rev 2003; 4:84–90.
104. Brook I, Gober AE. Dynamics of nasopharyngitis in children. Otolaryngol Head Neck Surg 2000; 122:696–700.
105. Brook I. Aerobic and anaerobic bacteriology of purulent nasopharyngitis in children. J Clin Microbiol 1988; 26:592–4.
106. Todd JK, Todd N, Damato J, Todd WA. Bacteriology and treatment of purulent nasopharyngitis: a double blind, placebo-controlled evaluation. Pediatr Infect Dis 1984; 3:226–32.
107. Sanders SS, Nelson GE, Sanders WE, Jr. Bacterial interference IV. Epidemiological determinants of the antagonistic activity of the normal flora against group A streptococci. Infect Immun 1977; 16:599–606.
108. Sprunt K, Redman W. Evidence suggesting importance of role of interbacterial inhibition in maintaining a balance of normal flora. Ann Intern Med 1968; 68:579–87.
109. Bernstein JM, Sagahtaheri-Altaie S, Dryjd DM, Wactawski-Wende J. Bacterial interference in nasopharyngeal bacterial flora of otitis-prone and non-otitis-prone children. Acta Otorhinolaryngol Belg 1994; 48:1–9.
110. Murray PR, Rosenblatt JE. Bacterial interference by oropharyngeal and clinical isolates of anaerobic bacteria. J Infect Dis 1976; 134:281–5.
111. Faden H, Zaz MJ, Bernstein JM, Brodsky L, Stanievich J, Ogra PL. Nasopharyngeal flora in the first three years of life in normal and otitis-prone children. Ann Otol Rhin Laryngol 1991; 100:612–5.
112. Feigin RD, Cherry JD. Textbook of Pediatric Infectious Diseases. 5th ed. Philadelphia: WB Saunders Company, 2004.
113. Butterton JR, Clawson-Simons J. Hymenoptera uvulitis. N Engl J Med 1987; 317:1291.
114. DeNavasquez S. Acute laryngitis and septicemia due to *H. influenzae* type b. Br Med J 1942; 2:187–8.
115. Li KI, Kiernan S, Wald ER. Isolated uvulitis due to *Haemophilus influenzae* type b. Pediatrics 1984; 74:1054–7.
116. Wynder SG, Lampem RM, Shoemaker ME. Uvulitis and *Haemophilus influenzae* b bacteremia. Pediatr Emerg Care 1986; 2:23–5.
117. Brook I. Uvulitis caused by anaerobic bacteria. Pediatr Emerg Care 1997; 13:221.
118. Gorfinkel HJ, Brown R, Kabins SA. Acute infectious epiglottitis in adults. Ann Intern Med 1969; 70:289–94.
119. Kotloff KL, Wald ER. Uvulitis in children. Pediatr Infect Dis 1983; 2:392–3.

17 | Infections of the Head and Neck

ABSCESSES OF THE HEAD AND NECK, GENERAL CONSIDERATIONS

Staphylococcus aureus and Group A beta-hemolytic streptococci (GABHS) were established as the predominant pathogens in abscesses of the head and neck in most studies done until 1970 (1). However, when methodologies suitable for recovery of anaerobic bacteria were used, these organisms were found to predominate especially in infections that originated from sites where these organisms are the predominant flora (i.e., dental, sinus, and tonsillar infections) (2,3). The recovery of anaerobes from abscesses and other infections of the head and neck is not surprising because anaerobic bacteria outnumber aerobic bacteria in the oral cavity by a ratio of 10:1 (4). Furthermore, these organisms were recovered from chronic upper respiratory infections such as otitis and sinusitis, and from periodontal infections (1).

PERITONSILLAR RETROPHARYNGEAL AND PARAPHARYNGEAL ABSCESSES

Peritonsillar, retropharyngeal, and parapharyngeal abscesses are deep neck infections that are generally secondary to contiguous spread from local sites. They share some clinical features, but also have distinctive manifestations and complications (Table 1). They all are potentially life threatening if not recognized early.

A peritonsillar abscess (or quinsy) occurs much more often in childhood than is generally recognized, but it is seldom diagnosed until tonsillectomy is performed and peritonsillar fibrosis discovered. Peritonsillar abscess consists of suppuration outside the tonsillar capsule and is situated in the region of the upper pole and involves the soft palate. Infection begins in the intratonsillar fossa, which lies between the upper pole and the body of the tonsil, and eventually extends around the tonsil. A quinsy usually is unilateral; rarely it occurs bilaterally (5).

Tonsillar abscess is uncommon and implies an abscess within the tonsil following retention of pus within a follicle to give pain and dysphagia. Retropharyngeal abscess is generally a disease of early childhood, caused by extension of an oral cavity suppuration to the retropharyngeal lymph glands (Table 1).

Anatomy

There are three major clinically important spaces between the deep cervical fascia. The parapharyngeal (or lateral pharyngeal, or pharyngomaxillary) space is in the upper neck, above the hyoid bone, between the pretracheal fascia of the visceral compartment medially and the superficial fascia, which invests the parotid gland, internal pterygoid muscle, and mandible laterally. It is an inverted cone, with the skull at the jugular foramen forming the base, and the hyoid bone the apex.

The second space is within the submental and submandibular triangles, and is situated between the mucosa of the floor of the mouth and the superficial layer of deep fascia of the regions.

The third space is the retropharyngeal space, which extends longitudinally downward from the base of the skull to the posterior mediastinum; posterior boundary is the prevertebral fascia and anterior boundary is the posterior portion of the pretracheal fascia. It is connected to the parapharyngeal space, where its lateral boundary is the carotid sheaths.

TABLE 1 Clinical Features of Peritonsillar, Retropharyngeal, and Lateral Pharyngeal Abscesses

	Usual age	Sites of origin	Location	Clinical findings	Complications/extension site	Management
Peritonsillar abscess	Adolescents, adults	Tonsillitis	Tonsillar capsule and space below superior constrictor muscle	Swelling of one tonsil, uvullar displacement; trismus, muffled voice	Spontaneous rupture and aspiration; contiguous spread to pterygomaxillary space	Antibiotics, drainage
Retropharyngeal abscess	Less than 4 years	Pharyngitis, dental infection trauma	Between posterior pharynx and prevertebral fascia	Unilateral posterior pharyngeal bulging; neck, hyperextension drooling, respiratory distress	Spontaneous rupture and aspiration; contiguous spread to posterior mediastinum, parapharyngeal space	Antibiotics, drainage; artificial airway
Lateral pharyngeal abscess	More than 8 years, adolescents, adults	Tonsillitis otitis media, mastoiditis, parotitis, dental manipulation	Anterior and posterior pharyngomaxillary space	Anterior compartment: swelling of the parotid area; trismus; tonsil prolapse/tonsillar fossa Posterior compartment: septicemia; minimal pain or trismus	Carotid erosion; airway obstruction; intracranium, lung, contiguous spread to mediastinum; septicemia	Antibiotics, drainage, artificial airway

Microbiology

Most deep neck abscesses are polymicrobial infections; the average number of isolates is five (range 1–10) (5–12). Predominant anaerobic organisms isolated in peritonsillar (8–12), lateral pharyngeal (7,12), and retropharyngeal (9,12) abscesses are *Prevotella, Porphyromonas, Fusobacterium,* and *Peptostreptococcus* spp.; aerobic organisms are GABHS, *S. aureus,* and *Haemophilus influenzae.* Anaerobic bacteria can be isolated from most abscesses whenever appropriate techniques for their cultivation have been employed (1), while GABHS is isolated in only about one-third of cases (8,10). More than two-thirds of deep neck abscesses contain beta-lactamase–producing bacteria (BLPB) (7,8). Retropharyngeal cellulitis and abscess in young children are more likely to have pathogenic aerobic isolates (Groups A and B streptococci, *S. aureus*), alone or in combination (13,14). *Fusobacterium necrophorum* is especially associated with deep neck infections that cause septic thrombophlebitis of great vessels and metastatic abscesses (Lemierre disease) (15,16). Rarely, *Mycobacterium tuberculosis* (17), atypical mycobacteria, or *Coccidioidis immitis* (18) is recovered.

Finegold (1) provided a thorough review of the literature summarizing many studies of the bacteriology of peritonsillar and retropharyngeal abscess. Hansen (19) who studied 153 aspirates from peritonsillar abscesses, recovered 151 anaerobes, including anaerobic gram-negative bacteria (AGNB), anaerobic gram-negative cocci, and fusiform bacilli. Hallander et al. (20) isolated anaerobic bacteria from 26 of 30 patients. Isolates included *Bacteroides,* fusobacteria, peptostreptococci, microaerophilic cocci, *veillonellae,* and bifidobacteria. Sprinkle et al. (21) recovered anaerobes from four of six individuals with peritonsillar abscess. Anaerobes only were isolated in one instance, and the others yielded mixed aerobic and anaerobic flora. Lodenkämper and Stienen (22) recovered *Bacteroides* spp. from six patients with retrotonsillar abscess, and Baba et al. (23) isolated anaerobic gram-positive cocci from four patients. Ophir et al. (24) isolated eight *Bacteriodes* spp. from 62 patients.

Several single-case reports described the recovery of anaerobes in peritonsillar abscess. Prévot (25) recovered *Ramibacterium pseudoramosum.* Alston (26) obtained *Bacteroides necrophorus.* Beerens and Tahon-Castel (27) recovered *Bacteroides funduliformis* and *Fusiformis fusiformis.* Gruner isolated *Actinomyces* spp. (28) and Rubinstein et al. (29) and Oleske et al. (30) isolated fusobacteria.

Anaerobes were isolated from all 16 aspirates of peritonsillar abscess in 16 children (8). There were 91 anaerobic and 32 aerobic isolates (Table 2). The predominant isolates were: pigmented *Prevotella* and *Porphyromonas* spp., anaerobic gram-positive cocci, *Fusobacterium* spp., gamma-hemolytic streptococci, alpha-hemolytic streptococci, GABHS, *Haemophilus* spp., clostridia, and *Staphylococcus aureus.* BLPB were found in 11 (68%) patients. These included all three isolates of *S. aureus,* eight (35%) of the 23 isolates of *Prevotella melaninogenica,* and two (40%) of the five isolates of *Prevotella oralis.*

The microbiology of 34 aspirates of peritonsillar abscesses in adults (31) yielded 107 bacterial isolates (58 anaerobic and 49 aerobic and facultative), accounting for 3.1 isolates/specimen (1.7 anaerobic and 1.4 aerobic and facultatives). Anaerobes only were present in six

TABLE 2 Bacteria Isolated in 16 Children with Peritonsillar Abscesses

Aerobic and facultative isolates	No. of isolates	Anaerobic isolates	No. of isolates
Gram-positive cocci (total)	27	Anaerobic cocci	22
Group A beta-hemolytic streptococci	4	Gram-positive bacilli (total)	12
Staphylococcus aureus	3	*Clostridium* sp.	3
Gram-negative bacilli (total)	5	Gram-negative bacilli (total)	57
Haemophilus influenzae	4	*Fusobacterium* sp.	15
Total no. of aerobes	32	*Bacteroides* sp.	14
		Pigmented *Prevotella* and *Porphyromonas* spp.	23
		Prevotella oralis	5
		Total no. of anaerobes	91

Note: Only the important pathogens are listed in detail. The total number of the groups of organisms is represented.
Source: From Ref. 8.

patients (18%), aerobic and facultatives in two (6%), and mixed aerobic and anaerobic flora in 26 (76%). Single bacterial isolates were recovered in four infections, two of which were GABHS and two were anaerobic bacteria. The predominant bacterial isolates were *S. aureus* (6 isolates), AGNB (21 isolates, including 15 pigmented *Prevotella* and *Porphyromonas* spp.), *Peptostreptococcus* spp. (16) and GABHS (10). BLPB were recovered from 13 (52%) of 25 specimens tested.

Jousimies-Somer et al. (32) studied samples from 124 patients with peritonsillar abscess. A total of 98% of the specimens yielded bacteria. Of the 550 isolates (mean, 4.4/patient), 143 were aerobes and 407 were anaerobes. Aerobes were isolated from 86% of patients-alone in 20 cases and together with anaerobes in 87. The most common aerobic isolates were GABHS (isolated from 45% of patients), *Streptococcus milleri* group (27%), *H. influenzae* (11%), and viridans streptococci (11%). Anaerobes were isolated from 82% of the samples and as a sole finding from 15. *F. necrophorum* and *Prevotella melaninogenica* were both isolated from 38% of patients, *Prevotella intermedia* from 32%, *Peptostreptococcus micros* from 27%, *Fusobacterium nucleatum* from 26%, and *Actinomyces odontolyticus* from 23%. The rate of previous tonsillar and peritonsillar infections was lowest (25%) among patients infected with GABHS and highest (52%) among those infected with *F. necrophorum* ($p < 0.01$). Recurrences and/or related tonsillectomies were more common among patients infected with *F. necrophorum* than among those infected with GABHS (57% vs. 19%; $p < 0.0001$) or with *Streptococcus milleri* group (43% vs. 19%; $p < 0.05$).

Mitchelmore et al. (33) evaluated aspirated from 53 peritonsillar abscesses. In 45 samples (85%), cultures were positive: seven yielded organisms consistent with an aerobic infection, mainly GABHS (5 of 7), and 38 yielded anaerobes. *Peptostreptococcus micros* and *S. milleri* were the predominant isolates in this group. Samples from ten patients (19%) grew one or more BLPB.

Myerson (34) described a case of anaerobic retropharyngeal abscess that yielded AGNB and hemolytic streptococci. Recovered aerobes were *Streptococcus viridans* and *Staphylococcus epidermidis*. Prévot (25) recovered *Sphaerophorus gonidiaformans* from a retropharyngeal abscess. Ernst (35) isolated *B. funduliformis* among other organisms from a retropharyngeal abscess. Janecka and Rankow (36) reported the recovery of *Bacteroides* and anaerobic streptococci from a patient with a retropharyngeal gas-forming abscess. Heinrich and Pulverer (37) recovered *P. melaninogenica* from three patients with parapharyngeal abscess.

Aspiration of retropharyngeal abscesses in 14 children (9) yielded anaerobes in all patients. Anaerobes were the only isolates in two patients (14%) and were mixed with aerobes in 12 (86%). There were 78 anaerobic isolates (5.6/specimen; Table 3). The predominant anaerobes were *Bacteroides*, *Peptostreptococcus*, and *Fusobacterium* spp. There were 26 aerobic isolates (1.9/specimen). The predominant aerobes were alpha- and gamma-hemolytic streptococci, *S. aureus*, *Haemophilus* spp., and GABHS. Sixteen BLPB were recovered from 10 patients (71%).

TABLE 3   Bacteria Isolated in 14 Children with Retropharyngeal Abscesses

Aerobic and facultative isolates	No. of isolates	Anaerobic isolates	No. of isolates
Gram-positive cocci (total)	22	Anaerobic cocci (total)	25
Group A beta-hemolytic streptococci	3	*Peptostreptococcus* spp.	18
Staphylococcus aureus	5 (5)	Gram-positive bacilli (total)	7
Gram-negative bacilli (total)	4 (1)	Gram-negative bacilli	
Haemophilus influenzae type B	3 (1)	*Fusobacterium* sp.	14
Total no. of aerobes	26 (7)	*Bacteroides* spp.	11 (1)
		Pigmented *Prevotella* and *Porphyromonas* spp.	18 (6)
		Prevotella oralis	3 (2)
		Total no. of anaerobes	78 (9)

Numbers in parentheses are the numbers of beta-lactamase-producing organisms.
Source: From Ref. 9.

Coulthard and Isaacs (38) studied 31 children with retropharyngeal abscess, 17 (55%) were 12 months old or less and 10 (32%) less than six months. Isolates included growths of *S. aureus* (25%), *Klebsiella* spp. (13%), GABHS (8%), and anaerobes (38%).

Pathogenesis

Similarity exists in the microbiology, and subsequently the antimicrobial therapy of deep neck abscesses. The microbiology of deep neck abscesses reflect the host's oropharyngeal (peritonsillar and pharyngeal lateral abscess) or nasopharyngeal (retropharyngeal abscess) flora. The bacteriology of specific space infections generally is associated with the bacterial flora of the originating focus. The oropharyngeal flora is comprised of over 350 different aerobic and anaerobic bacterial species; the number of anaerobic bacteria exceeds that of aerobic bacteria by a ratio of 10:1 to 100:1 (4). Most anaerobic bacteria recovered from clinical infections are found mixed with other organisms (39) and generally express their virulence in chronic infections. Polymicrobial infections are known to be more pathogenic for experimental animals than are those involving single organisms (39).

Elevated antibody levels to *F. nucleatum* and *P. intermedia*, known oral pathogens was found in children who had peritonsillar abscess or cellulitis, suggesting a pathogenic role for these organisms in these infections (40). Antibody titers to these organisms were measured by enzyme-linked immunosorbent assay in 17 patients with peritonsillar cellulitis and 19 with peritonsillar abscess patient as well as in 32 control patients. Serum levels in the patients were determined at day one and 42 to 56 days later. Significantly higher antibody levels to *F. nucleutum* and *P. intermedia* were found in the second serum sample of patients with peritonsillar cellulitis or abscess, as compared to their first sample or the levels of antibodies in controls.

Management

Management of tonsillar, peritonsillar, and retropharyngeal abscesses is similar. Systemic antimicrobial therapy should be given in large doses whenever the diagnosis is made.

If treatment is started within the first 24 to 48 hours following the onset of pain, the condition may resolve by fibrosis without abscess formation. If the patient is not seen until pus has formed, or if the antibiotic therapy fails to relieve the condition, then the abscess must be drained. In tonsillar and peritonsillar abscesses, the tonsils should be removed six to eight weeks following the abscess especially in those with a history of recurrences of tonsillitis or abscess. However, this is not always necessary in children. Ophir et al. (24) demonstrated the ability to manage on an outpatient basis, most patients with peritonsillar abscess, after needle aspiration of the abscess. However, another study reported greater rate of recurrences in patients treated with needle aspiration (41).

Surgical drainage is still the therapy of choice. The recovery of aerobic and anaerobic BLPB from most abscesses mandates the use of antimicrobial agents effective against these organisms. Antimicrobial agents with expected efficacy include cefoxitin, a carbapenem (i.e., imipenem or meropenem), tigecycline the combination of a penicillin (i.e., ticarcillin) and a beta-lactamase inhibitor (i.e., clavulanate), chloramphenicol, or clindamycin. Antimicrobial therapy can abort abscess formation if given at an early stage of the infection. However, when pus is formed, antimicrobial therapy is effective only in conjunction with adequate surgical drainage.

SPECIFIC FEATURES OF EACH ABSCESS

Peritonsillar Abscess (Quinsy)

Peritonsillar abscess is the most common deep head and neck infection. It generally occurs in adolescents and adults as a complication of repeated episodes of bacterial tonsillitis; rarely it can occur as a secondary complication of viral infection, such as Epstein–Barr (EB) virus mononucleosis. The infection penetrates the tonsillar capsule into the space between the superior constrictor muscle and the tonsillar capsule. The most common location is the superior pole of the tonsil.

Diagnosis and Clinical Manifestations

The abscess generally is preceded by acute pharyngotonsillitis. An afebrile interval of a few days can occur, or fever caused by the primary infection persists (Table 1). Quinsy usually is unilateral; rarely it occurs bilaterally (5). The patient can be apprehensive and pale, and the temperature and pulse rate rise, often preceded by rigor. There is difficulty in swallowing or speaking. Pain increases in severity, radiates to the ear, and causes trismus due to spasm of the pterygoid muscle. The breath has a foul odor. Saliva may dribble from the mouth because of pain on swallowing. The tonsil is swollen and inflamed, but the soft palate does not bulge. The uvula is edematous and pushed toward the opposite side; the affected tonsil usually is hidden by the swelling but can have some mucopurulent secretions on its surface. Ipsilateral cervical lymph nodes are enlarged and tender.

With the development of a peritonsillar abscess there is acute pain on one side of the throat and considerable constitutional disturbance. If not reversed by antibiotic therapy, or surgical drainage, the abscess can leak slowly or burst in about a week's time. This can lead to aspiration and pneumonia. Computerized tomography (CT) and intraoral ultrasound are helpful in distinguishing between abscess and cellulitis (42,43).

Bilateral abscess formation is unusual and more difficult to diagnose since the classic signs of congestion on the affected side of the palate, and edema of the uvula with a shift to the opposite side, are absent (5).

Obtaining adequate specimens for cultures from the abscess is important, as a variety of organisms can be recovered. Specimens are best collected at the time of surgical drainage or through needle aspiration. Throat swab or swabs obtained after drainage are inappropriate as they can be contaminated by oropharyngeal flora. Specimens should be transported promptly in media or transport systems supportive of growth of both aerobic and anaerobic bacteria; specimens should be inoculated and incubated to optimize recovery of these organisms.

Treatment

Needle aspiration or incision and drainage of the abscess under local or generalized anesthesia, combined with administration of parenteral antimicrobial therapy is the therapy of choice. Hospitalization and general anesthesia are required in younger children. Occasionally, outpatient treatment is possible (24,44). Emergency tonsillectomy also is an option. Patients with peritonsillar abscess and a history of recurrent tonsillitis should be considered for tonsillectomy after the acute episode subsides (45).

RETROPHARYNGEAL ABSCESS

The potential space between the posterior pharyngeal wall and prevertebral fascia contains two paramedial chains of lymph glands that disappear by puberty. These lymphatics drain the nasopharynx, posterior paranasal sinuses and adenoids. Lymph nodes can become infected during purulent infections in the regions of drainage, which can lead to their suppuration (46).

Retropharyngeal abscess generally follows bacterial pharyngitis or nasopharyngitis. Rarely it is an extension of vertebral osteomyelitis; a complication of endoscopy, dental procedure, or other medical/surgical trauma; or secondary to wound infection following penetrating injury of the posterior pharynx.

Diagnosis and Clinical Manifestations

The patient generally has had acute pharyngitis or nasopharyngitis, when there is abrupt onset of high fever and difficulty swallowing associated with drooling, dysphagia, neck pain and hyperextension, and dyspnea (Table 1). Anterior bulging of the posterior pharyngeal wall usually is present, frequently to one side of the midline. Nasal obstruction can follow and/or signs of difficulty breathing can dominate the clinical picture. Cervical lymphadenopathy usually is present.

The oropharynx can be examined carefully, only in a cooperative patient, by a skilled examiner using indirect (mirror) hypopharyngeal inspection and digital palpation. The patient should be in the Trendelenburg position; there must be provision for adequate suction equipment in the event that the abscess ruptures.

A lateral radiograph of the nasopharynx and neck can identify the retropharyngeal mass. An abscess (or other mass) is present if the retropharyngeal soft tissue is more than one-half of the width of the adjacent vertebral body, with the child's neck extended. Air, air-fluid level, or foreign body should be looked for. Chest radiograph is performed to identify extension into the mediastinum. CT with contrast can sometimes distinguish neck cellulitis from deep neck abscess and delineates extension of abscess, and involvement of vascular structures (42,43); the study is not necessary in typical cases.

Differential diagnosis includes cervical osteomyelitis, meningitis, Pott's disease and calcified tendinitis of the longus colli muscle.

Treatment

Management includes drainage of the abscess and intravenous administration of antibiotics. Most abscesses can be drained by peroral incision and suction, which carries a small risk of aspiration. External incision is required rarely, when the abscess is extended longitudinally, or when fever persists after peroral drainage. When risk of airway obstruction is great, tracheostomy may be needed.

Complications

Untreated abscesses can rupture spontaneously into the pharynx causing catastrophic aspiration. Other complications are extension of infection laterally to the side of the neck, or dissection into the posterior mediastinum through facial planes and the prevertebral space. Death can occur from aspiration, airway obstruction, erosion into major blood vessels, or extension to the mediastinum.

LATERAL PHARYNGEAL ABSCESS

The lateral pharyngeal (pharyngomaxillary) space is divided into two compartments by the styloid process. The anterior portion is close to the tonsillar fossa medially, and internal pteryoid muscle laterally. The posterior compartment contains the carotid sheath and cranial nerves. Involvement of these structures determines the clinical manifestations and complications of abscesses in these spaces (46).

Clinical Manifestations

Infection of the lateral pharyngeal space can be the result of tonsillitis, pharyngitis, otitis media, mastoiditis (Bezold abscess), parotitis, or dental infections (usually of the mastication space) (Table 1).

With infection in the anterior compartment, there is usually high fever and chills, tender swelling below the angle of the mandible, induration and erythema of the side of the neck, and trismus. Most patients are acutely ill, have odynophagia, dysphagia, and mild dyspnea. A bulge in the lateral pharyngeal wall can be observed but the tonsil is normal in size and relatively uninflamed. Torticollis toward the side of the abscess (due to muscle spasm) is found often as is cervical lymphadenitis (CL). The classical triad of pharyngomaxillary abscess occurs only in anterior compartment syndrome and includes: (*i*) tonsillar and tonsillar fossa prolapse, (*ii*) trismus, and (*iii*) swelling of the parotid area. Infection in the posterior compartment is characterized by signs of septicemia, with minimal pain or trismus. Swelling can often be overlooked because it is deep behind the palatopharyngeal arch. Indirect laryngoscopy can reveal ipsilateral obliteration of the pyriform sinus. A tender high cervical mass can be palpated, which is ill-defined initially and fluctuant later.

Complications occur especially from infection in the posterior compartment and include respiratory distress, laryngeal edema, airway obstruction, septicemia, pneumonia, septic thrombosis of the internal jugular vein with metastatic abscesses (Lemierre syndrome), intracranial extension (causing meningitis, brain abscess, cavernous and lateral sinus thrombosis), and erosion of the carotid artery. Carotid artery erosion can cause bleeding from the external auditory canal. Additionally, dissection of the abscess through the junction of the cartilaginous external canal and bone can cause suppurative otorrhea. Extension of the infection inferiorly along the carotid sheath or posteriorly into the retropharyngeal space can lead to mediastinitis. CT or magnetic resonance imaging (MRI) delineates affected structures and vascular complications.

Treatment

Treatment requires drainage of the lateral neck in conjunction with high doses of appropriate antimicrobial therapy, intravenously. An external excision below the angle of the jaw is preferred as it provides access to the carotic artery, which should be ligated in case of arterial erosion. Surgical drainage is best performed after localization of infection, unless hemorrhage or respiratory obstruction necessitates earlier intervention. Disease progress must be monitored closely; tracheostomy may be required prophylactically. Airway obstruction due to laryngeal edema can develop abruptly.

Complications

If not treated either by antibiotics or by surgery the abscess may burst or leak slowly in about a week. Asphyxia from direct pressure or from sudden rupture of the abscess and also hemorrhage are the major complications of these infections.

Surgical drainage and antimicrobial therapy of these abscesses are essential for the prompt recovery and prevention of complications such as bacteremia, aspiration pneumonia, and lung abscess after spontaneous rupture.

ACUTE SUPPURATIVE PAROTITIS AND SIALADENITIS

Sialadenitis, an acute infection of the salivary glands, can occur in any of the glands. The parotid gland is the salivary gland most commonly affected by inflammation. Parotitis can present as an acute single or multiple recurrent episodes. Acute suppurative parotitis may arise from a septic focus in the mouth, such as chronic tonsillitis or dental sepsis, and may be found in patients taking tranquilizer drugs or antihistamines, both of which tend to suppress saliva excretion.

It occurs mostly in children younger than two month and in elderly persons who are debilitated by systemic illness or previous surgical procedures, although persons of all ages may be affected (47). Other predisposing factors include dehydration, immunosuppression, malnutrition, neoplasms of the oral cavity, tracheostomy, immunosuppression, sialectasis, ductal obstruction, and medications that diminish salivary flow such as antihistamines and diuretics (47,48).

The mode of spread of organisms into the parotid gland may be through a combinations of factors that enhance ascention of oral bacteria through the Stensen's duct. These include the decreased secretory function that occurs in the dehydrated or starving patient (49). Another possible mode of transmission of organisms is through transitory bacteremia especially in the neoatal period.

Microbiology

S. aureus is the most common pathogen associated with acute bacterial parotitis; however, streptococci (including *Streptococcus pneumoniae*) and aerobic gram-negative bacilli (including *Escherichia coli*) have also been reported (47,48). Aerobic gram-negative organisms are often seen in hospitalized patients. Organisms less frequently found are Arachnia, *H. influenzae*, *Treponema pallidum*, cat-scratch bacillus (Bartonella spp.), and *Eikenella corrodens* (50).

Mycobacterium tuberculosis and atypical mycobacteria are rare causes of parotitis (51). Several reports describe anaerobic isolates from parotid infections (52–60). However, the true incidence of anaerobic bacteria in suppurative parotitis was rarely determined because most studies did not employ proper techniques for their isolation.

Brook and Finegold reported two children with acute suppurative parotitis (57). In one case, the cultures yielded mixed culture of *P. intermedia* and alpha-hemolytic streptococci. In the other child, no aerobes were recovered and the specimen yielded growth of *F. nucleatum* and *Peptostreptococcus intermedius*. Of interest is that both of these patients were institutionalized mentally retarded children and one had Down's syndrome. Notably, children with Down's syndrome have a striking incidence of severe periodontal disease and have a greater prevalence of *P. melaninogenica* in the gingival sulcus in comparison with normal children (61).

Sussman recovered *Gaffkya anaerobia* from recurrently infected parotic gland (58). *Actinomyces israelii* and *Actinomyces eriksonii* also have been isolated (50,55).

Brook et al. studied 23 aspirates of pus from acute suppurative parotitis (62). A total of 36 bacterial isolates (20 anaerobic and 16 aerobic and facultative) were recovered, accounting for 1.6 isolates/specimen (0.9 anaerobic and 0.7 aerobic and facultative). Anaerobic bacteria only were present in 10 (43%) patients, aerobic and facultatives in 10 (43%), and mixed aerobic and anaerobic flora in 3 (13%). Single bacterial isolates were recovered in nine infections, six of which were *S. aureus* and three were anaerobic bacteria. The predominant bacterial isolates were *S. aureus* (8), AGNB, and *Peptostreptococcus* spp. (5).

There are several reports of recovery of anaerobes from infections of other salivary glands. Baba et al. (23) recovered a *Peptococcus* in pure culture from a purulent submaxillary gland infection. Brook (63) studied 47 aspirates of pus from acute suppurative sialadenitis, 32 from parotid, nine from submandibular and six from sublingual glands. Polymicrobial flora was isolated from 17 (64%) of these infections and the predominant aerobes were *S. aureus* and *H. influenzae* while the commonest anaerobes were AGNB and *Peptostreptococcus* spp. Brook (64) recovered anaerobes from two newborns with suppurative sialadenitis. *Peptostreptococcus magnus*, *P. intermedia*, and GABHS were isolated from one newborn and *P. melaninogenica* and *F. nucleatum* from the other. Complete recovery occurred following surgical drainage and antimicrobial therapy.

Pathogenesis

Although acute parotitis due to anaerobic bacteria has been rarely reported, its occurrence is not surprising. Both clinicopathologic correlations in humans and experimental studies in dogs have shown that bacteria can ascend Stensen's duct from the oral cavity and thus infect the parotid glands (50). Improved techniques for isolation and identification of anaerobic bacteria have shown that the flora of the mouth is predominantly anaerobic, and normal adults harbor about 10^{11} microorganisms per gram of material in gingival crevices (4). Saliva contains many genera of anaerobic bacteria including *Peptostreptococcus*, *Veillonella*, *Actinomyces*, *Propionibacterium*, *Leptotrichia*, pigmented *Prevotella* and *Porphyromonas*, *Bacteroides*, and *Fusobacterium* spp. Diminution in salivary flow could allow the ascent of any of the indigenous bacterial flora, thereby triggering acute parotitis (50).

Pigmented *Prevotella* and *Porphyromonas* spp. are the most common AGNB found in oral flora and, like *Peptostreptococcus* spp., are frequently isolated from odontogenic orofacial infections (1). The paucity of reports of involvement of such organisms in bacterial infections of the parotid gland probably indicates that anaerobic cultures have not been done, or that inadequate anaerobic transport or culture techniques accounted for failure to recover such organisms.

Diagnosis

Acute suppurative parotitis is characterized by the sudden onset of an indurated, warm, erythematous swelling of the cheek extending to the angle of the jaw. Acute bacterial parotitis usually is unilateral, the gland becomes swollen and tender, and patients frequently have toxemia with marked fever and leukocytosis. The orifice of the parotid duct is red and pouting, and pus may be seen exuding, or may be produced by gentle pressure on the duct. Pus rarely points externally because of the dense fibrous capsule of the gland.

The pathogenic process associated with suppurative parotid infection may lead to profound dehydration, delirium, high fever, bacteremia, and organ system failure.

Acute suppurative parotitis should be differentiated from viral parotitis (mumps), which usually is endemic and produces no pus. Other viruses that can cause parotitis include human immunodeficiency virus (HIV), enteroviruses, Epstein–Barr (EB)-virus, parainfluenza, influenza, cytomegalo virus, and lymphocytic choriomeningitis virus. Noninfectious disorders that may be associated with parotid swelling include collagen-vascular disease, cystic fibrosis, alcoholism, diabetes, gout, uremia, sarcoidosis, ectodermal dysplasia syndromes, familial dysautonomia, sialolithiasis, benign and malignant tumors, metal poisoning, and drug related disorders. Nonparotid swelling that may stimulate parotitis include lymphoma, lymphangitis, cervical adenitis, external otitis, dental abscess, *Actinomyces* not evolving the parotid, and cysts.

Suppurative parotitis is differentiated from these disorders by the ability to produce purulent material at the orifice of Stensen's duct by applying pressure over the gland. Occlusion of the orifice may, however, prevent the expression of pus. Tumors are generally unevenly swollen, and tenderness is variable.

Anaerobic infection of the buccal space (such as Ludwig's angina) not evolving the parotid have to be differentiated from parotitis. *Actinomyces* may have chronic exudate with sulfur granules and is frequently encountered with dental caries. Elevated white blood cells and sedimentation rate and serum amylase or urine diastase are generally seen in suppurative parotitis. Roentgenogram may reveal the presence of sialolith, and sialogram may demonstrate destruction of ductules or spherical dilation suggestive of suppurative illness (50). CT-sialography is an important tool in diagnosis of tumors (65).

Expression of the pus from the parotid gland and performance of Gram stain may support suppurative infection. Specimens for anaerobic culture should not be taken from Stensen's duct because oropharyngeal contamination is certain.

Needle aspiration of the involved gland may yield the causative organism. If no pus is aspirated, introduction of sterile saline and subsequent aspiration may yield material. The aspirates should be cultured for aerobic as well as anaerobic bacteria, fungi, and mycobacteria. Surgical exploration and drainage may be indicated for diagnosis as well as for therapy. If infection is not found, search should be made for noninfectious causes of parotic swelling previously mentioned.

Management

Maintenance of adequate hydration and administration of parenteral antimicrobial therapy are essential. The choice of antibiotics depends on the etiologic agent. Most cases respond to antimicrobial therapy; however, some inflamed glands may reach a stage of abscess formation that requires surgical drainage. Broad antimicrobial therapy is indicated to cover all possible aerobic and anaerobic pathogens, including adequate coverage for *S. aureus*, GABHS, and beta-lactamase–producing AGNB. The presence of methicillin-resistant staphylococci may mandate the use of vancomycin or linezolid. Clindamycin, cefoxitin, a carbapenem (i.e. imipenem, meropenem), tigecycline, the combination of metronidazole and a macrolide, or a penicillin plus beta-lactamase inhibitor, provide adequate coverage for anaerobic as well as aerobic bacteria.

Maintenance of good oral hygiene, adequate hydration, and early and proper therapy of bacterial infection of the oropharynx may reduce the occurrence of suppurative parotitis.

CERVICAL LYMPHADENITIS

CL is characterized by an inflammation of one or more lymph nodes in the neck. Usually involved are the anterior cervical, the submandibular, or the posterior cervical nodes. Although reactive inflammation of lymphatic tissue is usually in response to an infectious agent, an immunologic process without local infection or certain malignancies may produce similar histologic or clinical picture. In most pediatric cases, lymph node inflammation is generally a result of generalized reticuloendothelial system response. On the other hand, in adults, most cervical lymphadenopathy is likely to represent malignancy.

Microbiology

Infectious CL can be either acute unilateral or bilateral, and chronic (subacute). Because of the high frequency of CL in children, most microbiological studies were done in this age group. The most common causes of bilateral CL in children are viruses. However, the adenitis appears and resolves quickly without treatment. The most common viruses are EB, cytomegalovirus, herpes simplex, adeno virus, enterovirus, roseola, and rubella. Other pathogens include *Mycoplasma pneumoniae* and *Corynobacterium diphtheria*. The most common bacterial organisms causing acute unilateral infection associated with facial trauma or impetigo are *S. aureus* and GABHS (66–70). Other rare aerobic pathogens are *S. pneumoniae* and gram-negative rods. Other causes include *Bartonella henselae, Francisella tularensis, Pasteurella multocida, Yersinia pestis, Actinobacillus actinomycetemcomitans, Burkholderia gladioli, M. tuberculosis*, and non-TB *Mycobacterium* spp. (71–73). The presence of dental or periodontal disease suggests anaerobic bacteria (67,74). Adenitis in newborns is often related to Group B streptococci (75). Many of the investigations that attempted to evaluate the etiology of CL failed to use methodologies for the recovery of anaerobic bacteria (66,68–70). This probably accounted for the many sterile cultures obtained in these studies. Anaerobes such as AGNB (68) and *Peptostreptococcus* spp. (66,76) occasionally have been isolated.

Several reports described the recovery of anaerobes from cervical adenitis. Barton and Feigin (68) who studied 74 children, isolated four *Peptostreptococcus* spp. However, the microbiological techniques used in that study probably were not optimal for the recovery of anaerobes. Bradford and Plotkin (76) have reported the recovery of anaerobes from two children, one with alpha-hemolytic streptococci, *Bacteroides* spp., and *Peptostreptococcus* spp. and the other with *Bacteroides* spp.

Three studies that employed methodologies for recovery of anaerobes demonstrated the importance of these organisms in CL (67,74,77). Brook (67) studied 53 children who presented with CL (Table 4). Bacterial growth was noted in 45 children (85%). A total of 66 bacterial isolates (35 aerobes and 31 anaerobes) were recovered. Aerobes alone were recovered from 27 aspirates (60%), anaerobes alone from eight aspirates (18%), and mixed aerobic and anaerobic bacteria from nine specimens (20%). BLPB were recovered in 15 of the 45 (33%) specimens. Only 15% of the cultures in this study showed no bacterial growth. The large number of sterile

TABLE 4 Bacterial Isolates Recovered from 45 Aspirates Obtained from Children with Cervical Lymphadenitis

Aerobic and facultative isolates	No.	Anaerobic isolates	No.
Gram-positive cocci		Gram-positive cocci	
Alpha-hemolytic streptococci	4	*Peptostreptococcus* spp.	9
Group A beta-hemolytic streptococci	8	Gram-negative cocci	
Group C streptococci	2	*Veillonella parvula*	2
Staphylococcus aureus	14	Gram-positive bacilli	
Staphylococcus epidermidis	3	*Propionibacterium acnes*	5
Gram-negative bacilli		*Bifidobacterium* spp.	2
Klebsiella pneumoniae	1	*Lactobacillus* sp.	1
Escherichia coli	2	Gram-negative bacilli	
Mycobacterium scrofulaceum	1	*Fusobacterium nucleatum*	4
Total	35	*Bacteroides* spp.	2
		Prevotella melaninogenica	3
		Prevotella oris-buccae	1
		Bacteroides ureolyticus	1
		Porphyromonas asaccharolyticus	1
		Total	31

Source: From Ref. 67.

lymph node cultures in past studies (24% to 35%) may be related to the failure of isolation of fastidious organisms.

Roberts and Linsey (74), who recovered organisms in 35 nodes, grew mycobacterial species in 22 cultures and bacteria in 11 cultures, five of which were anaerobic.

Brook et al. reported the microbiology of needle aspirates from 40 inflamed cervical lymph glands in adults (77). Forty-two bacterial, 11 mycobacterial and six fungal isolates were isolated. Aerobes only were recovered in 11 (27.5%), anaerobes alone in five (12.5%) and mixed aerobic and anaerobic bacteria in seven (17.5%). *Mycobacterium* spp. were recovered in 11 (27.5%) and fungi in six (15%). The recovery of anaerobes was associated with dental infection. Eighteen aerobic bacteria were isolated and the predominant ones were *S. aureus* (8 isolates) and GABHS (4). Twenty-four anaerobic bacteria were recovered and the predominant ones were: *Prevotella* spp. (6), *Peptostreptococcus* spp. (5), *Propionibacterium acnes* (4) and *Fusobacterium* spp. (3).

Most of the time, anaerobes were recovered as part of a polymicrobial infection in all of the above studies (67,74,77). Recovery of these organisms is not surprising because anaerobic bacteria outnumber aerobic organisms in the oropharynx by 10:1 and frequently are recovered from infection adjacent to the oral cavity (4).

Pathogenesis

Most organisms that cause skin or oropharynx mucous membrane infections can invade the lymph nodes, draining those sites (66–70). Many organisms cause a regional CL, whereas others invade the cervical nodes as part of a more generalized lymphadenitis or systemic infection. Invasion occurs commonly at the site of pharyngitis or tonsillitis. Other entry sites for pyogenic adenitis are periapical dental abscess (usually producing a submandibular adenitis), impetigo of the face, infected acne, or otitis externa (usually producing preauricular adenitis). The problem is most prevalent among preschool children.

The lymphatic system of the cervical area serves as a line of defense against infections of the upper respiratory tract, teeth or the soft tissues of the face and scalp. Microorganisms that invade these glands are trapped and destroyed by phagocytic cells. The lymphatic chains in the neck include Waldeyer's ring (which includes the adenoids and tonsils), a collar of satellite lymph gland rings that surrounds them and a deep and superficial jugular chain (75). The cervical lymph glands that are commonly affected include the superficial and deep cervical, tonsillar, submandibular, submental, occipital, nucchal, and mastoid nodes. All these nodes are linked to each other in a consistent pattern.

As the inflammation progresses, the size of the glands increases because of edema, infiltration of neutrophilic leukocytes, and formation of necrosis or microabscesses (75). These changes are observed clinically by enlargement of the nodes, tenderness, warmth and redness. If the infection progresses, suppuration and abscess formation occurs. Rapid purulent reaction is often seen by pyogenic organisms such as *S. aureus* or GABHS, while slower formation of abscesses is generally seen in conditions associated with delayed cellular immune response such as mycobacterial, fungal, and cat-scratch disease (74).

Mycobacterial infection or scrofula is uncommon in the pediatric age group. However, these agents as well as fungi are more often found in older individuals (78), while *M. tuberculosis* accounts for most cases of scrofula in adults (71). Atypical mycobacteria (*Mycobacterium avium-intracellulare*, *Mycobacterium fortuitum*, and *Mycobacterium scrofulaceum*) account for most cases in children (79).

Cat-scratch disease is generally a self-limited disease that follows a scratch or a bite from a cat and is caused by *B. henselae* and *Bartonella clarridgeiae* (80).

CL, as part of generalized lymphadenopathy, can be associated with a retroviral infection related to the HIV, the cause of acquired immune deficiency syndrome (AIDS) (81). Opportunistic organisms such as *M. avium-intracellulare*, *M. fortuitum* and cytomegalovirus or malignancies such as lymphoma or Kaposi's sarcoma have been often present in the nodes of these patients (82).

The predominant anaerobes recovered were anaerobic gram-positive cocci and AGNB. These organisms are inhabitants of the oral pharyngeal cavity and have been recovered also from various upper and lower respiratory infections (1). The isolation of these anaerobic and aerobic organisms, all of which are part of the normal mouth flora, from lymph nodes aspirates suggests the oropharynx as the major port of entry into the lymphatic system for these organisms.

No significant correlation was found between the anaerobic bacteria isolated from CL aspirate and the age, gender, history, prior antibiotic therapy, or clinical presentation (67). The only exception was the presence of a higher prevalence of dental caries and dental abscesses in children from whom anaerobic bacteria were recovered (10 of 17 with anaerobes) than in those with aerobes (3 of 36) ($p < 0.05$) (67).

Diagnosis

The patients generally present with a swollen neck and high fever. The mass is often the size of a walnut or even an egg; it is taut, firm, and exquisitely tender. If left untreated, the mass may develop an overlying erythema.

The white count usually is about 20,000/cu mm with a shift to the left. A tuberculin skin test should be done and a throat culture obtained. Each tooth should be examined for a periapical abscess and percussed for tenderness.

The differential diagnosis should include evaluation for all causes of CL mentioned, including bacterial (beta-hemolytic streptococci, anaerobes), viral (infectious mononucleosis, mumps), cat-scratch disease, atypical mycobacteria, Kawasaki disease, sarcoidosis, tumors (sarcoma, leukemia, lymphoma, or Hodgkin's disease), tumors that do not involve lymph glands and cysts (thyroglossal, cystic hygroma or bronchial cleft).

Differentiation between infectious and noninfectious origin is of paramount importance. Infected cysts or ducts, hematomas of the sternocleidomastoid muscle in newborns can mimic CL. The duration of swelling and its location serves as an aid to diagnosis. Tumors and congenital anomalies are generally present for weeks, and the latter are often in the midline. Sinus tract are often seen in cysts. A history of cat contact may suggest cat-scratch disease. An immunofluorescent antibody assay (IFA) for *B. henselae* antibodies and polymerase chain reaction (PCR) testing are available. A history of dental or periodontal infection or dental manipulation may suggest involvement of anaerobic bacteria.

Detailed medical testing to ascertain skin lesions, animal exposure, dental problems, contact with tuberculosis, and recent travel, may provide essential information. Physical examination should include evaluation of the oropharyngeal and dental systems, skin and mucous membranes, spleen, and liver as well as other body systems.

Palpation of the mass to determine its location and consistency and motility are helpful. Ultrasound examination may assist in determining whether the lesion is cystic or solid (83). Appropriate laboratory tests such as serum amylase can assist in diagnosis. Radiological dental studies can detect a potential source of infection.

Establishment of the infection's etiology is important whenever the infection does not resolve within a few days. Aspiration of the lesion may provide important clues. Only inflamed lymph nodes should be aspirated, but these need not be fluctuant. The largest or most fluctuant node should be selected, and the skin cleansed and anesthetized. An 18- or 20-gauge needle attached to 20-mL syringe should be used, and if no material is obtained, 1 to 2 mL of saline should be injected and reaspirated. The aspirate should be inoculated for aerobic and anaerobic bacteria, fungi, and mycobacteria. Gram and acid fast strains should be done. Intradermal skin test for tuberculosis and atypical mycobacteria should be applied. Additional studies that are generally done, if no improvement occurrs following antistaphylococcal therapy, include erythrocyte sedimentation rate (ESR), chest roentgenogram and serological tests for toxoplasmosis, EB and HIV viruses, cytomegalovirus, coccidioidomycosis, histoplasmosis, tularemia, brucellosis and syphilis. A Gen-Probe *M. tuberculosis* direct test (Gen-Probe, Inc., San Diego, CA) can be used for rapid detection of Mycobacteria. If the diagnosis remains in doubt, excision biopsy should be performed. This should be submitted for the above studies as well as viral cultures, histology, and Giemsa, periodic acid-Schiff, and methenamine silver stains.

Management

Local heat may be of value for symptomatic relief in mild cases. Most of the cases of CL require no specific therapy as they are the sequellae of viral pharyngitis or stomatitis. Empiric therapy should provide adequate coverage for *S. aureus* and GABHS. Oral therapy should include penicillinase-resistant penicillins such as cloxacillin, dicloxacillin, or the combination of amoxicillin and a beta-lactamase inhibitor, such as clavulanic acid. The presence of methicillin-resistant staphylococci may mandate the use of vancomycin, linezolid, or tigecycline. Parenteral therapy may be required in toxic patients. Patients allergic to penicillin can be treated with a macrolide or clindamycin. Therapy should be given for at least 14 days. The presence of beta-lactamase–producing anaerobic as well as aerobic bacteria, especially in patients who have received penicillin, is known to be high (84). In these patients, antimicrobials effective against these organisms are indicated. These include clindamycin, the combination of a penicillin and a beta-lactamase inhibitor, or the combination of a macrolide and metronidazole.

A lack of clinical improvement after 36 to 48 hours requires a reassessment of therapy. Culture results may guide the selection of therapy.

Early treatment with antibiotics prevents most cases of pyogenic adenitis from progressing to suppuration. Once fluctuation occurs, however, antibiotic therapy alone is generally insufficient. When fluctuation or pointing is present, the abscess should be incised and drained. Surgical evacuation of the abscess is helpful in promoting resolution.

If cat-scratch disease or mycobacterial infection is suspected, incision and drainage should be avoided since chronically draining cutaneous fistulae often develop following such a procedure (85). Close aspiration, however, facilitates the resolution of cat-scratch disease. Therapy with rifampin, trimethoprim–sulfamethoxazole, or gentamicin should be considered in cat-scratch disease directed at *B. henselae*. Total surgical removal is the most effective therapy for nontuberculous mycobacterial CL (85). Therapy with antimycobacterial therapy is usually initiated until the organisms are identified as atypical mycobacteria. This includes the administration of rifampin and isoniazid. When atypical mycobacteria are recovered, these drugs are generally discontinued; however, therapy is continued for 9 to 12 months if *M. tuberculosis* is identified.

Early appropriate medical, surgical, and dental therapy of the conditions predisposing for CL can prevent the development of the infection. Such therapy includes dental care of caries or abscesses, therapy of fulminant oropharyngeal infections such as otitis and tonsillitis, and proper management of impetigo and other face and scalp infections. Prevention of exposure to contagious diseases such as tuberculosis and decreased exposure to pets that may transmit toxoplasmosis and cat-scratch disease may reduce the acquisition of these infections.

Complications

Complications include cellulitis, bacteremia, sepsis, toxin-related symptoms (in case of streptococci or staphylococci), internal jugolar vein thrombosis, pulmonary emboli or disseminated septic emboli, mediastinitis and pericarditis. These can occur if treatment is delayed.

ACUTE SUPPURATIVE THYROIDITIS

Acute suppurative thyroiditis (AST) is far less common, than the clinical types of subacute thyroiditis and Hashimoto's thyroiditis. Although infections of the thyroid are rare, they are potentially life-threatening. The symptoms and signs of AST may mimic those of a variety of noninfectious inflammatory conditions. Recognition of the clinical and bacteriological features of these infections is essential for prompt management.

Microbiology

S. aureus, GABHS, *Staphylococcus epidermidis*, and *S. pneumoniae* are, in descending order of frequency, the organisms most often isolated from AST (86–88). Other aerobic organisms are *Klebsiella* spp., *H. influenzae*, *S. viridans*, *Salmonella* spp., and Enterobacteriaceae.

Other rare agents include *M. tuberculosis* (89), atypical mycobacteria, *Aspergillus* spp., *C. immitis*, Candida, *T. pallidum*, and *Echinococcus* spp. (86–88). Viral agents have also been associated with subacute thyroiditis including measles, influenza, enterovirus adenovirus, echovirus, mumps, St. Louis encephalitis, and EB virus. Other implicated infections include malaria, Q fever and cat-scratch disease.

Yu et al. (88) presented a review of 191 patients seen between 1980 and 1997, where 130 microorganisms isolated, of which 74% were in pure culture. Gram-positive aerobes were most frequently found (39%), followed by: gram-negative aerobes (25%), fungi (15%); anaerobes (12%, mostly in mixed culture), and mycobacteria (9%). The most common causative pathogens were Streptococci, Staphylococci, *Pneumocystis carinii*, and mycobacteria. In contrast to the review by Berger et al. who summarized 224 published cases seen from 1900 to 1980 (86), no cases of syphilitic or parasitic thyroiditis were reported. The earlier review included cases from the pre-antibiotic era and had higher associated mortality (12.1%), whereas mortality in the later review (3.7%) was seen mostly in patients with AIDS and *P. carinii* or underlying malignancy. *P. carinii* thyroiditis is an entity almost exclusively seen with the advent of AIDS (90).

Anaerobic bacteria also may cause thyroiditis (86–88,91–95). Abe and colleagues (95) reported two children with recurrent episodes of AST. Anaerobic bacteria such as AGNB and *Peptostreptococcus* spp. were identified as causative agents. *E. corrodens* and *Actinomyces* spp. have also been reported (86,95,96). Polymicrobial infection (2–5 organisms) was observed in about a third of the patients (97).

Because methodologies for recovery of anaerobic bacteria were not uniformly used in all past reports, the true role of these organisms is unknown. Their recovery in AST was associated with postabortal sepsis, subphrenic abscess, and perforation of the esophagus (86–88).

Pathogenesis

The infrequent occurrence of AST has been attributed to several factors: its high concentration of iodine, rich supply of blood and lymphatics, and its unique anatomical isolation. Because the thyroid is encapsulated and without direct communication with neighboring structures, it may also be resistant to infection by direct extension from contiguous organs (86). A testimony of the gland's resistance to infection is the rare occurrence of post-surgical thyroid infection (98).

Various routes of infection have been suggested: hematogenous (91,92), direct spread from a adjacent site (93), a thyroglossal cyst or fistula (94), or a perforated esophagus (99). A predisposing factor to infection is the presence of previous diseased areas of the thyroid, such as goiter or adenomata, which are especially prevalent in females (92,99). A preceeding infection has been observed occasionally in other sites in the body. In recent series of AST, about one quarter of the patients were immunocompromised; half of these had AIDS (88).

The anaerobes recovered from inflamed thyroid are part of oral flora (4), and may, therefore, reach the gland in the same fashion as the aerobic pathogens. The recovery of these organisms as the only isolate of inflamed gland suggests that anaerobic bacteria may play an important role in the pathogenesis of AST, and they indicate the need for clinical awareness of these anaerobic bacteria as potential causes of this disease.

Diagnosis

AST is characterized by pain, firm swelling in the anterior aspect of the neck that moves on swallowing and develops over days to a few weeks with or without fever, tenderness, local warmth, fever, erythema, dysphagia, dysphonia, hoarseness, and concurrent pharyngitis in the majority of cases (86). Other signs related to pressure upon the neck muscle include limitation of cervical extension and involuntary depression of the chin upon swallowing (97). Subsequent fluctuance may develop later. The duration of symptoms before diagnosis ranges from 1 to 180 days (mean 18 days). The infection may involve both lobes or a single lobe or only the thyroidal isthmus. AST can occur as part of a cellulitis in the neck or because of infection of a cyst in a multinodular goiter.

The infection may extend locally and systemically. Death may occur, especially if therapy is delayed or is inappropriate. Death can be a result of pneumonia, tracheal obstruction or perforation, metastatic infection, sepsis, mediastinitis, pericarditis, and rupture of thyroid abscess.

Residua of the infection are rare and include vocal cord paralysis, transitory hypothyroidism that may require replacement therapy, myxedema, disruption of regional sympathetic nerves, and recurrent infection.

Differentiation from other more common thyroid conditions such as goiter or adenoma can be difficult, especially in the early stage of the disease. Subacute thyroiditis may have similar local signs, but systemic manifestations are not as severe. Leukocytosis may occur but is infrequent and mild in degree. Subacute thyroiditis generally subsides with time, whereas untreated AST generally will result in signs of increasing toxicity (97,100).

Local and systemic signs are generally present in acute bacterial infection but are often absent in mycobacterial illness. Fungal, gummatous, and parasitic thyroiditis are usually first diagnosed at surgery.

Laboratory investigations can assist in the diagnosis. The leukocyte count is elevated. The serum thyroxine (T_4), triiodothyronine (T_3), and thyroid-stimulating hormone (TSH) are generally normal. However, thyroid function tests may show mild increases in T_3 and T_4 caused by hormone release from the inflamed gland (100). On scintiscan, there may be some depression of radioiodine uptake in a portion of the thyroid, but radioactive iodine uptake usually is normal. Thyroid radionuclide scanning may not visualize the organ with diffuse inflammation, although "patchy" uptake or a "cold" area may be present with localized or less severe involvement (97). Ultrasonography and CT may be used to exclude the possibility of cervical abscess outside the thyroid capsule (95).

Patients often have leukocytosis and an elevated ESR or C-reactive protein. An ultrasound of the neck often reveals unilobular swelling, and is very useful in detecting local abscesses formation, spread to contiguous structures or defining the anatomy if surgical exploration is planned (101). Furthermore, sonography assists in the differentiation of AST from other causes of anterior neck pain and fever and allows radiographically guided drainage of a thyroid abscess, if present. CT/MRI scans of the neck are usually not required unless the ultrasound has failed to clarify the diagnosis, or if the clinical course suggests extension of a thyroid abscess to other areas of the mediastinum. Lateral soft tissue radiographs of the neck will show evidence of tissue edema, and the tracheal air column may be deviated or compressed. The presence of anaerobic infection may be associated with the presence of soft-tissue gas, and foul-smelling pus (94).

Diagnosis can be facilitated by needle aspiration of the neck mass and Gram stain of the specimen (100,102).

Aspirated material should be processed in a manner similar to that discussed in the section on CL.

Management

AST requires immediate parenteral antibiotic therapy before abscess formation begins. An appropriate antibiotic may be selected on the basis of the results of Gram stain of the aspirated pus. Alterations in therapy can be made when final culture and sensitivities results are reported. Because of the wide range of different bacteria that can be involved in this infection, a broad coverage of antimicrobial agents is indicated, at least until culture results are available.

The choice of antimicrobial agent is similar to the one discussed in the section on parotitis. Most of the anaerobes recovered from this infection are susceptible to penicillin; however, some resistant strains may occur among growing number of AGNB.

Operative therapy is indicated when antibiotics fail to control sepsis promptly, as evidenced by leukocytosis, continued fever, and progressive signs of local inflammation. Surgical drainage should be performed if clinical examination or radiographic findings by ultrasound/CT scan are consistent with an abscess or if there is evidence of gas formation. If extensive necrosis or persistence of infection inspite of antibiotics is demonstrated, lobectomy may be required (97,100–102). Debridement of necrotic tissue should be performed and the wound allowed to heal by secondary intention.

The prognosis following appropriate medical and surgical therapy is excellent. Hypothyroidism rarely occurs and the thyroid function tests return to normal with eradication of infection (97,100,102).

Control of the conditions known to predispose the infection is important and should include management of any preexisting thyroid pathology, such as goiter and adenomas, and prevention of extension of infection to adjacent structures.

Complications

Transient or rarely prolonged hypothyroidism can occur in cases with severe, diffuse inflammation and necrosis of the gland and may require L-thyroxine replacement. Other local complications include abscess formation: vocal cord paralysis, abscess rupture or extension into adjacent sites and organs (anterior mediastinum, trachea, esophagus), thrombosis of the internal jugular vein (Lemiere's syndrome), and extrinsic compression of the trachea (103).

INFECTED NECK CYSTS

Cysts of the neck are usually painless, insensitive, and slow-growing. Some may be present at birth, and others appear as late as middle age. These cysts include thyroglossal duct cyst, cystic hygroma, brachial cleft cyst, laryngocele, and dermoid cyst (104). All of these cysts can become inflamed and cause local infection.

Thyroglossal Duct Cyst

Thyroglossal duct cyst is the commonest congenital mass and is almost always located in the midline (104). This type of cyst results from embryologic anomalies in the descent of the thyroid gland. The thyroid forms high in the neck at the base of the tongue and hyoid bone and, as growth proceeds and the neck enlarges, it descends to the lower part of the neck. If the cyst retains its attachment to the tongue it is called a thyroglossal duct, and any cystic space in this duct is a thyroglossal duct cyst. The duct always joins the base of the tongue by passing behind the hyoid bone, and thus thyroglossal duct cysts are always found below the hyoid bone in the midline or occasionally just to the left of the midline. The cyst moves on swallowing and on protruding the tongue because it is attached to the thyroid gland.

The cyst can become infected and cause a tender, red swelling in the midneck. When infected, the cyst is best treated with antibiotics until the acute infection subsides. During the quiescent phase, these cysts are treated by surgical resection of the cyst and the entire length of tract. Malignant thyroid tumors, usually of the papillary carcinoma variety, have been reported within thyroglossal duct tissue.

Cystic Hygroma (Lymphangioma)

This is the rarest of all neck swellings. This cyst develops from the jugular lymph sac when it fails to communicate with the thoracic duct or the internal jugular vein (104). About half of the cysts are present since birth, and the remainder develops during childhood. The swelling, which may attain a very considerable size, is predominantly found in the posterior triangle of the neck, but may extend to the hypopharynx and larynx. The cyst is smooth, firm, fluctuant, not bound, and it transilluminates. Histologically, it consists of a multilocular cyst enclosing clear lymph within thin walls. It can cause compression of the trachea or difficulty in swallowing. Removal of a small cyst is not difficult but poses problems of access and of complete removal if the hypopharynx and larynx are involved. In such instances, there is an appreciable recurrence rate. When infection or sudden hemorrhage into the tissue occurs, there may be a sudden increase in the cyst's size.

Branchial Cyst

The cyst represents the remnants of the first branchial cleft. It may occasionally open to the lateral wall of the pharynx on the palatopharyngeal fold or in the floor of the external auditory meatus at the junction of its cartilaginous and bony parts (104). This type of cyst usually appears at the anterior border of the sternomastoid muscle at the junction of its middle and upper thirds. It is cystic and quite mobile, and its fluid contains cholesterol crystals. Treatment includes complete removal.

Laryngocele

Laryngocele is a remnant of the primitive air sac and presents at the side of the neck over the thyroid membrane. It may be easily inflated and emptied of air, and it shows a characteristic radiographic appearance. Treatment consists of complete surgical removal of the cyst. Sometimes the mouth of the sac becomes blocked, and infection develops and presents similar to that of a pyocele.

Dermoid Cyst

Dermoids can occur anywhere along lines of fusion, and in the neck they are almost invariably found above the hyoid bone in close relation to the mylohyoid muscle. They are midline swellings, which move on swallowing and on protruding the tongue because they are intimately related to the muscle fibers forming the base of the tongue (104).

Enlargement within the mouth may cause feeding problems, and should the cyst enlarge into the hypopharynx, respiration may be hampered. Microscopically, this cyst resembles a dermoid elsewhere in the body, having a thick fibrous capsule and containing hairs and epithelial debris which may discharge through the sinus. Removal should be either through the floor of the mouth or via a submental incision, depending upon the situation of the sinus.

Etiology and Pathogenic Consideration

The organisms that can cause secondary infection of these cysts can originate from either the skin or oral pharynx mucous surfaces. Blocking of these cysts by dried secretions predisposes them to infection by prevention of the evacuation of their contents. *S. aureus* and GABHS are the predominant aerobic isolates, while pigmented *Prevotella* and *Porphyromonas* spp., and *Peptostreptococcus* spp., all part of the oral flora, are the predominant anaerobes (105–107). We have recovered these organisms from three congenital cysts (two bronchial and one thyroglossal cyst) in one report (2). We evaluated 24 infected neck cysts, as part of a study of 231 epidermal cysts (105). Aerobic bacteria were recovered in 13 (54%) instances, anaerobes only in eight (33%), and mixed aerobic and anaerobic bacteria were found in three (13%). The predominate aerobic organisms were *S. aureus* (11 isolates) and GABHS (5). The most frequent anaerobes were *Peptostreptococcus* spp. (7), and AGNB (7).

Diagnosis

Swelling associated with redness, local warmth, and enlargement of the regional lymph glands generally evolves acute infection. Pressure on surrounding tissue, including the trachea and esophagus can also occur. Systemic signs are usually rare.

The infection may extend to adjacent structures and if suppuration occurs, drain into the facial planes or into the oropharynx or the trachea. Systemic dissemination is rare.

Infections at other adjacent sites such as the cervical lymph glands, parotid and thyroid glands must be excluded. Noninfectious enlargement of the cysts usually is not painful and may be caused by fluid retention or malignant transformation. The patient's history may provide useful information. A precipitating factor such as blowing may suggest laryngocele.

Meticulous physical examination, including a search for the cyst's orifice, transillumination, radiological and scanning studies, may be helpful. Aspiration of the infected site may lead to exact diagnosis of the infection's etiology. Aspirated material should be processed as previously described for CL to identify aerobic and anaerobic bacteria, mycobacteria, and fungi. Biopsy or complete surgical removal following subsidement of the acute inflammation may provide histologic–pathologic diagnosis to exclude malignant transformation that may also be associated with infection. Pulsating masses necessitate an angiography.

Therapy

Antimicrobial therapy should be directed at the eradication of the predominant organisms causing secondary cyst infection. The choice of antibiotics is similar to the one described in the section on parotitis. Most acute cases respond to antimicrobial therapy; however, when suppuration occurs, surgical drainage may be required. Complete surgical removal may be delayed until resolution of the acute inflammation.

Prevention can be achieved by surgical removal of cysts before acquisition of infection, or removal of those recurrently infected.

REFERENCES

1. Finegold SM. Anaerobic Bacteria in Human Disease. New York: Academic Press, 1977.
2. Brook I. Microbiology of abscesses of the head and neck in children. Ann Otol Rhinol Laryngol 1987; 96:429–33.
3. Brook I, Finegold SM. Aerobic and anaerobic bacteriology of cutaneous abscesses in children. Pediatrics 1981; 67:891–5.
4. Socransky SS, Manganiello SD. The oral microbiota of man from birth to senility. J Periodontal 1971; 42:485–96.
5. Brook I, Shah K. Bilateral peritonsillar abscess: an unusual presentation. South Med J 1981; 74:514–5.
6. Herzon FS, Martin AD. Medical and surgical treatment of peritonsillar, retropharyngeal, and parapharyngeal abscesses. Curr Infect Dis Rep 2006; 8:196–202.
7. Sakae FA, Imamura R, Sennes LU, Araujo Filho BC, Tsuji DH. Microbiology of peritonsillar abscesses. Rev Bras Otorrinolaringol 2006; 72:247–51.
8. Brook I. Aerobic and anaerobic bacteriology of peritonsillar abscess in children. Acta Paediatr Scand 1981; 70:831–8.
9. Brook I. Microbiology of retropharyngeal abscesses in children. Am J Dis Child 1987; 141:202–4.
10. Jokipii AMM, Jokipii L, Sipila P, et al. Semiquantitative culture results and pathogenic significance of obligate anaerobes in peritonsillar abscesses. J Clin Microbiol 1988; 26:957–61.
11. Floodstrom A, Hallander HO. Microbiological aspects of peritonsillar abscesses. Scand J Infect Dis 1976; 8:157–60.
12. Dodds B, Maniglia AJ. Peritonsillar and neck abscesses in the pediatric age group. Laryngoscope 1988; 98:956–9.
13. Asmar BI. Bacteriology of retropharyngeal abscess in children. Pediatr Infect Dis J 1990; 9:595–6.
14. Asmar BI. Neonatal retropharyngeal cellulitis due to group B streptococcus. Clin Pediatr 1987; 26:183–5.
15. Hughes CE, Spear RK, Shinabarger CE, et al. Septic pulmonary emboli complicating mastoiditis: Lemierre's syndrome. Clin Infect Dis 1994; 18:633–5.
16. Moreno S, Altonzano JG, Pinilla B, et al. Lemierre's disease: postanginal bacteremia and pulmonary involvement caused by *Fusobacterium necrophorum*. Rev Infect Dis 1989; 2:319–24.
17. Neumann JL, Schlueter DP. Retropharyngeal abscess as the presenting feature of tuberculosis of the cervical spine. Am Rev Respir Dis 1974; 110:508–11.
18. Barratt GE, Koopmann CF, Coulthard SW. Retropharyngeal abscess. A ten year experience. Laryngoscope 1984; 94:455–63.
19. Hansen A. Nogle undersøgelser over gram-negative aerobe ikke-spore-dannende bacterier isolerede fra peritonsillere abscesser hos mennesker. Copenhagen: Ejnar Munksgaard, 1950.
20. Hallander HO, Floodstrom A, Holmberg K. Influence of the collection and transport of specimens on the recovery of bacteria from peritonsillar abscesses. J Clin Microbiol 1975; 2:504–9.
21. Sprinkel PM, Veltri RW, Kantor LM. Abscesses of the head and neck. Laryngoscope 1974; 84:112–8.
22. Lodenkämper H, Stienen G. Importance and therapy of anaerobic infections. Antibiotic Med Clin Ther 1955; 1:653–60.
23. Baba S, Mamiya K, Suzuki A. Anaerobic bacteria isolated from otolaryngologic infections. Jpn J Clin Pathol 1971; 19:35–9.
24. Ophir D, Bawnik J, Poria Y, Porat M, Marshak G. Peritonsillar abscess. A prospective evaluation of outpatient management by needle aspiration. Arch Otolaryngol Head Neck Surg 1988; 114:661–3.
25. Prévot AR. Biologies des maladies dués aux anaerobies. Paris: Éditions Medicales Flamarion, 1955.
26. Alston JM. Necrobacillosis in Great Britain. Br Med J 1955; 2:1524–8.

27. Beerens H, Tahon-Castel M. Infections humaines à bactéries anaerobies nontoxigènes. Brussels: Presses Acad Eur, 1965.
28. Gruner OPN. Actinomyces in tonsillar tissue: a histological study of tonsillectomy material. Acta Pathol Microbiol Scand 1969; 76:239–44.
29. Rubenstein E, Onderdonk AB, Rahal J, Jr. Peritonsillar infection and bacteremia caused by *Fusobacterium gonidiaformans*. J Pediatr 1974; 85:673–5.
30. Oleske JM, Starr SE, Nahmias AJ. Complications of peritonsillar abscess due to *Fusobacterium necrophorum*. Pediatrics 1976; 57:570–1.
31. Brook I, Frazier EH, Thompson DH. Aerobic and anaerobic microbiology of peritonsillar abscess. Laryngoscope 1991; 101:289–92.
32. Jousimies-Somer H, Savolainen S, Makitie A, Ylikoski J. Bacteriologic findings in peritonsillar abscesses in young adults. Clin Infect Dis 1993; 16(Suppl. 4):S292–8.
33. Mitchelmore IJ, Prior AJ, Montgomery PQ, Tabaqchali S. Microbiological features and pathogenesis of peritonsillar abscesses. Eur J Clin Microbiol Infect Dis 1995; 14:870–7.
34. Myerson MC. Anaerobic retropharyngeal abscess. Ann Otol Rhinol Laryngol 1932; 41:805–8.
35. Ernst O. Zur bedetung des *Bacteroides funduliformis* als infektions-errerger. Z Hyg 1961; 132:352–9.
36. Janecka IP, Rankow RM. Fatal mediastinitis following retropharyngeal abscess. Arch Otolaryngol Head Neck Surg 1971; 93:630–3.
37. Heinrich S, Pulverer G. Uber den Nachweis des *Bacteroides melaninogenicus* in Krankheitsprozessen bei Mensch und Tier. Z Hyg 1960; 146:341–9.
38. Coulthard M, Isaacs D. Retropharyngeal abscess. Arch Dis Child 1991; 66:1227–30.
39. Brook I, Hunter V, Walker RI. Synergistic effects of anaerobic cocci, *Bacteroides*, *Clostridia*, *Fusobacteria*, and aerobic bacteria on mouse and induction of substances abscess. J Infect Dis 1984; 149:924–8.
40. Brook I, Foote PA, Jr., Slots J. Immune response to anaerobic bacteria in patients with peritonsillar cellulitis and abscess. Acta Otolaryngol 1996; 116:888–91.
41. Wolf M, Even-Chen I, Kronenberg J. Peritonsillar abscess: repeated needle aspiration versus incision and drainage. Ann Otol Rhinol Laryngol 1994; 103:554–7.
42. Friedman NR, Mitchell RB, Pereira KD, Younis RT, Lazar RH. Peritonsillar abscess in early childhood. Presentation and management. Arch Otolaryngol Head Neck Surg 1997; 123:630–2.
43. Scott PM, Loftus WK, Kew J, Ahuja A, Yue V, van Hasselt CA. Diagnosis of peritonsillar infections: a prospective study of ultrasound, computerized tomography and clinical diagnosis. J Laryngol Otol 1999; 113:229–32.
44. Lamkin RH, Portt J. An outpatient medical treatment protocol for peritonsillar abscess. Ear Nose Throat J 2006; 85:658–60.
45. Parker CGS, Tami TA. The management of peritonsillar abscess in the 90s: an update. Am J Otolaryngol 1992; 12:286–8.
46. Echevvarria J. Deep neck infections. In: Schlossberg D, ed. Infections of the Head and Neck. New York: Springer, 1987:168–84.
47. Krippaehne WW, Hunt TK, Dunphy JE. Acute suppurative parotitis: a study of 161 cases. Ann Surg 1962; 156:251–7.
48. Spiegel R, Miron D, Sakran W, Horovitz Y. Acute neonatal suppurative parotitis: case reports and review. Pediatr Infect Dis J 2004; 23:76–8.
49. Baurmash HD. Chronic recurrent parotitis: a closer look at its origin, diagnosis, and management. J Oral Maxillofac Surg 2004; 62:1010–8.
50. Brook I. Diagnosis and management of parotitis. Arch Otolaryngol Head Neck Surg 1992; 118:469–71.
51. Tunkel DE. Atypical mycobacterial adenitis presenting as a parotid abscess. Am J Otolaryngol 1995; 16:428–32.
52. Shevky M, Kohn C, Marshall MS. *Bacterium melaninogenicum*. J Lab Clin Med 1934; 19:689–94.
53. Heck WE, McNaught RC. Periauricular *Bacteroides* infection, probably arising in the parotid. JAMA 1952; 149:662–3.
54. Beigelman PM, Rantz LA. Clinical significance of *Bacteroides*. Arch Intern Med 1949; 84:605–8.
55. Coleman RM, Georg LK. Comparative pathogenicity of *Actinomyces naeslundii* and *Actinomyces israelii*. Appl Microbiol 1969; 18:427–32.
56. Anthes WH, Blaser MJ, Reller LB. Acute suppurative parotitis associated with anaerobic bacteremia. Am J Clin Pathol 1981; 75:260–2.
57. Brook I, Finegold SM. Acute suppurative parotitis caused by anaerobic bacteria: report of two cases. Pediatrics 1978; 62:1019–20.
58. Sussman SJ. *Gaffkya anaerobia* infection and recurrent parotitis. Clin Pediatr 1986; 25:323–4.
59. Lewis MA, Lamey PJ, Gibson J. Quantitative bacteriology of a case of acute parotitis. Oral Surg Oral Med Oral Pathol 1989; 68:571–5.
60. Guardia SN, Cameron R, Phillips A. Fatal necrotizing mediastinitis secondary to acute suppurative parotitis. J Otolaryngol 1991; 20:54–6.

61. Meskin LH, Farsht EM, Anderson DL. Prevalence of *Bacteroides melaninogenicus* in the gingival crevice area of institutionalized trisomy 21 and cerebral palsy patients and normal children. J Periodontol 1968; 39:326–8.

62. Brook I, Frazier EH, Thompson DH. Aerobic and anaerobic microbiology of acute suppurative parotitis. Laryngoscope 1991; 101:170–2.

63. Brook I. Aerobic and anaerobic microbiology of suppurative sialadenitis. J Med Microbiol 2002; 51:526–9.

64. Brook I. Suppurative sialadenitis associated with anaerobic bacteria in newborns. Pediatr Infect Dis J 2006; 25:280.

65. Yousem DM, Kraut MA, Chalian AA. Major salivary gland imaging. Radiology 2000; 216:19–29.

66. Munck K, Mandpe AH. Mycobacterial infections of the head and neck. Otolaryngol Clin North Am 2003; 36:569–76.

67. Brook I. Aerobic and anaerobic bacteriology of cervical adenitis in children. Clin Pediatr 1980; 19:693–6.

68. Barton LL, Feigin RD. Childhood cervical lymphadenitis: a reappraisal. J Pediatr 1974; 84:846–52.

69. Yamauchi T, Ferrieri P, Anthony BFL. The aetiology of acute cervical adenitis in children: serological and bacteriological studies. J Med Microbiol 1980; 13:37–43.

70. Scobie WG. Acute suppurative adenitis in children: a review of 964 cases. Scott Med J 1969; 14:352–4.

71. Ridder GJ, Boedeker CC, Technau-Ihling K, Grunow R, Sander A. Role of cat-scratch disease in lymphadenopathy in the head and neck. Clin Infect Dis 2002; 35:643–9.

72. Poropatich C, Tuazon CU, Wilson W. Suppurative cervical adenitis caused by *Actinobacillus actinomycetemcomitans*. Oral Surg Oral Med Oral Pathol 1990; 69:727–8.

73. Graves M, Robin T, Chipman AM, Wong J, Khashe S, Janda JM. Four additional cases of *Burkholderia gladioli* infection with microbiological correlates and review. Clin Infect Dis 1997; 25:838–42.

74. Roberts FJ, Linsey S. The value of microbial cultures in diagnostic lymph-node biopsy. J Infect Dis 1984; 149:162–5.

75. Gosche JR, Vick L. Acute, subacute, and chronic cervical lymphadenitis in children. Semin Pediatr Surg 2006; 15:99–106.

76. Bradford BJ, Plotkin SA. Cervical adenitis caused by anaerobic bacteria. J Pediatr 1976; 89:1060.

77. Brook I, Frazier EH. Microbiology of cervical lymphadenitis in adults. Acta Otolaryngol 1998; 118:443–6.

78. Freidig EE, McClure SP, Wilson WR, Banks PM, Washington JA, II. Clinical–histologic–microbiologic analysis of 419 lymph node biopsy specimen. Rev Infect Dis 1986; 8:322–8.

79. Lai KK, Stottmeier KD, Sherman IH, McCabe WR. Mycobacterial cervical lymph-adenopathy: relation of etiologic to age. JAMA 1984; 251:1286–8.

80. Bass JW, Vincent JM, Person DA. The expanding spectrum of Bartonella infections: II. Catscratch disease. Pediatr Infect Dis J 1997; 16:163–79.

81. Kamani N, Lightman H, Leiderman I, Krilov LR. Pediatric acquired immunodeficiency syndrome-related complex: clinical and immunologic features. Pediatr Infect Dis J 1988; 7:383–8.

82. Butt AA. Cervical adenitis due to *Mycobacterium fortuitum* in patients with acquired immuno-deficiency syndrome. Am J Med Sci 1998; 315:50–5.

83. Kelly CS, Kelly RE, Jr. Lymphadenopathy in children. Pediatr Clin North Am 1998; 45:875–88.

84. Brook I, Gober AE. Emergence of beta-lactamase-producing aerobic and anaerobic bacteria in the oropharynx of children following penicillin chemotherapy. Clin Pediatr 1984; 23:338–41.

85. Hazra R, Robson CD, Perez-Atayde AR, Husson RN. Lymphadenitis due to nontuberculous mycobacteria in children: presentation and response to therapy. Clin Infect Dis 1999; 28:123–9.

86. Berger SA, Zonszein J, Villamena P, Mittman N. Infectious diseases of the thyroid gland. Rev Infect Dis 1983; 5:108–22.

87. Jeng LB, Lin JD, Chen MF. Acute suppurative thyroiditis: a ten year review in a Taiwanese hospital. Scand J Infect Dis 1994; 26:297–300.

88. Yu EH, Ko WC, Chuang YC, et al. Suppurative *Acinetobacter baumanii* thyroiditis with bacteremic pneumonia: case-report and review. Clin Infect Dis 1998; 27:1286–90.

89. Bulbuloglu E, Ciralik H, Okur E, Ozdemir G, Ezberci F, Cetinkaya A. Tuberculosis of the thyroid gland: review of the literature. World J Surg 2006; 30:149–55.

90. Golshan MM, McHenry CR, de Vente J, et al. Acute suppurative thyroiditis and necrosis of the thyroid gland: a rare endocrine manifestation of acquired immunodeficiency syndrome. Surgery 1997; 121:593–6.

91. Chi H, Lee YJ, Chiu NC, et al. Acute suppurative thyroiditis in children. Pediatr Infect Dis J 2002; 21:384–7.

92. Gaafar H, El-Garem F. Acute thyroiditis with gas formation. J Laryngol Otol 1975; 89:323–7.

93. Ogawa E, Katsushima Y, Fujiwara I, Iinuma K. Subacute thyroiditis in children: patient report and review of the literature. Pediatr Endocrinol Metab 2003; 16:897–900.

94. Bussman YC, Wong ML, Bell MJ, Santiago JV. Suppurative thyroiditis with gas formation due to mixed anaerobic infection. J Pediatr 1977; 90:321–2.

95. Abe K, Taguchi T, Okuno A, Matsuura N, Takebayashi K, Sasaki H. Recurrent acute suppurative thyroiditis. Am J Dis Child 1978; 132:990–1.
96. Cheng AF, Man DW, French GL. Thyroid abscess caused by *Eikenella corrodens*. J Infect 1988; 16:181–5.
97. Rich EJ, Mendelman PM. Acute suppurative thyroiditis in pediatric patients. Pediatr Infect Dis J 1987; 6:936–40.
98. Fewins J, Simpson CB, Miller FR. Complications of thyroid and parathyroid surgery. Otolaryngol Clin North Am 2003; 36:189–206.
99. Yung BC, Loke TK, Fan WC, Chan JC. Acute suppurative thyroiditis due to foreign body-induced retropharyngeal abscess presented as thyrotoxicosis. Clin Nucl Med 2000; 25:249–52.
100. Slatosky J, Shipton B, Wahba H. Thyroiditis: differential diagnosis and management. Am Fam Physician 2000; 61:1047–52 (see also 1054).
101. Naik KS, Bury RF. Imaging the thyroid. Clin Radiol 1998; 53:630–9.
102. Shah SS, Baum SG. Diagnosis and management of infectious thyroiditis. Curr Infect Dis Rep 2000; 2:147–53.
103. Lough DR, Ramadan HH, Aronoff SC. Acute suppurative thyroiditis in children. Otolaryngol Head Neck Surg 1996; 114:462–5.
104. Acierno SP, Waldhausen JHT. Congential cervical cysts, sinuses and fistulae. Otolaryngol Clin North Am 2007; 40:161–76.
105. Brook I. Microbiology of infected epidermal cysts. Arch Dermatol 1989; 125:1658–61.
106. Ohata C, Komatani M, Shirabe H, Takagi K, Kawatsu T. Bacteriological analysis of epidermal cysts. Skin Research 1996; 38:305–9.
107. Nishijima S, Higashida T, Oshima S, Nakaya H. Bacteriology of epidermoid cysts. Jpn J Dermatol 2003; 113:165–8.

18 | Actinomycosis

Actinomycosis is an uncommon, chronic, bacterial infection that induces both suppurative and a granulomatous inflammation. Localized swelling with suppuration, abscess formation, tissue fibrosis, and draining sinuses characterize this disease. The infection spreads contiguously forming often draining sinuses that extrude characteristic but not pathognomonic "sulfur granules." Infections of the oral and cervicofacial regions are most common; however, any site in the body can be infected. Other regions that are often affected are the thoracic region, abdomino-pelvic region, and the central nervous system (CNS). Musculoskeletal and disseminated disease can also be rarely seen.

ETIOLOGY

Actinomycetes of the genera *Actinomyces*, *Propionibacterium*, or *Bifidobacterium* act as the principal pathogens. However, 98% to 99% of actinomycoses are caused by non-spore forming anaerobic, or microaerophilic bacterial species of the genus *Actinomyces*, family *Actinomycetaceae*, order *Actinomycetales*. Of the 30 *Actinomyces* species, eight may cause disease in humans: the strictly anaerobic *Actinomyce israelii*, *Actinomyce gerencseniae* (formerly known as *Actinomyces israelii serovar*), *Actinomyce odontolyticus*, *Actinomyce naeslundii*, *Actinomyce meyeri*, *Actinomyce viscosus*, *Actinomyce pyogenes*, and *Actinomyce georgiae*. *Actinomyces israelli* is the most common species causing human disease. *Propionibacterium propionicum* (formerly known as *Arachnia propionica*) and *Bifidobacterium dentium* (formerly known as *Actinonyces eriksonii*) are also associated with clinically indistinguishable infection (1). The organisms are filamentous, branching, gram-positive, pleomorphic non-spore-forming, non-acid-fast anaerobic or microaerophilic bacilli. *Actinomyces* are fastidious bacteria that require enriched culture media, may be aided in growth by 6% to 10% ambient CO_2, It takes 3 to 10 or more days to grow them in culture. Characteristically, *Actinomyces* species appear as "molar tooth" colonies on agar, or as "bread-crumb" colonies suspended in broth media. They are prokaryotes with cell walls that contain both muramic acid and diaminopimelic acid. Most actinomycotic infections are polymicrobial, involving other aerobic and anaerobic bacteria. The most common co-isolates depend on the infection site and are *Actinobacillus actinomycetemcomitans*, *Eikenella corrodens*, *Bacteroides*, *Fusobacterium*, *Capnocytophaga*, aerobic and anaerobic *streptococci*, *Staphylococcus*, and *Enterobacteriaceae*.

EPIDEMIOLOGY

The agents of *Actinomyces* are members of the endogenous mucous membrane flora in the oral cavity, gastrointestinal tract, bronchi, and female genital tract. No external environmental reservoir such as soil or straw has been documented, and there is no person-to-person transmission of the pathogenic *Actinomyces* species. Infection can occur in all age groups however, it is rarely seen in children or in patients older than 60 years (1). Most cases are encountered in individuals in the middle decades of life. A male-to-female infection ratio of 3:1 is reported in most series. The explanation for this ratio is the poorer oral hygiene and augmented oral trauma in males. The annual reported incidence in the U.S.A. is fewer than

100 cases. However, because of the fastidious nature of the organism, the true incidence is likely much higher.

PATHOGENSESIS AND PATHOLOGY

Actinomyces species are agents of low pathogenicity and require disruption of the mucosal barrier to cause disease. Actinomycosis usually occurs in immunocompetent persons but may afflict persons with diminished host defenses. Oral and cervicofacial diseases commonly are associated with dental caries and extractions, gingivitis and gingival trauma, infection in erupting secondary teeth, chronic tonsillitis, otitis or mastoiditis, diabetes mellitus, immuno-suppression, malnutrition, and local tissue damage caused by surgery, neoplastic disease, or irradiation. Pulmonary infections usually arise after aspiration of oropharyngeal or gastro-intestinal secretions. Gastrointestinal infection frequently follows loss of mucosal integrity, such as with surgery, appendicitis, diverticulitis, trauma, or foreign bodies (1). The use of intrauterine contraceptive devices (IUDs) was linked to the development of actinomycosis of the female genital tract. The presence of a foreign body in this setting appears to trigger infection. Other predisposing factors are steroid use, immunosuppression, and human immunodeficiency viral infections (2).

Other bacterial species that often are co-pathogens to *Actinomyces* species may assist in the spread of infection by inhibiting host defenses and reducing local oxygen tension. Once the organism is established locally, it spreads to surrounding tissues that ignore tissue planes in a progressive manner, leading to a chronic, indurated, suppurative infection often with draining sinuses and fibrosis, especially in pelvic and abdominal infection. The fibrotic walls of the mass prior to suppuration are "wooden" in nature, and may be confused with a neoplasm. Hematogenous spread can be fulminant, but is rare.

The infection tendency is to spread without regard for anatomical barriers, including fascial planes and lymphatic channels. *Actinomyces* grow in microscopic or macroscopic clusters of tangled filaments surrounded by neutrophils. Plasma cells and multinucleated giant cells often are observed with lesions, as may be large macrophages with foamy cytoplasm around purulent centers. When visible, these clusters are pale yellow and exude through sinus tracts; they are called "sulfur granules" (originally called "drusen"). These granules (1 to 2 mm in diameter) are made of aggregates of organisms and contain calcium phosphate. A central purulent loculation surrounds the granules. Their centers have a basophilic staining property, with eosinophilic rays terminating in pear-shaped "clubs." One to six granules can be present per loculation, and up to 50 loculations can be present in a lesion.

CLINICAL MANIFESTATION

Cervicofacial

This is the most common form of actinomycosis (1). The infection is generally odontogenic in origin, and evolves as a chronic or subacute painless or painful soft-tissue swelling or mass involving the submandibular or paramandibular region. However, the submental and retro-mandibullar spaces, tempomandibullar joint and cheek can be involved. The swelling may have ligneous consistency caused by tissue fibrosis. Depending on the composition of the concomitant synergistic flora, the onset of actinomycosis may be acute, subacute, or chronic. When *Staphylococcus aureus* or beta-hemolytic streptococci are involved, an acute painful abscess or a phlegmatous cellulitis may be the initial manifestation. The chronic form of the disease is characterized by painless infiltration and induration that usually progress to form multiple abscesses and draining sinus tracts discharging pus that may contain sulfur granules in up to 25% of instances. Periapical infection, trismus, fever, pain, and leukocytosis may be present. The infection can extend to the carotid artery, tongue, sinuses, ears, mastoid, orbit, salivary glands, pharynx, masseter muscle, thyroid, larynx, trachea, or thorax (3). Bone (most commonly the mandible) may be invaded from the adjacent soft tissue leading to periostitis or osteomyelitis. Cervical spine or cranial bone infection may lead to subdural empyema and invasion of the CNS. The differential diagnosis includes tuberculosis (scrofula), fungal infections, nocardiosis, suppurative infections by other organisms, and neoplasm.

Thoracic

This is an indolent, slow process involving the pulmonary parenchyma and pleural space. This form accounts for 15% to 30% of actinomycosis cases and often results from aspiration of infective material from the oropharynx, and rarely following esophageal perforation, by extension into the mediastinum from the neck, or by spread from an abdominal site, and hematogenous spread to the lung (4). It often spreads from pneumonic focus across lung fissures to involve the pleura and the chest wall, with eventual fistula formation and drainage containing sulfur granules. The mediastinum, pericardium, and myocardium can also rarely be affected. Granules rarely are present in the sputum. The incidence of this complication, as well as the destruction of thoracic vertebrae and adjacent ribs, has declined in the antibiotic era.

The complaints of patients with thoracic actinomycosis are nonspecific. The most common are chest pain, a productive cough, dyspnea, weight loss, and fever. Anemia, mild leukocytosis, and an elevated sedimentation rate are relatively common. There often is a history of underlying lung disease, and patients rarely present in an early stage of infection. The pulmonary lesion is either a mass lesion or pneumonitis and may resemble tuberculosis, especially when cavity formation occurs, and blastomycosis, which may destroy ribs posteriorly but rarely forms sinuses. Nocardiosis, bronchogenic carcinoma, cryptococcosis, aspiration pneumonia, pulmonary infection, and lymphoma can also mimic thoracic actinomycosis. Pleural thickening, effusion, or emphysema is common.

Abdominal

This is a chronic, localized, inflammatory process that often occurs weeks, months, or years after the integrity of the gastrointestinal mucosa is broken by surgery for acute appendicitis with perforation, or for perforated colonic diverticulitis, or by emergency surgery on the lower intestinal tract after trauma. Occasionally, abdominal actinomycosis may manifest without identifiable predisposing factors. The ileocecal region is involved most frequently (usually following appendicitis with perforation), with the formation of a mass lesion. The infection extends slowly to contiguous organs, especially the liver, and may involve retroperitoneal tissues, the spine, or the abdominal wall. Hepatic, renal, and splenic disseminations are uncommon complications (5). Persistent draining sinuses may form, and those involving the perianal region can simulate Crohn's disease or tuberculosis. The extensive fibrosis of actinomycotic lesions, presenting to the examiner as a mass, often suggests tumor. A frequent finding on computed tomography (CT) is an infiltrative mass with dense inhomogeneous contrast medium enhancement. Constitutional symptoms and signs are nonspecific; the most common are fever, diarrhea or constipation, weight loss, nausea, vomiting, pain, and sensation of mass.

Pelvic

This condition is observed in patients who present with prolonged use of IUDs, usually for longer than two years. Pelvic actinomycosis may also occur from extension of intestinal infection, commonly from indolent ileocecal disease (2). Manifestations of infection may range from a chronic vaginal discharge to pelvic inflammatory disease with tubo-ovarian abscesses or pseudomalignant masses (see chapter 24). Patients generally present with abnormal vaginal bleeding or discharge, abdominal or pelvic pain, menorrhagia, fever, and weight loss.

Endometritis is the earlier form of the infection, followed by tubo-ovarian abscesses. Extension to the uterus, bladder, rectal area, abdominal wall, peritoneum, pelvic bones, thorax, and systemic sites can also occur.

Central Nervous System

Infections of the CNS are very rare and generally manifest as single or multiple encapsulated brain abscesses that appear as ring-enhancing lesions with thick wall that may be irregular or nodular on CT with intravenous contrast material and are indistinguishable from those caused by other organisms (6). Rarely, solid nodular or mass lesions termed actinomycetomas or actinomycotic granulomas are found. Headache and focal neurological signs are the most common finding. Most actinomycotic infections of the CNS are thought to be seeded hematogenously from a distant primary site; however, direct extension of cervicofacial disease is well recognized. Sinus formation is not a characteristic of CNS disease. The rare meningitis caused by *Actinomyces* is chronic and basilar in location, and the pleocytosis usually is lymphocytic. Thus, it may be misdiagnosed as tuberculous meningitis.

DIAGNOSIS

A combination of appropriate microbiological and pathological studies is essential for proper diagnosis. A high index of suspicion should be communicated to the microbiology diagnostic laboratory, along with material from draining sinuses, from deep-needle aspiration, or from biopsy specimens. It is important to avoid antimicrobial therapy prior to obtaining a specimen. Anaerobic culture is required, and no selective media are available to restrict overgrowth of the slow-growing *Actinomyces* by associated microflora. The presence, in pus or tissue specimens, of non-acid-fast, gram-positive organisms with filamentous branching is very suggestive of the diagnosis. The characteristic morphology of sulfur granules and the presence of gram-positive organisms within are helpful. In tissue sections stained with hematoxylin and eosin, sulfur granules are round or oval basophilic masses with a radiating arrangement of eosinophilic terminal "clubs." However, *Actinomyces* species are infrequently visible in sections stained with hematoxylin and eosin; visualization is facilitated by special stains such as Grocott-Gomori methenamine silver, *p*-aminosalicylic acid, McCallen-Goodpasture, and Brown-Brenn. Multiple biopsy sections from different tissue levels are recommended to improve histopathologic diagnosis. The granules must be distinguished from similar structures that are sometimes produced in infections and that are caused by *Nocardia*, *Monosporium*, *Cephalosporium*, *Staphylococcus* (botryomycosis), and others. *Actinomyces* and *Arachnia* generally can be differentiated from other gram-positive anaerobes by means of growth rate (slow), by catalase production (negative, except *A. viscosus*), and by gas–liquid chromatographic detection of acetic, lactic, and succinic acids produced in peptone–yeast–glucose broth. Direct fluorescent antibody conjugates and immunofluorescence testing can be used but are not readily available to clinical microbiology laboratories.

Imaging methods such as conventional radiography, CT, and magnetic resonance imaging do not provide a specific diagnosis but allow more accurate definition of the dimensions and extension of the infection.

TREATMENT

Prolonged antimicrobial therapy (i.e., 6–12 months) has typically been recommended for patients with all clinical forms of actinomycosis, to prevent disease recrudescence. However, individualization of courses of therapy is recommended, where the duration of antibiotics depends on the initial burden of disease, the site of infection, and the clinical and radiologic response to treatment. Adequate drainage is indicated if abscesses are present.

Penicillin G is the drug of choice for treating an infection caused by any of the *Actinomyces*. It is given in high dosage over a prolonged period, because the infection has a tendency to recur. Most deep-seated infections can be expected to respond to intravenous penicillin G, 10 to 20 million units/day given for two to six weeks, followed by an oral phenoxypenicillin in a dosage of 2 to 4 g/day. A few additional weeks of oral penicillin therapy may suffice for uncomplicated cervicofacial disease; complicated cases and extensive pulmonary or abdominal disease may require treatment for 12 to 18 months. Little evidence exists of acquired resistance to penicillin G by *Actinomyces* during prolonged therapy. Alternative first-line antibiotics include erythromycin, chloramphenicol and clindamycin. First-generation cephalosporins, ceftriaxone, and imipenem also have been employed successfully. Metronidazole, aminoglycosides, ciprofloxacin, tetracycline, and antifungal drugs are not active against these organisms (7). In vitro antibiotic sensitivity testing of *Actinomyces* is difficult, and the results may not be predictive of antibiotic activity in vivo.

The need to use combination antibiotic therapy to attack microorganisms that are isolated in association with *Actinomyces* has not been established. However, since many of these organisms are known pathogens, coverage is desirable for them as well. This is especially important in lower abdominal infections. Surgical removal of infected tissue may also be necessary in some cases, especially if extensive necrotic tissue or fistulas are present, if malignancy cannot be excluded, and if large abscesses cannot be drained by percutaneous aspiration. When well-defined IUD-related symptoms and Papanicolaou smears demonstrate *Actinomyces* by specific fluorescent-labeled antibody, the IUD should be removed. Antibiotic administration for a two-week period may be indicated. More serious infections require prolonged therapy.

PROGNOSIS

The availability of antibiotics has greatly improved the prognosis for all forms of actinomycosis. At present, cure rates are high and neither deformity nor death is common.

REFERENCES

1. Smego RA, Jr., Foglia G. Actinomycosis. Clin Infect Dis 1998; 26:1255–61.
2. Lippes J. Pelvic actinomycosis: a review and preliminary look at prevalence. Am J Obstet Gynecol 1999; 180:265–9.
3. Oostman O, Smego RA. Cervicofacial actinomycosis: diagnosis and management. Curr Infect Dis Rep 2005; 7:170–4.
4. Mabeza GF, Macfarlane J. Pulmonary actinomycosis. Eur Respir J 2003; 21:545–51.
5. Wagenlehner FM, Mohren B, Naber KG, Mannl HF. Abdominal actinomycosis. Clin Microbiol Infect 2003; 9:881–5.
6. Smego RA, Jr. Actinomycosis of the central nervous system. Rev Infect Dis 1987; 9:855.
7. Smith AJ, Hall V, Thakker B, Gemmell CG. Antimicrobial susceptibility of Actinomyces species with 12 antimicrobial agents. J. Antimicrob Chemother 2005; 56:407–9.

19 | Mediastinitis

Mediastinitis is a life-threatening condition with extremely high mortality if recognized late or treated improperly (1). The mediastinum contains essential and vital structures and organs. These include the thymus, trachea, bronchi, esophagus, aorta and aortic arch, pericardium, heart lymph nodes, and nerve tisssue. Although mediastinal infections are rare, they may be life threatening. Acute and chronic forms of the infection are recognized (2).

PATHOGENESIS

Infection of the mediastinum is always a secondary event, which determines its etiology. Most cases of mediastinitis occur following cardiovascular surgery (1,2). Risk factors for the development of mediastinitis following cardiovascular surgery include the following: bilateral internal mammary artery grafts, diabetes mellitus, emergency surgery, external cardiac compression, obesity, postoperative shock, especially when multiple blood transfusions are required, prolonged bypass and operating room time, re-exploration following initial surgery, sternal wound dehiscence, and surgical technical factors (3).

Esophageal perforation is the second most common cause of mediastinitis (4). The causes of esophageal perforation include the following: erosion of esophageal wall by malignancy, foreign bodies, instrumentation from endoscopes during diagnostic or therapeutic procedures, placement of nasogastric or feeding tubes, spontaneous esophageal rupture, and trauma, mostly blunt trauma to the chest or abdomen. Other causes of mediastinitis are tracheobronchial perforation, due to either penetrating or blunt trauma or instrumentation during bronchoscopy, descending infection following surgery of the head and neck, great vessels, or vertebrae, progressive odontogenic infection (i.e., Ludwig angina), mediastinal extension of lung infection, extension from paravertebral abscess or osteomyelitis of the sternum or ribs, extension from mediastinal or cervical lymph nodes and chronic fibrosing mediastinitis due to granulomatous infections and blood-borne infection (1–3).

The origin of bacterial pathogens causing the infection following open-heart operations is unknown in most patients (1,2). Possible sources are areas of sternal osteomyelitis or sternal instability that leads eventually to sternal separation and migration of bacteria into deeper tissues. Inadequate mediastinal drainage in the operating room may also contribute to the development of a deeper chest infection. The patient's own skin or oropharyngeal flora as well as external bacteria in the local surgical environment can be a source of infection.

Mediastinitis that follows cardiac surgery, blood-borne infection, extension from paravertebral abscess or osteomyelitis of the sternum or ribs and extension from mediastinal or cervical lymph nodes are not likely to be caused by anaerobic bacteria (5,6). Anaerobes are extremely rare in post-cardiac surgery. However, perforation of the esophagus, extension of retropharyngeal abscess, suppurative parotitis (7), cervical cellulitis (8), or abscess of dental origin (9,10) that are usually caused by anaerobes of oral origin are very likely to involve mixed aerobic–anaerobic oral flora. Since anaerobic bacteria are part of the normal oral flora, their presence in mediastinitis associated with exposure to oropharyngeal bacterial flora is not surprising. Similar anaerobic bacteria are also found in mediastinitis due to extension of pulmonary, pleural, and pericardial infections or secondary to deep and post-surgical neck infections (11).

MICROBIOLOGY

Staphylococcus aureus, Staphylococcus epidermidis, Enterobacteriaceae, *Enterobacter cloacae, Enterococcus* spp., *Pseudomonas* spp., *Proteus* spp., *Haemophilus* spp., *Corynobacterium xerosis, Mycoplasma* spp., nontuberculous mycobacterium, and *Nocardia, Aspergillus, and Candida* spp. are the predominant pathogens recovered after cardiovascular surgery (12,13). These organisms can also be recovered mixed with anaerobic bacteria whenever polymicrobial infection is present. Histoplasmosis and tuberculosis are the most common identifiable causes of chronic mediastinitis (Table 1).

The major bacteria recovered from infections originating from the oral flora are Group A streptococci and oral anaerobic bacteria. These include pigmented *Prevotella* and *Porphyromonas, Fusobacterium,* and *Peptostreptococcus* spp. (14). There are also a few cases that reported involvement of *Bacteroides fragilis* group (15).

The role of anaerobic bacteria in mediastinitis was not established by prospective studies and the data in the literature is based mostly on several case reports.

Ferzil et al. (16) reported a 17-year-old female who developed anaerobic mediastinitis that complicated infectious mononucleosis. They recovered *S. aureus, Streptococcus constellatus, Streptococcus milleri,* and *Prevotella melaninogenica.* Several reports described the concomitant recovery of *Clostridium* spp. including *Clostridium perfringens* in mediastinitis secondary to esophageal perforation (17). Guardia et al. (7) reported a case of fatal necrotizing mediastinitis secondary to acute suppurative parotitis. The infection was the result of synergistic necrotizing cellulitis caused by mixed aerobic and anaerobic bacteria. The causative isolates were *E. coli, Enterococcus Escherichia* spp., *B. fragilis, C. perfringes, P. melaninogenica,* and *Candida albicans.* Isaacs et al. (18) reported a case of a 34-year-old woman with an upper respiratory infection who developed a para, retropharyngeal, and mediastinal abscesses. *Peptostreptococcus* and *Bacteroides* spp. were isolated from the infected sites.

Murray and Finegold (14) reported two cases of anaerobic mediastinitis and summarized the literature that included additional 18 cases reported between 1930 and 1981. The predominant origin of the infection in these patients were odontogenic (in 7 instances),

TABLE 1 Predominant Organisms Recovered from Mediastinitis

Aerobic bacteria
    Staphylococcus aureus
    Staphylococcus epidermidis
    Streptococcus pyogenes
    Microaerophillic streptococcus
    Enterococcus spp.
    Haemophilus spp.
    Enterobacteriaceae
    Enterobacter cloacae
    Klebsiella pneumoniae
    Pseudomonas spp.
    Proteus spp.
    Corynobacterium xerosis
Anaerobic bacteria
    Peptostreptococcus spp.
    Clostridium spp.
    Bacteroides spp.
    Pigmented *Prevotella and Porphyromonas* spp.
    Fusobacterium spp.
Other organisms
    Mycoplasma spp.
    Nontuberculous mycobacterium
Fungi
    Nocardia spp.
    Aspergillus spp.
    Candida spp.
    Histoplasma spp.

oral abscess (in 3), pleural fluid (in 2), and trauma (in 2). Polymicrobial flora was found in all but one case and the predominant anaerobic bacteria isolated from these patients were *Bacteroides*, *Peptostreptococcus*, pigmented *Prevotella*, and *Fusobacteeium* spp. Moncada et al. (19) reported five cases of mediastinitis caused by anaerobes, originating from odontogenic and deep cervical infections; two of these were in children.

Wheatley et al. (20) reported two cases of descending necrotizing mediastinitis due to anaerobic bacteria, in which infection arising from the oropharynx spreads to the mediastinum. They also reviewed the English language literature on this disease from 1960 to 1990 summarizing 43 additional cases. Polymicrobial aerobic–anaerobic flora was present in 30 of the 36 (83%) cases where the microbiological result was given; anaerobes only in one (3%) and aerobes alone in five (14%).

Brook and Frazier studied the microbiologic and clinical characteristics of 17 adults with mediastinitis (21). Aerobic or facultative bacteria were present only in three patients (18%), anaerobic bacteria only in seven (41%), and mixed aerobic–anaerobic flora in seven (41%). There were a total of 42 isolates, 13 aerobic or facultative, and 29 anaerobic bacteria, an average of 2.5/specimen. Anaerobic bacteria predominated in infections that originated from esophageal perforation and orofacial, odontogenic, and gunshot sources. The predominant aerobes were alpha-hemolytic Streptococcus (3 isolates), *S. aureus* (2), and *Klebsiella pneumoniae* (2). The predominant anaerobes were *Prevotella* and *Porphyromonas* spp. (8), *Peptostreptococcus* spp. (7), and *B. fragilis* group (3). This study highlights the polymicrobial aerobic–anaerobic nature of mediastinitis.

DIAGNOSIS

Esophageal perforation can be associated with acute or delayed symptoms. Perforation can also occur following mechanical obstruction by foreign bodies that induce necrosis. Perforation may occur following esophageal surgery. Abrupt onset of neck and chest pain, dyspnea, tachycardia, hypotension, chills, fever, and leukocytosis are generally observed. Subcutaneous emphysema is seen when the perforation site is at the level of the cricopharyngeal muscle and in proximal perforation.

Postoperative patient generally presents with fever, high pulse, and complaints suggestive of a sternal wound infection. Most patients present with mediastinitis within two weeks of surgery. However, a delay of months is occasionally seen. Patients usually complain of increasing sternal pain, draining wound site, and progressive redness. Infants may present with irregular breathing characterized by an inspiratory halt with resumption of inspiration after a brief rest (22).

Chest radiography may show widened mediastinum, subcutaneous and mediastinal emphysema, and pleural effusions (2,15). Basilar or retrocardiac infiltrates may be observed. Foreign bodies may be detected by plain films, computed tomography, magnetic resonance imaging, or fluoroscopy. Mediastinal emphysema is suggestive of an esophageal perforation as well as other conditions such as perforations of tracheobronchial tree or penetration of air following surgical procedures in the upper respiratory tract. Esophageal dye studies are the most useful in cases of suspected esophageal perforation. If no extravasation is observed, barium is given to provide better definition of the esophageal wall. Fiberoptic bronchoscopy is performed when a perforated airway is suspected as the cause of the mediastinitis.

Purulent drainage, erythema, tenderness, fever and leukocytosis, and occasionally sternal instability can be present in mediastinitis secondary to sternotomy wound infection. No symptoms may accompany chronic mediastinitis and the lesion may be only detected by chest radiographs.

Systemic signs of sepsis strongly suggest mediastinal involvement as compared to superficial wound infection. Compression of adjacent structures (esophagus, tracheobronchial tree, or superior vena cava) may be present. Other features are low-grade fever, weight loss, and anemia. Diagnostic and therapeutic surgical exploration may be warranted. Appropriate cultures for aerobic and anaerobic bacteria of blood, pleural fluid wound site, or surgical specimen including mediastinal pacing wires should be taken. Any sternal drainage should be sent for Gram stain and culture for aerobic and anaerobic bacteria as well as fungi. This helps to establish a diagnosis and to tailor antimicrobial therapy. Diagnosis of tuberculosis and histoplasma can be established by tuberculin skin test and histoplasma serology. Proper cultures for tuberculosis and histoplasma should be performed.

Bacteremia is found in almost 60% of patients with postoperative mediastinitis (23). Mortality rate is high, especially if diagnosis and therapy are delayed.

MANAGEMENT

Treatment includes surgical intervention, antimicrobial therapy, and supportive measures. Maintaining the airway, monitoring the vital signs, and administering parenteral fluids are essential (24). Surgical correction of perforations, debridement of wound infection, mediastinal irrigation, and excision of chronic lesions are an integral part of management. In severe infection, it may be necessary to leave the wound open, until subsequent secondary closure (25). Topical use of granular sugar was suggested as a mean to heal refractory severe infection (26).

Prophylactic antibiotics should be administered prior to surgical sternotomy usually with a first generation cephalosporin. Coverage for anaerobic bacteria is not indicated. Selection of antimicrobials for the treatment of mediastinitis is determined by bacteriologic studies. Often no pathogen is recovered, and antimicrobial therapy is empiric. Such treatment should be effective against the oral aerobic and anaerobic flora as well as *S. aureus*. Treatment effective against anaerobic bacteria should be administered to those where exposure to oral flora might have occurred (i.e., after perforation of the esophagus, extension of retropharyngeal abscess, suppurative parotitis or cervical cellulitis, or abscess of dental origin). There is generally no need or empyrical antianaerobic antimicrobial agents in post-surgical mediastinitis, unless exposure to oral flora has occurred. Antimicrobials also effective against enteric bacteria are important in mediastinitis secondary to sternal wound.

Vancomycin or linezolid are effective against gram-positive anaerobes and methicillin-resistant *S. aureus*. Clindamycin or the combination of metronidazole plus a beta-lactamase resistant penicillin carbapenems (i.e., imipenem, meropenem, ertapenem), tigecycline or the combination of a penicillin (amoxicillin, ampicillin, ticarcillin, or piperacillin) and a beta-lactamase inhibitor (clavulanic acid, sulbactam, or tazobactam) are adequate for anaerobes, Enterobacteriaceae, and *S. aureus*. Aminoglycosides, quinolones or a fourth generation cephalosporins (i.e., cefepime) are effective additives against aerobic gram-negative rods. Systemic antimicrobial therapy should be given for at least four to six weeks.

CONCLUSION

Mediastinitis is a life-threatening infection with a high mortality when it is recognized late or treated improperly. Mediastinitis caused by anaerobic bacteria often occurs after perforation of the esophagus, extension of retropharyngeal abscess, suppurative parotitis or cervical cellulitis, or abscess of dental origin. The anaerobes recovered from these infections are often of oral origin and involve mixed aerobic–anaerobic oral flora. The management of mediastinitis evolves directing appropriate antimicrobial therapy against the potential bacterial pathogens.

REFERENCES

1. Balkan ME, Oktar GL, Oktar MA. Descending necrotizing mediastinitis: a case report and review of the literature. Int Surg 2001; 86:62–6.
2. El Oakley RM, Wright JE. Postoperative mediastinitis: classification and management. Ann Thorac Surg 1996; 61:1030–6.
3. Robicsek F. Postoperative sterno-mediastinitis. Am Surg 2000; 66:184–92.
4. Kiernan PD, Hernandez A, Byrne WD, et al. Descending cervical mediastinitis. Ann Thorac Surg 1998; 65:1483–8.
5. Mitjans MS, Sanchis JB, Padro XB, et al. Descending necrotizing mediastinitis. Int Surg 1969 2000; 85:331–5.
6. Kerschner JE, Beste DJ, Conley SF, Kenna MA, Lee D. Mediastinitis associated with foreign body erosion of the esophagus in children. Int J Pediatr Otorhinolaryngol 2001; 59:89–97.

7. Guardia SN, Cameron R, Phillips A. Fatal necrotizing mediastinitis secondary to acute suppurative parotitis. J Otolaryngol 1991; 20:54–6.
8. Pignat JC, Haguenauer JP, Navailles B. Diffuse spontaneous cervical cellulitis caused by anaerobic bacteria. Rev Laryngol Otol Rhinol (Bord) 1989; 110:141–4.
9. Garcia-Consuegra L, Junquera-Gutierrez L, Albertos-Castro JM, Llorente-Pendas S. Descending necrotizing mediastinitis caused by odontogenic infections. Rev Stomatol Chir Maxillofac 1998; 99:199–202.
10. Tung-Yiu W, Jehn-Shyun H, Ching-Hung C, Hung-An C. Cervical necrotizing fasciitis of odontogenic origin: a report of 11 cases. Oral Maxillofac Surg 2000; 58:1347–52.
11. Sancho LM, Minamoto H, Fernandez A, Sennes LU, Jatene FB. Descending necrotizing mediastinitis: a retrospective surgical experience. Eur J Cardiothorac Surg 1999; 16:200–5.
12. Bor DH, Rose RM, Modlin JF, Weintraub R, Friedland GH. Mediastinitis after cardiovascular surgery. Rev Infect Dis 1983; 5:885–7.
13. L'Ecuyer PB, Murphy D, Little JR, Fraser VJ. The epidemiology of chest and leg wound infections following cardiothoracic surgery. Clin Infect Dis 1996; 22:424–9.
14. Murray PM, Finegold SM. Anaerobic mediastinitis. Rev Infect Dis 1984; 6:S123–7.
15. Howell HS, Printz RA, Pickleman JR. Anaerobic mediastinitis. Surg Gynecol Obstet 1976; 113:353–9.
16. Ferzli G, Worth M, Glaser JB. Mediastenitis complicating infectious mononucleosis. Infect Surg 1988; 5:310–2.
17. Salo JA, Savola JK, Toikkanen VJ, et al. Successful treatment of mediastinal gas gangrene due to esophageal perforation. Ann Thorac Surg 2000; 70:2143–5.
18. Isaacs LM, Kotton B, Peralta MM, Jr., et al. Fatal mediastinal abscess from upper respiratory infection. Ear Nose Throat J 1993; 72:620–2.
19. Moncada R, Warpeha R, Pickleman J, et al. Mediastinitis from odontogenic and deep cervical infection. Chest 1978; 73:497–500.
20. Wheatley MJ, Stirling MC, Kirsh MM, Gago O, Orringer MB. Descending necrotizing mediastinitis: transcervical drainage is not enough. Ann Thorac Surg 1990; 49:780–4.
21. Brook I, Frazier EH. Microbiology of mediastinitis. Arch Intern Med 1996; 156:333–6.
22. Feldman R, Gromisch DS. Acute suppurative mediastinitis. Am J Dis Child 1971; 121:79–81.
23. Munoz P, Menasalvas A, Bernaldo de Quiros JC, Desco M, Vallejo JL, Bouza E. Postsurgical mediastinitis: a case-control study. Clin Infect Dis 1997; 25:1060–4.
24. Losanoff JE, Jones JW, Richman BW. Primary closure of median sternotomy: techniques and principles. Cardiovasc Surg 2002; 10:102–10.
25. Iacobucci JJ, Stevenson TR, Hall JD, Deeb GM. Sternal osteomyelitis: treatment with rectus abdominis muscle. Br J Plast Surg 1989; 42:452–9.
26. Szerafin T, Vaszily M, Peterffy A. Granulated sugar treatment of severe mediastinitis after open-heart surgery. Scand J Thorac Cardiovasc Surg 1991; 25:77–80.

20 | Pulmonary Infections

Pulmonary infections due to anaerobic bacteria usually occur in individuals who are prone to aspiration of their oral secretions or gastric contents because of impaired cough reflex. This tendency can be due to tracheoesophageal malformations, central nervous system disorders, debilitation, and temporary or permanent altered consciousness (1). Neurologically impaired individuals are especially prone to develop lower respiratory tract infections that originate from their endogenous bacterial flora because of several predisposing factors (Table 1).

The management of pulmonary infections involves directing appropriate antimicrobial therapy against the potential bacterial pathogens. The importance of anaerobes in pulmonary infections due to aspiration is due to their predominance in the microflora of the oral mucous where they outnumber aerobic microorganisms by a ratio of 10:1 (2). Often, anaerobic organisms are present in combination with other facultative or aerobic organisms.

PATHOGENESIS

Aspiration Pneumonia and Lung Abscess

The aspiration of saliva and oropharyngeal secretions that contain many aerobic and anaerobic bacteria introduces these organisms into the lower respiratory tract (1). A breakdown of the normal host protective mechanisms predisposes to anaerobic infection and is the common denominator of patients who develop this infection.

Aspiration of food and vomitus is common in those who are prone to aspirate because of debilitation, dysphagia, alcoholism, nasogastric tube feeding, congenital malformations of the upper airways, central nervous system disorders such as seizures, and altered consciousness. If active or passive clearance of the aspirate is not achieved, there is a short latent period of several hours before the onset of pneumonia. Poor oral hygiene, gingivitis, and periodontitis, as well as therapy with diphenylhydantoin contribute to poor oral hygiene and promote the development of pneumonia in those who aspirate.

The initial lesion following aspiration is pneumonitis, which has a relatively insidious onset and involvement of dependent segments of the lung. If left untreated, tissue necrosis may in some cases, that fail to resolve, lead to abscess formation or empyema after one to two weeks. Excavation may lead to solitary lung abscess or multiple small areas of necrosis of the lung, with or without air-fluid levels (necrotizing pneumonia). However, lung abscess can develop without a documented aspiration.

Empyema

Empyema is defined as the presence of pus in the pleural cavity and represents an effusion containing great numbers of polymorphonuclear leukocytes and fibrin. Acute empyema is generally secondary to infection at another site, most commonly a pulmonary infection. Empyema generally is an internal extension of pneumonia or lung abscess; oral, retropharyngeal, or skin abscess (3); and mediastinal lymph nodes or paravertebral abscess or external introduction of organisms related to trauma or surgery. Predisposing conditions unique to children are cerebral palsy, hypogammaglobulinemia, Down's syndrome, congenital heart disease, and prematurity (4).

TABLE 1 Factors Predisposing Individuals to Develop Lower Respiratory Tract Infections Due to Endogenous Anaerobic Bacterial Flora

Impaired mechanical defenses due to
Neurologic injury (i.e., depressed cough reflex, altered consciousness, seizures)
Intubation or tracheostomy
Debilitation
Dysphagia
Alcoholism
Nasogastric tube
Feeding malformations
Constant recumbent position
Change in oropharyngeal flora
Repeated administration of antibiotics
Gingivitis due to anticonvulsion therapy
Poor oral hygiene, gingivitis, periodontitis
Long-term hospitalization and response to hospital flora
Impaired immunological defenses in some genetic disorders (i.e., Down's syndrome)
Delay in recognition of acute illness because of the patient's inability to complain

MICROBIOLOGICAL TECHNIQUES

Materials that are appropriate for anaerobic cultures should be obtained using a technique that bypasses the normal oropharyngeal flora. Special transport media that protect the specimen from exposure to oxygen are most useful (1). Specimens should be obtained for all types of anaerobic pulmonary infections, especially those that are serious and/or fail to respond to empiric therapy.

Unacceptable or inappropriate specimens can be expected to yield normal flora also and, therefore, have no diagnostic value. The most appropriate lower respiratory specimen is a percutaneous transtracheal aspirate (TTA), tracheal aspirate obtained through protected double-lumen catheter or by lung puncture. Collection of materials from the pleural fluid and closed abscesses is also acceptable. Throat or nasopharyngeal swabs, sputum or bronchoscopic specimens, and material from superficial wounds or abscesses not collected properly to exclude surface contamination should not be cultured for anaerobic bacteria.

MICROBIOLOGY

Similar genera of anaerobes are isolated from pulmonary infections in children (6–8) and adults (1,3,5,9) and include pigmented *Prevotella* and *Porphyromonas*, *Bacteroides*, *Fusobacterium*, and *Peptostreptococcus* spp. (Table 2). Many anaerobic gram-negative bacilli (AGNB) can produce the enzyme beta-lactamase. Organisms of the *Bacteroides fragilis* group, which are most frequently involved in intra-abdominal infections, can also be isolated in lower respiratory infections. Prompt identification of these organisms can assist in the initiation of appropriate antimicrobial therapy.

Aspiration Pneumonia and Lung Abscess

Studies involving adult patients and using the TTA method show anaerobes in 70% to 90% of cases of pneumonitis, necrotizing pneumonia, and lung abscess (1,3,5,9). Anaerobes, either alone or in combination with aerobes, have been recovered from approximately 80% of lung abscesses (9). The anaerobes most frequently isolated are pigmented *Prevotella* and *Porphyromonas*, *Fusobacterium nucleatum*, anaerobic gram-positive cocci, microaerophilic cocci, and *B. fragilis* (which can be found in 10–20% of the patients). The major aerobic pathogens that are usually isolated mixed with anaerobic bacteria are *Staphylococcus aureus*, *Klebsiella pneumoniae*, and *Pseudomonas aeruginosa*.

Brook and Finegold (6,7,10), who utilized TTA, evaluated 74 children with aspiration pneumonia: 52 patients with pneumonitis, 12 with necrotizing pneumonia, and 10 with lung abscess. Anaerobic bacteria were recovered in 90% of aspirates. Cultures yielded an average

TABLE 2 Predominant Aerobic and Anaerobic Organisms Recovered in Aspiration Pneumonia, Lung Abscess, and Empyema in Children

Anaerobic bacteria	Aerobic and facultative bacteria
Anaerobic cocci	Gram-positive cocci
Peptostreptococcus spp.	*Streptococcus pneumoniae*
Veillonella spp.	Alpha-hemolytic streptococci
Microaerophilic streptococci	Group A, beta-hemolytic streptococci
Gram-positive bacilli	*Staphylococcus aureus*
Bifidobacterium spp.	*Staphylococcus epidermidis*
Gram-negative bacilli	Gram-negative bacilli
Fusobacterium nucleatum	*Proteus* spp.
Fusobacterium spp.	*Pseudomonas aeruginosa*
Pigmented *Prevotella* and *Porphyromonas* spp.	*Klebsiella pneumoniae*
Bacteroides ureolyticus	*Escherichia coli*
Prevotella oris-buccae	*Serratia marcescens*
Prevotella oralis	*Citrobacter* spp.
Bacteroides spp.	*Enterobacter* spp.
Bacteroides fragilis group	*Haemophilus influenzae*
	Haemophilus parainfluenzae
	Eikenella corrodens

of 4.9 organisms/patient (2.7 anaerobes and 2.2 aerobes). The predominant aerobic and facultative bacteria were *P. aeruginosa*, *Streptococcus pneumoniae*, *Escherichia coli*, *K. pneumoniae*, and *S. aureus*. The main anaerobes were *Peptostreptococcus* spp., pigmented *Prevotella* and *Porphyromonas* spp., *F. nucleatum*, *B. fragilis* group, and *Bacteroides* spp. Fusobacteria and gram-negative enteric rods were more frequently isolated in children younger than four years and *B. fragilis* group was absent in children younger than two years. Many of the organisms produced beta-lactamase. These include all *S. aureus* and *B. fragilis* group, and about half of pigmented *Prevotella* and *Fusobacterium* spp.

Empyema

The aerobic and anaerobic microbiology of empyema in adults were studied in 197 patients (11) Three hundred forty-three organisms (216 aerobic or facultative and 127 anaerobic organisms) were isolated. Aerobic bacteria were isolated in 127 (64%) patients, anaerobic bacteria in 25 (13%), and mixed aerobic and anaerobic bacteria in 45 (23%). The predominant aerobic or facultative organisms were *S. pneumoniae* (70 isolates), *S. aureus* (58), *E. coli* (17), *K. pneumoniae* (16), and *Haemophilus influenzae* (12). The predominant anaerobes were pigmented *Prevotella* and *Porphyromonas* spp. (24), *B. fragilis* group (22), anaerobic cocci (36), and *Fusobacterium* spp (20). Beta-lactamase–producing bacteria (BLPB) were recovered in 49 (38%) out of 128 tested specimens. Most patients from whom *S. pneumoniae* and *H. influenzae* were recovered had pneumonia, and most patients with *S. aureus* had pneumonia, aspiration pneumonia, and lung abscesses. The recovery of anaerobic bacteria was mostly associated with the concomitant diagnosis of aspiration pneumonia and lung, subdiaphragmatic, dental, and oropharyngeal abscesses. These data highlight the importance of anaerobic bacteria in selected cases of empyema.

The organisms isolated from empyema in children are *S. aureus*, *S. pneumoniae*, *H. influenzae* type b, *Streptococcus pyogenes*, *K. pneumoniae*, *Mycoplasma pneumoniae* (5,11), and anaerobic bacteria (8,12). A reduction in the proportion of *S. aureus* and *H. influenzae* and an increase in *S. pneumoniae* was noted in the U.S.A. since the early 1990s (13).

Fajardo and Chang (12) retrospective evaluated 104 children with pleural empyema and recovered anaerobes in five. All these patients were older than 10 years and had pneumonia. Polymicrobial infection occurred in four and the recovered anaerobes were *Peptostreptococcus* spp. (3 isolates), *Bacteroides* spp. (2), and *F. nucleatum* (1).

Brook studied the microbiology of empyema in 72 institutionalized neurologically impaired children (12). Ninety-three organisms, 60 aerobic or facultative and 33 anaerobic, were found. Aerobic bacteria were isolated in 48 (67%) patients, anaerobic bacteria in 17 (24%), and mixed aerobic and anaerobic bacteria in 7 (10%). The predominant aerobic or facultative bacteria were *H. influenzae* (15 isolates), *S. pneumoniae* (13), and *S. aureus* (10). The predominant anaerobes were similar to those found in aspiration pneumonia (7) or lung abscesses (6) and were gram-negative bacilli (15, including 7 *B. fragilis* group and 5 pigmented *Prevotella* and *Porphyromonas* spp.), *Peptostreptococcus* spp. (9), and *Fusobacterium* spp. (6). As was found also in adults (11) most cases of *S. pneumoniae* and *H. influenzae* were associated with pneumonia, while the recovery of anaerobic bacteria was linked to the diagnosis of aspiration pneumonia, lung abscess, subdiaphragmatic abscess, and dental or oropharyngeal abscess.

DIAGNOSIS

Aspiration Pneumonia and Lung Abscess

A sudden onset of fever, chills, rapid respiration, cough, vomiting and diarrhea, abdominal distention, and elevated peripheral white blood cells are the commonest manifestations. Rarely, apnea and hypotensive shock are observed. The onset of the infection is sometimes more insidious than acute non-aspiration pneumonia. Chemical pneumonitis due to aspiration is generally not accompanied by fever. Weeks to months of malaise, low-grade fever, and cough, with significant weight loss and anemia, may precede consolidation and abscess formation. Examination may reveal dyspnea with frequent expiratory grunts, dilated nostrils, flushed cheeks, cyanosis, rales, diminished breath sounds, dullness, and prolonged expiration. The presence of a pneumonic process in a posterior upper lobe or superior lower lobe suggests the presence of aspiration and lung abscess. Cavitation with an air-fluid level establishes the diagnosis.

Empyema

Fever, sweating, chest pain, anemia, leukocytosis, and weight loss are the presenting signs. Pleural effusion can be diagnosed on physical and radiological examination. Lateral decubitus X rays and fluoroscopy may be helpful. Ultrasonography may be more helpful than computed tomography in evaluating fibrinous organization of the effusion. The pleural fluid findings are generally not organism specific. The fluid obtained through thoracentesis should be studied for volume, specific gravity, color, pH, consistency, odor, total protein content, glucose, lactic acid, red and white cell count, Gram and acid-fast stains, wet mount for fungi, mycobacteria, and aerobic and anaerobic cultures. Foul smell may suggest the presence of anaerobic bacteria.

The presence of an infection has been associated with a protein concentration above 3 g/100 mL, glucose lower than 60 mg/dL, a specific gravity higher than 1.018, low pH level (equal to or less than 7.1, or equal to or above 0.3 than serum pH) (14), a lactic dehydrogenase level above 550 units and a lactic acid level higher than 47 mg/100 mL. (15). However, the levels of lactic acid may also be elevated in the presence of malignancy in the pleura. The presence of a large number of mononuclear cells may indicate a granulomatous infection.

Pleural fluid and blood cultures frequently are sterile in those who have been previously treated with antibiotics. In these patients, antigen detection using latex particle agglutination, counterimmunoelectrophoresis, or coagglutination methods on pleural fluid, blood, and urine can help establish a specific etiology. Antigens can still be detected in pleural fluid for several days after initiation of therapy.

MANAGEMENT

Antimicrobial therapy is of utmost importance. The selection of antimicrobial agents is based on age, history, physical examination and radiographic findings, and by the organism recovered from reliable sources (i.e., blood, properly collected sputum, or pleural fluid). Guidelines for the selection of antimicrobial therapy are presented in the section "Principles of Antimicrobial Therapy".

Aspiration Pneumonia and Lung Abscess

The duration of treatment varies and depends on the type of pulmonary involvement and may need to be up to six weeks especially in lung abscess. Prolonged therapy can prevent relapse. In uncomplicated instances, therapy is continued until clinical improvement, the patient has been afebrile for five to seven days, and has shown improvement on chest roentgenogram. Of note is that radiographic changes can lag up to 10 days behind clinical improvement. Those with necrotizing pneumonia and lung abscess may require longer courses of therapy than those with pneumonitis (6). In addition to effective antimicrobial therapy, anaerobic pleuropulmonary infections may require drainage. Bronchoscopy may be helpful in relieving obstruction. Because lung abscess and necrotizing pneumonitis can drain spontaneously through postural drainage, surgical evacuation is not necessary if diagnosis is made early and appropriate therapy is instituted.

Empyema

Surgical drainage and administration of appropriate antimicrobial agents are the mainstay of therapy. Drainage of the pleural space can help in allowing full lung re-expansion, reduce respiratory distress, and prevent the formation of a thick peel that restricts lung expansion. Several techniques are effective in achieving adequate pleural fluid drainage. The specific method used depends primarily on the stage of the infection and the patient's response to therapy.

During the early exudative phase of small parapneumonic effusions, one or more needle aspirations often provide adequate drainage and establish the microbial etiology. However, if the patient remains toxic and fluid accumulates rapidly, closed drainage by intercostal catheter may be required. The majority of patients with empyema are managed with intercostal tube drainage. Open drainage during the early phase of the infection is potentially dangerous and can result in lung collapse. Although continuous closed chest tube drainage is the preferred method during the fibrinopurulent phase, treatment with thoracenteses alone is also an option (16). Delay in instituting effective drainage may result in pleural fluid loculations and further fluid thickening. If loculation occurs and/or thick peel forms, then intercostal tube drainage is inadequate. Closed intercostal drainage with suction may be effective, but open drainage with rib resection is often required. Utilization of immediate infusion through the inserted tube of tissue plasminogen activator or urokinase may be employed in severe cases (17). Thoracoscopy with removal of adhesions plus drainage is also an option in those who do not respond to medical therapy. Decortication, removal of the entire empyema, is often more effective in allowing the expansion of the lung in chronic empyema.

PRINCIPLES OF ANTIMICROBIAL THERAPY

Appropriate management of mixed pulmonary aerobic and anaerobic infections requires the administration of antimicrobials that are effective against both the aerobic and anaerobic components of the infection (1,5,18). When such a therapy is not given, the infection may persist and more serious complications may occur (1,5,18).

The appropriate antimicrobial choice depends on the susceptibility of the organisms to antimicrobials. Unfortunately, the susceptibility of anaerobic bacteria to antimicrobial agents has become less predictable. Resistance to several antimicrobial agents by *B. fragilis* group and other AGNB has increased over the past three decades (19). Although routine susceptibility testing of all anaerobic isolates is unnecessary, it is important to perform susceptibility testing of isolates recovered from sterile body sites or those that are clinically important and have variable or unique susceptibility (20). Testing should be limited to those anaerobes isolated from blood cultures, pulmonary infections, and those isolated in pure culture. In addition to susceptibility testing, screening of AGNB for the production of the enzyme beta-lactamase may be helpful. Such screening can rapidly provide information regarding the organism's penicillin susceptibility. However, occasional bacterial strains may resist beta-lactam antibiotics through mechanisms other than the production of beta-lactamase.

When choosing antimicrobials for the therapy of polymicrobial pulmonary infections, their aerobic and anaerobic antibacterial spectrum should be considered. An attempt should be made to cover most or at least the most predominant organisms (with the heaviest growth in culture), with a single agent or a combination of agents. Some antimicrobials have a limited range of activity. Metronidazole is active only against anaerobes, and aminoglycosides and the "older"quinolones (i.e., ciprofloxacin) are mostly effective against Enterobacteriaceae. None of these agents can be administered as a single agent for the therapy of mixed infection. Others such as a penicillin plus a beta-lactamase inhibitor or a carbapenem have a wider spectrum of activity against Enterobacteriaceae and anaerobes.

Antimicrobial therapy may be guided by Gram stain of appropriate material but should not be withheld pending culture results in severely ill patients. Penicillin G may no longer be effective in the treatment of pleuropulmonary infections when BLPB are present. Two studies in adults showed clindamycin (which is more effective against anaerobic BLPB) to be more effective than penicillin in the treatment of lung abscesses in adults (21,22). A recent retrospective study illustrates the superiority of antimicrobials effective against penicillin-resistant anaerobic bacteria (ticarcillin–clavulanate or clindamycin) as compared to an antibiotic without such coverage (ceftriaxone) in the therapy of aspiration or tracheostomy-associated pneumonia in 57 children (23).

Antimicrobial therapy is directed at the major pathogens. Antimicrobials that are effective against penicillin-resistant anaerobic organisms are clindamycin, cefoxitin, chloramphenicol, metronidazole, the "newer" quinolones (i.e., moxifloxacin), a carbapenem (i.e., imipenem, meropenem, ertapenem), tigecycline or the combination of a penicillin plus a beta-lactamase inhibitor. Penicillin should be added to metronidazole to cover microaerophilic and anaerobic streptococci. Coverage against Enterobacteriaceae or *P. aeruginosa* may require the addition of an aminoglycoside, a quinolone, or a wide-spectrum cephalosporin (i.e., cefepime). When antistaphylococcal coverage is needed, a penicillinase-resistant penicillin (i.e., oxacillin), vancomycin, tigecycline, or linezolid should be administered. The last three agents are also effective against methicillin resistant staphylococci.

Therapy of community-acquired aspiration pneumonia is generally with clindamycin or combination of a penicillin plus a beta-lactamase inhibitor. In hospital-acquired aspiration pneumonia, coverage against Enterobacteriaceae or *P. aeruginosa* is also required by adding an effective agent or using a carbapenem.

REFERENCES

1. Finegold SM. Anaerobic Bacteria in Human Disease. New York: Academic Press, 1977.
2. Gibbons RJ. Aspects of the pathogenicity and ecology of the indigenous oral flora of man. In: Ballows A, Dehaan RM, Dowell VR, Guze LB, eds. Anaerobic Bacteria: Role in Disease. Springfield, IL: Thomas, 1974:267–85.
3. Bartlett JC, Gorbach SL, Thadepalli H, Finegold SM. Bacteriology of empyema. Lancet 1974; 1:338–40.
4. Freij BJ, Kusmiesz H, Nelson GD, McCracken GH. Parapneumonic effusions and empyema in hospitalized children: a retrospective review of 227 cases. Rev Infect Dis 1984; 3:578–91.
5. Levison ME. Anaerobic pleuropulmonary infection. Curr Opin Infect Dis 2001; 14:187–91.
6. Brook I, Finegold SM. Bacteriology and therapy of lung abscess in children. J Pediatr 1979; 94:10–2.
7. Brook I, Finegold SM. Bacteriology of aspiration pneumonia in children. Pediatrics 1980; 65:1115–20.
8. Brook I. Microbiology of empyema in children and adolescents. Pediatrics 1990; 85:722–6.
9. Bartlett JG, Finegold SM. Anaerobic pleuropulmonary infections. Medicine 1972; 51:413–50.
10. Brook I. Percutaneous transtracheal aspiration in the diagnosis and treatment of aspiration pneumonia in children. J Pediatr 1980; 96:1000–3.
11. Brook I, Frazier EH. Aerobic and anaerobic microbiology of empyema. A retrospective review in two military hospitals. Chest 1993; 103:1502–7.
12. Fajardo JE, Chang MJ. Pleural empyema in children: a nationwide retrospective study. South Med J 1987; 80:593–6.
13. Hardie W, Boukulic R, Garcia VF, et al. Pneumococcal pleural empyemas in children. Clin Infect Dis 1996; 22:1057–63.
14. Bryant RE, Salmon CJ. Pleural empyema. Clin Infect Dis 1996; 22:747–64.
15. Brook I. Lactic acid in pleural fluids. Respiration 1981; 40:344–8.
16. Doski JJ, Lou D, Hicks BA, et al. Management of parapneumotic collections in infants and children. J Pediatr Surg 2000; 35:265–70.

17. Kornecki A, Sivan Y. Treatment of loculated pleural effusion with intrapleural urokinase in children. J Pediatr Surg 1997; 32:1473–5.
18. Bartlett J. Treatment of community-acquired pneumonia. Chemotherapy 2000; 46(Suppl. 1):24–31.
19. Cuchural GJ, Jr., Tally FP, Jacobus NV, et al. Susceptibility of the *Bacteroides fragilis* group in the United States: analysis by site of isolation. Antimicrob Agents Chemother 1988; 32:717–22.
20. Rosenblatt J. Brook I clinical relevance of susceptibility testing of anaerobic bacteria. Clin Infect Dis 1993; 16(Suppl. 4):S446–8.
21. Levison ME, Mangura CT, Lorber B, et al. Clindamycin compared with penicillin for the treatment of anaerobic lung abscess. Ann Inter Med 1983; 98:466–71.
22. Gudiol F, Manresa F, Pallares R, et al. Clindamycin vs. Penicillin for anaerobic lung infections, high rate of penicillin failures associated with penicillin-resistant *Bacteroides melaninogenicus*. Arch Inter Med 1990; 150:2525–9.
23. Brook I. Treatment of aspiration or tracheostomy-associated pneumonia in neurologically impaired children: effect of antimicrobials effective against anaerobic bacteria. Inter J Pediatr Otolary 1996; 35:171–7.

21 | Other Chest Infections

INFECTIONS IN PATIENTS WITH CYSTIC FIBROSIS

Microbiology

The bacteria most often isolated from children suffering from cystic fibrosis (CF) are *Pseudomonas aeruginosa* and *Staphylococcus aureus*. Only a few studies attempted to identify anaerobic bacteria in the lower respiratory tract of patients with CF (1,2). One study attempted to report the number of anaerobes in selected sputum samples from patients with CF by sputum liquefication (3). When cultured by a semiquantitative method, 26 (24%) of 109 sputum specimens from 21 CF patients contained greater than 10^5 cfu of anaerobes/mL. Anaerobes were isolated from repeated sputum specimens from five patients. The anaerobes most often isolated were *Prevotella disiens*, pigmented *Prevotella* and *Porphyromonas* spp., and anaerobic gram-positive cocci. Anaerobes were isolated more often from sputum liquefied by sonication than from unliquefied sputum, suggesting that they were unlikely to be oropharyngeal contaminants. Baran and Cordier (4) used transtracheal aspiration (TTA) in children with CF and reported a good correlation between the organisms isolated in the sputum and TTA. However, anaerobic culture techniques were not employed in this study.

Several studies suggested the possible role of anaerobes in conjunction with aerobic bacteria in the pulmonary infectious process in CF. Thomassen et al. (2), recovered anaerobes from lung tissue or lung aspirates in two patients. The isolates were two *Bacteroides* spp. and one each of an anaerobic cocci and *Propionibacterium acnes*.

Brook and Fink (1) obtained six TTA and expectorated sputum specimens from four children with CF. Differences between the bacteria isolated in TTA and sputum aspirates were present in all instances. Six isolates were recovered from both sites (three *P. aeruginosa*, two *S. aureus*, and one *Aspergillus flavus*). Five aerobes were recovered only from the sputum and not from TTA (two *Klebsiella pneumoniae* and one each of *P. aeruginosa*, *Escherichia coli*, and *Proteus mirabilis*). Nine organisms were isolated only from TTA (two each of *Veillonella parvula* and alpha-hemolytic streptococci, and one each of *Bacteroides fragilis*, *Prevotella melaninogenica*, *Lactobacillus* spp., *Haemophilus influenzae*, and gamma-hemolytic streptococci). The recovery of anaerobes from four of the six TTA specimens suggests their possible role in pulmonary infection in CF.

Diagnosis

Although the number of the patients with CF studied so far is small, a few conclusions can be drawn relating to the efficacy of TTA and lung aspirates in the diagnosis and management of pulmonary infection in these patients. Judicious use of these procedures can circumvent therapy with unnecessary antimicrobials. Utilization of TTA and lung aspirates can prompt specific therapy directed against organisms that otherwise would not be optimally treated, because they are either not isolated in the sputum or, if recovered, are considered to be contaminants.

Management

As anaerobic organisms are part of the normal oropharyngeal flora and would contaminate any expectorated sputum specimen, TTA, lung aspirates, or double lumen brush catheter specimens are adequate for their cultivation. The role of these bacteria in the pathogenesis of the pulmonary infection in patients with CF is not yet clear. Adequate treatment of these infections is complex and often refractory to various antimicrobials. The ineffectiveness of antimicrobial therapy against the anaerobic component of the infection may account for that failure in some cases. These bacteria are part of the mouth flora and can reach the lower respiratory tract following aspiration.

The significance of the presence of multiple aerobic and anaerobic organisms in the TTA of CF patients has to be determined on a case-by-case basis. Many of the anaerobes recovered from infected lungs of CF patients are known pulmonary pathogens (5). These include *B. fragilis*, pigmented *Prevotella* and *Porphyromonas* spp., and anaerobic cocci. Data in other pleuropulmonary infections suggest that effective therapy against most of the bacteria present, including anaerobes, is important for complete cure of the infection.

Many of the anaerobes isolated in patients with CF are resistant to penicillins. These include the *B. fragilis* group and many strains of pigmented *Prevotella* and *Porphyromonas* spp. (6). Further studies are warranted to evaluate whether therapy should also be directed against these organisms; this would necessitate the use of agents such as clindamycin, chloramphenicol, metronidazole, cefoxitin, a carbapenem (i.e. imipenem, meropenem), or the combination of a penicillin plus a beta-lactamase inhibitor. These agents should be used in conjunction with antimicrobials directed against aerobic pathogens such as *P. aeruginosa* and *S. aureus* whenever they are present. Fluoroquinolones have a broad spectrum of activity against gram-positive, gram-negative, mycobacteria, and atypical organisms and some of the newer one (moxifloxacin) are also effective against anaerobes. They have excellent oral bioavailability, with good tissue penetration, and long elimination half-lives. The experience with fluoroquinolones in children has been limited because of concerns about arthropathy. However, there has not been a definitive fluoroquinolone-associated case of arthropathy described in the literature (7). The use of these agent in patients with CF has shown them to be effective (8).

COLONIZATION AND INFECTION FOLLOWING TRACHEOSTOMY AND INTUBATION AND USE OF VENTILATORY TUBES

Bacterial colonization of the tracheobronchial tree almost always follows tracheal intubation after tracheostomy (9) and use of ventilatory tubes (10). Wound infection of the tracheostomy site frequently occurs following prolonged use of the tracheostomy. It is sometimes difficult to evaluate the clinical significance of the isolation of pathogenic bacteria from tracheal cultures of patients with tracheostomy, differentiate between colonization or clinical infection (11), and assess various factors influencing the acquisition of those bacteria.

Microbiology

The specific microbial causes of ventilator-associated pneumonia (VAP) are many and varied. Most cases of VAP are caused by bacterial pathogens that normally colonize the oropharynx and gastrointestinal tract, or that are acquired via transmission by health care workers from environmental surfaces or from other patients. Common pathogens include *Pseudomonas* species and other highly resistant aerobic gram-negative bacilli, staphylococci, Enterobacteriaceae, streptococci, and *Haemophilus* spp. (11). Antibiotic-resistant pathogens such as *Pseudomonas* and *Acinetobacter* species, and methicillin-resistant strains of *S. aureus* are much more common after prior antibiotic treatment or prolonged hospitalization or mechanical ventilation, and when other risk factors are present. The bacterial pathogens responsible for VAP also vary depending on patient characteristics and in certain clinical circumstances, such as in acute respiratory distress syndrome or following tracheostomy, traumatic injuries, or burns. But these differences appear to be primarily due to the duration of mechanical ventilation and/or degree of prior antibiotic exposure of these patients.

The causes of VAP can vary considerably by geographic location (even between units in the same hospital), emphasizing the importance of local epidemiologic and microbiologic data. Atypical bacteria, viruses, and fungi also have been implicated as causes of VAP, but these pathogens have not been studied systematically and their role is presently unclear. The role of anaerobes in pediatric patients intubated for prolonged periods has been studied (12).

Serial tracheal cultures were obtained from 27 patients who required tracheostomy and prolonged intubation for periods ranging from 3 to 12 months. Tracheal cultures yielded pathogenic aerobic and anaerobic bacteria. Of the 1508 isolates (969 aerobes and 539 anaerobes) recovered from 444 tracheal aspirates, the most common were *K. pneumoniae*, *S. aureus*, pigmented *Prevotella* and *Porphyromonas* spp., *Peptostreptococcus* spp., *Fusobacterium nucleatum*, and *B. fragilis* group. This accounts for 2.2 aerobes and 1.2 anaerobes isolates/specimen. Twenty-one (78%) patients yielded both aerobic and anaerobic bacteria from the tracheal aspirates, and from six patients (22%), only aerobes were isolated.

All of the patients became colonized with aerobic or anaerobic bacteria (or both). Twenty-four (89%) of the patients developed chronic tracheobronchitis with recurrent episode(s) of pneumonia.

Eleven of the patients had one or two episodes of pneumonia in one year, seven had three to five episodes, and six had more than five episodes. There were 68 episodes of pneumonia in those 24 patients (2.8 episodes/patient). In about half of the episodes, a change in the bacterial flora occurred during the episodes of pneumonia, with the appearance of new pathogens. Although all of the patients responded favorably to antimicrobial therapy, the bacterial pathogens usually persisted or were replaced by others.

All the patients became colonized by more than two organisms. Peptostreptococci and pigmented *Prevotella* and *Porphyromonas* spp. were more frequently isolated during episodes of pneumonia than during periods when the patients were only colonized ($p < 0.05$). The data suggest that anaerobic bacteria are also a part of the bacterial flora causing colonization, tracheobronchitis, and pneumonia in children who require tracheostomy and prolonged intubation.

The microbiology of bronchial aspirates, using protective brush was evaluated in 10 children with VAP (10). Aerobic or facultative organisms only were isolated in one child, anaerobes only in three, and aerobic mixed with anaerobic bacteria in six. There were 10 aerobic or facultative and 17 anaerobic isolates. The predominant aerobes were *P. aeruginosa* (2 isolates) and *Klebsiella* spp. (2). The predominant anaerobes were pigmented *Prevotella* and *Porphyromonas* spp. (5), *Peptostreptococcus* spp., (4), *Fusobacterium* spp., and *B. fragilis* group (2 isolates each). All patients except one responded to antimicrobial therapy directed against the recovered isolates. The isolation of gram-negative aerobic and facultative bacteria such as *P. aeruginosa* and Enterobacteriaceae were simillar to the results obtained in adults (13,14).

Agvald-Ohman et al. (15) who studied 41 mechanically ventilated intensive care unit (ICU) patients found that those patients were heavily colonized in their lower airways by potential pathogenic microorganisms, including a high load of anaerobic bacteria. Anaerobes, mainly peptostreptococci and *Prevotella* spp., were isolated from subglottic and/or tracheal secretions in 59% of the patients.

Roberts et al. (16) who studied 26 mechanically ICU patients utilizing protected tracheal sampling methods found that anaerobic bacteria frequently colonize their lower respiratory tract and demonstrated their potential importance in VAP. Twenty-eight anaerobic strains were identified, with bacterial counts higher than 10^3 cfu/mL in 11 cases. Of the 15 patients colonized by anaerobes, 14 were also colonized by aerobic bacteria. Early onset colonization occurred in 16 of 22 patients colonized by aerobes and in 8 of 15 patients colonized by anaerobes. Five patients developed VAP following colonization (by anaerobic bacteria in two cases). In eight patients, colonization by anaerobic bacteria occurred despite antimicrobial therapy.

The microbiology of tracheostomy site wound infection is similar to the one of the bronchial aspirates of patients that developed tracheobronchitis and pneumonia. A study investigating 25 tracheostomy site wounds (17) found aerobic bacteria only in four wounds (16%), anaerobic bacteria only in two (8%), and mixed aerobic and anaerobic isolates in 19 patients (76%). A total of 145 isolates (72 aerobes and 73 anaerobes) were recovered, an average of 5.8 isolates/specimen. The most frequently occurring isolates were *Peptostreptococcus* spp., *Bacteroides* spp., alpha-hemolytic streptococci, *Fusobacterium* spp., and *P. aeruginosa*. Twenty-nine isolates recovered from 19 (72%) patients produced beta-lactamase. These included all isolates of *S. aureus* and *B. fragilis* group and four of 11 (36%) of pigmented *Prevotella* and *Porphyromonas* spp.

Pathogenesis

As anaerobes are part of the normal oral flora, their presence in the tracheal aspirates and tracheostomy site wounds of intubated patients is not surprising. The acquisition of normal oral flora organisms occurs in patients who undergo tracheostomy and intubation because of their inability to clear their secretions and their dependency on mechanical suctioning.

B. fragilis, which is not usually a part of the normal oral flora, was isolated from many of these patients; however, the occurrence of this pathogen in pleuropulmonary infections was noted especially in patients with poor oral hygiene (18). Peptostreptococci and pigmented *Prevotella* and *Porphyromonas* spp. were more frequently isolated from patients with pneumonia than from patients with colonization, suggesting the possible pathogenic role of these organisms.

Organisms that appeared in the tracheal secretions prior to the acquisition of pneumonia can be also present in episodes of pneumonia in half of the patients (12). However, newly acquired pathogens appear in many cases of pneumonia.

With the increase in prevalence of enteric gram-negative bacilli in the oropharyngeal flora of seriously ill hospitalized patients, these organisms became the most common cause of hospital-acquired pneumonia (19). Since tracheobronchitis and pneumonia generally follow the inhalation or aspiration of organisms present in the upper respiratory tract, the alteration of the pharyngeal flora of seriously ill patients may be an important first step in the pathogenesis of hospital-acquired pneumonia caused by enteric gram-negative bacilli.

Diagnosis

Colonization is defined as the isolation of a potential pathogen from tracheal cultures for at least four weeks, in the absence of purulent tracheobronchial secretions or clinical evidence of infection. Tracheobronchitis should be considered when purulent secretions appear, but when physical examination and chest films show no evidence of pneumonia. The diagnosis of pneumonia can be made only when unequivocal clinical and radiographic evidence of pulmonary parenchymal involvement is present and when a patient has leukocytosis and develops fever.

The presence of pneumonia was associated with longer duration of intubation, a high number of neutrophils and bacteria and elastic fibers in tracheal aspirates (19).

Management

The patient should be examined daily, with particular attention to the quantity and character of tracheal secretions. Chest films should be taken when indicated. The patient should be treated by postural drainage and frequent suctioning and cleaning of tracheostomy tubes, which should be changed once a week. Treatment should include antibiotic administration when pneumonia is suspected. The choice and changes in the therapy with antimicrobial agents are based on the patient's clinical condition and the results of the tracheal cultures. Routine cultures of the tracheal secretions for surveillance of aerobic and anaerobic bacteria would enable the clinician to monitor changes in the tracheal flora and facilitate the selection of appropriate antimicrobial therapy whenever the patient is infected. Repeated tracheal cultures for aerobic and anaerobic bacteria during the course of the pneumonia would allow for adjustment of the therapy if and when the bacteria present change or become resistant to the antibiotics used. Prophylaxis against acquisition of pneumonia is not recommended, since this would only facilitate the selection and acquisition of resistance by the bacteria, which would make it more difficult to treat the patients if and when they become infected.

The use of selective decontamination of the oral and gut flora is controversial. Aerosolized antimicrobials have not been shown to be consistently effective and may induce the development of bacterial resistance (20).

Antimicrobial therapy may be guided by Gram stain of appropriate material, but should not be withheld pending culture results in severely ill patients.

Discussion of the choice of antibiotics for anaerobes is included in the section on aspiration pneumonia (chap. 20). As enteric gram-negative bacilli were recovered mixed with other organisms in almost half of the cases studied, the institution of combined therapy of an aminoglycoside or other agents effective against these bacteria and one of the other drugs effective against anaerobes is recommended as an initial therapy of lower respiratory infection. Appropriate coverage for *S. aureus* may be indicated for wounds.

COLONIZATION IN INTUBATED NEWBORNS

Microbial colonization of the tracheobronchial tree generally follows tracheal intubation. It is difficult not only to differentiate between colonization and clinical infection, but also to try to assess the various factors that may influence the acquisition of these bacteria (10).

The newborn infant who presents with respiratory distress syndrome may require intubation for extended periods of time.

Microbiology

The bacteriology of tracheal aspirates from intubated newborns was studied in 127 newborns (21). Specimens were obtained twice weekly as long as the newborns were intubated. Each newborn had between one and eight specimens taken (average 1.7) for a total of 212 specimens. No bacterial or fungal growth was obtained from 65 specimens, whereas the 147 remaining specimens yielded 209 bacterial and fungal isolates accounting for 1.4 isolates/specimen. The total isolates recovered were 168 aerobes, 36 anaerobes, and 5 *Candida albicans*. Of this total, 101 specimens yielded one isolate, 36 two isolates, five specimens three isolates, four specimens four isolates, and one aspirate yielded five isolates. Seventyeight (61%) newborns received antimicrobial therapy. A higher incidence of positive cultures and the presence of more than one organism per culture were found in those infants not receiving antibiotics. More isolates per specimen were noted with increasing time of intubation. The rate of isolation of *S. aureus*, *P. aeruginosa*, and *K. pneumoniae* remained constant with increased length of intubation, the rate of recovery of *Staphylococcus epidermidis*, *Streptococcus viridans*, and *P. acnes* increased, and the rate of isolation of *E. coli* and other anaerobic organisms decreased.

Friedland et al. (22) demonstrated that bacterial colonization of an indwelling object in the neonatal airway increases with the duration of intubation. Furthermore, four days seem to represent a critical period in the formation of such colonization.

Anaerobic bacteria were found to play a role in three of the five cases of pneumonia that were diagnosed in intubated newborns (23). These three infants presented with premature rupture of membranes and developed neonatal pneumonia caused by organisms belonging to members of the *B. fragilis* group. In all three instances, the organisms were recovered from tracheal aspirates and in two from blood cultures as well. (see Chapter 6)

Pathogenesis

Data obtained in several studies (24,25) demonstrated the occurrence of microbial colonization immediately after intubation in 70% of newborns. The bacteria recovered from the first specimens obtained from newborns, which were taken immediately after intubation and usually within 24 hours after delivery, may reflect microbial contamination acquired upon passage through the birth canal. Organisms recovered at that time were primarily gram-positive cocci and *Bacteroides* spp. These bacteria tended to decrease in numbers and were replaced by organisms such as *S. viridans*, *S. epidermidis*, and *P. acnes*.

The use of systemic antibiotics in newborns can alter the bacterial flora of their respiratory tract, which may result in an overgrowth of aerobic gram-negative bacilli. It is noteworthy that organisms such as *S. aureus*, *P. aeruginosa*, and a variety of anaerobes tend to increase in numbers in chronically intubated older children and adults (12).

Since anaerobic bacteria are part of the normal flora of the cervix, their presence in tracheal aspirates of neonates is not surprising. Similar anaerobic bacteria were isolated from conjunctiva and gastric aspirates of newborns and represent acquisition during passage through the birth canal (26).

The microbial colonization of the trachea in intubated neonates with different aerobic and anaerobic bacteria could be due to their acquisition from the mother's cervical flora. Some of the acquired anaerobes can cause pneumonia in the newborn (see chap. 6) (23). The flora tends to decrease in proportion with time and is replaced by skin flora.

Diagnosis

Obtaining tracheal aspirate for culture and the Wright's staining is effective in defining infective and non-infective conditions in newborns with respiratory distress. Moreover, it seemed to be effective in early recognition of perinatal pneumonia caused by both aerobic and anaerobic bacteria. Although obtaining tracheal cultures by aspiration of material from an endotracheal tube that is used for ventilation is not ideal, it seemed to be a simple and safe procedure with almost no side effects or risks. Since anaerobes, along with facultative and aerobic bacteria, may play a role in perinatal pneumonia. This must be considered in devising therapeutic regimens.

The presence of polymorphonuclear leukocytes on Wright's stain of the aspirated material correlated with the presence of pathogenic organisms and an inflammatory process. In cases where pathologic examination was done, inflammatory changes were noted in the lungs; thus, the use of appropriate staining procedures provides another tool for determining the pathogenicity of the recovered bacteria. Additional evidence for the significance of the organisms in tracheal aspirates from babies with perinatal pneumonia was an accompanying bacteremia with at least one of the same organisms in two of the five patients studied by Brook et al. (23). Clinical signs of pneumonia should also alert the clinician to the presence of this infection.

Management

Whenever neonatal pneumonia is present, appropriate antimicrobial therapy should be administered. A penicillin derivative and one of the aminoglycosides or a third-generation cephalosporin are generally effective for treatment of infection or pneumonia in newborns. This combination will provide adequate coverage for the majority of organisms causing neonatal pneumonia such as gram-negative enteric rods and group B streptococci. While most anaerobic organisms are susceptible to penicillin G, members of the *B. fragilis* group, and growing number of pigmented *Prevotella* and *Porphyromonas* spp., and *Fusobacterium* spp. are known to be resistant to that agent. Discussion of the choice of antibiotics for anaerobes is included in the section on aspiration pneumonia (see chap. 20).

Due to the generally short duration of neonatal tracheal intubation, tracheal colonization generally does not present as a management problem. Prompt termination of the intubation will usually be followed by rapid resolution of the condition. The same caution in management as indicated in the management of older individuals (see previous section on long-term intubation) is required. This requires daily examination of the patient, with particular attention to the quantity and character of the tracheal secretion, frequent suctioning and cleaning of tubes, and change of tubes when indicated.

TRACHEITIS

Tracheitis is inflammation of the subglottic trachea, is due to multiple etiologies, and can extend to the intrathoracic trachea, bronchi, and lungs. Bacterial tracheitis can cause sudden, complete obstruction of the airway. Bacterial tracheitis can occur at any age or season, but it frequently mirrors the epidemiology of viral laryngotracheobronchitis (LTB).

Microbiology

Tracheitis can be part of an upper respiratory tract viral infection, a primary site of *Mycoplasma* infection, or a bacterial complication of viral LTB. It is difficult clinically to differentiate between acute tracheitis caused by influenza, adenovirus, or bacteria. Predominant pathogens of bacterial tracheitis are *S. aureus, Streptococcus pyogenes, H. influenzae,* and *Streptococcus pneumoniae* (27,28). Rare pathogens are *Moraxella catarrhalis* and anaerobic bacteria (*Peptostreptococcus, Prevotella,* and *Fusobacterium* spp.) (29).

Brook recovered 17 aerobic and facultative and 13 anaerobic bacteria from tracheal aspirated of 14 children with bacterial tracheitis (29). Aerobes only were present in six (43%) specimens, anaerobes only in three (21%), and mixed aerobic and anaerobic flora in five (36%). Polymicrobial flora was recovered in 10 of the 14 specimens. The predominant organisms were *S. aureus* (5 isolates), *H. influenzae* type b (4), *Peptostreptococcus* spp. (4), pigmented *Prevotella* and *Porphyromonas* (4), *Fusobacterium* spp. (2), and *M. catarrhalis* (2). Two organisms that were also isolated from the tracheal aspirates were recovered form the blood of two patients (one each of *H. influenzae* and *Prevotella intermedia*). Eleven beta-lactamase-producing organisms were isolated from nine patients. These included all isolates of *S. aureus* and *M. catarrhalis,* and two each of *H. influenzae* and *Prevotella* spp. The data confirm the predominance of *S. aureus* and *H. influenzae* in causing bacterial tracheitis in children and suggest a potential role for anaerobic bacteria.

Pathogenesis

Bacterial tracheitis almost always follows viral LTB and is characterized by sloughing of the epithelial lining of the trachea, and the presence of copious mucopurulent secretions. Frequently a pseudomembrane can organize, causing symptoms and radiographic appearance of a foreign body in the extra-thoracic trachea (27,28). The major pathology is at the level of the cricoid cartilage.

Diagnosis

The diagnosis of epiglottitis, LTB, or bacterial tracheitis is suspected because of the presence of signs of upper airway obstruction, such as inspiratory stridor, hoarseness, barking cough, and retractions (28). Bacterial tracheitis can follow LTB, measles, influenza, or less significant upper respiratory tract infections. It usually occurs as a viral infection wanes, with abrupt worsening, or new onset of fever and stridor. The patient is toxic appearing, agitated, and unable to improve air flow by any positional maneuver. Usual treatment for croup is ineffective, and suctioning copious thick purulent tracheal secretions affords only temporary relief. Establishment of artificial airway is of urgent importance in many cases (30).

Diagnosis is based on the clinical course of upper airway obstruction, evidence of bacterial infection (e.g., high fever and leukocytosis with neutrophilia and immature forms), and lack of classical findings of epiglottitis. Lateral neck radiograph shows edema of the subglottic trachea and in some cases partially adherent concretions of necrotic epithelium and inflammatory cells simulating a foreign body. Diagnosis is confirmed at bronchoscopy by observation of pseudomembranes and purulent secretions in the subglottic trachea (although severe viral LTB is sometimes difficult to differentiate). Gram stain and culture of secretions usually confirm etiology. Blood culture is positive in less than one-half of patients. Toxin-producing strains of *S. aureus* or *S. pyogenes* can cause systemic manifestations (31).

Differential Diagnosis

Differentiation among causes of infectious upper airway obstruction is facilitated by careful attention to history of the illness, physical findings, and context of the illness in the family and community. Lifesaving management depends on accurate diagnosis. Differentiation should be made between bacterial tracheitis and viral LTB, epiglottitis, and retropharyngeal abscess.

The recognition of acute epiglottitis and bacterial tracheitis is most important, since complete obstruction of the airway is likely to occur, sometimes suddenly and unexpectedly. Complete obstruction during LTB is less common, more gradual, and predictable.

Management

Maintenance of adequate respiratory exchange is of primary importance. This requires careful observation and monitoring for signs of increasing obstruction or fatigue. Antimicrobial agents effective against *S. aureus* and *H. influenzae*, and streptococci are required. Ceftriaxone is appropriate initial therapy. However, if Gram stain of tracheal secretion reveals neutrophils and gram-positive cocci only, nafcillin or vancomycin (for methicillin resistant staphylococci), especially for hospital-acquired infection, is appropriate. When culture of tracheal secretions reveals a pathogen, specific therapy can be chosen. Antibiotics are usually continued for 10 to 14 days; oral administration is appropriate after defervescence and extubation.

Culture for anaerobic bacteria should be performed only if the specimen is collected through the endotracheal tube during the intubation process. Intravenous fluids, oxygen, and humidity are generally provided. The recovery of anaerobic organisms from tracheal aspirates may require the administration of appropriate antimicrobial agents such as clindamycin, chloramphenicol, metronidazole, cefoxitin, the combination of a penicillin and a beta-lactamase inhibitor, a carbapenem (i.e., imipenem, meropenem), or tigecycline. Agents that are effective against *S. aureus* (i.e., beta-lactam-resistant penicillins, vancomycin or linezolid) and *H. influenzae* (second- and third-generation cephalosporins), are generally not effective against beta-lactamase-producing anaerobes.

Severe cases are managed in the same manner as in epiglottitis. Bronchoscopy is indicated to establish the diagnosis and often is therapeutic since it allows the removal of necrotic debris and inspissated secretions. Artificial airway is usually warranted. Mechanical ventilation may be needed, and sedation is often required for intubated patients. Frequent suctioning is important to prevent sudden obstruction of the endotracheal tube. Complicating bronchopneumonia is common. Extubation can be accomplished when mucosal edema and purulence decrease, usually requiring a longer time than for LTB. Most patients become afebrile within three to five days of appropriate therapy. Tracheostomy may be required if strictures or granulation tissue develop and cause obstruction.

Complications

Endotracheal tube plugging and accidental extubation with subsequent cardiorespiratory arrest are the most common causes of morbidity and mortality. Urgent removal and skillful reintubation are required. Frequent suctioning and careful securing of the airway are critical preventive measures. Other complications include pneumonia, atelectasis, pulmonary edema, septicemia, and retropharyngeal cellulitis. Subglottic stenosis is an infrequent sequela, occurring in less than 3% of patients.

REFERENCES

1. Brook I, Fink R. Transtracheal aspiration in pulmonary infection in children with cystic fibrosis. Eur J Respir Dis 1983; 64:51–7.
2. Thomassen MJ, Klinger JD, Badger SJ, van Heeckeren DW, Stern RC. Cultures of thoracotomy specimens confirm usefulness of sputum cultures in cystic fibrosis. J Pediatr 1984; 104:352–5.
3. Jewes LA, Spencer RC. The incidence of anaerobes in the sputum of patients with cystic fibrosis. J Med Microbiol 1990; 31:271–4.
4. Baran D, Cordier N. Usefulness of transtracheal puncture in the bacteriological diagnosis of lung infections in children. Helv Paediatr Acta 1973; 28:391–9.
5. Bartlett JG, Finegold SM. Anaerobic infections of the lung and pleural space. Am Rev Respir Dis 1974; 110:56–77.
6. Brook I, Calhoun L, Yocum P. Beta lactamase-producing isolates of *Bacteroides* species from children. Antimicrob Agents Chemother 1980; 18:164–7.
7. Jafri HS, McCracken GH, Jr. Fluoroquinolones in paediatrics. Drugs 1999; 58(Suppl. 2):43–8.
8. Richard DA, Nousia-Arvanitakis S, Sollich V, et al. Oral ciprofloxacin vs. intravenous ceftazidime plus tobramycin in pediatric cystic fibrosis patients: comparison of antipseudomonas efficacy and assessment of safety with ultrasonography and magnetic resonance imaging. Pediatr Infect Dis J 1997; 16:572–8.
9. Aass AS. Complications to tracheostomy and long term intubation: a follow-up study. Acta Anaesthesiol Scand 1975; 19:127–33.

10. Brook I. Pneumonia in mechanically ventilated children. Scand J Infect Dis 1995; 27:619–22.
11. Park DR. The microbiology of ventilator-associated pneumonia. Respir Care 2005; 50:742–63.
12. Brook I. Bacterial colonization tracheobronchitis and pneumonia, following tracheostomy and long-term intubation in pediatric patients. Chest 1979; 74:420–5.
13. Baughman RP, Thorpe JE, Staneck J, Rashkin M, Frame PT. Use of the protected specimen brush in patient with endotracheal or tracheostomy tubes. Chest 1987; 91:233–6.
14. Pollock HM, Hawkins EL, Bonner JR, Sparkman T, Bass JB, Jr. Diagnosis of bacterial pulmonary infections with quantitative protected catheter cultures obtained during bronchoscopy. J Clin Microbiol 1983; 17:255–9.
15. Agvald-Ohman C, Wernerman J, Nord CE, Edlund C. Anaerobic bacteria commonly colonize the lower airways of intubated ventilated intensive care unit (ICU) patients. Clin Microbiol Infect 2003; 9:397–405.
16. Robert R, Grollier G, Frat JP, et al. Colonization of lower respiratory tract with anaerobic bacteria in mechanically ventilated patients. Intensive Care Med 2003; 29:1062–8.
17. Brook I. Microbiological studies of tracheostomy site wounds. Eur J Respir Dis 1987; 71:380–3.
18. Karim RM, Momin IA, Lalani II, et al. Aspiration pneumonia in pediatric age group: etiology, predisposing factors and clinical outcome. J Pak Med Assoc 1999; 49:105–8.
19. Salata RA, Lederman MM, Shlaes DM, et al. Diagnosis of nosocomial pneumonia in intubated, intensive care unit patients. Am Rev Respir Dis 1987; 135:426–32.
20. Linden PK, Paterson DL. Parenteral and inhaled colistin for treatment of ventilator-associated pneumonia. Clin Infect Dis 2006; 43(Suppl. 2):S89–94.
21. Brook I, Martin WJ. Bacterial colonization in intubated newborns. Respiration 1980; 40:323–8.
22. Friedland DR, Rothschild MA, Delgado M, Isenberg H, Holzman I. Bacterial colonization of endotracheal tubes in intubated neonates. Arch Otolaryngol Head Neck Surg 2001; 127:525–8.
23. Brook I, Martin WJ, Finegold SM. Neonatal pneumonia caused by members of *Bacteroides fragilis* group. Clin Pediatr 1980; 19:541–4.
24. Sprunt K, Leidy G, Redman W. Abnormal colonization of neonates in an intensive care unit: means of identifying neonates at risk of infection. Pediatr Res 1978; 12:998–1002.
25. Brook I, Martin WJ, Finegold SM. Bacteriology of tracheal aspirates in intubated newborn. Chest 1980; 78:875–7.
26. Brook I, Barrett CT, Brinkman CR, III, Martin WJ, Finegold SM. Aerobic and anaerobic flora of maternal cervix and newborns conjunctiva and gastric fluid: a prospective study. Pediatrics 1979; 63:451–5.
27. Bernstein T, Brilli R, Jacobs B. Is bacterial tracheitis changing? A 14 year month experience in a pediatric intensive unit. Clin Infect Dis 1988; 27:458–62.
28. Orlicek SL. Management of acute laryngotracheo-bronchitis. Pediatr Infect Dis J 1998; 17:1164–5.
29. Brook I. Aerobic and anaerobic microbiology of bacterial tracheitis in children. Pediatr Emerg Care 1997; 13:16–8.
30. Graf J, Stein F. Tracheitis in pediatric patients. Semin Pediatr Infect Dis 2006; 17:11–3.
31. Burns JA, Brown J, Ogle JW. Group A streptococcal tracheitis associated with toxic shock syndrome. Pediatr Infect Dis J 1998; 17:933–5.

22 | Intra-abdominal Infections

Intra-abdominal infections generally occur after entry of enteric organisms into the peritoneal cavity through a defect in the intestinal wall or a viscus as a result of infarction, obstruction, or trauma. Abdominal, retroperitoneal, and visceral abscesses generally occur as a complication of local or generalized peritonitis, secondary to appendicitis, diverticulitis, necrotizing enterocolitis, pelvic inflammatory disease, and tubo-ovarian infection, surgery, or trauma.

SECONDARY PERITONITIS AND INTRA-ABDOMINAL ABSCESSES

Microbiology

Anaerobic bacteria are predominant in intra-abdominal infection because they are the main component of the gastrointestinal tract (GIT) flora, where they outnumber aerobic and facultative bacteria in the ratio of 1000 to 10,000 to one (1). The peritonitis that follows introduction of the enteric flora to the peritoneal cavity is usually a synergistic polymicrobial infection.

Secondary Peritonitis

Mixed aerobic and anaerobic flora is recovered in the peritoneal cavity following ruptured appendix (2), diverticula, or intestinal viscus (3) and from postoperative wound (4). Similar isolates are also isolated from liver, pelvic, and subphrenic abscesses, and blood cultures of these patients. The predominant aerobic bacteria are *Escherichia coli*, *Enterococcus faecalis*, *Klebsiella* spp., *Enterobacter* spp., and the main anaerobic bacteria are gram-negative bacilli (*Bacteroides fragilis* group and pigmented *Prevotella* and *Porphyromonas*), *Peptostreptococcus* and *Clostridium* spp.

Liver Abscess

Polymicrobial involvement is common, with *E. coli* and *Klebsiella pneumoniae* being the two most frequently isolated aerobic pathogens. Enterobacteriaceae are especially prominent when the infection is of biliary origin. Other organisms include *Actinomyces* spp., *Eikenella corrodens*, *Yersinia enterocolitica*, *Salmonella typhi*, and *Brucella melitensis*.

Anaerobes may be involved in at least half of cases of pyogenic liver abscess (5). The most prevalent anaerobes in liver abscess are anaerobic and microaerophilic streptococci (not true anaerobes), *Fusobacterium* spp., *B. fragilis* group, and pigmented *Prevotella* and *Porphyromonas* spp. A colonic source is usually the initial source of infection. *Staphylococcus aureus* abscesses usually result from hematogenous spread of organisms involved with distant infections, such as endocarditis. *Streptococcus milleri* has been associated with both monomicrobial and polymicrobial abscesses in patients with Crohn's disease. *S. aureus* and beta-hemolytic streptococci are also associated with trauma; *Enterococcus* spp., *K. pneumoniae*, and *Clostridium* spp. with biliary disease; and *Bacteroides* and *Clostridium* spp. with colonic disease (Table 1).

Amebic liver abscess is most often due to *Entamoeba histolytica*. Fungal abscesses primarily are due to *Candida albicans* and occur in individuals with prolonged exposure to antimicrobials, hematologic malignancies, solid-organ transplants, and congenital and acquired immunodeficiency. Abscesses due to *Aspergillus* spp. have been reported.

TABLE 1 Correlation Between the Microbiology of 48 Liver Abscesses and Predisposing Conditions (in parenthesis—number of abscesses)

Organisms isolated	Biliary disease		Colonic disease		Hematogenous seeding (4)	Trauma (4)	Pancreatitis (2)	Recent gastric or duodenal surgery (7)	Unknown (8)	Total (48)
	Benign (5)	Malignant (5)	Benign (9)	Malignant (4)						
Aerobic										
Alpha-hemolytic streptococci		1	1	1				1	1	5
Beta-hemolytic streptococci[a]			1					1	1	3
Enterococcus spp.	4				1	2	1			8
Staphylococcus aureus		2					1 (1)	1 (1)		4 (2)
Escherichia coli		1 (1)[b]	2	2 (1)	1 (1)	3 (1)		2 (1)		11 (5)
Klebsiella pneumoniae	1	2 (2)					1		1	5 (2)
Pseudomonas aeruginosa						1		1		2
Proteus mirabilis				1					1	2
Serratia marcescens				1				1	1	3
Subtotal	5	6 (3)	4	5 (1)	2 (1)	6 (1)	3 (1)	7 (2)	5	43 (9)
Anaerobic										
Peptostreptococcus spp.	2	3	3	1	1 (1)	1	1	3	3	18 (1)
Microaerophilic streptococci	2	2	3	1	2	1		1		12
Propionibacterium acnes					1		1	1		3
Veillonella parvulla			1	1		1				3
Clostridium spp.	2	1	3	2 (2)	1	1				10 (2)
Fusobacterium spp.				2 (1)	2			2 (1)	4	10 (2)
Bacteroides spp.	1		3	2 (1)	1		1	2	3 (2)	13 (3)
Prevotella spp.					1	1		1	1	4
Subtotal	7	6	13	9 (4)	9 (1)	5	3	10 (1)	11 (2)	73 (8)
Total	12	12 (3)	17	14 (5)	11 (2)	11 (1)	6 (1)	17 (3)	16 (2)	116 (17)

[a] Group A (2 isolates), Group F (one isolate).
[b] Organisms recovered from blood.
Source: Ref. 5.

Spleenic Abscess

Abscess microbiology can be monomicrobial, polymicrobial, or sterile. Bacterial pathogens most commonly cause unilocular abscesses. Mycobacterial, fungal, or protozoan infections are detected less commonly overall but are most frequently seen in patients who are immunosuppressed. The predominant aerobic and facultative isolates are *E. coli*, *S. aureus*, *Proteus mirabilis*, *Enterococcus* spp., and *K. pneumoniae* (5,6). The predominant anaerobes were *Peptostreptococcus* spp., *B. fragilis* group, *Fusobacterium* spp. and *Clostridium* spp. *S. aureus*, *K. pneumoniae*, and *Enterococcus* spp. are mostly associated with endocarditis, *E. coli* with urinary tract and abdominal infection, *B. fragilis* group and *Clostridium* spp. with abdominal infection and *Fusobacterium* spp. with respiratory infection (Table 2).

Retroperitoneal Abscess

The infection is often polymicrobial. The predominant aerobic and facultative isolates are *E. coli*, *K. pneumoniae*, *Enterococcus* spp., and *S. aureus* (7). The predominant anaerobes are *Peptostreptococcus* spp., *B. fragilis* group, *Prevotella* spp., and *Clostridium* spp. The number of anaerobes/site generally outnumbered the number of aerobic or facultative and is especially high in pelvic abscesses. Certain trends in recovery of organisms according to abscess site were noted (Table 3). *S. aureus* was more commonly isolated from pancreatic and retrofascial abscesses. *K. pneumoniae* and *Pseudomonas aeruginosa* were commonly recovered from pancreatic abscesses, *Neisseria gonorrhoeae* and streptococcus group B were only isolated from pelvic retroperitoneal sites. *Prevotella bivia* and *Prevotella disiens* were mostly recovered from pelvic abscesses. *Clostridium* spp. and *Fusobacterium nucleatum* predominated in anterior retroperitoneal sites. *Propionibacterium acnes* was mostly isolated from vascular graft infection. No differences in recovery rates were noted among *B. fragilis* group, *Peptostreptococcus* spp., and *E. coli* isolates. The number of aerobic and facultatives was especially high in pancreatic abscesses (PA; Table 3).

PATHOGENESIS

The dynamics and changes in the microbial flora of the GIT influence the nature and severity of infections after perforation. The number of microorganisms increases at the distal portions of the GIT. At the stomach and upper bowel there are 10^4 organisms/g or less, at the lower ileum the number increases up to 10^8 organisms/g, and the colon it reaches up to 10^{11} organisms/g (1), most of which are anaerobes. The changes in the number of intestinal bacteria account for some of the differences in peritoneal cavity cultures after perforations. An average of three isolates/specimen and about 10^7 organisms/g were recovered in perforation of the small intestine, and 26 bacterial isolates and 10^{12} organisms/g were found in specimens of colonic perforation. A synergistic relationship exists between the aerobic and anaerobic bacteria in intra-abdominal infections (8). The presence of the higher number of organisms in the distal portion of the colon can explain why infection developed in 45% of patients with descending-colon injuries as compared with only 13% in other colon sites (9).

Peritonitis is defined as inflammation of the serosal membrane lining the abdominal cavity and the organs within it. Peritoneal infections are classified as primary (i.e., spontaneous), secondary (i.e., related to a pathologic process in a visceral organ), or tertiary (i.e., persistent or recurrent infection after adequate initial therapy).

The most common etiology of primary peritonitis is spontaneous bacterial peritonitis (SBP) due to chronic liver disease. Approximately 10% to 30% of all patients with liver cirrhosis who have ascites develop over time bacterial peritonitis. The infection results from translocation of bacteria across the gut wall or mesenteric lymphatics and, less frequently, from hematogenous seeding.

Secondary peritonitis (SP) and intra-abdominal abscesses generally occur because of the entry of enteric microorganisms into the sterile peritoneal cavity through a defect in the wall of the intestine or other viscus as a result of perforation due to appendicitis, diverticulitis, gastric, and duodenal ulcer disease, inflammatory bowel disease, volvulus, obstruction, cancer, infarction, strangulation of the small bowel, gastrointestinal surgery, or direct trauma.

TABLE 2 Correlation Between the Microbiology of 29 Splenic Abscesses and Predisposing Conditions (number of abscesses)

Organisms	Endocarditis (6)	Urinary tract infection (3)	Intra-abdominal focus (7)	Respiratory tract (3)	Trauma (3)	Hemoglobinopathy (1)	Cancer/ chemotherapy (4)	Unknown (2)	Total (29)
Candida albicans							2(1)		2(1)
Aerobic bacteria									
Alpha-hemolytic streptococci	1(1)[a]	1							2(1)
Beta-hemolytic streptococci				1					1
Enterococcus spp.	2(2)		1						3(2)
Staphylococcus aureus	2(2)				1			1(1)	4(3)
Escherichia coli		3(1)	2(1)						5(2)
Klebsiella pneumoniae	2(1)			1(1)					3(2)
Pseudomonas aeruginosa							1(1)		1(1)
Proteus mirabilis		2			1				3
Salmonella typhi						1			1
Subtotal	7(6)	6(1)	3(1)	2(1)	2	1	1(1)	1(1)	23(11)
Anaerobic bacteria									
Peptostreptococcus spp.	1		4	2(1)	2		1	1	11(1)
Microaerophilic *Streptococcus*	1			1					2
Propionibacterium acnes			1			1	1		3
Veillonella parvula					1				1
Clostridium spp.			2(1)		1				3(1)
Fusobacterium spp.				2(1)				1	3(1)
Bacteroides fragilis group			4(2)				1		5(2)
Prevotella spp.			1	1			1		3(4)
Subtotal	2		12(3)	6(2)	4	1	4	2	31
Total	9(6)	6(1)	15(4)	8(3)	6	2	7(1)	3(1)	56(17)

[a] Organisms also recovered from blood.
Source: From Ref. 2.

TABLE 3   Aerobic and Anaerobic Bacteria Isolated from 161 Retroperitoneal Abscesses (in parenthesis—number of abscesses)

	Anterior retroperitoneal (n=109)						Posterior retroperitoneal (perinephric) (8)	Retrofascial space (iliopsoas) (21)	Pelvic retroperitoneal (23)	Total (161)
	Esophageal (5)	Duodenal (4)	Pancreatic (n=46)	Vascular graft (n=15)	Lower GI (n=29)	Unknown (n=10)				
Aerobic bacteria										
Staphylococcus aureus			6			1		3	1	11
Staphylococcus Epidermidis			2			1			2	5
Alpha-streptococci	1		3		4	1	1	5	2	17
Gamma-streptococci		1	4		2	2	1	2	1	13
Group A streptococci									1	1
Group B streptococci									3	3
Enterococcus spp.	1	1	11		3			1	2	19
Enterobacteriaceae (other)			6		4	2	2	2	4	20
Neisseria gonorrhoeae									4	4
Escherichia coli			18	2	19	7	3	8	3	60
Serratia marescens			3		1	1		1		6
Klebsiella pneumoniae	2	1	12		2	1		1	1	20
Enterobacter spp.			4	1		1		1	1	8
Proteus spp.			3	1	1	1			2	8
Pseudomonas aeruginosa			5		1	2			1	9
Subtotal	4	3	77	4	37	20	7	24	28	204

(Continued)

TABLE 3 (*Continued*) Aerobic and Anaerobic Bacteria Isolated from 161 Retroperitoneal Abscesses (in parenthesis—number of abscesses)

	Anterior retroperitoneal (n=109)					Unknown (n=10)	Posterior retroperitoneal (perinephric) (8)	Retrofascial space (iliopsoas) (21)	Pelvic retroperitoneal (23)	Total (161)
	Esophageal (5)	Duodenal (4)	Pancreatic (n=46)	Vascular graft (n=15)	Lower GI (n=29)					
Anaerobic bacteria										
Peptostreptococcus spp.	3	2	29	8	9	5		4	35	95
Veillonella parvula	1		6		1			1	1	10
Bifidobacterium spp.			2					2		4
Eubacterium spp.			1		1	1		1	2	6
Propionibacterium acnes			4	5		1			3	13
Clostridium spp.			3	1	4	1	1		2	12
Clostridium perfringens			4		2	1	1	1	1	10
Fusobacterium nucleatum			2		1	2		1		6
Fusobacterium spp.	1		3		1	1		2	1	8
Bacteroides spp.			4		1		2	1	3	12
Bacteroides fragilis group	1	2	17	5	20	5	3	8	5	66
Prevotella spp.	2	2	6		2	2	2	2	4	22
Porphyromonas spp.	1				1	1			1	4
Subtotal	9	6	81	19	43	20	9	23	58	268
Total	13	9	158	23	80	40	16	47	86	472

Source: From Ref. 7.

In women, localized peritonitis can occurs in the pelvis from an infected fallopian tube or a ruptured ovarian cyst.

Tertiary peritonitis (TP) is a persistent or recurrent infection following apparently adequate treatment of SBP or SP, often without the original visceral organ pathology. TP usually present with an abscess, or phlegmon, with or without fistulization. It often develops in patients with significant preexisting comorbidities or the immunocompromised. Patients with TP have longer stay in the ICU and hospital, and higher organ dysfunction scores, and mortality rates (50–70%) (10).

Peritonitis can also be caused by introduction of a chemically irritating material, such as gastric acid from a perforated ulcer or bile from a perforated gall bladder or a lacerated liver. In children, peritonitis is associated primarily with appendicitis, but may occur with intussusception, volvulus, incarcerated hernia, or rupture of a Meckel's diverticulum. Although less common in pediatrics, peritonitis also may occur as a complication of intestinal mucosal disease, including peptic ulcers, ulcerative colitis, and pseudomembraneus enterocolitis.

Intra-abdominal infections in the neonatal period generally are a complication of necrotizing enterocolitis but may be associated with meconium ileus or spontaneous rupture of the stomach or intestines. Following perforation, the peritonitis usually is a synergistic infection in which more than one organism is involved.

Intra-peritoneal abscesses are the most common of all abdominal abscesses. The most common causes are: (*i*) perforation of a diseased viscus, which includes peptic ulcer perforation, (*ii*) perforated appendicitis and diverticulitis, (*iii*) gangrenous cholecystitis, (*iv*) mesenteric ischemia with bowel infarction, and (*v*) pancreatitis or pancreatic necrosis progressing to PA. Other causes include necrotizing enterocolitis, pelvic inflammatory disease, tubo-ovarian infection, abdominal surgery, or trauma.

The most common source of pyogenic liver abscess is biliary tract disease. Obstruction of the bile flow by biliary stone disease, obstructive malignancy, stricture, and congenital diseases is followed by bacterial proliferation. The abscesses usually are multiple with a biliary source. Appendicitis currently causes about 10% of liver abscess. Infections in organs in the portal bed can result in a localized septic thrombophlebitis, followed by septic emboli that become the nidus for microabscess that usually coalesce into a solitary lesion.

Several mechanisms for splenic abscess exist. Prior splenic insult in addition to bacteremia is required for a splenic abscess to occur. The spread of organisms can be hematogenic or contiguous. Contiguous spread includes spread from gastric or colonic perforations, pancreatic pseudocysts, and subphrenic abscesses. This is the least common mechanism. The most common predisposing causes of splenic abscess are pyogenic infection, splenic trauma, hemoglobinopathies and contiguous disease processes extending to the spleen (11). The recovery of anaerobes correlates with a predisposing factor that allows the dissemination of anaerobic bacteria from another infectious site to the spleen (11). These infections can be either chronic respiratory infections caused by anaerobic bacteria, such as peritonsillar abscess or chronic mastoiditis, or abdominal infection.

Retroperitoneal space abscesses are often insidious and difficult to diagnose and cause a high rate of morbidity and mortality. The retroperitoneal infections can occur at various sites posterior to the peritoneum (12). These include four spaces: anterior retroperitoneal (containing the esophagus, duodenum, pancreas, bile duct, portal and splenic veins, appendix, ascending and descending colon, and rectosigmoid), posterior retroperitoneal (or perinephric, containing the kidneys, ureters, gonadal vessels, aorta, inferior cava, and lymph nodes), retrofascial (or iliopsoas, containing the twelfth rib, spine, and paraspinous muscle), and pelvic retroperitoneal (containing the prevesical, retrovesical presacral, and perirectal spaces).

DIAGNOSIS

Secondary Peritonitis

Fever, diffuse abdominal pain, nausea, and vomiting are characteristic symptoms. Signs of peritoneal inflammation, including rebound tenderness, abdominal wall rigidity, and decrease in bowel sounds are observed. These may be later followed by shock, toxemia, restlessness and irritability, a higher temperature, an increase in the pulse rate, chills and convulsions.

An elevated blood leukocyte count in excess of 12,000 with a predominance of polymorphonuclear forms is often present. Abdominal roentgenograms may reveal free air in the peritoneal cavity, evidence of ileus or obstruction and obliteration of the shadow of the psoas muscle. Computed tomography (CT) scanning and ultrasonography can improve the diagnostic accuracy of appendicitis.

Intra-abdominal Abscess

The manifestations of intra-peritoneal abscess that complicate appendicitis are progressive and persistent (>36 hours) abdominal symptoms, localized peritonitis, systemic toxicity, and a palpable mass on rectal examination, or when right lower quadrant mass is palpated following illness longer than five days. Pelvic abscesses can be palpated on rectal examination. Vague upper abdominal pain and pulmonary or pleural symptoms often suggest a subphrenic location.

Liver abscesses generally present with fever accompanied by chills, malaise, sweats and aching pain and tenderness over the liver or epigastrium. Leukocytosis, anemia, hypergamma-globulinemia, elevated alkaline phosphatase, and other liver enzymes, and positive blood culture are often present. Splenic abscesses are characterized by fever, abdominal pain that is generalized or localized to the left upper quadrant.

Air fluid level outside the intestinal lumen, localized ileus, or right lower quadrant mass suggest an appendiceal abscess; presence of a soft tissue mass, loss of psoas shadow, or displacement of the ureter or bladder can suggest the presence of retroperitoneal abscess. Subphrenic abscesses are often associated with pleural effusions.

The best imaging procedure for the diagnosis of abdominal abscesses is CT (13). Ultrasonically guided fluid collection and abscess drainage are routine procedures in diagnosis and treatment of abdominal abscesses. CT and fluoroscopy with contrast often give invaluable information. Magnetic resonance imaging (MRI) and gallium (Ga-67) scan may be useful in detecting abdominal abscesses.

Roentgenographic studies for abscesses may show elevation, change in contour, and reduced mobility of the diaphragm. Left lobe liver abscess may deform the barium- or gas-filled stomach, or displace the duodenal cap. Pleural effusion or thickening also may be observed, and occasionally a gas-fluid level may be noted inside the liver.

MANAGEMENT

The mainstay of therapy is stabilization of the patient by correcting fluid and electrolyte deficiencies with parenteral fluids, alleviation of intestinal obstruction with nasal suction, and controlling the infection with antibiotics.

The treatment of abdominal infection always should include surgical correction and drainage. The surgical intervention should be performed as soon as possible, preferably when patient is stabilized. The medical therapy should supplement the surgical approach by attempting to eradicate both aerobic and anaerobic microorganisms.

Management of pyogenic *intra-peritoneal* abscess includes adequate drainage mainten-ance of fluid, nutritional and electrolyte status, and systemic antimicrobials.

The effective management is influenced by the location and number of abscesses. In instances of acute appendicitis associated with an abscess, the initial approach usually includes percutaneous drainage of the abscess, medical therapy that includes antibiotic therapy, followed by appendectomy at a later time. Percutaneous aspiration of pyogenic abscesses can aid in the diagnosis and provides guidance in the selection of the proper antibiotic therapy (14).

Open surgical drainage is rarely necessary, because of the use of ultrasound and better imaging techniques. However, if the patient's condition is unstable, or the patient does not respond to antimicrobial therapy, open surgical drainage should be performed.

Solitary large *liver abscesses* should be drained. However, small abscesses generally resolve after several weeks of antimicrobial therapy, as long as any biliary obstruction has been relieved. Multiple *splenic* abscesses usually respond to several weeks of antimicrobial therapy alone. However, splenectomy or abscess drainage by laparotomy or percutaneously is the therapy of choice for large abscesses and those that do not resolve with antimicrobial therapy.

The proper management of mixed aerobic and anaerobic infections requires the administration of antimicrobials effective against both aerobic and anaerobic components of the infection (15). If such therapy is not delivered, the infection may progress and serious complications may develop.

Antibiotics effective against *B. fragilis* group include clindamycin, cefoxitin, metronidazole, the combination of a penicillin (e.g., piperacillin) plus a beta-lactamase inhibitor (e.g., tazobactam), the carbapenems (e.g., imipenem, meropenem, ertapenem) tigecycline, and the newer quinolones (i.e., moxifloxacin). Susceptibility testing of the organisms should be done in serious infections.

Therapy directed at the Enterobacteriaceae includes aminoglycosides, fourth generation cephalosporin; (e.g., cefepime and ceftazidine) and quinolones. Triple-agent therapy includes also ampicillin to cover *Enterococcus* spp. is advocated by some (15).

Single-agent therapy with either cefoxitin, moxifloxacin, a carbapenem, tigecycline or a penicillin plus a beta-lactamase inhibitor is as effective as combination therapies. The advantage of single-agent therapy is avoiding the ototoxicity and nephrotoxicity of aminoglycosides and may also be less expensive. Single agent may, however, may not always be effective against hospital-acquired resistant bacteria. If *S. aureus* is present in an abscess, anti-staphylococcal agents should be used.

Antimicrobials, especially when used without surgical drainage, should be administered for at least six to eight weeks. A shorter course, of four to six weeks, may be used when good surgical drainage has been achieved.

PROPHYLACTIC ANTIBIOTICS

Administration of prophylactic antimicrobial therapy prior to surgery ensures adequate tissue levels of antimicrobial agents effective against all potential aerobic and anaerobic pathogens. The site of perforation also will direct the choice of antimicrobial therapy. In perforation of the upper part of the GIT that does not involve, Enterobacteriaceae and *B. fragilis* group, a first-generation cephalosporin such as cefazolin would suffice. However, in perforation of the lower intestinal canal or in those with perforation of the upper GIT, which are at risk of harboring these pathogens, antimicrobials effective against *Enterobacteriaceae* and *B. fragilis* group should be given as prophylaxis, as well as for therapy.

COMPLICATIONS

Complications of peritonitis include septic shock, respiratory failure, retroperitoneal or intra-abdominal abscesses, small bowel obstruction from adhesions, fistula, and postsurgical wound infection. Complication of abscesses includes multiple organ failure. An abdominal abscess can rarely rupture or hemorrhage into the peritoneal cavity, causing peritonitis.

PANCREATIC ABSCESS

A PA is a collection of pus resulting from tissue necrosis, liquefaction, and infection. PA is a late complication of acute necrotizing pancreatitis (ANP), occurring more than four weeks after the initial attack. Infected necrosis refers to bacterial contamination of necrotic pancreatic tissue in the absence of abscess formation (16).

Pathophysiology

PA forms through various mechanisms, including fibrous wall formation around fluid collections, penetrating peptic ulcers, and secondary infection of pseudocysts. Patients are at risk for sepsis and death as mortality rate approaches 100% if surgical intervention and drainage are not performed.

Microbiology

The organisms isolated from ANP and PA are aerobic and anaerobic bacteria of enteric origin. The aerobic and facultatives include *E. coli*, *K. pneumoniae*, *E. faecalis*, *S. aureus*, *P. aeruginosa*, *P. mirabilis*, and *Streptococcus* spp. The anaerobes are gram-negative anaerobic bacilli, *Clostridium* spp. and *Candida* spp. (16,17). Translocation of enteric bacterial flora accounts for many cases of pancreatic infection.

Diagnosis

Physical findings are nonspecific and include abnormal vital signs consistent with sepsis, abdominal guarding, and rebound tenderness. The presence of prolonged pancreatitis, hemodynamic instability, fever, failure of medical therapy, or the presence of fluid collections suggests the possibility of necrosis and potentially, abscess formation. Collection of pancreatic fluid for via CT-guided needle biopsy can establish the bacterial or fungal etiology (18). Abdominal contrast-enhanced CT; ultrasound, either endoscopic or transabdominal; and MRI are potential modes for imaging pancreatic necrosis or abscess.

Management

Surgical drainage followed by placement of indwelling drains is the procedure of choice. CT-guided drainage is an option in those who cannot tolerate an open procedure. Systemic antimicrobials effective against the commonly recovered aerobic and anaerobic should be administrated (see previous section). Carbapenems are active against all likely pathogens and penetrate well into pancreatic tissue. Other antibiotics that have been shown to be efficacious in ANP include amikacin, cefuroxime, ceftazidime, and metronidazole (19).

Complications

These include recurrent pancreatitis, bowel obstruction, fistula formation, and death.

CHOLANGITIS

Acute cholangitis is bacterial infection of the biliary tract that can cause significant morbidity and mortality. Choledocholithiasis, neoplasm, stricture biliary tract manipulations and interventions, and stents are the most common cause of biliary tract obstruction resulting in cholangitis.

Microbiology

The bile is normally sterile. In the presence of obstruction, the incidence of infection increases. Polymicrobial infections are present in two-thirds of patients. The predominant bacteria were *E. coli*, *Enterococcus* spp., *Klebsiella* spp., *Enterobacter* spp., *Clostridium* spp., and *B. fragilis* group (20).

Diagnosis

Physical examination may reveal fever, icterus, jaundice, pruritus, acholic or hypocholic stools, and right upper quadrant tenderness. Leukocytosis, hyperbilirubinemia and elevated alkaline phosphatase levels, transaminases and serum amylase are common. Blood culture can be positive in about half of the patients.

Noninvasive diagnostic techniques include sonography, which is the recommended initial imaging modality. Standard CT, helical CT cholangiography, and magnetic resonance cholangiography often add important information regarding the type and level of obstruction. Endoscopic sonography is a more invasive means of obtaining high-quality imaging, and endoscopic or percutaneous cholangiography offers the opportunity to perform a therapeutic procedure at the time of diagnostic imaging. Endoscopic modalities currently are favored over percutaneous procedures because of a lower risk of complication (21).

Management

Many patients with acute cholangitis respond to antibiotic therapy; however, patients with severe or toxic cholangitis may not improve and may require emergency biliary drainage. Administration of broad-spectrum intravenous antibiotics (see previous section) and correction of fluid and electrolyte imbalances constitute essential medical care for cholangitis.

The elevated biliary pressures caused by an obstruction may impair with the biliary secretion of antibiotics. Treatment may require decompression and drainage of the biliary system. Percutaneous transhepatic biliary drainage is another possible nonsurgical method of biliary drainage. For patients with severe cholangitis, endoscopic drainage is the current approach. Overall prognosis depends on the severity of the illness at the time of presentation and the cause of the biliary obstruction. Increased mortality is observed in patients with hypotension, acute renal failure, liver abscess, cirrhosis, high malignant strictures, female gender, and advanced age.

REFERENCES

1. Gorbach SL. Intestinal microflora. Gastroenterology 1971; 60:1110–29.
2. Brook I. A 12 year study of aerobic and anaerobic bacteria in intra-abdominal and postsurgical abdominal wound infections. Surg Gynecol Obstet 1989; 169:387–92.
3. Brook I. Aerobic and anaerobic microbiology in intra-abdominal infections associated with diverticulitis. J Med Microbiol 2000; 49:827–30.
4. Sanderson PJ, Wren MWP, Baldwin AWF. Anaerobic organisms in postoperative wounds. J Clin Pathol 1979; 32:143–7.
5. Brook I, Frazier EH. Microbiology of liver and spleen abscesses. J Med Microbiol 1998; 47:1075–80.
6. Westh H, Reines E, Skibsted L. Splenic abscess: a review of 20 cases. Scand J Infect Dis 1990; 22:569–73.
7. Brook I, Frazier EH. Aerobic and anaerobic microbiology of retroperitoneal abscesses. Clin Infect Dis 1998; 26:938–41.
8. Brook I, Hunter V, Walker RI. Synergistic effects of anaerobic cocci, Bacteroides, Clostridium, Fusobacterium, and aerobic bacteria on mouse mortality and induction of subcutaneous abscess. J Infect Dis 1984; 149:924–8.
9. Mandal AK, Thadepalli H, Matory E, Lou MA, O'Donnell VA, Jr. Evaluation of antibiotic therapy and surgical techniques in areas of homicidal wounds of the colone. Am Surg 1984; 50:254–7.
10. Malangoni MA. Evaluation and management of tertiary peritonitis. Am Surg 2000; 66:157–61.
11. Chang KC, Chuah SK, Changchien CS, et al. Clinical characteristics and prognostic factors of splenic abscess: a review of 67 cases in a single medical center of Taiwan. World J Gastroenterol 2006; 12:460–4.
12. Brook I. Intra-abdominal, retroperitoneal, and visceral abscesses in children. Eur J Pediatr Surg 2004; 14:265–73.
13. Klatchko BA, Schwartz SI. Diagnostic and therapeutic approaches to pyogenic abscess of the liver. Surg Gynecol Obstet 1989; 168:332–6.
14. Gohl J, Gmeinwieser J, Gusinde J. Intraabdominal abscesses. Intervention versus surgicaltreatment. Zentralbl Chir 1999; 124:187–94.
15. Bohnen JM, Solomkin JS, Dellinger EP, Bjornson HS, Page CP. Guidelines for clinical care: anti-infective agents for intra-abdominal infection. A Surgical Infection Society policy statement. Arch Surg 1992; 127:83–9.
16. Baron TH, Morgan DE. Acute necrotizing pancreatitis. N Engl J Med 1999; 340:1412–7.
17. Brook I. Microbiological analysis of pancreatic abscess. Clin Infect Dis 1996; 22:384–5.
18. Shankar S, van Sonnenberg E, Silverman SG, Tuncali K, Banks PA. Imaging and percutaneous management of acute complicated pancreatitis. Cardiovasc Intervent Radiol 2004; 27:567–80.
19. Wyncoll DL. The management of severe acute necrotising pancreatitis: an evidence-based review of the literature. Intensive Care Med 1999; 25:146–56.
20. Brook I. Aerobic and anaerobic microbiology of biliary tract disease. J Clin Microbiol 1989; 27:2373–5.
21. Hanau LH, Steigbigel NH. Acute (ascending) cholangitis. Infect Dis Clin North Am 2000; 14:521–46.

23 | Urinary Tract and Genitourinary Suppurative Infections

Anaerobes have been involved in many different types of urinary tract infection (UTI). The types of infections of the urinary tract in which anaerobes have been involved include para- or periurethral cellulitis or abscess, acute and chronic urethritis, cystitis, acute and chronic prostatitis, prostatic and scrotal abscesses, periprostatic phlegmon, ureteritis, periureteritis, pyelitis, pyelonephritis, renal abscess, scrotal gangrene, metastatic renal infection pyonephrosis, perinephric abscess, retroperitoneal abscess, and other infections.

URINARY TRACT INFECTION

Acute UTI may be limited to the lower urinary tract, but persistent or recurrent cases often progress to involve the renal pelvis and parenchyma, producing pyelonephritis.

Microbiology

Most bacterial UTI have been ascribed to large groups of gram-negative aerobic or facultative anaerobic bacilli, including *Escherichia, Klebsiella, Aerobacter, Proteus,* and *Pseudomonas* species. Other organisms usually not considered pathogenic, such as *Staphylococcus epidermidis,* may also be responsible. The clinical significance of other specific groups of organisms including the obligate anaerobe, many strains of which are present in the fecal, vaginal, and cervical flora, has received even less attention in urinary tract disease in adults and children (1–3).

Several reports describe the recovery of anaerobes in UTI in adults (1), but many lack sufficient clinical bacteriologic detail to judge the reliability of the data; however, there are a good number of well-documented reports of infections of all types in adults.

The types of UTI in which anaerobes have been involved include para- or periurethral cellulitis or abscess, acute and chronic urethritis, cystitis, acute and chronic prostatitis, prostatic and scrotal abscesses, periprostatic phlegmon, ureteritis, periureteritis, pyelitis, pyelonephritis, renal abscess, scrotal gangrene, metastatic renal infection pyonephrosis, perinephric abscess, retroperitoneal abscess, and other infections (3–5). Moberg and Nord (6), and Eggert-Kruse et al. (7) have observed a marked increase in the number of anaerobic bacteria in urine voided after prostatic massage of infertile men.

The anaerobes recovered in these studies (1,4–7) were gram-negative bacilli (including *Bacteroides fragilis* and pigmented *Prevotella* and *Porphyromonas* spp.), *Clostridium* spp. (including *Clostridium perfringens*), anaerobic gram-positive cocci, and *Actinomyces* spp. In many cases, they were recovered mixed with coliforms or streptococci.

Brook (2) recovered anaerobic bacteria from five young females with UTI: three had pyelonephritis and two had cystitis. Two of the patients had a history of prior recurrent UTI. Urine samples were collected using suprapubic aspiration. The anaerobic organisms recovered were three isolates of *B. fragilis* and one each of *Prevotella melaninogenica, Peptostreptococcus asaccharolyticus,* and *Bifidobacterium adolescentis*. Mixed infection was present in three patients. In two patients, *B. fragilis* was present with *Escherichia coli* and in the other patient, two anaerobes were present. All patients were treated with antimicrobial agents for 10 to 14 days and responded well to therapy. Two of the patients had a recurrence of UTI with aerobic organisms recovered from their urine within six to eight months.

Pathogenesis

Acute UTI may be limited to the lower urinary tract, but persistent or recurrent cases often progress to involve the renal pelvis and parenchyma, producing pyelonephritis.

The source of bacteria-causing UTI usually is the patient's fecal flora. As anaerobes are part of the fecal flora, it is not surprising to find them in some cases of UTI. Congenital anomalies of the urinary tract, especially those that obstruct the flow of urine, predispose to UTI. Foreign bodies, urethral catheters, and nephrolithiasis also predispose to infection. Most UTIs, however, are not related to a structural or functional abnormality. The consistently higher incidence in girls beyond infancy may result from the short female urethra; the usual route of infection is an ascending one from external genitalia rather than a hematogenous one.

The periurethral region of healthy females probably forms a barrier against UTI, and the bacterial flora at that region has been found to influence the acquisition of infections (8). Anaerobes were found to constitute 95% of the total colony-forming units (cfu) of organisms per square centimeter of the periurethral area of healthy females (9).

The colonization of the urethra with anaerobic bacteria in adolescent males was related to sexual activity (10). A higher prevalence of potential uropathogens was found in the subpreputial space in uncircumcised young men as compared with circumcised individuals (11). Pure culture of facultative gram-negative rods was more common in uncircumcised males, and Streptococci, strict anaerobes and genital mycoplasmas were found almost exclusively in uncircumcised males. The presence of anaerobes in the periurethral region in females, and the urethra in males, may explain the mode of infectivity of these organisms.

Anaerobes may also gain access to the urinary tract, other than the urethra, by the ascending route, by direct extension from adjacent organs, such as the uterus or bowel, or by way of the bloodstream. Bran et al. (12) showed that urethral trauma may introduce organisms from the urethra to the bladder. Alling and colleagues (13) demonstrated that patients with indwelling urethral catheters have a high incidence of anaerobes recovered from urine. Sapico et al. (14) have shown that, on occasion, patients with indwelling Foley catheters will show anaerobes along with aerobes and facultative organisms.

The growth conditions for anaerobes may be at times favorable in the urinary tracts of patients. Requirements are the availability of nutrients (15) and oxygen tension low enough to permit the growth of certain anaerobic bacteria. A low oxygen tension may be found when facultative anaerobes or aerobes are present, which consume the available oxygen for their growth and so create ideal conditions. Once introduced into the bladder or other parts of the urinary tract, certain anaerobes are capable of growing well in the urine (16).

The low medullary blood flow, plasma skimming, and countercurrent flow all promote decreased oxygen supply to the medullary tissues, thus assisting the growth of anaerobes in cases of pyelonephritis. Medullary tissues derive their metabolic energy from anaerobic glycolysis to a greater extent than does cortical tissue. Anaerobic glycolysis of the inner medulla is relatively unaffected by the hypertonic environment of the medulla (16). The state of dehydration further disposes a patient to anaerobic UTI, because the oxygen tension of the urine is sharply decreased in the dehydrated patient (17).

Diagnosis

Symptoms may be absent, particularly in the chronic form of the disease. Onset may be gradual or abrupt. Fever may be as high as 40.3°C (104.5°F), accompanied by chills. Urinary frequency, urgency, incontinence, dysuria, prostration, anorexia, and pallor may occur. Vomiting may be projectile. There may be irritability and sometimes convulsions.

Signs include dull or sharp pain or tenderness in the kidney area or abdomen. Hypertension and evidence of chronic renal failure may be present in long-standing and severe cases. Jaundice may occur, particularly in early infancy. Anemia is found in cases of long-standing infection. Leukocytosis is usually in the range of 15,000 to 35,000/cu mm.

The diagnosis of acute pyelonephritis should be based on at least two consecutive positive urine cultures showing growth, and on a history of fever, chills, flank pain, nausea and vomiting, frequency, urgency, dysuria, and elevated sedimentation rate (above 30 mm/hr).

Diagnosis of lower UTI (cystitis) should be based on at least two consecutive positive urine cultures and signs of urgency and dysuria.

The presence of more than 10^5 cfu/mL urine is a widely held standard for diagnosing UTI. This is based on observations over 40 years ago (18), in adult women with a clinical diagnosis of pyelonephritis. In women with the acute urethal syndrome, bladder infection was documented by suprapubic aspirate or urethral catheter specimens when concurrent midstream cultures had colony counts as low as 10^2 cfu/mL (19). Colony counts of 50,000 cfu/mL or greater from specimens of catheterized urine obtained from children less than two years of age with fever were the most common characteristics of infection in children (20).

Leukocyte esterase, nitrite reaction, and microscopic examination for white cells and bacteria in both unstained and Gram-stained urine specimens often are performed. The sensitivity of the first two tests is less than 75% (21). However, when used on freshly voided specimens, a positive nitrite test is highly predictive of UTI (22).

The early detection of pyelonephritis and its differentiation from cystitis is of great clinical importance. Numerous studies have attempted to differentiate between lower and upper UTI in adults and children (18–23). In addition to the evaluation of symptoms and signs such as fever and flank pain, several other methods have been proposed for determining the level of UTI (23–27), but no single method is both simple and reliable. Ureteric catheterization is an invasive and unjustifiable procedure for those with acute UTI (24). The bladder washout technique (23) is less elaborate but requires trained personnel. In addition, the reliability of this test for diagnosing the level of involvement has been questioned (28). Identification of antibody-coated bacteria (26,27) is simple but has been found to have little value for young children (29).

Differences have been reported in urinary lactic dehydrogenase isoenzyme levels in the two types of infection (30).

Because the level of infection cannot be determined accurately with any of these tests, the best way to detect involvement of renal parenchyma seems to be the evaluation of clinical findings supplemented by a battery of laboratory tests.

Patients with proved UTI should be examined by abdominal ultrasonography, voiding cystotourethrography, or radionuclide cystogram and intravenous pyelography to identify anomalies of the urinary tract or vesicoureteral reflux. These studies should be delayed when possible until infection has been cleared for a few weeks. Renal cortical scintigraphy using technetium 99m dimercaptosuccinic acid can detect acute pyelonephritis. Radiologic studies of patients with anaerobic UTI show abnormalities that are indistinguishable from UTI caused by other bacteria.

Examination of the urine generally reveals pyuria. Slight or moderate hematuria occasionally occurs. There may be slight proteinuria. Pathogenic organisms and casts of all types may be present in the urine, but the urine may be normal for long periods of time.

As anaerobes are found as normal flora in the urethra, it is seldom satisfactory or reliable to obtain voided specimens for diagnosis of UTI caused by anaerobic bacteria. Suprapubic aspiration of the bladder is the best method for obtaining a culture. In the study reported by Finegold et al. (15), anaerobes were recovered from 14 of 100 random urine specimens. Relatively high counts of anaerobes were recovered in certain cases. In follow-up studies, these authors failed to recover any obligate anaerobes from 19 specimens of "urethral" urine, and "midstream" urine yielded anaerobes in mixed culture in 13 instances. The anaerobes recovered from the voided specimens clearly represented normal urethral flora. In this study, anaerobes were recovered in counts of 10^3 to 10^4/mL or greater on a number of occasions (15). Thus, even quantitative anaerobic culture is not helpful in distinguishing between infection and the presence of anaerobes as normal flora.

The report of Segura et al. (31) confirmed the validity of suprapubic bladder puncture for documentation of anaerobic UTI. In their study, suprapubic bladder aspirations were performed in two groups of patients: in one group aerobic cultures did not reveal organisms that were present in significant numbers on Gram stain, and a second group required suprapubic bladder aspiration for other reasons, such as an inability to void. Of 5781 patients studied, at least 1.3% with significant bacteriuria had anaerobic organisms involved. Of the 10 suprapubic bladder taps that were positive for anaerobes, there was one instance in which an anaerobe was recovered in pure culture; this was an isolate of *B. fragilis* in a patient with known renal tuberculosis. Five of the patients had two anaerobes recovered.

Possibly, with the improvements and simplification of the techniques of recovery of anaerobic organisms and proper methods of their collection and transportation to the laboratory, the yield of anaerobes in UTI may increase.

There is at present evidence suggesting the role of anaerobic organisms in UTI. It is therefore recommended that in symptomatic cases in which routine aerobic cultures fail to yield bacterial growth, and Gram stain shows bacteria to be present in the urine sediment, appropriate cultures for anaerobic bacteria be obtained.

Management

Increased fluid intake can assist in clearing the infection in the acute stage. Although there is no substantial evidence that routine surgical correction alters the course of recurrent UTI to any significant degree, repair of clearly obstructive lesions is indicated.

Eradication of infection with appropriate antibiotic therapy is of utmost importance. Acute uncomplicated infection, which is commonly caused by enteric organisms such as *E. coli*, generally is treated by oral sulfonamides, trimethoprim–sulfamethoxazole, ampicillin, or a quinolone (in adults). At least 10 days of therapy is required for patients with presumed pyelonephritis, reflux, or urinary tract abnormalities and for those who have not yet been evaluated radiographically. Those not suspected as having pyelonephritis or those with normal urinary tract (28,32) can be treated with antibiotics for 3 to 4 days.

The quinolones should not be routinely used in children because of these drugs' potential harmful effect on the cartilage. However, their use may be considered whenever resistance to other antimicrobials exists. Acutely, ill patients may be treated with intravenously administered drug—one of the antibiotics mentioned above or an aminoglycoside such as gentamicin. The recovery of aerobic or facultative anaerobic organisms from the urine of a patient with UTI does not exclude the possibility of the concomitant presence of an anaerobe.

A prolonged course of urinary tract antisepsis (two to six months or longer) may be indicated, especially for repeated infections. Repeated urinalysis and culture should be obtained 48 hours after starting treatment and at intervals of one to two months for at least a year.

The recovery of anaerobes in UTI may have important implications for the choice of antimicrobial agents. Most anaerobic organisms are sensitive to penicillin and cephalosporins. Most anaerobes, however, are resistant to sulfonamides, and all are highly resistant to aminoglycosides. Furthermore, *B. fragilis* and growing number of strains of *Prevotella* and *Porphyromonas* are also resistant to penicillin and cephalosporins (33).

The recovery of anaerobes requires the choice of an agent that is effective against these organisms. Penicillin or cephalosporins can be used against most anaerobic organisms; however, the recovery of penicillin-resistant organisms requires administration of appropriate antimicrobial agents such as clindamycin, chloramphenicol, ticarcillin, cefoxitin, metronidazole, carbapenems (i.e., meropenem, imipenem), tigecycline, or the combination of a penicillin and a beta-lactamase inhibitor. Some of the newer quinolones have extended coverage against anaerobic bacteria (i.e., moxifloxacin).

Complications

In patients with uncomplicated cystitis or pyelonephritis, treatment ordinarily results in complete resolution of symptoms. Cystitis may occasionally result in upper tract infection or bacteremia, especially during instrumentation. Cases of anaerobic bacteremia following urologic procedures have been reported (14). Repeated symptomatic UTI in patients with obstructive uropathy, neurogenic bladder, structural renal disease, or diabetes more often progresses to chronic renal disease. Untreated UTI can progress to renal abscess, pyonephrosis, perinephric, or retroperitoneal abscess. Anaerobes have been recovered in each of these disease states (Table 1) (34).

TABLE 1 Bacteriologic Characterization of 103 Suppurative Genitourinary Infection

Urinary tract (male and female)

	Kidney abscess	Perinephric abscess	Bladder abscess	Periurethral abscess	Labial infection
Number of specimens	6	3	2	7	4
Types of bacterial growth					
Aerobes only	—	—	—	1	1
Anaerobes only	2	—	1	1	1
Aerobes and anaerobes	4	3	1	5	2
Bacterial isolates specimens					
Aerobes	0.7	1.3	1.0	0.9	0.7
Anaerobes	3	1.7	3.5	2.0	1.0
Total	3.7	3	4.5	2.9	1.7

Genital tract (female)

	Bartholin's cyst abscess	Labial cyst abscess	Vulvar abscess	Vaginal abscess
Number of specimens	26	2	4	4
Types of bacterial growth				
Aerobes only	2	—	—	—
Anaerobes only	5	1	3	3
Aerobes and anaerobes	19	1	1	1
Bacterial isolates specimens				
Aerobes	0.9	0.2	0.2	0.7
Anaerobes	1.7	2.0	2.5	2.5
Total	2.6	2.2	2.7	3.2

Genital tract (male)

	Scrotal cyst abscess	Penile abscess	Scrotal abscess	Testicular abscess	Prostate abscess	Infected hydrocele	Scrotal infection	Penile infection	All sites
Number of specimens	3	7	15	6	3	2	3	6	103
Types of bacterial growth									
Aerobes only	—	—	2	—	1	—	—	—	7
Anaerobes only	—	5	3	4	—	—	2	3	34
Aerobes and anaerobes	3	2	10	2	2	2	1	3	62
Bacterial isolates specimens									
Aerobes	1.0	0.4	1.0	0.5	2.0	1.0	0.7	0.7	0.8
Anaerobes	1.3	1.7	1.9	1.3	1.3	2.0	2.0	1.3	1.8
Total	2.3	2.1	2.9	1.8	3.3	3.0	2.7	2.0	2.6

Source: From Ref. 34.

GENITOURINARY SUPPURATIVE INFECTIONS: PERINEPHRIC AND RENAL ABSCESSES

Perinephric and renal abscesses are rare (34–41). The newer imaging methods allow for an earlier diagnosis and a more accurate anatomic identification, as well as enabling a less invasive therapeutic approach.

Microbiology

Most suppurative genitourinary infections involve anaerobic bacteria. Brook (34) studied 103 patients, 29 of them younger than 18 years old (55 males and 48 females), with localized suppurative genitourinary tract infections (Table 1). The infections in males included scrotal abscess, scrotal cyst abscess, scrotal wound, penile abscess, penile wound, testicular abscess, infected hydrocele, prostate abscess, kidney abscess, perinephric abscess, and periuretheral abscess. The 48 females had Bartholin's cyst abscess, vulvar abscess, vaginal abscess and labial wound, labial cyst abscess, kidney abscess, perinephric abscess, periurethral abscess, and bladder abscess. Anaerobic bacteria only were present in 34 (33%) specimens, aerobic bacteria only were present in 7 (7%), and mixed aerobic and anaerobic flora were present in 62 (60%). A total of 275 isolates (189 anaerobic and 86 aerobic) were recovered, an average of 2.6 isolates/specimen (1.8 anaerobes and 0.8 aerobes). The predominant anaerobes recovered were *Bacteroides* spp. (103 isolates) and anaerobic cocci (53). The most frequently recovered aerobes were *E. coli* (26), *Staphylococcus aureus* (10), and *Proteus* spp. (8). These findings have important implications regarding the culturing techniques of these infections and for the selection of antimicrobials for their management.

The organisms that predominate in perinephric and renal abscesses are *S. aureus*, *Enterobacteriaceae* (especially *E. coli* and including *Salmonella* spp.), *Pseudomonas* spp., *Enterococcus* spp., coagulase-negative staphylococci, *Streptococcus* spp., *Actinomyces* spp., Fungi and *Mycobacterium tuberculosis* (35,38,42,43). Anaerobic bacteria were rarely reported from pediatric cases of these abscesses. In contrast to studies in children, anaerobic bacteria were recovered in up to a quarter of cases of perinephric and renal abscesses in adults (1,35,40,44).

Brook (39) reported isolation of anaerobic bacteria of oral or gastrointestinal origin from a series of 10 children, 6 with perinephric and 4 with renal abscesses. In 9 of 10 children, polymicrobial infections were described. A total of 20 organisms (2.0/specimen), 8 aerobic or facultative and 12 anaerobic, were recovered in the abscess specimens. The predominant isolates were *B. fragilis* group (7 isolates), *E. coli* (4), and *S. aureus* (2). Organisms similar to those recovered in the abscesses were also isolated in the blood in seven cases and in the urine in four cases. Thirteen beta-lactamase-producing organisms were found in nine cases. These included all seven isolates of *B. fragilis* group and two isolates of *S. aureus*, the single isolate of *P. melaninogenica*, and three of the four *E. coli* isolates.

Pathogenesis

Most abscesses occur in otherwise healthy individuals, but certain recognized factors increase the risk. These include: urinary tract conditions (infection, anomalies such as reflux and obstruction, urinary tract stones, neurogenic bladder, polycystic disease, tumor, and peritoneal dialysis), primary infection elsewhere with subsequent seeding (originating from skin, dental, cardiac, respiratory, genital, abdominal, gastrointestinal, intravascular catheter, and intravenous drug abuse), surgery (of the urinary tract including transplantation, and abdominal), immunodeficiency states, trauma to kidney, and diabetes mellitus (36–52).

Hematogenous infection is usually caused by *S. aureus* originating from the skin or another location of infection or appearing spontaneously (1,4,13). Abscess that follows UTI is generally caused by Enterobacteriaceae.

Perinephric abscesses are generally caused by Enterobacteriaceae. Bacteria invade the perinephric space by direct extension from an intrarenal abscess or by vesicoureteral reflux, urinary tract obstruction or surgery of the urinary tract or abdomen. Perinephric abscesses may also originate from hematogenous seeding by *S. aureus* from a distant primary site.

The recovery of anaerobes correlates with a predisposing factor that allows dissemination of anaerobic bacteria from another infectious site to the kidney and perinephric area

(1,4,34,39,44). Local spread of such organisms can be from a perforated viscus, or through hematogenous spread from the upper respiratory tract or dental sites (39). The anaerobic organisms isolated from those abscesses are similar to these that colonize the mucous membranes of the site of origin. This association may enable the clinician to initiate empiric antimicrobial therapy, even before abscess drainage. Anaerobic bacteria that originate from the oral cavity (i.e., *Prevotella* spp.) were recovered in renal abscesses associated with respiratory infections, whereas gut flora organisms (i.e., *B. fragilis* group) were found in abscesses that were associated with an abdominal origin.

The role of anaerobic bacteria in perinephric abscesses was especially apparent in association with obstruction leading to urinary extravasation (44,53,54), renal transplantation (55), perforation of the colon (56), and in a necrotic tumor (57,58). Anaerobes were found in renal abscesses adults in association with seeding during anaerobic bacteremia, or in association with altered renal architecture (44), where stasis and necrosis of tissue are important factors. Similarly, associated conditions were also found in the children (39). However, in contrast to adults (44), renal stones were not observed in the children (39).

Diagnosis

Symptoms are generally nonspecific and include lethargy, decreased appetite, weight loss, nausea, and vomiting. They are typically associated with fever and with unilateral pain in the flank or abdomen or tenderness in the costovertebral angle (35,37–39,42,45–49,52). However, pain can be referred to other sites. Their duration is generally one to three weeks prior to diagnosis. Other findings may be scoliosis due to splinting of the affected side, pain on bending to the other side, and chest abnormalities, such as reduced respiratory excursion, lower ribs tenderness, pulmonary dullness, lowered breath sounds and rales on the abscess side.

Dysuria or frequency is common when the abscess is preceded by a UTI. A mass can be palpated in about 5% of patients and is more likely found in infants. An abscess should be suspected in patients who had any of the predisposing conditions especially if they fail to respond to therapy of pyelonephritis.

Laboratory findings include elevated white blood count and erythocyte sedimentation rate. Microscopic pyuria and, positive urine culture can be found in about half of the patients each, and positive blood culture in 34%.

A sample of abscess content should be obtained by aspiration or at the time of surgery for Gram stain and culture. Culture and stain for aerobic and anaerobic bacteria, fungi, and mycobacteria should be obtained.

Ultrasonography is initially performed in those who are unresponsive to antibiotic treatment for pyelonephritis. However, ultrasonography and renal cortical scintigraphy may not distinguish between abscess, and uncomplicated pyelonephritis unless there is a distinctively rimmed, round mass with central liquefaction. Enhanced computed tomography is the most reliable imaging modality for diagnosis of renal and perinephric abscesses (59).

Serial renal ultrasound is performed to document progress in those recovering from a renal abscess. However, it must be recognized that resolution of the ultrasonographic abnormality lags behind clinical and laboratory improvement, and often takes months to resolve.

Management

Medical management alone using an intravenous antibiotic is the initial therapeutic approach. Percutaneous drainage, open surgical drainage, or nephrectomy may be indicated if this fails.

Empiric antibiotic therapy should initially include agents effective against *S. aureus* and Enterobacteriaceae. A pencillinase-resistant penicillin such as nafcillin or oxacillin, plus an aminoglycoside is an adequate combination. An antimicrobial effective against methicillin resistant *S. aureus* (i.e. vancomycin, linezolid) may be needed.

Although beta-lactamase-resistant penicillins (i.e., nafcillin) are active against *S. aureus*, they are not effective against beta-lactamase-producing anaerobic bacteria (33). Similarly, third-generation cephalosporins (i.e., cefotaxime) although effective against Enterobacteriaceae, do not provide adequate coverage against these organisms.

As many of the anaerobic bacteria recovered in these abscesses in adults (13,34,41) and children (38,39) are resistant to penicillins through the production of beta-lactamase (33), antimicrobials effective against these organisms should be utilized in treating perinephric and renal abscesses in which these organisms are suspected or isolated. These antimicrobials include metronidazole, chloramphenicol, clindamycin, carbapenem (i.e., imipenem, meropenem ertapenem), tigecycline, cefoxitin, and the combination of a penicillin and a beta-lactamase inhibitor (i.e., ticarcillin or amoxicillin plus clavulanate) (33,60).

Addition or replacement of an antimicrobial ineffective against anaerobes with an agent with anti-anaerobic activity should be considered, especially with underlying chronic obstructive disease or typical infection in other sites. Therapy should be adjusted according to the results from culture of the abscess. Therapy directed at the spectrum of potential pathogens should not be reduced based upon the blood or urine culture results only, as these do not always correlate with recovery of isolates from abscess specimens (35,39,40).

The length of parenteral therapy depends on the clinical response and whether percutaneous or surgical drainage is performed. At least two weeks of therapy is appropriate in conjunction with drainage of the abscess in those with uncomplicated infection. Without drainage, six weeks or more of therapy may be needed (61). Aspiration is usually performed with ultrasonographic guidance (62,63). Therapeutic drainage can be performed without significant morbidity which avoids the need for open drainage under general anesthesia.

Surgical drainage is done when antimicrobial therapy and percutaneous drainage fail. Open surgical drainage was previously used when an abscess ruptured into an adjacent space. Presently, however, a percutaneous approach usually provide adequate drainage. Nephrectomy is performed only for those with massive abscess where the involved kidney is unlikely to stay functional.

Complications

Complications include loss of renal function, extension of the infection into the kidney, or perinephric space, causing more tissue destruction and organ dysfunction, and rupture into an adjacent space (pulmonary, abdominal). Bacteremia can result in spread of the infection to other sites.

REFERENCES

1. Finegold SM. Anaerobic Bacteria in Human Disease. New York: Academic Press, 1977.
2. Brook I. Urinary tract infection caused by anaerobic bacteria in children. Urology 1980; 16:596–8.
3. Kumazawa J, Kiyoara H, Narahashi K, Hidaka M, Momose S. Significance of anaerobic bacteria isolated from the urinary tract. I. Clinical studies. J Urol 1974; 112:257–60.
4. Bartlett GJ, Gorbach SL. Anaerobic bacteria in suppurative infections of the male genitourinary system. J Urol 1981; 125:376–8.
5. Mazuecos J, Aznar J, Rodriguez-Pichardo A, et al. Anaerobic bacteria in men with urethritis. J Eur Acad Dermatol Venereol 1998; 10:237–42.
6. Moberg PJ, Nord CE. Anaerobic bacteria in urine before and after prostatic massage of infertile men. Med Microbiol Immunol 1985; 174:25–8.
7. Eggert-Kruse W, Rohr G, Strock W, Pohl S, Schwalbach B, Runnebaum B. Anaerobes in ejaculates of subfertile men. Hum Reprod Update 1995; 1:462–78.
8. Fair WR, Timothy MM, Millar MA, Stamey TA. Bacteriologic and hormonal observations of the urethra and vaginal vestibule in normal, premenopausal women. J Urol 1970; 104:426–31.
9. Bollgren I, Kallenius G, Nord CE. Periurethral anaerobic microflora of healthy girls. J Clin Microbiol 1979; 10:419–24.
10. Chambers CV, Shafer MA, Adger H, et al. Microflora of the urethra in adolescent boys. Relationships to sexual activity and nongonococcal urethritis. J Pediatr 1987; 110:314–21.
11. Serour F, Samra Z, Kushel Z, Gorenstein A, Dan M. Comparative periurethral bacteriology of uncircumcised and circumcised males. Genitourin Med 1997; 73:288–90.
12. Bran JL, Levinson ME, Kaye D. Entrance of bacteria into the female urinary bladder. N Engl J Med 1972; 286:626–9.

13. Alling B, Brandberg A, Seeberg S, Svanborg A. Aerobic and anaerobic microbial flora in the urinary tract of geriatric patients during long-term care. J Infect Dis 1973; 127:34–9.
14. Sapico FL, Wideman PA, Finegold SM. Aerobic and anaerobic bladder urine flora of patients with indwelling urethral catheters. Urology 1976; 7:382–4.
15. Finegold SM. Significance of anaerobic and capnophilic bacteria isolated from the urinary tract. In: Kass EM, ed. Progress in Pyelonephritis. 1st ed. Philadelphia: F.A. Davis, 1965:159.
16. Oxygen tension of the urine and renal function. N Engl J Med 1963; 269:159 (Editorial).
17. Leonhardt KO, Landes RR. Urinary oxygen pressure in renal parenchymal and vascular disease. Effects of breathing oxygen. JAMA 1965; 194:345–50.
18. Kass EH. Horatio at the orifice: the significance of bacteriuria. J Infect Dis 1978; 138:546–57.
19. Stamm WE, Counts GW, Running KR, et al. Diagnosis of coliform infection in acutely dysuric women. N Engl J Med 1982; 307:463–8.
20. Hoberman A, Wald ER, Reynolds EA, et al. Pyuria and bacteriuria in urine specimens obtained by catheter from young children with fever. J Pediatr 1994; 124:513–9.
21. Lohr JA. Use of routine urinalysis in making a presumptive diagnosis of urinary tract infection in children. Pediatr Infect Dis J 1991; 10:646–50.
22. Lohr JA, Portilla MG, Geudus TG, et al. Making a presumptive diagnosis of urinary tract infection by using a urinalysis performed in an on-site laboratory. J Pediatr 1993; 122:22–5.
23. Fairley KP, Carson NE, Gutch RC, et al. Site of infection in acute urinary-tract infection in general practice. Lancet 1971; 2:615–8.
24. Hewstone AS, Whitaker J. The correlation of ureteric urine bacteriology and homologous antibody titer in children with urinary infection. J Pediatr 1969; 70:540–3.
25. Steele RW. The epidemiology and clinical presentation of urinary tract infections in children 2 years of age through adolescence. Pediatr Ann 1999; 28:653–8.
26. Thomas V, Shelokov A, Forland M. Antibody-coated bacteria in the urine and the site of urinary-tract infection. N Engl J Med 1974; 290:588–90.
27. Andersen HJ, Jacobsson B, Larsson H, Winberg J. Hypertension, asymmetric renal parenchymal defect, sterile urine, and high *E. coli* antibody titre. Br Med J 1973; 3:14–8.
28. Rushton HG. Urinary tract infections in children. Epidemiology, evaluation, and management. Pediatr Clin North Am 1997; 44:1133–69.
29. Hellerstein S, Kennedy E, Nussbaum L, Rice K. Localization of the site of urinary tract infections by means of antibody-coated bacteria in the urinary sediments. J Pediatr 1978; 92:188–93.
30. Devaskar U, Montgomery W. Urinary lactic dehydrogenase isoenzymes IV and V in the differential diagnosis of cystitis and pyelonephritis. J Pediatr 1978; 93:789–91.
31. Segura JW, Kelalis PP, Martin WJ, Smith LH. Anaerobic bacteria in the urinary tract. Mayo Clin Proc 1972; 47:20–3.
32. Moffatt M, Embree J, Grimm P, Lau B. Short-course antibiotic therapy for urinary tract infections in children. Am J Dis Child 1988; 142:57–61.
33. Hecht DW. Anaerobes: antibiotic resistance, clinical significance, and role of susceptibility testing. Anaerobe 2006; 12:115–21.
34. Brook I. Anaerobic bacteria in suppurative genitourinary infection. J Urol 1989; 141:889–93.
35. Edelstein H, McCabe RE. Perinephric abscess in pediatric patients: report of six cases and review of the literature. Pediatr Infect Dis J 1989; 8:167–70.
36. Timmons JW, Perlmutter AD. Renal abscess: a changing concept. J Urol 1977; 119:299–301.
37. Wipperman CF, Schofer O, Beetz R, et al. Renal abscess in childhood: diagnostic and therapeutic progress. Pediatr Infect Dis J 1991; 10:446–50.
38. Rote AR, Bauer SB, Retik AB. Renal abscess in children. J Urol 1978; 119:254–8.
39. Brook I. The role of anaerobic bacteria in perinephric and renal abscesses in children. Pediatrics 1994; 93:261–4.
40. Yen DH, Hu SC, Tsai J, et al. Renal abscess: early diagnosis and treatment. Am J Emerg Med 1999; 17:192–7.
41. Kawashima A, Sandler CM, Ernst RD, Goldman SM, Raval B, Fishman EK. Renal inflammatory disease: the current role of CT. Crit Rev Diagn Imaging 1997; 38:369–415.
42. High KP, Quagliarello VJ. Yeast perinephric abscess: report of a case and review. Clin Infect Dis 1992; 15:128–33.
43. Santoro-Lopes G, Halpern M, Goncalves RT. Perinephric abscess caused by *Streptococcus agalactius* after renal transplantation. J Infect 2005; 51:e145–7.
44. Apostolopoulou C, Konstantoulaki S, Androulakakis P, Vatopoulou T, Varkarakis M. Isolation of anaerobic organisms from the kidney in serious renal infections. Urology 1982; 20:479–81.
45. Costas S, Rippey JJ, Van Blerk PJ. Segmental acute pyelonephritis. Br J Urol 1972; 44:399–404.
46. Segura JW, Kelalis PP. Localized renal parenchymal infections in children. J Urol 1973; 109:1029.
47. Klein DL, Filpi RG. Acute renal carbuncle. J Urol 1977; 118:912–5.
48. Sugao H, Takiuchi H, Sakurai T. Acute focal bacterial nephritis and renal abscess associated with vesicoureteral reflux. Urol Int 1988; 43:253–6.

49. Davis NS, Powell KR, Rabinowitz R. *Salmonella* renal abscess in a four-year-old child. Pediatr Infect Dis J 1989; 8:122–3.
50. Murphy JJ, Kohler FP. Reevaluation of modern antibacterial agents used for perirenal abscess. J Am Med Assoc 1959; 171:1287–92.
51. Dembry LM, Andriole VT. Renal and perirenal abscesses. Infect Dis Clin North Am 1997; 11:663–80.
52. Wunderlich HF, Bailen JL, Raff MJ, Melo JC. *Bacteroides fragilis* perinephric abscess. J Urol 1980; 123:601–2.
53. Kirchner FK, Turner BI. *Bacteroides ruminicola* pyonephrosis. Br J Urol 1982; 54:432.
54. Ribot S, Gal K, Goldblat MV, Eslami HH. The role of anaerobic bacteria in the pathogenesis of urinary tract infections. J Urol 1981; 126:852–3.
55. Fisher MC, Baluarte HJ, Long SS. Bacteremia due to *Bacteroides fragilis* after elective appendectomy in renal transplant recipients. J Infect Dis 1981; 143:635–8.
56. Murray NW, Molavi A. Perinephric abscess: an unusual presentation of perforation of the colon. Johns Hopkins Med J 1977; 140:15–8.
57. Graham BS, Johnson AC, Sawyers JL. Clostridial infection of renal cell carcinoma. J Urol 1986; 135:354–5.
58. Lenkey JL, Reece GJ, Herbert DL. Gas abscess transformation of hypernephroma. AJR 1979; 133:1174–6.
59. Levine E. Acute renal and urinary tract disease. Radiol Clin North Am 1994; 32:989–1004.
60. Snydman DR, Jacobus NV, McDermott LA, et al. Multicenter study of in vitro susceptibility of the *Bacteroides fragilis* group, 1995 to 1996, with comparison of resistance trends from 1990 to 1996. Antimicrob Agents Chemother 1999; 43:2417–22.
61. Roberts JA. Management of pyelonephritis and upper urinary tract infections. Urol Clin North Am 1999; 26:753–63.
62. Deyoe RL, Cronan JJ, Lambiase RE, Dorfman GS. Percotaneous drainage of renal and perirenal abscess: results in 30 patients. Am J Radiol 1990; 156:81–3.
63. Lambiase RE, Deyoe RL, Cronan JJ, Dorfman GS. Percotaneous drainage of 335 consecutive abscess: results of primary drainage with one year followup. Radiology 1992; 184:167–79.

24 | Female Genital Tract Infections

Female genital infections include vulvovaginitis (VV), vulvovaginal pyogenic infections (abscesses of Bartholin's and Skene's glands, infected labial inclusion cysts, labial abscesses, furunculosis, and hidradenitis), endometritis, pyometritis, salpingitis, pelvic inflammatory disease (PID), and tubo-ovarian (TOA) and pelvic abscess.

MICROBIOLOGY AND PATHOGENESIS

With only a few exceptions, such as Group A beta-hemolytic streptococci and sexually transmitted organisms, the bacterial pathogens involved in gynecologic infections reflect the normal microflora of the vagina and cervix. This flora is complex and includes obligate anaerobes such as gram-negative bacilli, *Peptostreptococcus* spp., aerobic gram-negative bacilli of the Enterbacteriaceae family, and aerobic as well as microaerophilic streptococci.

Many studies have documented that the vagina and cervix of healthy females harbor an indigenous microflora (1). The normal vaginal flora is fairly homogeneous and consists of aerobic and anaerobic bacteria (2). The aerobic components include lactobacilli, Group B and D streptococci, *Staphylococcus epidermidis*, *Staphylococcus aureus*, and gram-negative enteric rods such as *Escherichia coli* (2).

The recovery of anaerobes from the vaginal canal varies and depends on the adequacy of methods used for their isolation (2). Different strains of anaerobes were recovered in 49% to 92% of female subjects. Anaerobic cocci were reported in 7% to 57% of the cultures, predominantly *Peptostreptococcus asaccharolyticus* and *Peptostreptococcus anaerobius*.

Anaerobic gram-negative bacilli (AGNB) were isolated from most of the cultures; their isolation rates were between 57% and 65%. The predominant strains were *Prevotella bivia*, *Prevotella disiens*, *Bacteroides fragilis* group, pigmented *Prevotella* and *Porphyromonas* spp. and *Prevotella oralis*. Although the last two species are generally confined to the oral cavity, they could also be recovered from the cervical flora. *Veillonella* organisms were recovered from 27% of the cultures, *Bifidobacterium* spp. from 10% to 72%, and *Eubacterium* spp. from 15%. *Clostridium* spp. were recovered from 17%; these were isolates of *Clostridium bifermentans*, *Clostridium perfringens*, *Clostridium ramosum*, and *Clostridium difficile* (2).

Normal variations in cervical-vaginal flora are related to the effects of age, pregnancy, and menstrual cycle (2). During early childhood, the normal flora is similar to that of adolescents or adults and includes Enterobacteriaceae and anaerobes. The prepubescent vagina is more supportive of growth of anaerobic bacteria, especially *Bacteroides* spp., than in adults (3). Also often recovered at that age group is *S. epidermidis*. In contrast yeasts and *Gardnerella vaginalis* are isolated in 10% of females (3). The microflora in females before puberty, during the child-bearing years, pregnancy, and after menopause are not uniform. Colonization with lactobacilli is low in prepubertal females and postmenopausal females and high in pregnant women as well as those in their reproductive years who are not pregnant.

In the premenarchal period the vaginal epithelium becomes corniform under the influence of the estrogens, and supports the growth by a variety of microorganisms. However, changes in the flora occur in the adolescent and adults during the menstrual cycle.

These host factors may greatly influence the composition of the microbiology of established pelvic infections. The concentration of obligate anaerobes, particularly *Bacteroides* spp., increases substantially in certain situations, as during the first half of the menstrual cycle, during the postpartum period, with pelvic malignancy or immunosuppression, and after pelvic infections.

Anaerobes can be cultured in 50% to 90% of females with a variety of genital infections and are the exclusive isolates in 20% to 50% (4). Obligate anaerobes are particularly common in closed space infections, such as TOA and vulvovaginal abscesses. The most common anaerobes found in these infections are AGNB (especially *P. bivia* and *P. disiens*) and anaerobic cocci. Although *B. fragilis* is cultured less frequently, it is more important in closed-space infections.

Anaerobes generally are not the only pathogens found, but are usually mixed with aerobes. The most common aerobic pathogens are members of the Enterobacteriaceae family, especially *E. coli*, and aerobic or microaerophilic streptococci.

SPECIFIC INFECTIONS

Vulvovaginitis

VV is considered to be a disturbance in vaginal flora rather than a true infection (6). Prepubertal females are particularly susceptible to bacterial VV because of anatomic, physiologic, and hygienic considerations (6) including the relative unprotected location of the vaginal introitus and its proximity to the anus, lack of estrogen-induced mucosal cornification, and the neutral to alkaline pH of the vagina (6). Behavioral factors include the tendency of some females to wipe the perineum from back-to-front, place contaminated hands and foreign bodies in the introitus and vagina, and use harsh soaps and bubble baths (6). The healthy, normal pH of 3.8 to 4.2 is largely dependent upon the presence of *Lactobacillus acidophilus*, that produces lactic acid and hydrogen peroxide (7).

In both specific and nonspecific VV, changes occur in the normal vulvovaginal flora that may induce inflammation. The specific organisms that cause infection in the prepubertal female are often respiratory, enteric, or sexually transmitted pathogens. The respiratory pathogens include Group A streptococcus, *Streptococcus pneumoniae*, *Neisseria meningitidis*, *S. aureus*, and *Haemophilus influenzae*. Other rare pathogens are Shigella (8), Yersinia (9), and Candida (6).

The three most common types of VV include nonspecific VV, or VV caused by candida, or trichomonas. Sexually acquired infections include *Neisseria gonorrhoeae*, *G. vaginalis*, *Trichomonas vaginalis*, *Chlamydia trachomatis*, herpes simplex virus, and *Condyloma accuminata*.

Bacterial vaginosis is the most prevalent infectious cause of vaginitis (6,10). It is a synergistic infection caused by a complex alteration in the microbial flora, with 100- to 1000-fold increase in the number of *G. vaginalis* organisms as well as anaerobic bacteria, a decrease in lactobacilli, and an increase in organic acids produced by the abnormal flora (11). *Mycoplasma hominis* is also associated with nonspecific vaginitis (11). Several investigations have shown an association between bacterial vaginosis and the development of acute PID. The microorganisms associated with bacterial vaginosis include anaerobes such as *P. bivia*, *Prevotella* spp., and *Peptostreptococcus* spp. (10), butyrate-producing *Peptostreptococcus* spp., a comma-shaped bacterium (12), and *Mobiluncus curtisii*, a curved motile anaerobic rod (12). The exact role of each of these organisms is unclear and requires more study. Other yet unknown triggers for bacterial overgrowth may exist.

Bacterial vaginitis is characterized by the presence of a gray to white homogenous thin discharge adherent to the vaginal wall, vaginal fluid pH greater than 4.5, a positive whiff test, and the presence of clue cell in 20% of all vaginal epithelial cells. An association has been demonstrated between sexual abuse and bacterial vaginitis (13).

Treatment of bacterial vaginosis attempts to restore the vaginal ecosystem. Loss of dominance of lactobacillus results in overgrowth of facultative and obligate symptom causing anaerobes. Therapy of specific VV should be prescribed according to offending pathogens with either oral or intravaginal cream. Two intravaginal preparations are currently available, clindamycin (2%) vaginal cream or metronidazole gel (0.75%) (14,15). Clindamycin cream is administered once a day, whereas metronidazole gel is administered twice daily. Oral metronidazole is an accepted treatment for bacterial vaginosis administered as a single dose (2 g) or 250 mg three times a day or 500 mg given orally twice a day for seven days (16).

Ampicillin, although less effective, is an alternative drug treatment during pregnancy. Concomitant treatment of the female's sexual partner is still under investigation. The response of patients to metronidazole, although this drug is not effective against any of the nonanaerobic bacteria, supports the role of the anaerobic bacteria in this infection. Furthermore, clindamycin therapy eradicated and/or decreased counts of major bacterial vaginosis-associated microflora such as *Gardnerella*, gram-negative and gram-positive anaerobes, and *M. hominis* and was correlated with cure in 22 of 24 (92%) women (17). Possibly the elimination of only the anaerobic component of the infection may help to modify the microbial flora and restore normal condition.

Vulvovaginal Pyogenic Infections

Vulvovaginal pyogenic infections include abscesses of Bartholin's and Skene's glands, infected labial inclusion cysts, labial abscesses, furunculosis, and hidradenitis (6). Most infections are related to both aerobic and anaerobic organisms arising from the normal vaginal and cervical flora. *N. gonorrhoeae* is responsible for approximately 10% of these infections. The majority of nonvenereal abscesses are caused by anaerobic bacteria.

Parker and Jones (18) recovered anaerobes in two-thirds of 75 patients with such infections. Similarly, Swenson and associates (19) recovered anaerobes from 10 of 15 patients with Bartholin's gland abscess. Anaerobic streptococci and *Bacteroides* spp. were cultured from these abscesses. The clinical course of such infections is indistinguishable from that associated with other pathogens (20).

Brook (21,22) summarized the microbiology of 40 vulvovaginal infections, including Bartholin's abscesses (26 cases), vulvar abscesses, vaginal abscesses and labial wounds (four each), and labial cyst abscesses (two). Aerobic bacteria only were recovered in four (10%), anaerobic bacteria only in 12 (30%), and mixed aerobic and anaerobic flora in 24 (60%) (Table 1). There were 32 aerobic and facultative isolates (0.8/site) of 71 anaerobes (1.8/site). The average number of isolates was the highest in vaginal abscesses. The predominant aerobic organisms were *E. coli*, *N. gonorrhoeae*, and *S. aureus*, and the most frequently isolated anaerobes were *Peptostreptococcus* and *Bacteroides* spp. Beta-lactamase–producing bacteria (BLPB) were isolated in 90% of the patients. The predominant BLPB were *B. fragilis* group and *Prevotella* and *Porphyromonas* spp., Enterobacteriaceae and *Staphylococcus* spp.

In diabetic patients, the inflammation can extend to deeper structures of the perineum, the lower extremities, or back and cause extensive necrosis (23). Other pathogens in addition to *Peptostreptococcus* spp. and *B. fragilis* are *S. aureus* and facultative streptococci, particularly *Streptococcus pyogenes*.

Therapy consists primarily of surgical drainage; antibiotics are of secondary importance (24). In the absence of bacteriological and antibiotic susceptibility data, initial selection of drugs should include those effective against both aerobic and anaerobic bacteria of vaginal–cervical origin. Broad-spectrum antibiotics such as ampicillin or the cephalosporins are often useful. If beta-lactamase–producing anaerobes are suspected, however, clindamycin, chloramphenicol, cefoxitin, metronidazole, a carbapenem, or a combination of a penicillin and a beta-lactamase inhibitor should be administered (24,25).

Endometritis and Pyometra

Endometritis and pyometra are seen more commonly in older females who suffer from cervical canal obstruction or carcinoma or following delivery. However, they can also be seen occasionally in adolescent females. Endometritis occurs when bacteria invade the uterine cavity, and pyometra develops when pus is collected within the uterus. Regardless of the etiology, anaerobes are predominant in endometritis and pyometra.

Hillier et al. (26) obtained endometrial biopsies for histologic and microbiologic study from 178 consecutive women with suspected PID, and 85 of them underwent laparoscopy to diagnose salpingitis. Histologic endometritis was confirmed in 117 (65%) women. Among women who underwent laparoscopy, salpingitis was present in 68% of those with and 23% of those without endometritis. Some but not all bacterial vaginosis-associated microorganisms were linked with

TABLE 1 Microbiology of 40 Vulvovaginal Pyogenic Infections

No. of cases	Bartholin's cyst abscess (26)	Labial cyst abscess (2)	Vaginal abscess (4)	Vulvar abscess (4)	Labial wound (4)	Total (40)
Aerobes						
Staphylococcus aureus	2			1	1	4
S. epidermidis		1			1	2
Enterococcus spp.			1			1
Neisseria gonorrhoeae	4		1			5
Diphtheroids					1	1
Lactobacillus spp.	3					3
Escherichia coli	6		1			7
Klebsiella pneumoniae	2					2
Proteus spp.	3					3
Acinetobacter spp.	1					1
Citrobacter spp.	2					2
Enterobacter spp.	1					1
Subtotal	24	1	3	1	3	32
Anaerobes						
Peptostreptococci spp.	12	2	1	1	1	17
Veillonella spp.	2					2
Eubacteria spp.	2					2
Propionibacterium acnes				3		3
Lactobacillus spp.	1					1
Clostridium spp.	1		1	1	1	4
Fusobacterium spp.	2					2
Bacteroides spp.	8		2	3		12
B. fragilis group	5		4	1	1	11
Prevotella and *Porphyromonas* spp.	6	1	2	1		10
Prevotella bivia	4	1		1	1	7
Subtotal	43	4	10	10	4	71
Total	67	5	13	11	7	103

Source: From Ref. 21.

endometritis. By logistic regression analysis, after adjustment for bacterial vaginosis, endometritis was associated with endometrial *N. gonorrhoeae*, *C. trachomatis* and AGNB. *Mycoplasma genitalium* is also associated with cervicitis and endometritis.

Carter and colleagues (27), who studied 133 patients with endometritis and pyometra, isolated obligate anaerobes from 75% of the patients. The most frequent anaerobic isolates were anaerobic streptoccocci and *Bacteroides* spp. Swenson and coworkers (19), studied 14 females with this diagnosis and recovered anaerobes from 13, often associated with facultative bacteria, but in pure culture in six. Muram et al. (28) recovered anaerobes only from five of 15 of their patients with pyometra, and mixed aerobic and anaerobic flora from seven.

Pyometra should be considered an abscess and treated promptly and vigorously with drainage of the uterine cavity followed by curettage to debride the necrotic tissue (29). The most serious fatal complication of these conditions is spread of the organisms from the uterus into the blood (6).

Antibiotics effective against aerobic and anaerobic bacteria should be given. This is especially important for patients with signs of systemic infection, such as fever, peritonitis, tachycardia, or leukocytosis. Appropriate specimens for cultures should be obtained prior to initiation of therapy. Combined therapy with an aminoglycoside or a third-generation cephalosporin and an agent against anaerobes (clindamycin, metronidazole, chloramphenicol, cefoxitin) or single-agent therapy with carbapenem (i.e., imipenem, meropenem) will be adequate in most patients. Evacuation of the uterus remains the mainstay of management, however.

ACUTE SALPINGITIS AND PELVIC INFLAMMATORY DISEASE

Pathogenesis and Microbiology

PID usually begins with cervical infection that is caused by *C. trachomatis, N. gonorrhoeae*, or both. Acute salpingitis and PID occur after extension of the infection from the lower parts of the female genital tract to higher structures. Organisms infecting the cervix can spread to involve the uterus and fallopian tubes in two ways: by causing a transient endometritis that extends to involve the endosalpinx or by reaching the tubes via lymphatic spread. Acute salpingitis and PID may be gonococcal or nongonococcal, according to the presence or absence of associated endocervical gonorrhea. Acute pelvic salpingitis and PID is predominantly a disease of young sexually active nonparous females.

The recovery of *N. gonorrhoeae* from the upper genital tract is variable. Many species of aerobes and anaerobes that are related to the normal vaginal flora can be isolated. Chlamydiae and mycoplasmae also have been implicated. It is generally suspected that sexually transmitted pathogens paves the way to polymicrobial aerobic–anaerobic PID and that the cervical bacteria travel through the endometrium and salpinges to the TOA junction (30). Presumably, it explains the rarity of pelvic infections during the full-term pregnancy. The isolation of gonococci from the endocervix does not necessarily account for upper genital tract disease. Moreover, the eradication of gonococci may not be an adequate treatment for acute salpingitis. The morbidity and sequelae of both gonococcal and nongonococcal salpingitis may be attributed to repeated ascending infection by the aerobic and anaerobic microorganisms that are secondary invaders.

The polymicrobial etiology of acute salpingitis is well documented (30–32). Culdocentesis and laparoscopy have revealed mixed aerobic and anaerobic bacterial flora in addition to gonococci in patients with acute salpingitis. The most frequent pathogens appear to be gonococci and anaerobic bacteria (most commonly *Peptostreptococcus* and *Bacteroides* spp.). Anaerobes are present in the upper genital tract during an episode of acute PID, with the prevalence dependent on the population under study (33). Vaginal anaerobes can facilitate acquisition of PID and cause tissue damage to the fallopian tube, either directly or indirectly through the host inflammatory response.

Brook studied 57 culdocenthesis aspirates of PID, 15 of which were in adolescent females (34). There were 93 anaerobes and 90 aerobes (1.6/specimen each). The predominant anaerobes were *Bacteroides* spp. (33, including 16 *B. fragilis* group) and anaerobic cocci (32). The predominant aerobes were Enterobacteriaceae (31), *N. gonorrhoeae* (13), *Streptococcus* spp. (16), and *S. aureus* (7). BLPB were isolated in 29 (51%) patients. These included all 16 of the *B. fragilis* group, 6 of 7 *S. aureus* and 7 of 31 Enterobacteriaceae.

A characteristic pattern has evolved from these studies. In approximately one-third of patients, only gonococci could be recovered from the intraabdominal site; another third had gonococci plus anaerobic and aerobic bacteria; and the final third had both aerobic and anaerobic bacteria, but not gonococci, recovered from their abdominal cavities (4,25,33). Animal studies demonstrated the synergistic relationship between *N. gonorrhoeae* and *Bacteroides* spp. (35). Mixture of aerobic bacteria and AGNB were inoculated subcutaneously and intrapentonealy in mice. The growth of each component of the mixed infection was enhanced when these were present together in a subcutaneous abscess in mice. Furthermore, the emergence of encapsulated strains was enhanced in these infections (35). This synergy may enable the organisms to cause more severe local and systemic damage to the host.

Of particular interest was the observed ability of encapsulated *N. gonorrhoeae* to induce the conversion of slightly encapsulated *Bacteroides* spp. to heavily encapsulated ones (35). This phenomenon may represent the events that occur after cervical *N. gonorrhoeae* infection, which may lead to tubal or pelvic inflammation. In this fashion a nonvirulent *Bacteroides* that is part of the normal vaginal flora can become virulent after exposure to *N. gonorrhoeae*; however, the *N. gonorrhoeae* that eventually did not survive in the abscess were able to induce encapsulation of the *Bacteroides* spp. Similarly, the conversion of nonencapsulated *N. gonorrhoeae* after coinoculation with an encapsulated *Bacteroides* isolate may explain the increased virulence of *N. gonorrhoeae* isolates recovered from the tubes or cul-de-sac (36,37).

C. trachomatis has also received attention as an etiologic agent in acute salpingitis. Studies show a 30% incidence of *Chlamydia* isolation from the fallopian tubes of patients with acute salpingitis (38). Serologic studies suggest that *C. trachomatis* is associated with 40% to 60% of acute salpingitis cases (39). The presence of the major outer-membrane protein of *C. trachomatis* was associated with chronic salpingitis and/or salpingitis isthmica nodosa with tubal occlusion (40).

Mycoplasmae have frequently been recovered from the lower genital tract of females with salpingitis and is associated serologically with salpingitis and tubal factor infertility (41). Hinonen and Miettnen recovered *C. trachomatis* significantly more frequently from the fallopian tubes among cases with severe PID (42), thus confirming role of *C. trachomatis* as the leading cause of PID in both laparoscopically mild and severe PID.

DIAGNOSIS

Acute PID causes fever, increased vaginal discharge, chills, malaise, anorexia, nausea, and severe bilateral lower abdominal pain. Adynamic ileus is present if associated pelvic peritonitis has occurred. Pelvic examination reveals a purulent discharge oozing from an inflamed cervical os, and exquisite cervical motion tenderness. The adnexal regions are tender and thickened, and an adnexal or cul-de-sac mass may be palpable if infection is recurrent or chronic. Criteria for clinical diagnosis of PID were published by the Center for Disease Control (CDC) (Table 2) (43). The CDC recommends the use of three minimum criteria and optional, additional criteria for the diagnosis of PID.

PID must be differentiated from other acute lower abdominal processes such as acute appendicitis, pelvic endometrosis, ovarian tumors, rupture of an ovarian cyst, or a ruptured ectopic pregnancy. Diagnosis of acute salpingitis and PID should also include visual confirmation of tubal inflammation by such procedures as colposcopy and laparoscopy. Although laparoscopy is considered the gold standard for diagnosis, it is seldom indicated clinically or practical. Laparoscopy may miss endometritis or mild salpingitis. Ultrasonographic studies are nonspecific, but can reveal fluid in the uterus or cul-de-sac, increased adnexal volume, and hydrosalpinx. Definitive diagnosis can be made by demonstrating endometritis on endometrial biopsy TOA or thickened, fluid-filled tubes on radiographic studies, and laparoscopic findings suggesting PID.

Although an accurate bacteriologic diagnosis is of great importance, the relative inaccessibility of pelvic structures and the likelihood of external contamination of cultures obtained through the vagina limits the value of such cultures, especially for anaerobes. Procedures such as colposcopy, laparoscopy, or culdocentesis to obtain culture specimens can increase diagnostic accuracy. Material obtained for culture should be Gram stained and cultured aerobically and anaerobically.

TABLE 2 Criteria for Clinical Diagnosis of PID

Minimum criteria
   Lower abdominal tenderness
   Bilateral adnexal tenderness
   Cervical motion tenderness
Additional criteria to increase specificity
   Routine
      Oral temperature $>38.3°C$ ($>100.9°F$)
      Abnormal cervical or vaginal mucopurulent   discharge
      Presence of abundant numbers of white blood cells (WBCs) on saline microscopy of vaginal secretions
      Elevated erythrocyte sedimentation rate or C-reactive protein
      Evidence of cervical infection with *Neisseria gonorrhoeae* or *Chlamydia trachomatis*
   Definitive criteria
      Histopathologic evidence on endometrial biopsy
      Transvaginal sonography or magnetic resonance imaging techniques showing thickened, fluid-filled tubes with or without
         free pelvic fluid or tubo-ovarian complex, or Doppler studies suggesting pelvic infection (e.g., tubal hyperemia)
      Laparoscopy abnormalities consistent with PID

Abbreviations: PID, pelvic inflammatory disease.
Source: From Ref. 43.

MANAGEMENT

The threshold of suspicion for the diagnosis and empiric treatment of PID should be low. Salpingitis and PID are managed primarily with antimicrobial therapy. This can be achieved by penicillin plus probenecid, ampicillin, or tetracycline. In areas where resistance of gonococci to penicillin has been observed, spectinomycin can be used. Surgical intervention may be required if the patient fails to respond to medical therapy.

Adolescents are at particularly high risk for future reproductive complications because of their tendency not to complete prescribed treatment regimens. Severely ill patients should therefore be admitted to the hospital, particularly if an adnexal mass or peritonitis is present.

Several investigations have shown an association between bacterial vaginosis and the development of acute PID (10). The microorganisms associated with bacterial vaginosis include anaerobes such as *P. bivia*, other *Prevotella* spp. and *Peptostreptococcus* spp. The studies that have demonstrated the presence of bacterial vaginosis-associated bacteria in addition to the sexually transmitted organisms (*N. gonorrhoeae* and *C. trachomatis*) suggest that treatment of acute PID must be broad-spectrum in nature and effective against anaerobic bacteria as well as *N. gonorrhoeae* and *C. trachomatis*.

Early treatment of PID has been shown to reduce the effects of the infection on the fallopian tubes (25) and decrease the incidence of serious sequela. Antimicrobial therapy should be aimed at the eradication of both aerobic and anaerobic bacterial pathogens as well as *C. trachomatis*. Agents effective against the anaerobic pathogens are metronidazole, clindamycin, cefoxitin, a carbapenem (i.e., imipenem, meropenem), and the combination of a penicillin and a beta-lactamase inhibitor (44). Antimicrobials effective against the gram-positive aerobic pathogens *N. gonorrhoeae* and *C. trachomatis* are macrolides, (e.g. azithomycin) and penicillins. Aminoglycosides or third-generation cephalosporins are effective against gram-negative enterics.

There is no single agent that can provide complete coverage. Therefore, combination therapy has been advocated. A combination therapy that is often used is cefoxitin and doxycycline (Table 3). While cefoxitin provides adequate coverage against anaerobic gram negative bacilli, doxycycline is directed against *N. gonorrhoeae* and *C. trachomatis*. The combination of clindamycin and gentamicin also provides coverage for AGNB, and *C. trachomatis* (46). The combination of metronidazole and a macrolide possesses activity against AGNB, by metronidazole and against *C. trachomatis* and *N. gonorrhoeae* by the macrolide. The combination of metronidazole and a macolide (spiramycin) has been shown to be synergistic in mice against *P. bivia* and *B. fragilis*, alone or in mixed infection with *N. gonorrhoeae* (45).

Treatment regimens for PID must provide antimicrobial coverage for *N. gonorrhoeae*. *C. trachomatis*, anaerobes, streptococci, and gram-negative facultative bacteria (Table 3). When sexually transmitted pathogens are involved, sexual partners need to be treated. The CDC recommends several regimens for inpatient treatment and two regimens for outpatient treatment (Tables 4 and 5) (43). Parenteral Regimen A is continued for at least 48 hours after clinical improvement and should be followed by doxycycline 100 mg orally twice daily to conclude a 14-day course. Parenteral Regimen B is continued for at least 24 hours after clinical

TABLE 3 Antimicrobials Effective Against Organisms Causing Pelvic Inflammatory Disease

	Bacteroides spp.	*Enterobacteriaceae*	*Neisseria gonorrhoeae*	*Chlamydia*
Metronidazole	+++	−	−	−
Cefoxitin, Cefotetan	++	++	+++	−
Clindamycin	+++	−	±	+
Doxycycline	+	±	++	+++
Azithomycin	±	±	+++	++
A penicillin and beta-lactamase inhibitor	+++	++	++	−
Quinolone	+	+++	++	++

Key: −, no activity; ±, minimal activity; +, some activity; ++, good activity; +++, excellent activity.

TABLE 4   CDC Recommendations for the Parenteral Treatment of Pelvic Inflammatory Disease

Parenteral Regimen A
Cefotetan 2 g IV every 12 hr
Or
Cefoxitin 2 g IV every 6 hr
Plus
Doxycycline 100 mg IV or orally every 12 hr
Parenteral Regimen B
Clindamycin 900 mg IV every 8 hr
Plus
Gentamicin loading dose IV or IM (2 mg/kg of body weight), followed by a maintenance dose (1.5 mg/kg) every 8 hr. Single daily dosing may be substituted
Alternative Parenteral Regimens
Levofloxacin[a] 500 mg IV every 24 hr, or Ofloxacin 400 mg IV every 12 hr, or
With or without
Metronidazole 500 mg IV every 8 hr
Or
Ampicillin/Sulbactam 3 g IV every 6 hr
Plus
Doxycycline 100 mg IV or orally every 12 hr

[a] Not approved below the age of 18 years.
Abbreviations: CDC, Centers for Disease Control; IM, intramuscular; IV, intravenous.
Source: From Ref. 43.

improvement and followed by either doxycycline 100 mg orally twice daily or clindamycin 450 mg orally four times daily to conclude a 14-day course.

Both oral regimens provide good coverage against the likely pathogens of PID. Oral Regimen A provides better anaerobic coverage but is more costly. Although single-dose azithromycin is effective in the treatment of chlamydial cervicitis (47), its use in the treatment of PID remains controversial.

Patients with an intrauterine device (IUD) have a higher incidence of acute salpingitis, and the clinical presentation of infection in this group may be different (48). Unilateral adnexal infection occurs more frequently, and the infections may be more severe. In addition, serious *Actinomyces* infections generally are associated with this form of contraception (49). It is important to make a precise microbiologic diagnosis of pelvic actinomycosis, since penicillin or macrolides are the agents of choice, and prolonged therapy is necessary (49,50) (see Chapter 18).

TABLE 5   CDC Recommendations for the Oral Treatment of Pelvic Inflammatory Disease

Oral Regimen A
Ofloxacin[a] 400 mg orally twice a day for 14 day or Levofloxacin 500 mg orally once daily for 14 day
With or without
Metronidazole 500 mg orally twice a day for 14 day
Oral Regimen B
Ceftriaxone 250 mg IM once
Or
Cefoxitin 2 g IM plus probenecid 1 g orally in a single dose concurrently once
Or
Other parenteral third-generation cephalosporin (e.g., ceftizoxime or cefotaxime)
Plus
Doxycycline 100 mg orally twice a day for 14 day
With or without
Metronidazole 500 mg orally twice a day for 14 day

[a] Not approved below the age of 18 years.
Abbreviations: CDC, Centers for Disease Control; IM, intramuscular.
Source: From Ref. 43.

COMPLICATIONS

Peritonitis can result when microorganisms spill from the fimbriated ends of the fallopian tubes into the peritoneal cavity. Long-term sequelae are commonly observed following nongonococcal salpingitis. They include recurrent exacerbations, TOA, sterility, chronic pain, and dysfunctional bleeding.

Tubo-Ovarian and Pelvic Abscess

TOA is generally a consequence of salpingitis or PID of acute or chronic nature. Other conditions associated with pelvic abscess formation include endometritis, pyelonephritis, uterine fibroids, and malignancy in the pelvic area. Most pelvic abscesses are polymicrobial with preponderance of anaerobic bacteria, with *Bacteroides* spp. predominating, followed by peptostreptococci and rarely, clostridia. *P. bivia* and *P. disiens* are major pathogens in these infections (51); these pathogens possess virulence characteristics similar to the *B. fragilis* group (35).

Swenson and colleagues (19) recovered anaerobes from 8 of 10 pelvic abscesses, and these organisms were the exclusive pathogens in five patients. Similarly, Thadepalli (52) isolated anaerobes from all 13 patients with pelvic abscess; these organisms were the only isolates in nine patients. The specimens for culture were obtained in both studies either at operation or by culdocentesis, thereby avoiding contamination by the normal vaginal flora.

We studied 53 TOA, 13 of which were in adolescent females (34). The predominant aerobic bacteria were *N. gonorrhoeae* (18 isolates), Enterobacteriaceae (7), and *S. aureus* (4). The predominant anaerobes were AGNB (45 isolates, including 15 of the *B. fragilis* group, 12 pigmented *Prevotella* and *Porphyromonas* spp. and six *P. bivia*) and anaerobic cocci (34). BLPB were isolated in 31 (58%) patients. These included all 15 *B. fragilis* group, five of 12 pigmented *Prevotella* and *Porphyromonas* spp. and seven of 18 *N. gonorrhoeae*.

The bacteriology of TOA is somewhat different from that of other pelvic abscesses. Whereas pelvic abscesses are caused by mixed aerobic and anaerobic bacteria, exclusively anaerobic bacteria were found in nearly one-half of the cases of TOA. Patients with TOA most commonly present with lower abdominal pain or an adnexal mass(es). Fever and leukocytosis may be absent. Ultrasound, computed tomography scans and magnetic resonance imaging, laparoscopy, or laparotomy may be necessary to confirm the diagnosis (53–55). TOA may be unilateral or bilateral, regardless of IUD usage.

Slap et al. (56) attempted to determine whether the clinical features of PID differ in adolescents with and without TOA. Some clinical characteristics were found to help identify adolescents with acute PID who have TOA. These patients may have fewer signs of acute illness than those without TOA and may develop symptoms later in the menstrual cycle. A six variable model was developed that performed best in differentiating the TOA and non-TOA group: last menstrual period more than 18 days prior to admission, previous PID, palpable adnexal mass, white blood cell count greater than or equal to 10,500/mL, erythrocyte sedimentation rate greater than 15 mm/h, and heart rate greater than 90/min.

Rupture of a TOA causes severe pain referred to the site of involvement. Chills, fever, and signs of progressing peritonitis follow the onset of pain. Diarrhea may occur early but ceases as the peritonitis worsens. If large volumes of pus are released into the peritoneal cavity, infection may spread upward along the colonic gutters; subphrenic abscesses may form, causing pain in the shoulders.

Intravenous clindamycin, cefoxitin, or metronidazole in combination with an aminoglycoside or single-agent therapy with a carbapenem, or a beta-lactamase inhibitor plus a penicillin (i.e. piperacillin plus tazobactam), are suitable choices for therapy. If no clinical response occurs after 48 to 72 hours or if the abscess enlarges, sonographiclly guided aspiration or surgery is necessary, while antibiotic therapy is continued (57,58).

Surgery is also necessary with a TOA rupture. This is vital since the patient fatality rate approaches 90% with medical therapy alone. Rapid diagnosis of such an abscess is the key to a successful outcome (53).

REFERENCES

1. Gorbach SL, Menda KB, Thadepalli H, Keith L. Anaerobic microflora of the cervix in healthy women. Am J Obstet Gynecol 1973; 117:1053–5.
2. Larsen B. Vaginal flora in health and disease. Clin Obstet Gynecol 1993; 36:107–21.
3. Hammerschlag MR, Alpert S, Onderdonk AB, et al. Anaerobic microflora of the vagina in children. Am J Obstet Gynecol 1978; 131:853–60.
4. Ross J. Pelvic inflammatory disease. Clin Evid 2006; 15:2176–82.
5. Forslin L, Falk V, Danielson D. Changes in the incidence of acute gonococcal and non-gococcal salpingitis. Br J Vener Dis 1978; 54:247–50.
6. Zeger W, Holt K. Gynecological infections. Emerg Med Clin North Am 2003; 21:631–8.
7. Sobel JD. Individualizing treatment of vaginal canal. Am Acad Dermatol 1990; 23:572–6.
8. Murphy TV, Nelson JD. Shigella vaginitis: report of 38 patients and review of the literature. Pediatrics 1979; 63:511–6.
9. Watkins S, Quan L. Vulvovaginitis caused by *Yersinia enterocolitica*. Pediatr Infect Dis 1984; 3:444–5.
10. Sweet RL. Role of bacterial vaginosis in pelvic inflammatory disease. Clin Infect Dis 1995; 20(Suppl. 2):S271–5.
11. Emans JS. Vulvovaginitis in the child and adolescent. Pediatr Rev 1986; 8:12–9.
12. Spiegel CA, Eschenbach DA, Amsel R, Holmes KK. Curved anaerobic bacteria in bacterial (nonspecific) vaginosis and their response to antimicrobial therapy. J Infect Dis 1983; 148:817–22.
13. Hammerschlag MR, Cummings M, Doraiswamy B, Cox P, McCormack WM. Nonspecific vaginitis following sexual abuse in children. Pediatrics 1985; 75:1028–31.
14. Schmitt C, Sobel JD, Meriwether C. Bacterial vaginosis: treatment with clindamycin cream versus oral metronidazole. Obstet Gynecol 1992; 79:1020–3.
15. Bristoletti P, Fredricsson B, Hagstrom B, et al. Comparison of oral and vaginal metronidazole therapy for non-specific bacterial vaginosis. Gynecol Obstet Invest 1986; 21:144–9.
16. Swedberg J, Steiner JF, Deiss F, et al. Comparison of single dose vs. one-week of metronidazole for symptomatic bacterial vaginosis. JAMA 1985; 254:1046–9.
17. Hill GB, Livengood CH, III. Bacterial vaginosis-associated microflora and effects of topical intravaginal clindamycin. Am J Obstet Gynecol 1994; 171:1198–204.
18. Parker RT, Jones CP. Anaerobic pelvic infections and developments in hyperbaric oxygen therapy. Am J Obstet Gynecol 1966; 96:645–59.
19. Swenson RM, Michaelson TC, Daly MJ, Spaulding EH. Anaerobic bacterial infections of the female genital tract. Obstet Gynecol 1973; 42:538–41.
20. van Bogaert LJ. Management of Bartholin's abscess. World Health Forum 1997; 18:200–1.
21. Brook I. Anaerobic bacteria in suppurative genitourinary infections. J Urol 1989; 141:889–93.
22. Brook I. Aerobic and anaerobic microbiology of Bartholin's abscess. Surg Gynecol Obstet 1989; 169:32–4.
23. Roberts DB, Hester LL, Jr. Progressive synergistic bacterial gangrene arising from abscesses of the vulva and Bartholin's gland duct. Am J Obstet Gynecol 1972; 114:285–91.
24. Omole F, Simmons BJ, Hacker Y. Management of Bartholin's duct cyst and gland abscess. Am Fam Physician 2003; 68:135–40.
25. Ross J. Pelvic inflammatory disease. BMJ 2001; 322:658–9.
26. Hillier SL, Kiviat NB, Hawes SE, et al. Role of bacterial vaginosis-associated microorganisms in endometritis. Am J Obstet Gynecol 1996; 175:435–41.
27. Carter B. A bacteriologic and clinical study of pyometra. Am J Obstet Gynecol 1951; 62:793–7.
28. Muram D, Drouin P, Thompson FE, Oxorn H. Pyometra. Can Med Assoc J 1981; 125:589–92.
29. Henriksen E. Pyometra associated with malignant lesions of the cervix and the uterus. Am J Obstet Gynecol 1956; 72:884–6.
30. Eschenbach DA, Buchanan TM, Pollock HM, et al. Polymicrobial etiology of pelvic inflammatory disease. N Engl J Med 1975; 293:166–71.
31. Cunningham FG, Hauth JC, Strong JD, et al. Evaluation of tetracycline or penicillin and ampicillin for treatment of acute pelvic inflammatory disease. N Engl J Med 1977; 296:1380–3.
32. Soper DE, Brockwell NJ, Dalton HP, Johnson D. Observations concerning the microbial etiology of acute salpingitis. Am J Obstet Gynecol 1994; 170:1008–14.
33. Walker CK, Workowski KA, Washington AE, Soper D, Sweet RL. Anaerobes in pelvic inflammatory disease: implications for the Centers for Disease Control and Prevention's guidelines for treatment of sexually transmitted diseases. Clin Infect Dis 1999; 28(Suppl. 1):S29–36.
34. Brook I. The role of beta-lactamase–producing bacteria in obstetrical and gynecological infections. Gynecol Obstet Invest 1991; 32:44–50.
35. Brook I. Induction of subcutaneous and intraperitoneal abscesses in mice by *Neisseria gonorrhoeae* and *Bacteroides* sp. Am J Obstet Gynecol 1986; 155:424–9.
36. Draper DL, James JF, Brooks GF, Sweet RL. Comparison of virulence markers of peritoneal and fallopian tube isolates with endocervical *Neisseria gonorrhoeae* isolates from women with acute salpingitis. Infect Immun 1980; 27:882–8.

37. Mikamo H, Kawazoe K, Izumi K, Watanabe K, Ueno K, Tamaya T. Studies on the pathogenicity of anaerobes, especially *Prevotella bivia*, in a rat pyometra model. Infect Dis Obstet Gynecol 1998; 6:61–5.
38. Guaschino S, De Seta F. Update on *Chlamydia trachomatis*. Ann NY Acad Sci 2000; 900:293–300.
39. Paavonen J, Saikku P, Vesterinen E, Aho K. *Chlamydia trachomatis* in acute salpingitis. Br J Vener Dis 1979; 55:203–6.
40. Dieterle S, Rummel C, Bader LW, Petersen H, Fenner T. Presence of the major outer-membrane protein of *Chlamydia trachomatis* in patients with chronic salpingitis and salpingitis isthmica nodosa with tubal occlusion. Fertil Steril 1998; 70:774–6.
41. Taylor–Robinson D. *Mycoplasma genitalium* – an update. Int J STD AIDS 2002; 13:145–51.
42. Heinonen PK, Miettinen A. Laparoscopic study on the microbiology and severity of acute pelvic inflammatory disease. Eur J Obstet Gynecol Reprod Biol 1994; 57:85–9.
43. Workowski KA, Berman SM. Centers for disease control and prevention. Sexually transmitted diseases treatment guidelines. Clin Infect Dis 2007; 44(Suppl. 3):S73–6.
44. Hecht DW. Anaerobes: antibiotic resistance, clinical, significance, and the role of susceptibility testing. Anaerobe 2006; 12:115–21.
45. Brook I. Metronidazole and spiramycin effect on *Bacteroides* sp. *Staphylococcus aureus* abscess. J Antimicrobial Chemother 1987; 20:713–8.
46. Wasserheit JN, Bell TA, Kiviat NB, et al. Microbial causes of proven pelvic inflammatory disease and efficacy of clindamycin and tobramycin. Ann Intern Med 1986; 104:187–93.
47. Lau CY, Qureshi AK. Azithromycin versus doxycycline for genital chlamydial infections: a meta-analysis of randomized clinical trials. Sex Transm Dis 2002; 29:497–502.
48. Beerthuizen RJ. Pelvic inflammatory disease in intrauterine device users. Eur J Contracept Reprod Health Care 1996; 1:237–43.
49. Atad J, Hallak M, Sharon A, Kitzes R, Kelner Y, Abramovici H. Pelvic actinomycosis. Is long-term antibiotic therapy necessary? Reprod Med 1999; 44:939–44.
50. Taylor ES, McMillan JH, Greer BE, Droegemueller W, Thompson HE. The intrauterine device and tubo-ovarian abscess. Am J Obstet Gynecol 1975; 123:338–48.
51. Kirby BD, George WL, Sutter VL, Citron DM, Finegold SM. Gram negative anaerobic bacilli: their role in infection and patterns of susceptibility to antimicrobial agents. I. Little known *Bacteroides* sp. Rev Infect Dis 1980; 2:914–51.
52. Thadepalli H, Gorbach SL, Keith L. Anaerobic infections of the female genital tract: bacteriologic and therapeutic aspects. Am J Obstet Gynecol 1973; 117:1034–40.
53. Landers DV, Sweet RL. Current trends in the diagnosis and treatment of tuboovarian abscess. Am J Obstet Gynecol 1985; 151:1098–110.
54. Tukeva TA, Aronen HJ, Karjalainen PT, Molander P, Paavonen T, Paavonen J. MR imaging in pelvic inflammatory disease: comparison with laparoscopy and US. Radiology 1999; 210:209–16.
55. Apter S, Shmamann S, Ben-Baruch G, Rubinstein ZJ, Barkai G, Hertz M. CT of pelvic infection after cesarean section. Clin Exp Obstet Gynecol 1992; 19:156–60.
56. Slap GB, Forke CM, Cnaan A, et al. Recognition of tubo-ovarian abscess in adolescents with pelvic inflammatory disease. J Adolesc Health 1996; 18:397–403.
57. Perez-Medina T, Huertas MA, Bajo JM. Early ultrasound-guided transvaginal drainage of tubo-ovarian abscesses: a randomized study. Ultrasound Obstet Gynecol 1996; 7:435–8.
58. Caspi B, Zalel Y, Or Y, Bar Dayan Y, Appelman Z, Katz Z. Sonographically guided aspiration: an alternative therapy for tubo-ovarian abscess. Ultrasound Obstet Gynecol 1996; 7:439–42.

25 | Cutaneous and Soft-Tissue Abscesses and Cysts

CUTANEOUS ABSCESSES

Subcutaneous and cutaneous abscesses can be caused by polymicrobial aerobic and anaerobic pathogens. Although the primary treatment of these infections is generally through surgical drainage, knowledge of their microbiology permits institution of empiric antimicrobial therapy before the results of cultures are available.

Microbiology

The most common etiologic agents involved in skin and soft-tissue infections are *Staphylococcus aureus* and group A beta-hemolytic streptococci (GABHS) (1). These organisms frequently produce impetigo, furunculosis, cellulitis, and wound infections (2). Gram-negative enteric bacteria (i.e. *Enterobacter* spp. and *Escherichia coli*) are also recovered occassionally.

The predominant anaerobes are gram-positive cocci, gram-negative bacilli (including *Bacteroides fragilis* group and *Prevotella* and *Porphyromonas* spp.), and *Fusobacterium* spp. (1–3). Anaerobes predominated in infections of the vulvovaginal, buttocks, perirectal, finger, and head areas. Aerobic bacteria are prevalent in the neck, hand, leg, and trunk areas. Many of these infections are polymicrobial (Fig. 1).

The most prevalent aerobe, *S. aureus*, is recovered whenever abscesses originate from skin surfaces. It is, however, found less often from the buttocks, perirectal, and vulvovaginal areas. The infections at these latter sites generally originate from adjacent mucous membranes rather than skin. Among gram-negative aerobes, *Enterobacter* spp. are recovered mostly from the trunk and legs, while *E. coli* is recovered mainly from the vulvovaginal, buttocks, and perirectal areas.

Peptostreptococcus spp. that are normal skin inhabitants and part of the endogenous gastrointestinal flora (4) are also isolated from infections at all sites. *B. fragilis* group, which predominate in the feces, are cultured most frequently from abscesses of the perirectal area. Pigmented *Prevotella* and *Porphyromonas* spp., which occur in stools as well as in the oral cavity (2,4), are recovered from infections proximal to these sites and from the head and neck. Most strains of *B. fragilis* group and many strains of *Prevotella*, *Porphyromonas*, and *Fusobacterium* spp. are resistant to penicillin. Beta-lactamase–producing bacteria (BLPB) are recovered in about half of the abscesses (5).

Pathogenesis

Predisposing factors to abscess formation include trauma, obstruction of drainage, ischemia, chemical irritation, hematoma formation, accumulation of fluid, foreign bodies, and stasis in the vascular system.

The location of the abscess is of paramount importance in the selection of the organism that may be involved in the infection. Under appropriate conditions of lowered tissue resistance, almost any of the common bacteria can initiate an infectious process. Cultures from lesions frequently contain several bacterial species; as might be expected, the organisms found most frequently are the "normal flora" of these regions (Fig. 1).

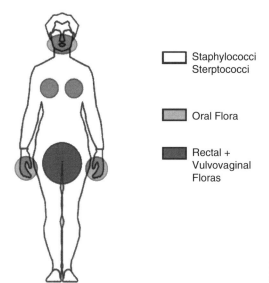

Staphylococci
Sterptococci

Oral Flora

Rectal +
Vulvovaginal
Floras

FIGURE 1 Distribution of organisms in abscesses, wounds, burns, and decubitus ulcers.

Aspirates from abscesses of the perineal and oral regions tend to yield organisms found in stool or mouth flora. Conversely, pus obtained from abscesses in areas remote from the rectum or mouth contain primarily constituents of the microflora indigenous to the skin (2–4).

Diagnosis

Skin and subcutaneous tissue infections are characterized by redness, tenderness, heat, and swelling. Associating lymphangitis is characterized by the presence of reddish streaks extending proximally and associated with tender enlargement of regional lymph nodes. Systemic symptoms may be mild, and include fever and malaise. Fluctuation in the abscess indicates that it is ready for drainage. Laboratory findings include leukocytosis, rapid sedimentation rate, and often positive blood cultures. Certain organisms can cause bacteremia more frequently, and manipulation, including surgical incision, of the abscess may be followed by transient bacteremia.

Pus or fluid obtained by aspiration or incision should be gram stained and cultured for aerobic and anaerobic bacteria.

X ray may detect localized collections of pus when free gas is present or when abnormal tissue density is observed. Ultrasound, computed tomography (CT), angiography, and radionuclide scans may be helpful (6).

Management

Surgical drainage is the treatment of choice. Although antimicrobials may prevent suppuration if given early or prevent spread of an existing abscess, they are not substituted for surgical drainage. Heat application can relieve the pain and speed suppuration and liquefaction.

Several antibiotics can be partially inactivated by pus and low pH (aminoglycosides and quinolones). The activity of antibiotics effective against multiplying organisms (i.e., beta-lactames) is impaired by the failure of bacteria to multiply in pus. Furthermore, phagocytosis is reduced in the cavity. Because of the combination of these factors, many abscesses are resistant to antimicrobial therapy.

Because anaerobes frequently are associated with cutaneous abscesses, especially in areas adjacent to mucosal surfaces, their presence should be anticipated if antimicrobial therapy is employed. Appropriate antimicrobial includes clindamycin, metronidazole, cefoxitin, tigecycline, a carbapenem (e.g., imipenem, meropenem, ertapenem), or a combination of a beta-lactamase inhibitor (i.e., clavulanic acid, tazobactam), and a penicillin (i.e., amoxicillin, ticarcillin, piperacillin). Linezolid, tigecycline, and vancomycin are administered for methicillin-resistant *S. aureus*.

Complications

The infection may spread locally or systemically. Local spread generally follows the path of least resistance along fascial planes. Lymphatic spread may lead to lymphangitis, lymphadenitis, or bubo. Involvement of veins may lead to infective thrombophlebitis, bacteremia, septic embolization, and systemic dissemination.

PARONYCHIA

Paronychia is an inflammation of the structure surrounding the nails. Paronychia, whether acute or chronic, results from a breakdown of the protective barrier between the nail and the nail fold. The entry of organisms into the moist nail crevice results in the bacterial or fungal (yeast or mold) colonization of the area. It is common in housewives, cleaners, nurses, children who suck their fingers, or others who often have their hands in water (7). Paronychia is more common in women than in men, with a female-to-male ratio of 3:1.

Microbiology and Pathogenesis

The bacteriology of paronychia is polymicrobial aerobic and anaerobic in three-fourth of the cases. The predominant aerobic organisms are *S. aureus*, *Streptococcus* spp., *Eikenella corrodens*, GABHS, *Klebsiella pneumoniae*, *Proteus* spp., *Pseudomonas aeruginosa*, and *Candida albicans*. The predominant anaerobes are gram-negative bacilli of oral origin (*Prevotella* and *Porphyromonas*), *Fusobacterium*, and *Peptostreptococcus* spp. BLPB are present in about half of the patients (8).

The anaerobic organisms isolated are part of normal oropharyngeal flora and may represent self-inoculation through nail biting and finger sucking of the patient's own mouth flora onto the finger. This phenomenon is parallel to the acquisition of infection following human bites and clenched fist injuries. In studies that applied methodology for cultivation of aerobic and anaerobic organisms in bite infections, anaerobic organisms were recovered from about half of the patients studied (9).

Acute paronychia usually results from a trauma that breaks down the physical barrier between the nail bed and the nail; this disruption allows the introduction of pathogens. Activities, such as nail biting, finger sucking, manicuring, or artificial nail placement, can also induce such trauma.

Chronic paronychia generally occurs in individuals whose hands are repeatedly exposed to moisture or have prolonged and repeated contact with irritants or chemicals. Especially susceptible are housekeepers, dishwashers, bartenders, and swimmers.

Diagnosis

Acute paronychia is manifested by erythema, fever, edema, and tenderness. There is less erythema in chronic paronychia, with a cushion-like thickening of the paronychial tissue. The nail plates may be thickened and discolored, with pronounced transverse ridges.

This condition begins as a subcuticular or intracutaneous infection with local exudate which eventually spreads under the fingernail base. Infection may follow the nail margin or extend beneath the nail and suppurate. Rarely, it penetrates deep into the finger, causing tendon necrosis and osteomyelitis. The chronically infected nail eventually becomes distorted.

When the exudate is purulent, a bacterial culture for aerobic and anaerobic bacteria is indicated. A microscopic examination in potassium hydroxide and culture for *Candida* and dermatophytes are helpful. A large amount of budding yeast on potassium hydroxide examination suggests that *Candida* may be of etiologic significance. A positive culture for *Candida* in the absence of a positive potassium hydroxide examination and clinical signs suggestive of candidiasis may indicate that the organism is a nonpathogen.

Management

An acute infection is treated with hot compresses or soaks of the affected finger three to four times per day and an appropriate systemic antibiotic. If the paronychia does not resolve or if it progresses to an abscess, it should be drained promptly. A purulent pocket should be opened cautiously with a scalpel. Infection extending along the tendon sheaths requires prompt surgical incision and drainage.

The initial treatment of chronic paronychia consists of the avoidance of inciting factors such as exposure to moist environments or skin irritants. Keeping the affected lesion dry is essential for proper recovery. Choice of footgear may also be considered. Mild cases of chronic paronychia may be treated with warm soaks. Chronic paronychia caused by dermatophytes that are sensitive to griseofulvin will respond readily to treatment with this agent. If *Candida* is present, nystatin or amphotericin-B lotion should be used, and occasionally either may be incorporated with the steroid. Oral therapy with antifungal agents (e.g., Ketoconazole) is useful if topical therapy failed (7).

Treatment effective against anaerobes of oral origin is warranted. When *S. aureus* is suspected, penicillin and a penicillinase-resistant penicillin should be used. Linezolid, tigecycline or vancomycin are indicated for methicillin-resistant *S. aureus*. The combination of a penicillin (i.e., amoxicillin, ticarcillin) and a beta-lactamase inhibitor (i.e., clavulanic acid) is effective. First-generation cephalosporins are not as effective as the above combination because of the resistance of some anaerobic bacteria and *E. corrodens*. Cefoxitin, a combination of a penicillin and a beta-lactamase inhibitor and the carbapenems are effective parenteral agents.

E. corrodens has unique susceptibility: it is susceptible to penicillin, ampicillin, azithromycin, and the quinolones but resistant to oxacillin, methicillin, nafcillin, and clindamycin, and occasionally resistant to cephalosporins.

The patient should avoid water, detergents, and chemicals, and dry their fingernail areas after washing. Sucking of fingers or nail biting should be avoided.

ANORECTAL ABSCESS

The classic locations of anorectal abscesses are: perianal (60% of all), ischiorectal (20%), intersphincteric (5%), supralevator (4%), and submucosal (1%). Perianal abscess is an infection of the soft tissues surrounding the anal canal, with formation of a discrete abscess cavity. The severity and depth of the abscess vary, and the abscess cavity is often associated with formation of a fistulous tract. The peak incidence of the abscesses is in the third to fourth decades of life and is more common in men than women. Perianal abscesses also occur in infants.

Microbiology

The infection is generally polymicrobial due to aerobic and anaerobic bacteria. The predominant anaerobes are gram-negative bacilli (including *B. fragilis* group and pigmented *Prevotella* and *Porphyromonas* spp.), gram-positive anaerobic cocci, *Fusobacterium*, and *Clostridium* spp. The predominant aerobes are *E. coli*, *S. aureus*, GABHS, *P. aeruginosa*, and *Proteus morganii* (10,11).

Pathogenesis

Perirectal abscesses and fistulas are anorectal disorders arising mainly from the obstruction of anal crypts. Infection of the static glandular secretions results in suppuration and abscess formation within the anal gland. The abscess typically forms initially within the intersphincteric space and then spreads along adjacent potential spaces. The abscess is initiated as a result of diarrhea or constipated that abrade the anal canal causing destruction of the normal mucosal barrier, allowing bacteria to invade perianal tissues and anal glands. Invading bacteria may be of stool or skin flora. If untreated, the abscess may burrow along the rectal sphincter, exiting next to the anus on the buttock, forming a fistula-in-ano. Alternatively, it may burrow through the musculature of the perirectal ring into the deeper tissues, forming an ischiorectal abscess. Predisposing condition includes ulcerative colitis, and primary, or secondary neutropenia.

Diagnosis

The clinical presentation correlates with the abscess anatomical location. Patients with perianal abscesses typically complain of dull perianal discomfort and pruritus. The pain often is exacerbated by movement and increased perineal pressure from sitting or defecation. Physical examination demonstrates a small, erythematous, well-defined, fluctuant, subcutaneous mass near the anal orifice.

Ischiorectal abscesses often present with systemic fevers, chills, and severe perirectal pain and fullness consistent with the more advanced nature of this process. External signs are minimal and may include erythema, induration, or fluctuance. On rectal examination, a fluctuant indurated mass can be encountered.

Intersphincteric abscesses are sometimes difficult to diagnose and present with rectal pain and localized tenderness on examination. Suspicion of an intersphincteric or supralevator abscess may require confirmation by CT scan, magnetic resonance imaging (MRI), or anal ultrasonography.

Management

Drainage is the mainstay. The abscess should be incised to prevent spread. Fistulous tracts must be opened and excised. Gram stain and cultures should be done. Administration of antimicrobials effective against anaerobic bacteria and enteric gram-negative rods is generally essential especially in the presence of a systemic inflammatory response, diabetes, or immunosuppression. The agents effective against anaerobes include: clindamycin, cefoxitin, chloramphenicol, or metronidazole. Aminoglycosides, quinolones, or third-generation cephalosporins provide coverage for gram-negative enteric rods. Single-agent therapy with cefoxitin, a carbapenem, tigecycline or the combination of a penicillin (such as ampicillin or ticarcillin), and a beta-lactamase inhibitor (such as sulbactam or clavulanic acid) may be adequate.

Complications

Complications include septicemia, anorectal fistulas, anal gangrene, and abscess recurrence.

PILONIDAL ABSCESS

Pilonidal sinus is a cyst which is a small midline closure defect that may that can collect debris and subsequent become inflamed. When it communicates with the subarachnoid space, it serve as a route of entry of bacteria into the central nervous system. It is more common in men than in women.

Microbiology and Pathogenesis

The infection is generally polymicrobial due mainly to enteric aerobic and anaerobic bacteria. Anaerobic isolates outnumbering aerobes at a ratio of 5:1 (12). The predominant anaerobic organisms are gram-negative bacilli (including *B. fragilis* group and pigmented *Prevotella* and *Porphyromonas* spp.), gram-positive anaerobic cocci, *Fusobacterium* spp., and *Clostridium* spp. The main aerobic organisms are *E. coli*, *Enterococcus* spp., *Proteus* spp., and *Pseudomonas* spp.

Diagnosis and Management

Physical findings dependent on the stage of disease. In the early stages, a sinus tract or pit is present in the sacrococcygeal region which can progress to midline edema or abscess. Examination of the abscess includes tenderness, fluctuance, warmth, purulent discharge, induration, or cellulitis. Fever and other systemic signs of infection are rare.

Surgical drainage is the therapy of choice. However, antimicrtobial therapy is needed. The choices of antimicrobial are similar to the one for perirectal abscess.

Complications

Complications include recurrence, systemic infection, abscess formation, squamous cell carcinoma, and verrucous carcinoma (13).

INFECTED EPIDERMAL CYSTS

Epidermal cysts are closed sacs with a definite wall that result from proliferation of surface epidermal cells. Production of keratin and lack of communication with the surface are responsible for cyst formation. Epidermal cysts can become infected and an abscess can develop.

Microbiology

The organisms known to cause most of epidermal cyst infections are *S. aureus*, GABHS, and anaerobic bacteria that originate from the normal flora adjacent to the site of cyst infection. Anaerobes are isolated in about half of the patients. The predominant anaerobic organisms are *Peptostreptococcus* spp. and gram-negative bacilli (including pigmented *Prevotella* and *Porphyromonas* spp. and *B. fragilis* group). The predominant aerobic or facultative bacteria are *S. aureus*, GABHS, and *E. coli.* (14,15). (See chapter 17).

S. *aureus* is the predominant isolate in infections in the trunk and extremities, but anaerobes are frequently isolated in cyst abscesses in rectal, vulvovaginal, head, and scrotal areas.

Management

Surgical drainage is the therapy of choice for an epidermal cyst abscess. However, recurrences are frequent because the keratin producing lining of the cyst is not removed. Administration of systemic antimicrobials may be indicated in selected severe cases, especially in immunocompromised patients or in instances where local or systemic spread of the infection has occurred.

Antimicrobial management of mixed infections requires the administration of antimicrobials effective against both aerobic and anaerobic bacterial components of the infection. Antimicrobials that provide coverage for *S. aureus* as well as the anaerobic bacteria include cefoxitin, clindamycin, a carbapenem, tigecycline, and the combination of beta-lactamase inhibitors and a penicillin. A combination of metronidazole and a beta-lactamase–resistant penicillin can be an alternative.

HIDRADENITIS SUPPURATIVA

Hidradenitis suppurativa (HS) is recurrent inflammation of the apocrine sweat glands, particularly those of the axilla, genital, and perianal areas. It can result in obstruction and rupture of the duct and secondary infection. The lesions generally drain spontaneously, with formation of multiple sinus tracts and with hypertrophic scarring. Although not initially infected, the lesions frequently become secondarily infected. Often, patients with HS also are afflicted with acne, pilonidal cysts, and chronic scalp folliculitis; thus, giving rise to the term follicular occlusion tetrad.

Microbiology and Pathogenesis

The infection is generally polymicrobial due mainly to aerobic and anaerobic bacteria of skin and proximal mucous membranes origin. Anaerobic bacteria alone or in combination with aerobic organisms were isolated from about two-thirds of patients. The predominant aerobic bacteria are *S. aureus* (isolated from about a third of cases), GABHS, microaerophilic streptococci, and *P. aeruginosa*. The most frequently isolated anaerobes are *Peptostreptococcus*, *Prevotella*, *Fusobacterium*, and *Bacteroides* spp. (16,17).

The anaerobes isolated from the patients are part of the flora of the oropharynx (*Prevotella* spp., *Fusobacterium* spp., *Peptostreptococcus* spp., and microaerophilic streptococci), gastrointestinal tract (*Bacteroides* spp., *Peptostreptococcus* spp.) (4), and skin (*Peptostreptococcus* spp.) and presumably reached the HS lesions from these sites.

Diagnosis

The primary lesions are reddish–purple nodules that gradually become fluctuant and drain. Irregular sinus tracts with repeated crops of lesions are formed; reparative processes are only partially successful. The involved areas show a mixture of burrowing, draining tracts, and ciccatricial scarring. In some, HI is associated with acne conglobata or dissecting cellulitis of the scalp that is often associated with spondyloarthropathy.

The patient can present with pain, multiple red, hard, raised nodules in areas where apocrine glands are concentrated. As suppuration progresses, surrounding cellulitis may emerge. Chronic recurrences result in palpable thick sinus tracts under the skin, which can turn into draining fistulas. In chronic condition, the multiple nodules can coalesced and be surrounded by a fibrous reaction resulting in scarred and unsightly appearance of the area.

HI can be a primary condition, but may be observed in association with: Crohn's disease, irritable bowel syndrome, Down syndrome, arthritis, Graves' disease or Hashimoto's thyroiditis, Sjögren's syndrome, and herpes simplex.

Culture of blood and any exudate and/or aspiration or drainage of larger nodules for aerobic and anaerobic bacteria should be obtained.

Management

Management is difficult and involves antimicrobial therapy, and moist heat locally to establish drainage in the initial phases of the infection. Large abscesses are surgically drained.

Gram's stain results may guide the clinician in selecting empiric antimicrobial therapy. However, the final choice of agents should be determined by the isolation of specific organisms, aerobes and anaerobes, and the results of sensitivity testing.

Initial empiric antimicrobial therapy should be effective against *S. aureus* as well as other potential aerobic and anaerobic pathogens. Antimicrobial agents active against *S. aureus* and anaerobic bacteria include clindamycin, a carbapenem, tigecycline, cefoxitin, and beta-lactamase inhibitor and penicillin combinations, and metronidazole with beta-lactamase–resistant penicillin. Cefoxitin and carbapenems also provide coverage against Enterobacteriaceae. However, agents active against Enterobacteriaceae (i.e., aminoglycosides, a quinolone, a fourth-generation cephalosporins) should be added when treating infections involving these bacteria.

PUSTULAR ACNE LESIONS

Acne vulgaris, a disorder of the pilosebaceous apparatus, is the most common skin disorder of the second and third decades of life.

Microbiology and Pathogenesis

Bacterial factors are important in the pathogenesis of acne. Acne is believed to be associated with *Propionibacterium acnes* (18). The improvement in acne patients treated with systemic antibiotics effective against *P. acnes*, as well as other organisms, support this concept.

The morphogenesis of acne lesions can be divided into two phases. The first phase is noninflammatory, during which keratin accumulates in affected follicles producing whiteheads (closed comedones), which have very small orifices, and blackheads (open comedones) which have distended orifices. The second is an inflammatory phase during which a variety of inflamed lesions may develop from a proportion of comedones.

P. acnes is known to be related with the inflammatory process in acne lesions (18), *Propionibacterium* spp. possess immunostimulatory mechanisms such as complement activation, stimulation of lysosomal enzyme release from human neutrophils, and production of serum-independent neutrophil chemotactic factors (19). Organisms other than *P. acne* may contribute to the inflammatory process. A recent study highlighted the polymicrobial nature of over two-thirds of culture positive pustular acne lesions and suggests the potential for pathogenic role of aerobic and anaerobic organisms other than *P. acnes* and *Staphylococcus* spp. in acne vulgaris (20). These include *Peptostreptococci* and anaerobic gram-negative bacilli such as *Porphyromonas* and *Prevotella* spp. (20).

Management

Antimicrobial therapy is a common adjuvant in the management of acne vulgaris. Topical or systemic antimicrobial agents effective against anaerobic bacteria including *P. acne* (i.e., clindamycin, macrolides and tetracylines) are beneficial. The empirical choice of antimicrobials may not always provide coverage for some of the resistant organisms that can be recovered from pustular acne lesions. Resistance of *P. acnes* to some of the topical antimicrobials has been increasing (21). Processing pustular specimens for aerobic and anaerobic bacteria can provide guidelines for adequate management of infected acne lesions.

REFERENCES

1. Finch R. Skin and soft-tissue infections. Lancet 1988; 1(8578):164–8.
2. Brook I, Frazier EH. Aerobic and anaerobic bacteriology of wounds and cutaneous abscesses. Arch Surg 1990; 125:1445–51.
3. Meislin HW, Lerner SA, Graves MH, et al. Cutaneous abscesses: anaerobic and aerobic bacteriology and outpatient management. Ann Intern Med 1977; 7:145–9.
4. Rosebury T. Microorganisms Indigenous to Man. New York: McGraw-Hill, 1962.
5. Brook I. Presence of beta-lactamase-producing bacteria and beta-lactamase activity in abscess. Am J Clin Pathol. 1986, 86;97–101.
6. John SD. Trends in pediatric emergency imaging. Radiol Clin North Am 1999; 37:995–1034.
7. Jebson PJ. Infections of the fingertip. Paronychias and felons. Hand Clin 1998; 14:547–55.
8. Brook I. Aerobic and anaerobic microbiology of paronychia. Ann Emerg Med 1990; 19:994–6.
9. Merriam CV, Fernandez HT, Citron DM, Tyrrell KL, Warren YA, Goldstein EJ. Bacteriology of human bite wound infections. Anaerobe 2003; 9:83–6.
10. Brook I, Martin WJ. Aerobic and anaerobic bacteriology of perirectal abscess in children. Pediatrics 1980; 66:282.
11. Brook I, Frazier EH. The aerobic and anaerobic bacteriology of perirectal abscesses. J Clin Microbiol 1997; 35:2974–6.
12. Brook I. Microbiology of infected pilonidal sinuses. J Clin Pathol 1989; 42:1140–2.
13. Gur E, Neligan PC, Shafir R, et al. Squamous all carcinoma in perineal inflammatory disease. Ann Plost Sung 1997; 38:653–7.
14. Brook I. Microbiology of infected epidermal cysts. Arch Dermatol 1989; 125:1658–61.
15. Nishijima S, Higashida T, Oshima S, Nakaya H. Bacteriology of epidermoid cysts. Jpn. J. Dermatol 2003; 113:165–8.
16. Highet AS, Warren RE, Weekes AJ. Bacteriology and antibiotic treatment of perineal suppurative hidradenitis. Arch Dermatol 1988; 124:1047–51.
17. Brook I, Frazier EH. Aerobic and anaerobic microbiology of axillary hidradenitis suppurativa. J Med Microbiol 1999; 48:103–5.
18. Burkhart CG, Burkhart CN, Lehmann PF. Acne: a review of immunologic and microbiologic factors. Postgrad Med J 1999; 75:328–31.
19. Kim J. Review of the innate immune response in acne vulgaris: activation of Toll-like receptor 2 in acne triggers inflammatory cytokine responses. Dermatology 2005; 211:193–8.
20. Brook I, Frazier EF, Cox ME, Yeager KJ. The aerobic and anaerobic microbiology of postular acnes. Anaerobe 1995; 1:305–7.
21. Leydenn JJ. Antibiotic resistance in topical treatment of acne vulgaris. Cutis. 2004; 73 (6 suppl) 6–10.

26 | Soft Tissue and Muscular Infections

Skin, soft tissue, and muscular infections are among the most common infections, and may sometimes lead to serious local and systemic complications. These infections can be potentially life-threatening infections that may have rapid progress. Their early recognition and proper medical and surgical management is therefore of primary importance.

Anaerobic infections of the skin and soft tissue frequently occur in areas of the body, which have been compromised or injured by foreign body, trauma, ischemia, malignancy, or surgery. Because the indigenous local microflora usually is responsible for these infections, anatomic sites that are subject to fecal or oral contamination are particularly at risk. These include wounds associated with surgery of the intestine or pelvic tract, human bites, decubitus ulcers in the perineal area, pilonidal cysts, omphalitis, and cellulitis around the fecal monitoring site (Fig. 1 in chap. 25).

Some of the clues to the anaerobic origin of such infections are putrid discharge, gas production, and extensive tissue necrosis with a tendency to burrow through subcutaneous and fascial planes.

Many wound and skin infections that complicate surgical operations or trauma are caused by mixed bacterial flora. Aerobic and anaerobic, gram-negative, and gram-positive organisms, whose origins are most often lesions or perforations of the gastrointestinal, respiratory, or genitourinary tracts, may be present in such infections, and they may exist synergistically. All clinical manifestations can be seen: cellulitis, abscess formation, thrombosis, necrosis, gangrene, and crepitus (1).

The majority of skin infections are associated with a mixed aerobic and anaerobic flora. There are, however, certain classic syndromes caused by specific anaerobes that have distinctive clinical presentations.

CLASSIFICATION AND DIAGNOSIS

Impetigo

Streptococcal impetigo manifests itself as appearance of small vesicles that rapidly pustulate and rupture. After the purulent discharge dries, a golden-yellow crust forms. The lesions remain superficial and do not ulcerate or infiltrate the dermis. Pain and scarring do not occur.

The bullous form of impetigo is due to *Staphylococcus aureus* (phage group II, usually type 71). The initial vesicles turn into fluid bullae that quickly rupture, leaving a moist red surface, which then generates "varnish-like" light brown crusts. Nikolsky sign and scarring do not occur.

The most severe form of *S. aureus* infection is staphylococcal scalded skin syndrome (SSSS), which is caused by a strain that produces exfoliative exotoxin, producing widespread bullae and exfoliation, with a positive Nikolsky sign (1). It starts abruptly, with fever, skin tenderness, and scarlatiniform rash. Bullae appear over two to three days, and are large and rupture promptly, leaving bright red skin surface.

Cellulitis

Cellulitis generally appears following trauma, with appearance of local tenderness, pain, and erythema. The area involved is red, hot, and swollen, with non-elevated borders, and is sharply demarcated streptococcal cellulitis following surgery can develop within 6 to 48 hours, be associated with hypotension, and a thin serous discharge. Regional lymphadenitis and bacteremia are common and can cause thrombophlebitis. The infection can spread rapidly in patients with dependent edema. Recurrent episodes of cellulitis of the lower extremities due to streptococci non-group A can occur in patients whose saphenous veins have been removed for coronary bypass (2). The patients often have systemic manifestation of fever; toxicity and chills; and edema, erythema, and tenderness along the saphenous venectomy site.

Infectious Gangrene (Gangrenous Cellulitis)

This is a rapidly progressive infection that involves extensive necrosis of the subcutaneous tissues and overlying skin. It includes several entities as follows:

1. Necrotizing fasciitis (NF; streptococcal gangrene)
2. Gas gangrene (clostridium myonecrosis) and anaerobic cellulitis
3. Progressive bacterial synergistic gangrene
4. Synergistic necrotizing cellulitis (perineal phlegmon) and gangrenous balanitis
5. Localized skin necrosis complicating cellulitis
6. Gangrenous cellulitis in the immunocompromised patient

Necrotizing Fasciitis
Streptococcal gangrene is an infection due to either group A, C, or G streptococci, initiated as an area of painful erythema and edema, which is followed in 24 to 72 hours by dusky skin, and yellowish to red-black fluid-filled bullae (3). The area is demarcated and is covered by necrotic eschar, surrounded by erythema resembling a third-degree burn. Unless treated a rapid progression occurs with frank cutaneous gangrene, accompanied sometimes by myonecrosis. Penetration along fascial planes can occur, followed by thrombophlebitis in the lower extremities, bacteremia at metastatic abscesses, and rapid death. Differentiation between cellulitis and NF is important. Cellulitis can be treated with antimicrobials alone while NF requires also surgical debridement of necrotic tissues.

Group A beta-hemolytic streptococcus (GABHS) infection can be associated with streptococcal toxic shock-like syndrome (TSLS) (4), which is manifested by fever, tachycardia, hypotension, multiorgan failure, and in 80% evidence of soft tissue infection (Table 1).

NF of the newborn, which involves the anterior abdominal wall, may extend to the flanks and the chest wall.

NF due to mixed anaerobic–aerobic flora is usually associated with endogenous source of the organisms, and presents in slightly different fashion. The involved area is first erythematous,

TABLE 1 Clinical Presentations of Soft Tissue Infections

	Necrotizing fasciitis (streptococcal gangrene)	Gas gangrene (clostridial myonecrosis)	Progressive bacterial synergistic gangrene	Synergistic necrotizing cellulitis	*Pseudomonas* gangrenous cellulitis
Fever	High	Moderate to high	Minimal or absent	Moderate	High
Systemic toxicity	Significant	Very significant	Minimal	Significant	Significant
Pain	Minimal	Significant	Significant	Significant	Mild
Crepitus	Absent	Present	Absent	Often present	Absent
Anaesthesia of lesions	Sometimes present	Absent	Absent	Absent	Sometimes present
Appearance of infection	Subcutaneous tissue and fascial necrosis. Overlying skin necrotic and dark	Significant edema. Yellow-brown discoloration of skin. Brown bullae. Necrotic area composed of green-black patches. Serosanguinous discharge	Necrotic central ulcer, dusky margin, and erythematous periphery	Crepitus cellulitis with foul-smelling, thick discharge from necrotic skin	Black/gray eschar dark discharge with surrounding erythema

swollen, hot, tender, painful, and has no sharp margin (5). Progression occurs within three to five days, with skin breakdown with bullae and cutaneous gangrene. The involved area becomes anesthetic because of small-vessel thrombosis that supplies the superficial nerves. The development of anesthesia can antedate the appearance of skin necrosis, and signifies the presence of NF and not simple cellulitis. Easy passage through an incision in the lesion along a plane with a probing hemostat is also diagnostic. Subcutaneous gas and foul smell are often present in polymicrobial infection, especially in those with diabetes. Systemic toxicity and elevated temperature are common. NF of the face, eyelids, neck, and lips (6–8) are rare but can be life threatening. Crepitus, severe pain, and necrosis of the epidermis and superficial fascia are evident. The infection can spread rapidly to other areas in the neck.

Gas Gangrene, Anaerobic Cellulitis
In clostridial anaerobic cellulitis, the onset is gradual after a few days of incubation, and is in a form of minimal local pain and swelling and no systemic toxicity. This distinguishes the process from true gas gangrene. A thin, dark, sometimes foul-smelling discharge and extensive tissue gas formation manifesting crepitus is seen. The clinical presentation of non-clostridial anaerobic cellulitis is similar to clostridial cellulitis.

Progressive Bacterial Synergistic Gangrene
The infection generally starts as a local area of tenderness, swelling, and erythema, which subsequently ulcerates. The painful ulcer enlarges and is surrounded by violaceous zone that fades into pink edematous border. Left untreated, the ulcer enlarges and may burrow through tissue emerging in distant sites (Meleney's ulcer) (9).

Synergistic Necrotizing Cellulitis
This infection in the form of Fournier's gangrene, starts as cellulitis, adjacent to the entry point, and involves the deep fascia. Pain, fever, and systemic toxicity occur. Swelling and crepitus of the scrotum increases, and gangrene develops. Abdominal wall involvement can be especially rapid in diabetics.

Gangrenous Cellulitis in the Immunocompromised Host
Cellulitis in the immunocompromised can be caused by expected pathogens as well as opportunistic ones. *Pseudomonas aeruginosa* is the major pathogen causing a sharply demarcated necrotic area with black eschar and surrounding erythema that may evolve from initial hemorrhagic bulla. *Rhizopus* spp. can be indolent, with slowly enlarging black ulcer, or may be rapidly progressive. The lesion has a central anesthetic black necrotic area with surrounding violaceous cellulitis and edema (10). Ulcerative or nodular lesions due to opportunistic organisms can develop in immunocompromised patients after trauma.

Secondary Bacterial Infections Complication Skin Lesions

Diabetic foot infections are divided into non-limb–threatening and limb-threatening. Non-limb–threatening infections are superficial, lack systemic toxicity, have minimal cellulitis that extends <2 cm from port of entry, and if ulceration is present it does not extend through the skin, and does not show signs of ischemia. Limb-threatening infections are associated with ischemia, have more extensive cellulitis, lymphangitis is present, and the ulcers penetrate through the skin into the subcutaneous tissue. Epidermal cysts in the chest, trunk, extremities, and vulvovaginal and scrotal areas can also become severely infected (11). Other skin lesions that can be secondarily infected with bacteria are the following: scabies (12), eczema herpeticum (13), psoriasis (14), poision ivy (15), diaper dermatitis (16), kerion (17), and atopic dermatitis (18).

MICROBIOLOGY

Impetigo

Most cases of impetigo and cellulitis are attributed to *S. aureus* and GABHS alone or in combination (Table 2) (19). A retrospective study investigated both the aerobic and anaerobic

TABLE 2   Bacterial Etiology

Impetigo and cellulitis, diabetic, and chronic skin ulcers
   Streptococcus group A
   Staphylococcus aureus
   Anaerobic oral flora (*Prevotella, Fusobacterium*, and *Peptostreptococcus* spp.)
   around oral area and head and neck
   Colonic flora: Enterobacteriaceae and anaerobes (i.e., *Escherichia coli* and
   Bacteroides fragilis group) around rectum and lower extremity
Necrotizing fasciitis
   Streptococcus group A (rarely also group C or E)
   S. aureus
   Enterobacteriaceae
   Enteric or oral anaerobes
Gas gangrene and crepitus cellulitis
   Clostridium perfringens and other *Clostridium* spp.
Progressive bacterial gangrene
   Peptostreptococcus spp.
   Microaerophilic streptococci
   Proteus spp.
Myositis
   S. aureus
   Streptococcus groups A, B, C, and G
   Enterobacteriaceae
   Yersinia entercolitica
   Pseudomonas spp.
   Aeromonas spp.
   Clostridium spp. (especially *perfringens*)
   Peptostreptococcus spp.
   Bacteroides spp.

microbiology of nonbullous impetigo in 40 children (20). Aerobic or facultative anaerobic bacteria only were present in 24 patients (60%), strict anaerobic bacteria only in 5 patients (12.5%), and mixed anaerobic–aerobic flora was present in 11 patients (27.5%). Sixty-four isolates were recovered: 43 aerobic or facultative and 21 anaerobic. The predominant aerobic and facultative bacteria were *S. aureus* (29 isolates) and GABHS (13). The predominant anaerobes were *Peptostreptococcus* spp. (12), pigmented *Prevotella* spp. (5), and *Fusobacterium* spp. (2). Single bacterial isolates were recovered in 17 patients (42.5%), 13 of which were *S. aureus*. *S. aureus* alone or mixed with GABHS or *Peptostreptococcus* spp. were isolated from all body sites. Mixed flora of *Peptostreptococcus* spp. with *Prevotella* or *Fusobacterium* spp. was mostly found in infections of the head and neck, while *Escherichia coli* mixed with *Bacteroides fragilis* and *Peptostreptococcus* spp. were isolated from infection of the buttocks area.

Cellulitis

GABHS is the major and *S. aureus* is a minor cause of the classic erysipelas. Streptococci other than group A were isolated in lower extremity cellulitis involved in post-saphenous venectomy (groups C, G, and B) (2) and in neonatal cellulitis. Cellulitis due to *Streptococcus pneumoniae* through bacteremic route were also described (21). Enterobacteriaceae and fungi (*Cryptococcus neoformans*) were recovered from cellulitis in the immunocompromised host. *E. coli* was recovered from children with nephrotic syndrome who developed cellulitis (22). *Aeromonas hydrophila* is recognized as a cause of cellulitis after laceration that occurred when swimming in fresh water and *Vibrio* spp. can infect wounds sustained in saltwater (23). Bacteremia and cellulitis due to *Vibrio vulnificus* may follow ingestion of raw oysters, especially in patients with alcoholic cirrhosis (24). *P. aeruginosa* is the major pathogen in bacteremia-associated cellulitis in the immunocompromised host.

The microbiology of cellulitis and its correlation with the site of infection was investigated in 278 swab and 64 needle aspirate specimens (25). Aerobic or facultative bacteria only were present in 138 (53%) of swab samples, anaerobic bacteria only in 69 (27%), and mixed aerobic–anaerobic flora in 52 (20%). In total, there were 582 isolates, 247 aerobic or facultative and 335 anaerobic bacteria (2.2 isolates/specimen). The predominance of certain isolates in different anatomical sites correlated with their distribution in the normal flora adjacent to the infected site. The highest recovery rates of anaerobic bacteria were from the neck, trunk, groin, external genitalia, and leg areas. Aerobes outnumbered anaerobes in the arm and hand. The predominant aerobes were *S. aureus*, GABHS, and *E. coli*. The predominant anaerobes were *Peptostreptococcus* spp., *B. fragilis* group, *Prevotella* spp., *Porphyromonas* spp., and *Clostridium* spp. Certain clinical findings correlated with the following organisms: swelling and tenderness with *Clostridium* spp., *Prevotella* spp., *S. aureus*, and GABHS; regional adenopathy with *B. fragilis* group; bollous lesions with Enterobacteriaceae; gangrene and necrosis with *Peptostreptococcus* spp., *B. fragilis* group, *Clostridium* spp., and Enterobacteriaceae; foul odor with *Bacteroides* spp.; and gas in tissues with *Peptostreptococcus* spp., *B. fragilis* group, and *Clostridium* spp. Certain predisposing conditions correlated with the following organisms: trauma with *Clostridium* spp.; diabetes with *Bacteroides* spp., Enterobacteriaceae, and *S. aureus*; and burn with *P. aeruginosa*.

Necrotizing Fasciitis

There are two main bacterial causes of NF: *Streptococcus pyogenes* (GABHS) and synergistic infection due to facultative and anaerobic bacteria. Streptococcal gangrene is due to either groups A, C, or G streptococci. However, GABHS can be recovered mixed also with other organisms. The predominant organisms present in synergistic infection, including those of the male genital area, Enterobacteriaceae, *S. aureus*, *Peptostreptococcus* spp., *Clostridium* spp., *Fusobacterium* spp., and *B. fragilis* group.

The most common GABHS recovered in recent outbreaks have been M1/T1 or M12/T12 types that contained pyrogenic exotoxin A or C genes (26).

Brook and Frazier (8) studied the microbiological and clinical characteristics of 83 patients with NF. Bacterial growth was noted in 81 of 83 (98%) specimens from the patients. Aerobic or facultative bacteria only were recovered in 8 (10%) specimens, anaerobic bacteria only in 18 (22%) specimens, and mixed aerobic–anaerobic flora in 55 (68%) specimens. In total, there were 375 isolates, 105 aerobic or facultative bacteria and 270 anaerobic bacteria (4.6 isolates/specimen). The recovery of certain bacteria from different anatomical locations correlated with their distribution in the normal flora adjacent to the infected site. Anaerobic bacteria outnumbered aerobic bacteria at all body sites, but the highest recovery rate of anaerobes was in the buttocks, trunk, neck, external genitalia, and inguinal areas. The predominant aerobes were *S. aureus*, *E. coli*, and GABHS. The predominant anaerobes were *Peptostreptococcus* spp., *Prevotella* spp., *Porphyromonas* spp., *B. fragilis* group, and *Clostridium* spp. Certain clinical findings correlated with some bacteria: edema with *B. fragilis* group, *Clostridium* spp., *S. aureus*, *Prevotella* spp., and GABHS; gas and crepitation in tissues with Enterobacteriaceae and *Clostridium* spp.; and foul odor with *Bacteroides* spp. Certain predisposing conditions correlated with some organisms: trauma with *Clostridium* spp.; diabetes with *Bacteroides* spp., Enterobacteriaceae, and *S. aureus*; and immunosuppression and malignancy with *Pseudomonas* spp. and Enterobacteriaceae.

A smaller study evaluated specimens obtained from eight children with NF (27). A total of 21 isolates were recovered, 13 anaerobic and 8 aerobic or facultatives. The facultative organism GABHS was present alone in two (25%) instances, and mixed aerobic and anaerobic bacteria were isolated in six (75%). The predominant isolates were *Peptostreptococcus* spp. (6 isolates, including 3 *Peptostreptococcus magnus*), GABHS (4), *B. fragilis* group (3), *Clostridium perfringens* (2), *E. coli* (2), and *Prevotella* spp. (2). Organisms similar to the ones isolated from the NF aspirates were recovered in the blood of all patients except one. These included GABHS (3 isolates), *B. fragilis* group (2), *E. coli* (1), *P. magnus* (1), and *C. perfringens* (1). All patients underwent surgical fasciotomy, and four required skin grafting. Antimicrobials were administered to all children. Despite extensive resection and intense supportive therapy, three patients died from sepsis accompanied by shock, acidosis and disseminated intravascular coagulation. These findings illustrate the polymicrobial aerobic–anaerobic flora of NF in children.

Gas Gangrene and Crepitant Cellulitis

C. perfringens is the most common *Clostridium* spp. causing the infection. *Clostridium septicum* and other species (*Clostridium novyi, Clostridium bifermentans, Clostridium histolyticum, Clostridium sordellii,* and *Clostridium fallax*) have also been recovered. Occasionally, the clostridium is recovered mixed with other aerobic and anaerobic bacteria.

Progressive Bacterial Synergistic Gangrene

Anaerobic or microaerophilic streptococci can be recovered from the advanced margin of the lesion, while *S. aureus* and sometimes gram-negative aerobic bacilli (especially *Proteus* spp.) can be isolated from the ulcerated area.

Diabetic and Other Chronic Superficial Skin Ulcers and Subcutaneous Abscesses

Decubitus ulcers can be colonized and infected by a variety of aerobic and anaerobic bacteria. The distribution of organisms depends on the location of the ulcer. While GABHS and *S. aureus* can be isolated in all body sites, organisms of oral flora origin (*Fusobacterium* spp., pigmented *Prevotella* and *Porphyromonas*, and *Peptostreptococcus* spp.) can be isolated in ulcers and wounds proximal to that site, while organisms of colonic or vaginal flora origin (*B. fragilis* group, *Clostridium* spp., *Peptostreptococcus* spp., and Enterobacteriaceae) can be recovered from lesions proximal to the perianal area (28). This principle applies to recovery of organisms in other skin and soft tissue wounds and abscesses (28,29); secondarily infected wounds and skin lesions caused by scabies (12); superficial thrombophlebitis (30); decubitus ulcers (31); diaper dermatitis (16); atopic dermatitis (18); kerion lesions (17); secondarily infected eczema herpeticum (13), psoriasis lesions (14), and poison ivy (15). Foot infections in diabetic patients are infected with *S. aureus*, group B *Streptococci, Enterococcus* spp., Enterobacteriaceae, and other gram-negative aerobic bacteria, as well as peptostreptococci and *B. fragilis* group (32,33).

Myositis

S. aureus is the predominant cause of tropical and nontropical infection (34). GABHS and other groups (B, C, and G), as well as *S. pneumoniae* and *Streptococcus anginosus* can be recovered. Gram-negative aerobic and facultatives have also been rarely recovered. These include Enterobacteriaceae, *Yersinia enterocolitica, Pseudomonas* spp., *Haemophilus influenzae, Neisseria gonorrhoeae,* and *Aeromonas* spp.

   Anaerobic bacteria such as *Bacteroides, Fusobacterium, Clostridium,* and *Peptostreptococcus* spp. have also been recovered in studies where proper methods for their isolation were employed in adults (35) and children (36). Pyogenic myositis can be classified into several major groups according to the organisms recovered: GABHS necrotizing myositis, clostridial myonecrosis (gas gangrene), and non-clostridial (crepitant) myositis. *C. perfringens* accounts for 80% to 95% of cases, *C. novyi* for 10% to 40%, and *C. septicum* for 5% to 15%. Rarely other clostridial species can be isolated: *C. bifermentans, C. fallax,* and *C. histolyticum*. Other organisms such as *E. coli*, Enterococci, and *Enterobacter* spp. can also be recovered mixed with *Clostridium* spp. Non-clostridial myositis can be divided into subgroups: anaerobic streptococcal myonecrosis—which is a mixed infection of GABHS or *S. aureus* with *Peptostreptococcus* spp.; synergistic non-clostridial anaerobic myonecrosis—due to polymicrobial flora; infected vascular gangrene—due to Bacteroides and other anaerobes plus *Proteus* spp.; and *A. hydrophila*—myonecrosis. Psoas abscess is generally due to *S. aureus* or polymicrobial aerobic–anaerobic flora.

PATHOGENESIS

Soft tissue and muscular infections frequently occur in areas of the body, which have been compromised or injured by foreign body, trauma, ischemia, malignancy, or surgery. Because the indigenous local microflora usually is often responsible for these infections, anatomic sites that are subject to fecal or oral contamination are particularly at risk. These include wounds associated with surgery of the intestinal tract, pelvis, human bites, decubitus ulcers in the perineal area, pilonidal cysts, omphalitis, and cellulitis around the fetal monitoring site.

Skin and Subcutaneous Infection

Predisposing conditions to progressive bacterial synergistic gangrene include (Table 3) surgery and draining sinus; to synergistic necrotizing cellulitis—diabetes, to streptococcal gangrene—diabetes, myxedema, and prior abdominal surgery; to clostridial myonecrosis (gas gangrene)—trauma, to necrotizing cutaneous mucormycosis—diabetes and corticosteroids therapy; to *Pseudomonas* gangrenous cellulitis—burns, and immunosuppression; and to pyoderma gangrenosum—ulcerative collitis and rheumatoid arthritis.

The acquisition of a potential pathogen as part of the skin flora such as GABHS generally antedates the emergence of impetigo by about 10 days (37). This organism can also colonize the nasopharynx in about a third of the patients with skin infection. Infection caused by GABHS may follow minor trauma such as abrasion or insect bite, especially during the hot and humid summer period. In contrast, facial impetigo occurring in cooler climates is generally a result of a contiguous spread from the nasopharynx.

Impetigo due to *S. aureus*, however, generally follows nasal colonization that is later followed by skin colonization (38). Trauma, or an underlying skin lesion (ulcer, furuncle), predisposes to the development of cellulitis. Rarely bloodborne spread can cause the infection. Cellulitis due to non-GABHS streptococci can develop in patients whose saphenous veins were used for coronary artery bypass (2). Cellulitis due to group streptococci and Enterococcus spp. can occur in patients with lower extremity lymphedema secondary to radical pelvic surgery, radiation therapy, or neoplasm of the pelvic lymph nodes (39,40). Cellulitis due to waterborne organisms can be caused after laceration sustained in fresh water (*A. hydrophila*) (41) and saltwater (*Vibrio* spp.) (24).

Gangrenous cellulitis generally follows introduction of the invading organism to the infected site. It can also develop from extension of the infection from deeper sites to the subcutaneous and skin tissues. This can follow intestinal surgery where clostridial myonecrosis develop, or when perirectal abscess dissects the perineal area to cause phlegmon.

Progressive bacterial synergistic gangrene following abdominal surgery is more common when wire sutures are used, in cases of ileostomy or colostomy, and at the exit of a fistulous tract adjacent to chronic ulceration in an extremity (9,42).

Gangrenous cellulitis can also start at a site of a metastatic infection due to bacteremia. An example is clostridial myonecrosis due to *C. septicum*, which originated from a colonic malignancy, or in *Aspergillus* or *Pseudomonas* gangrenous cellulitis.

A compromised patient is more susceptible to skin and subcutaneous infections caused by a variety of organisms, many of which do not cause infection in the normal host. Mucormycotic gangrene can develop in diabetic patients, those who receive immunosuppressive therapy or sustain an extensive burn wound. This infection occurs more frequently in conjunction with local factors such as fistulous tracts, ileostomy stomas, and open fracture sites. Infection with *Rhizopus* spp. can follow the use of an elastic bandage contaminated with the spores (10). Patients with chronic renal failure (with secondary hyperparathyroidism), those who are in chronic dialysis, or have extensive calcification of small arteries, can develop skin and subcutaneous fat necrosis (43). Skin lesions (such as eczematous dermatitis, traumatic lesions, etc.) can become secondarily infected, causing minimal-to-extensive infections (12–18).

Diabetic foot and other superficial skin ulcers can also become infected. The nature of the ulcer, which includes tissue necrosis and extensive undermining, and its location near mucous membrane orifices (anal, vaginal, or oral) that is colonized with aerobic and anaerobic flora, enables the adjacent flora to invade the ulcers. Infection in diabetic patients generally follows minor trauma in individuals with neuropathy and arterial vascular insufficiency. It then may progress to cellulitis, soft tissue necrosis, and osteomyelitis with a draining sinus.

Clostridial anaerobic cellulitis is most often caused by *C. perfringens* that is usually introduced into subcutaneous tissues through a contaminated or inadequately debrided

TABLE 3 Risk Factors for Soft Tissue and Muscular Infections

Skin and subcutaneous infection
Progressive bacterial synergistic gangrene
Surgery, draining sinus trauma
Synergistic necrotizing cellulitis
Diabetes, trauma
Streptococcal gangrene
Trauma, diabetes, myxedema, abdominal surgery, steroid and nonsteroidal
anti-inflammatory, varicella
Clostridial myonecrosis (gas gangrene)
Diabetes, corticosteroid therapy, trauma
Necrotizing cutaneous mucormycosis
Diabetes, corticosteroid therapy
Bacterial pseudomonal gangrenous cellulitis
Burns, immunosuppression
Pyoderma gangrenosum
Ulcerative colitis, rheumatic fever

wound. The source of the infection can also be a preexisting infection especially of the perineum, abdominal wall, buttocks, and lower extremities that can become contaminated with fecal flora. The presence of necrotic tissue or foreign material in the wound enhances infection with *Clostridium* spp. The source of *C. septicum* cellulitis in patients with leukemia and granulocytogenia (44), is bacteremia which originate from intestinal erosions.

NF due to GABHS, can occur after trauma, burn, childbirth, insect bite, muscle strain, penetrating wounds and splinters, surgery (especially in patients with diabetes, peripheral vascular disease, varicella infection, cirrhosis), and nonsteroidal anti-inflammatory and corticosteroid therapy (45). Predisposition to Fournier's gangrene, which is a form of NF in the male genitals, include local trauma, diabetes, paraphimosis, periurethral extravasation of urine, and perirectal or perianal infection and surgery in the area (i.e., herniorrhaphy, circumcision) (46). The infection can extend to the abdominal wall, especially in patients with diabetics, obesity, advanced age, and cardiorenal disease.

Trauma often predisposes to NF of the periorbital or facial areas, and oral, pharyngeal, or dental infection predisposes to cervical infection. NF in the newborn is often a complication of omphalitis. NF in older individuals can affect any body part. The portal of entry is usually a site of trauma, laparotomy in the presence of peritoneal soiling, or other surgical procedure, IM injections and IV infusions, local hypoxia, perirectal abscess, and decubitus ulcers in patients with intestinal perforation. Predisposing conditions include diabetes mellitus, alcoholism, and intravenous drug abuse (8).

Some subcutaneous infections, mostly subcutaneous abscesses, often in children, are a manifestation of osteomyelitis. This is as a result of a rupture of a subperiosteal abscess into the subcutaneous tissue. A draining sinus can be caused by chronic osteomyelitis. Bacteremia or endocarditis can predispose to metastatic pyogenic infection in the subcutaneous tissues in the form of an abscess.

Myositis

Infectious myositis caused by bacteria can invade from contiguous sites such as skin and subcutaneous abscesses, ulcers, penetrating wounds, and osteomyelitis; or through hematogenous spread. Trauma is a common cause in children (36,47). Vascular insufficiency in an extremity can also facilitate the process. However, primary muscle abscess can also occur in the absence of a predisposing site of infection (48). No conclusive evidence exists, which relate tropical pyomyositis causality to predisposing conditions unique to the tropics (i.e., filariasis, malaria, arbovirus). However, about two-thirds of tropical myositis cases have predisposing condition that includes diabetes, alcoholism, corticosteroid therapy, immunosuppressive therapy, hematological illnesses, and human immunodeficiency virus (HIV) infection (34,48).

The increased susceptibility of HIV patients to pyomyositis is believed to be due to the combination of the underlying cell-mediated immunodeficiency, defective neutrophils activity, and the potential of muscle injury (HIV myopathy, anti-retroviral associated mitochondrial myopathy, and concomitant bacterial infection). Clostridial myonecrosis usually follows muscle injury and contamination by dirt or during surgery. Contamination of the muscle can occur as a result of compound fracture penetrating war wounds (49), surgical wounds, especially following bowel or biliary tract surgery, arterial insufficiency of an extremity (50), and rarely after parenteral injection of medication, especially epinephrine in oil.

Spontaneous, nontraumatic gas gangrene is mostly due to *C. septicum*, which spreads by bacteremic route. Intestinal abnormalities that include necrotizing enterocolitis; volvulus; colon cancer; diverticulitis and bowel infarction; and leukemia, neutropenia, and diabetes mellitus are the major predisposing conditions.

Psoas abscess generally develops as a result of spread from an adjacent structure, either as an extension of intra-abdominal infection (appendicitis, diverticulitis, Crohn's disease), perinephric abscess, or infected retroperitoneal hematoma. It can also originate from vertebral tuberculosis or *S. aureus* osteomyelitis. Osteomyelitis of the ilium or septic arthritis of the sacroiliac joint can produce iliacis or psoas abscess.

DIAGNOSIS

The recovery of fastidious organisms depends on employment of proper methods for collection, transportation of specimen, and cultivation of organisms. Since many potential pathogens are part of the normal skin or mucous membrane flora, specimens should be obtained using methods of collection that will bypass the normal skin and mucous membrane flora. Therefore, disinfecting the skin, obtaining deep tissue, or surgically obtained aspirates will yield reliable specimens (51). A study compared the skin swab and needle aspirate methodology to establish the aerobic and anaerobic microbiology of perianal cellulitis in 10 children (52). This study demonstrated the superiority of needle aspirates in establishing the microbiology of the infection. Complete or partial concordance in microbiology between skin swabs and needle aspirates was present in six instances. In four instances, isolates recovered from needle aspirates were not isolated from the skin surface.

Radiological studies of soft tissue can reveal the presence of free gas in the tissue. This can assist in the differentiation between NF due to either streptococcal or mixed polymicrobial aerobic–anaerobic infection, and also signify the presence of gas-forming bacteria in other types of necrotic infections. A feathery linery pattern of gas can be observed in infected muscles in clostridial myonecrosis.

The presence of osteomyelitis as a cause of subcutaneous abscess or sinus tract can be discovered by radiological and radionuclide scanning studies. Plain radiograph can show osteopenia or osteolytic lesions, periosteal elevation, and periosteal new bone formation. Sclerotic lesions can be seen when the infection has been present for longer than a month.

Radionuclide scanning is useful in early diagnosis of osteomyelitis. Technetium-labeled methylene diphosphonate isotope is used most frequently, since its uptake by infected bone is enhanced with increased osteoblastic activity. In some cases, decreased uptake can be observed, reflecting compromised vascular supply to the bone.

Radionuclide (^{67}Ga) scanning can be used in the diagnosis of pyomyositis. It shows diffuse uptake in the involved area, but does not differentiate intramuscular abscess from necrotizing myositis or NF.

Computed tomography (CT) can show low-density areas with muscle loss, and a surrounding rim of contrast enhancement typical of pyomyositis. Magnetic resonance imaging (MRI) can detect alteration in soft tissue and is particularly useful in differentiating cellulitis from pus and abscess formation. MRI can show enlargement of involved muscles and areas of signal attenuation suggestive of fluid collection. Sonography or CT can be used to guide diagnostic aspiration.

CT scanning is the most rapid and sensitive method to diagnose psoas and iliacus muscle infection. It can show diffuse enlargement of the involved muscle, and may demonstrate the presence of gas within the muscle suggesting the presence of an abscess (53). The technique of SPECT/CT imaging is capable of co-localizing inflammatory signals with musculo-skeletal and internal structures. MRI is more sensitive in showing early inflammatory changes prior to development of frank abscess cavity and can show enlarged muscles. However, some infections can develop very rapidly, to life-threatening systemic illness, and definitive diagnosis of the nature and extent of necrotic fasciitis or myositis is made only on surgical exploration.

MANAGEMENT

Certain clinical conditions require prompt and urgent action. This is needed in SSSS, when a widespread rapid progressing bullae and exfoliation occurs, which starts abruptly, accompanied with fever, skin tenderness and scarlatiniform rash. Fluid replacement and antimicrobials should be given without delay. TSLS manifested by fever, tachycardia, hypotension, and multiorgan failure also requires urgent care.

Rapid surgical and medical responses are indicated in cellulitis that progresses into thrombophlebitis and bacteremia. Similarly, urgent intervention is needed in any of the infectious gangrenes (gangrenous cellulitis) which are rapidly progressive infection that involves extensive necrosis of the subcutaneous tissues and overlying skin. Special attention to progression should be given to NF where penetration along facial planes can occur, followed by thrombophlebitis in the lower extremities, bacteremia and metastatic abscesses, systemic toxicity, and rapid death. The development of local anesthesia can antedate the appearance of skin necrosis, and signifies the presence of NF and not simple cellulitis. Abdominal wall involvement can progress especially rapidly in diabetics with synergistic necrotizing cellulitis. Special attention should be given to the immunocompromised host with gangrenous cellulitis.

NF of the face, eyelids, neck, and lips can be life threatening. Crepitus, severe pain, and necrosis of the epidermis and superficial fascia are evident, which heralds a rapid spread to other areas in the neck.

Surgical Treatment

Treatment of infectious gangrene and gangrenous cellulitis consists of immediate surgical drainage with longitudinal incisions extending throughout the deep fascia and beyond the gangrenous and undermined areas (3). Areas of cutaneous necrosis should be excised and nonviable fascia should be debrided. Wide excision of the tissues should extend well into the normal tissue.

Surgical management of diabetic foot and decubitus ulcers includes unroofing of encrusted areas and wound probing to determine the extent of tissue destruction and potential bone involvement. Open ulcers should be carefully packed with sterile gauze moistened in one strength betadine or with normal saline, three times a day. Surgical debridement and drainage should be performed in those with deep tissue necrosis or suppuration (54). Infected cysts and subcutaneous abscesses should be promptly surgically drained. In cases where myositis is suspected, surgical exploration is important in order to determine the presence of muscle involvement.

In cases of NF, immediate surgical debridement is mandatory. Extensive incisions throughout the skin and subcutaneous tissue should be made, proceeding beyond the area of involvement until normal flora is reached. Necrotic fascia and fat should be excised, and the wound should be left open. An additional second procedure is often needed within 24 hours, to ensure the adequacy of the initial debridement (55).

In patients with pyomyositis, an emergency surgical exploration is warranted. This is done in order to define the nature of the infective process (crepitant cellulitis vs. gas gangrene), which is done by direct examination of the involved muscles. Furthermore, the surgical intervention is needed to perform appropriate debridement.

Immediate performance of extensive surgery is necessary to treat gas gangrene. The muscles involved should be removed, and fasciotomies to decompress and drain the swollen fascial compartment are performed. Complete amputation may sometimes be necessary.

Antimicrobial Therapy

Intensive surgical and medical therapy that includes the administration of intravenous fluids and management of septic shock are the hallmarks of treatment (55). Antimicrobial therapy is an essential element in the management of skin, soft tissue, and muscle infection. Establishing the bacterial etiology and the bacterial susceptibility initially by Gram stain, and later by culture, can allow for selection of proper antimicrobial therapy. Often, however, the initial therapy is empiric, based on epidemiological, historical, and clinical features.

In cases where streptococcal etiology is suspected, parenteral penicillin is used. If staphylococcal infection is suspected, or when no initial clue for etiology is available, a penicillinase-resistant penicillin (e.g., oxacillin) is given. Macrolides or vancomycin can be used in penicillin allergic individuals, and an aminoglycoside, or quinolone, or a third-generation cephalosporin (i.e., ceftazidime, cefepime) can be given when a gram-negative aerobe bacilli is suspected. Recently, there have been an increase in the isolation of methicillin-resistant *S. aureus* (MRSA). Patients with serious staphylococcal infections should therefore be initially started on agents active against MRSA until susceptibility results are available. Vancomycin, daptomycin, linezolid, tigecycline, and quinupristin/dalfopristin can be administered to treat these infections.

In infections that involve *Clostridium* spp., the combination of penicillin and clindamycin is recommended. This is based on in-vivo and in-vitro data of showing greater efficacy of the combination to each agent alone (56,57). Since many of the infections are polymicrobial aerobic–anaerobic in nature, coverage against these organisms is often necessary.

The gram-negative anaerobic bacilli, *Prevotella* spp., and *Fusobacterium* spp. previously susceptible to penicillins have been shown in the last decade to have increased rates of resistance to these and other antimicrobial agents. The production of the enzyme beta-lactamase is one of the main mechanisms of resistance to penicillins by many gram-negative anaerobic bacilli, including members of the *B. fragilis* group. Complete identification and testing for antimicrobial susceptibility and beta-lactamase production are therefore essential for the management of infections caused by these bacteria.

Antimicrobial therapy for mixed aerobic and anaerobic bacterial infections is required when polymicrobial infection is suspected (50). Antimicrobial agents that generally provide coverage for *S. aureus* as well as anaerobic bacteria include cefoxitin, clindamycin, carbapenem (i.e., imipenem, meropenem), and the combinations of a beta-lactamase inhibitor (i.e., tozobactam) and a penicillin (i.e., piperacillan) and the combination of metronidazole plus a beta-lactamase-resistant penicillin. Cefoxitin, the carbapenems, tigecycline, and a penicillin plus beta-lactamase inhibitor also provide coverage against Enterobacteriaceae. However, agents effective against these organisms (i.e., aminoglycosides, fourth-generation cephlosporins, and quinolones) should be added to the other agents when treating infections that include these bacteria.

Hyperbaric oxygen (HBO) therapy for clostridial myonecrosis is controversial (50). HBO increases the normal oxygen saturation in the infected wounds by a thousand fold, leading to a bacteriocidal effect, improved polymorphonuclear cells function, and enhanced wound healing (58). No controlled studies were done, and the published reports do not provide evidence of beneficial effect. The potential toxicity of HBO is also of concern. The most important limitation of utilizing HBO therapy is the lack of availability of appropriate hyperbaric chambers in most hospitals. Transportation of a seriously ill patient to a facility with a hyperbaric unit is hazardous, and the separation from immediate care for the unstable patient is risky. Transportation should not be done prior to extensive surgical debridement. However, the use of HBO should be considered when the involved tissue cannot be completely excised surgically, as may be the case in paraspinal or abdominal wall sites.

An additional mode of therapy is the negative pressure therapy or vacuum assisted closure. This is a very effective method of reducing bacterial load by removal of infected tissue debris and wound fluid (59).

REFERENCES

1. Stanley JR, Amagai M. Pemphigus, bullous impetigo, and the staphylococcal scalded-skin syndrome. N Engl J Med 2006; 355:1800–10.
2. Karakas M, Baba M, Aksungur VL, et al. Manifestation of cellulitis after saphenous venectomy for coronary bypass surgery. J Eur Acad Dermatol Venereol 2002; 16:438–40.
3. Cha JY, Releford BJ, Jr., Marcarelli P. Necrotizing fasciitis: a classification of necrotizing soft tissue infections. J Foot Ankle Surg 1994; 33:148–55.
4. Stevens DL. Invasive group A streptococcus infections. Clin Infect Dis 1992; 14:2–11.
5. Lally KP, Atkinson JB, Woolley MM, et al. Necrotizing fasciitis: a serious sequela of omphalitis in the newborn. Ann Surg 1984; 199:101–3.
6. Rapoport Y, Himelfarb MZ, Zikk D, et al. Cervical necrotizing fasciitis of odontogenic origin. Oral Surg Oral Med Oral Pathol 1991; 72:15–8.
7. Margolis RD, Cohen KR, Loftus MJ, et al. Nonodontogenic β-hemolytic necrotizing fasciitis of the face. J Oral Maxillofac Surg 1989; 47:1098–102.
8. Brook I, Frazier EH. Clinical and microbiological features of necrotizing fasciitis. J Clin Microbiol 1995; 33:2382–7.
9. Husseinzadeh N, Nahas WA, Manders EK, et al. Spontaneous occurrence of synergistic bacterial gangrene following external pelvic irradiation. Obstet Gynecol 1984; 63:859–62.
10. Wilson CB, Siber GR, O'Brien TF, et al. Phycomycotic gangrenous cellulitis. Arch Surg 1976; 111:532–8.
11. Brook I. Microbiology of infected epidermal cysts. Arch Dermatol 1989; 125:1658–61.
12. Brook I. Microbiology of secondary bacterial infection in scabies lesions. J Clin Microbiol 1995; 33:2139–40.
13. Brook I, Frazier EH, Yeager JK. Microbiology of infected eczema herpeticum. J Am Acad Dermatol 1998; 38:627–9.
14. Brook I, Frazier EH, Yeager JK. Microbiology of infected pustular psoriasis lesions. Int J Dermatol 1999; 38:579–81.
15. Brook I. Microbiology of infectal poison ivy dermatitis. Br J Dermatol 2000; 142:943–6.
16. Brook I. Microbiology of secondarily infected diaper dermatitis. Int J Dermatol 1992; 31:700–2.
17. Brook I, Frazier EH, Yeager JK. Aerobic and anaerobic microbiology of kerions. Pediatr Infect Dis J 1995; 14:326–7.
18. Brook I, Frazier EH, Yeager JK. Microbiology of infected atopic dermatitis. Int J Dermatol 1996; 35:791–3.
19. Dagan R, Bar-David Y. Double-blind study comparing erythromycin and mupirocin for treatment of impetigo in children: implications of a high prevalence of erythromycin-resistant *Staphylococcus aureus* strains. Antimicrob Agents Chemother 1992; 36:287–90.
20. Brook I, Frazier EH, Yeager JK. Microbiology of nonbulbous impetigo. Pediatr Dermatol 1997; 14:192–5.
21. Mujais S, Uwaydah M. Pneumococcal cellulitis. Infection 1983; 11:173–4.
22. Asmar BI, Bashour BN, Fleischmann LE. *Escherichia coli* cellulitis in children with idiopathic nephrotic syndrome. Clin Pediatr 1987; 26:592–4.
23. Bonner JR, Coker AS, Berryman CR, et al. Spectrum of *Vibrio* infections in a gulf coast community. Ann Intern Med 1983; 99:464–669.
24. Arnold M, Woo ML, French GL. *Vibrio vulnificus* septicemia presenting as spontaneous necrotizing cellulitis in a woman with hepatic cirrhosis. Scand J Infect Dis 1989; 21:727–31.
25. Brook I, Frazier EH. Clinical features and aerobic and anaerobic characteristics of cellulitis. Arch Surg 1995; 130:786–92.
26. Demers B, Simor AE, Vellend H, et al. Severe invasive group A streptococcal infections in Ontario, Canada: 1987–1991. Clin Infect Dis 1993; 16:792–800.
27. Brook I. Aerobic and anaerobic microbiology of necrotizing fasciitis in children. Pediatr Dermatol 1996; 13:281–4.
28. Brook I, Finegold SM. Aerobic and anaerobic bacteriology of cutaneous abscess in children. Pediatrics 1981; 67:891–5.
29. Meislin HW, Lerner SA, Gravis MH, et al. Cutaneous abscesses: aerobic and anaerobic bacteriology and outpatient management. Ann Intern Med 1977; 97:145–50.
30. Brook I, Frazier EH. Aerobic and anaerobic microbiology of superficial suppurative thrombophlebitis. Arch Surg 1996; 131:95–7.
31. Brook I. Microbiological studies of decubitus ulcers in children. J Pediatr Surg 1991; 26:207–9.
32. Sapico FL, Witte JL, Canawati HN, et al. The infected foot of the diabetic patient: quantitative microbiology and analysis of clinical features. Rev Infect Dis 1984; 6(Suppl. 1):S171–6.
33. Wheat LJ, Allen SD, Henry M, et al. Diabetic foot infections: bacteriologic analysis. Arch Intern Med 1986; 146:1935–40.
34. Christin L, Sarosi GA. Pyomyositis in North America: case reports and review. Clin Infect Dis 1992; 15:668–77.

35. Brook I, Frazier EH. Aerobic and anaerobic microbiology of infection after trauma. Am J Emerg Med 1998; 16:585–91.
36. Brook I. Pyomyositis in children, caused by anaerobic bacteria. J Pediatr Surg 1996; 31:394–6.
37. Ferrieri P, Dajani AS, Wannamaker LW, et al. Natural history of impetigo. I. Site sequence of acquisition and familial patterns of spread of cutaneous streptococci. J Clin Invest 1972; 51:2851–62.
38. Dillon HC. Impetigo contagiosa: suppurative and non-suppurative complications. I. Clinical bacteriologic, and epidemiologic characteristics of impetigo. Am J Dis Child 1968; 115:530–41.
39. Chmel H, Handy M. Recurrent streptococcal cellulitis complicating radical hysterectomy and radiation therapy. Obstet Gynecol 1984; 63:862–4.
40. Bouma J, Dankert J. Recurrent acute leg cellulitis in patients after radical vulvectomy. Gynecol Oncol 1988; 25:50–7.
41. Gold WL, Salit IE. *Aeromonas hydrophila* infections of skin and soft tissue: report of 11 cases and review. Clin Infect Dis 1993; 16:69–74.
42. Meleney FL. Bacterial synergy in disease processes with a confirmation of the synergistic bacterial etiology of a certain type of progressive gangrene of the abdominal wall. Ann Surg 1931; 44:961–81.
43. Demitsu T, Okada O, Yoneda K, Manabe M. Lipodermatosclerosis- report of three cases and review of the literature. Dermatology 1999; 199:271–3.
44. Moses AE, Hardan I, Simhon A, et al. *Clostridium septicum* bacteremia and diffuse spreading cellulitis of the head and neck in a leukemic patient. Rev Infect Dis 1991; 15:525–7.
45. Currie BJ. Group A streptococcal infections of the skin: molecular advances but limited therapeutic progress. Curr Opin Infect Dis 2006; 19:132–8.
46. Iorianni P, Oliver GC. Synergistic soft tissue infections of the perineum. Dis Colon Rectum 1992; 35:640–4.
47. Brook I. Aerobic and anaerobic microbiology of infections after trauma in children. Am J Emerg Med 1998; 15:162–7.
48. Small LN, Ross JJ. Tropical and temperate pyomyositis. Infect Dis Clin North Am 2005; 19:981–9.
49. Hart GB, Lamb RC, Strauss MB. Gas gangrene. J Trauma 1983; 23:991–1000.
50. Finegold SM. Anaerobic Bacteria in Human Disease. New York: Academic Press, 1977.
51. Jousimies-Somer HR, Summanen P, Baron EJ, Citron DM, Wexler HM, Finegold SM. Wadsworth-KLT Anaerobic Bacteriology Manual. 6th ed. Belmont, CA: Star Publishing, 2002.
52. Brook I. Microbiology of perianal cellulitis in children: comparison of skin swabs and needle aspiration. Int J Dermatol 1998; 371:922–4.
53. Gordin F, Stamler C, Mills J. Pyogenic psoas abscesses: noninvasive diagnostic techniques and review of the literature. Rev Infect Dis 1983; 5:1003–11.
54. Kravitz SR, McGuire JB, Shaarma S. The treatment of diabetic foot ulcer; reviewing the literature and surgical algorithm. Adv Skin Wound Care 2007; 20:227–37.
55. Hartoch RS, McManus JG, Knapp S, Buettner MF. Emergency management of chronic wounds. Emerg Med Clin North Am 2007; 25:203–21.
56. Stevens DL, Maier KA, Laine BM, et al. Comparison of clindamycin, rifampin, tetracycline, metronidazole, and penicillin for efficacy in prevention of experimental gas gangrene due to *Clostridium perfringens*. J Infect D.S. 1987; 155:220–8.
57. Stevens DL, Baine BM, Mitten JE. Comparison of single and combination antimicrobial agents for prevention of experimental gas gangrene caused by *clostridium perfringerns*. Antim Agents Chemo Ther 1987; 31:312–6.
58. Jallai N, Whithey S, Butler PE. Hyperbasic oxygen as adjuvunt therapy in the management of recrotizing fasciitis. Am J Surg 2005; 189:462–6.
59. Egington MT, Brown KR, Seabrook GR, Towne JB, Cambria RA. A prospective randomized evaluation of negative-pressure wound dressing for diabetic foot wounds. Ann Vasc Surg 2003; 17:645–9.

27 | Burn Infections

Burn wounds are a common form of injury. Fortunately, most burns are minor and are easily treated by cleansing and applying protective creams and dressings. Each year, however, a large number of individuals are seriously burned and require hospitalization and comprehensive treatment.

Burn injuries are the third cause of accidental death in children in the U.S.A. Of the approximately 360,000 individuals hospitalized for burn therapy and 3000 who die from burn injuries in the U.S.A. each year, one-third are children (1). The most serious and common complication of burns is infection. A third-degree burn is more likely to be associated with severe infection than is a partial thickness burn. Infection may be localized to the site of the burn or may be manifested as an overwhelming general sepsis.

Burn wound sepsis is a major cause of death among patients of all ages and is especially high in children (2). Sepsis is characterized by progressive bacterial proliferation within the burned tissue, invasion into adjacent tissues, and systemic dissemination (3).

The surface of every burn wound is contaminated to some degree by bacteria (3). Therefore, most burn centers routinely monitor surface bacterial growth, allowing the determination of the effect of therapy and prediction of the bacterial strains that may be involved in sepsis.

MICROBIOLOGY

Microorganisms usually gain access to burns directly because microbiota are normally present on the skin, and the skin is the interface with the outside world. The source of colonization of the burn wound usually is the patient's own endogenous flora as well as environmental organisms (4). These organisms can reach the wound directly through the skin or the blood stream. Soon after a burn injury, surface cultures may reveal multiple organisms. Within three to five days, the wound will become colonized by one or two specific organisms that have survived the competition with other microorganisms or have proven particularly resistant to burn wound therapy.

The progression of invasion by various organisms in the individual burn patient may parallel the course of the historical progression of predominance and control of various bacteria: during the 1940s and 1950s, beta-hemolytic streptococcus was the predominant pathogen. With the development of sulfonamides and penicillin, the threat of this organism was obviated. Subsequently, the infectious threat became penicillin-resistant *Staphylococcus aureus*. The eventual development of the penicillinase-resistant synthetic penicillins and the cephalosporins permitted control of penicillinase-producing *S. aureus*. During the late 1950s, however, gram-negative facultative anaerobes and strict aerobes (*Pseudomonas aeruginosa* and other *Pseudomonas* spp., and *Enterobacter*, *Proteus* and *Klebsiella* spp.) emerged as the dominant pathogens and today constitute the greatest septic threat to the burn patient. The problem is further complicated by the emergence of fungal organisms such as *Candida albicans* and *Candida tropicalis* in response to control of gram-negative species by antibacterial agents (5). *S. aureus* has regained prominence in the past 30 years. Septicemia is often related to *P. aeruginosa* infection. Other organisms that can cause sepsis are *Staphylococcus epidermidis*, *Acinetobacter*, *Serratia*, *Aeromonas*, *Candida*, *Mucor* spp., *Aspergillus*, *Geotrichum*, and *Cryptococcus* spp. Viral invasion of the burned area also can occur with herpes simplex and varicella viruses.

A number of case reports describe the involvement of anaerobes in burn wounds. These reports were summarized by Murray and Finegold (6). Clostridial wound infections were reported in 23 burns, especially those associated with severe burns. Clinical tetanus was described after burns (7), which illustrates the potentials for anaerobic burn wound infection. Nonclostridial anaerobic infections are less common. There are six such documented infections, mostly of *Bacteroides* spp. and anaerobic cocci.

A report (8) summarized data obtained from a prospective study of the flora of burn surfaces in 180 children, applying aerobic and anaerobic microbiological methodology. The data reflected a longitudinal evaluation of the mode of colonization at different anatomic sites and described the effect of antimicrobial agents administered to these children.

Specimens were obtained twice a week; from each patient between one and 21cultures had been taken. A total of 392 specimens were collected. Aerobic bacteria alone were present in 225 specimens (71%) and anaerobic bacteria alone were present in 26 (8%). Mixed aerobic and anaerobic bacteria were present in 68 burn specimens (21%).

A total of 551 isolates (419 aerobes and 132 anaerobes) were recovered, accounting for 1.7 isolates/specimen (1.3 aerobes and 0.4 anaerobes). The predominant aerobic isolates were *S. epidermidis*, *S. aureus*, alpha-hemolytic streptococcus, *Pseudomonas* spp., and *Enterococcus* spp. The predominant anaerobic isolates were *Propionibacterium acnes*, anaerobic gram-positive cocci, and gram-negative bacilli (including *Prevotella* and *Porphyromonas* spp., and *Bacteroides fragilis*).

Blood cultures were drawn from 45 children. Four of these children showed bacterial growth of one of each of the following isolates: *S. aureus*, *Escherichia coli*, *Peptostreptococcus asaccharolyticus*, and *B. fragilis*. The recovery of anaerobes from the blood illustrates the potential invasiveness of these organisms.

The number of isolates per specimen was higher in the oral and anal areas (3.2 and 2.8) than in the extremities and trunk (1.8 and 0.9). Gram-negative enteric rods and *Enterococcus* spp. were recovered more frequently from the anal area. *S. aureus*, *S. epidermidis*, and *P. acnes* were more frequently recovered from extremities. Anaerobic gram-negative bacilli and *Fusobacterium nucleatum* were more frequently recovered from the anal and oral areas. Specimens from burns of the anal and oral region tended to yield organisms found in the stool or mouth flora, respectively (9). Specimens obtained from burns in areas remote from the rectum or mouth grew primarily the microflora indigenous to the skin. With the exception of *P. acnes*, multiple anaerobic organisms usually were recovered from the anal and oral areas, whereas fewer anaerobic organisms were present at other sites. The high rate of recovery of anaerobes in the anal and oral areas is of particular interest and could be related to the introduction of stool and oral flora, which is predominantly anaerobic, to the burn site (Fig. 1, Chapter 25).

All children were treated with local application of Silvadene cream, and antimicrobial therapy was administered to 128 children. Statistical analysis showed no correlation between the bacteria isolated and the administration of antimicrobial agents.

Wang et al. (10) studied 102 burn wound specimens obtained from 34 patients for anaerobic cultures. Fifteen specimens from eight patients showed growth of anaerobic bacteria and 12 species were found. The predominant anaerobes were *Prevotella melaninogenica*, *Peptostreptococcus* spp., *B. fragilis*, and other strains of *Bacteroides* and *Peptostreptococcus*. They were mostly found in electric burn wounds and burn wounds affecting the perianal and oral areas. Wounds with anaerobic infection usually appeared gaseous, necrotic, and ischemic with foul odor. Of 19 blood samples from 10 patients, two were positive, Bacteroides was recovered in one sample, and *Peptostreptococcus* and *Serratia* spp. were isolated in the other.

Zhang (11) analyzed 158 specimens from deep necrotic burn tissues and exudates under burned subeschar, and blood, and found that more anaerobes were isolated from deep necrotic tissues and foul smelling exudates of subeschar. Most isolates were mixed with aerobes (97.1%) and of the 43 strains of anaerobes, Clostridium accounted for 18 and Bacteroides for 17. Other isolates included *F. nucleatum*, *Peptostreptococcus* spp., and *Veillonella parvula*.

Huang et al. (12) performed aerobic and anaerobic blood culture in 127 patients with extensive burns. The incidence rate of anaerobic septicemia was 20%, 61 strains (9 species) of anaerobes were isolated, and 20 (77%) were mixed infection of aerobes and anaerobes. The predominant anaerobes were *Peptostreptococcus* spp. (38%) and *B. fragilis* (36%).

Mousa (13) studied 127 patients for aerobic, anaerobic, and fungal burn wound infections. A total of 377 isolates were recovered (239 aerobes, 116 anaerobes, and 22 fungi). Aerobic bacteria alone were present in 49 patients (39%). Anaerobic bacteria alone were present in four patients (3.2%). *Candida* spp. alone was present in one patient (0.8%). Mixed aerobic and/or anaerobic bacteria and/or fungi were present in 73 patients (57.5%). The predominant isolates recovered in descending order of frequency were *P. aeruginosa*, *S. aureus*, *Bacteroides* spp., *Klebsiella* spp., and *Peptostreptococcus* spp. There were 70 patients (55%) infected with anaerobic bacteria. The rate of recovery of anaerobes was higher in patients with open wound dressing (73%) than in those with occlusive wound dressings (42%) ($p<0.01$). Seventeen patients presented with septic shock, 15 of them (88%) yielding positive anaerobic cultures. *Bacteroides* spp. were isolated from 14 patients with septic shock, and were recovered from the four patients who had anaerobic infection alone.

The incorporation of the microbiological data about the recovery of anaerobes in patients with burn, suggests the following progression of dominant infectious organisms: beta-hemolytic streptococci and then *S. aureus* may be early controllable threats. As the burn wound becomes established (after the first week postinjury), there is an increasing frequency of colonization by aerobic and facultative gram-negative organisms. The site of the burn can also affect the colonizing bacteria, whereas anaerobes belonging to the *Prevotella* and *Porphyromonas* spp. and *Fusobacterium* spp. can be found in burns in the oral and the anal areas. Later in the course of the infection (three to four weeks postinjury), the wound may become colonized by fungal organisms, most often by *C. albicans*. Frequently, a synergistic colonization of the wound may occur, with two organisms existing apparently to mutual benefit. The combination could be between different aerobes as well as between aerobes and anaerobes. A frequently occurring combination is that of a *Pseudomonas* and enterococcus. The combination appears to have a greater invasive potential than *Pseudomonas* alone.

PATHOGENESIS

The burn wound itself creates the most obvious defect in the body's defense against infection. The protective barrier of skin, the body's first line of defense, is damaged or destroyed, and a point of entry for bacteria is established. The larger the burn wound, the greater is the incidence of sepsis and mortality. The threat of septicemia persists until the burn wound is entirely healed and the skin resumes its protective function.

The burn victim has profound humoral and cellular defense system deficiencies. Alterations in the inflammatory response include reduced chemotaxis, diminished ability of the neutrophils to phagocytose, and thereby kill offending bacteria, a decrease in opsonin, an antibody that renders the bacteria susceptible to phagocytosis, and decreases in T suppressor cells, fibronectin, gamma-globulin, lymphocyte stimulator interleukin-2 and macrophage activity (14–17). Immunosuppression of burn patients greatly increases their susceptibility to infection.

With a full-thickness eschar of necrotic tissue serving as the culture medium, the concentration of bacteria may increase above 10^5 microorganisms/gram viable tissue; at this point, the local resistance factors are overwhelmed and systemic invasion occurs, with perivascular infiltration and lymphatic spread.

Although the source of contamination of the burn wound in most instances is the endogenous flora, the potential of cross contamination exists, and preventive measures should be carefully followed. The most common sources of cross-contamination are the hands of hospital personnel, the hydrotherapy unit, parenteral catheter, and urinary catheter. The burn wound can be susceptible to infection with anaerobic bacteria because of its necrotic, avascular qualities. Because anaerobes are predominant in the gastrointestinal and oral flora (9), they might colonize the burn wound, especially in burns adjacent to the oral and anal areas.

The failure to use anaerobic methodology may account for the lack of recovery of anaerobes in previous studies of the flora of burns. The recovery of these organisms from burns is not surprising, since anaerobes are part of the normal flora of the mucous membranes and skin of each individual (9,18) and participate in many of the infectious processes adjacent to those areas.

P. acnes, the predominant anaerobic isolate, is a normal inhabitant of the skin. However, it can on occasion cause bacteremia or shunt infections (18,19). Gram-positive anaerobic cocci are normal skin inhabitants and part of the normal fecal flora (9). They have also been isolated from intraabdominal abscesses (20). They were isolated as frequently from abscesses of the perineal region as *Bacteroides* spp.

B. fragilis, a predominant anaerobe in the feces (9), was cultured most frequently from burns of the anal area. *P. melaninogenica*, which occurs in stool as well as in the oral cavity (9), was most frequently recovered from the oral region. Most strains of *B. fragilis* and growing numbers of *Prevotella*, *Porphyromonas*, and *Fusobacterium* spp. are resistant to penicillin (21).

The data presented (8,10–12) demonstrate that anaerobes can colonize burn wounds, and can be associated with burn sepsis.

DIAGNOSIS

The signs of infection in a burn may be minimal, especially in the early stages. Local infection is recognized only by frequent inspection. An area of purulence or inflammation at the edge of the eschar may be the only sign. Systemic manifestations of sepsis include fever, tachycardia, acute respiratory distress, adynamic ileus, gastrointestinal hemorrhage, cardiovascular changes including septic shock, petechiae, and occasionally, evidence of other metastatic foci of infection. Deterioration of the patient's mental faculties may accompany a worsening of the vital signs.

The diagnosis of infection in a burn wound depends on an awareness of the possibility of this complication. Approaches to diagnosis should include frequent inspection of the site of the burn for purulent exudate, cracks in the eschar, evidences of cellulitis, and cultures of blood, the wound, and any exudates. Since the surface of every burn wound is contaminated to some degree by bacteria, most burn centers continually monitor surface growth of bacteria. Monitoring allows the anticipation of which bacterial strain(s) may be involved in wound sepsis. The burn wound can be the primary focal point for subsequent invasive infection of incipient bacteremia. Monitoring bacterial growth is a significant part of the overall treatment of the severely burned patient. Without topical antibacterials, the progress of burn wound infection from simple colonization to general invasive infection may be rapid.

The presence of organisms in the burn wound does not always indicate sepsis. However, dress changes and surgical wound debridement have been associated with bacteremia in 7.7% to 65% of episodes (22,23). Burn wound sepsis occurs only with the invasion of viable tissue. If surface cultures obtained with wet swab indicate colonization of the wound by any pathogenic organisms, wound biopsies may be done for quantitative culture or histologic examination. Either a growth of greater than 10^5 microorganisms per gram of tissue or the demonstration of organisms within viable tissue is diagnostic of invasive sepsis.

Sensitivities to antibiotics should be determined for all organisms cultured in septic patients. These sensitivities will guide the selection of antibiotic, and therapy can be initiated before the onset of systemic signs and symptoms of septicemia. Treatment of positive cultures with specific antibiotics during wound colonization does not guarantee the prevention of sepsis but may select for the emergence of resistant organisms.

MANAGEMENT

Prevention of Wound Sepsis

A primary objective in the management of burns and prevention of wound sepsis is construction of a barrier between the burned area and the environment. Topical antimicrobial and aggressive and early debridement therapies are a mainstay of burn treatment and have substantial impact on the rate of wound infection and septicemia. Although topical agents do not sterilize the wound, the numbers of colonizing organisms decrease, reducing the risk of bacterial invasion of the underlying tissue (24). The 0.5% silver nitrate soaks used with great benefit in the past have been largely replaced by topical creams of silver sulfadiazine–silver nitrate combination, which are easier to use and do not require dressing (25). Silver nitrate soaks are very effective against *Pseudomonas* and a variety of other organisms as well. Ten percent of mafenide hydrochloride cream is effective against *Pseudomonas* organisms, but causes pain and an acidosis related to carbonic anhydrase inhibition.

Mafenide acetate cream is used currently to minimize the problem of acidosis, and it is effective in diminishing mortality from burn wound sepsis (24). Although mafenide application causes severe local pain, it appears to be the best drug for patients with extensive burns involving thick eschar, because mafenide penetrates eschar to a greater degree than other topical agents. Mafenide is effective against most gram-positive organisms and is particularly effective against the *Clostridium* spp. Mafenide also possesses a broad-spectrum activity against gram-negative rods.

Silver sulfadiazine was found to be very effective against *Pseudomonas* as well as Enterobacteriaceae, *S. aureus*, anaerobes and fungi without producing pain or significant metabolic toxicity (25). Some data suggest the in vitro inhibition of *Herpesvirus huminis*. Povidone-iodine ointment is a useful agent. It diffuses well through the eschar, is nontoxic, and has a wide spectrum. It is important to remember that despite the effectiveness of the various topical antibacterial agents, invasive burn wound sepsis still occurs, particularly in patients with large-burn injuries.

Other topical agents include Silverton dressing (releasing nanocrystalline silver), bactroban, myostatin and other topical antimicrobials (i.e., nitrofurazone, bacitracin) (24).

General Supportive Measures

The survival of patients with major burns depends upon appropriate resuscitation for burn shock, maintenance of nutrition, adequate pulmonary care, and the ability to control infection (24,26). In patients with wound sepsis, general supportive measures are essential to maintain vital organ functions until the sepsis is controlled. The goals of the supportive measures are to prevent respiratory insufficiency and cardiovascular collapse and to alleviate the adynamic ileus.

Systemic Antibiotics

In the past, streptococcal cellulitus was a frequent early complication of burn injury and, therefore, intravenous penicillin was recommended to be given on a prophylactic basis for the first three to five days postburn (27). However, the use of early prophylactic antibiotics may not prevent infection and may be harmful and establish resistant flora (28). It is, therefore, recommended that systemic antimicrobial agents should be administered only when systemic infection is strongly suspected and should be based on the information gained whenever possible from bacteriologic cultures. Because anaerobic bacteria frequently are associated with burns especially in areas adjacent to the mucous membrane surfaces, the physician should consider their presence when a local or systemic invasive involvement by these organisms is present.

Using appropriate aerobic and anaerobic microbiological techniques in monitoring the bacterial colonization of burns can help the physician select proper therapy if complications occur. The presence of penicillin-resistant anaerobic bacteria may warrant the administration of appropriate antimicrobials for the organisms, including such agents as clindamycin, chloramphenicol, cefoxitin, metronidazole, a carbapenem, or the combination of a beta-lactamase inhibitor and a penicillin. Local debridement of the wound should be done with application of local therapy of silver sulfadiazine 1%, mafenide acetate, or aqueous silver nitrate 0.5% (28).

In cases of invasive burn wound sepsis or septicemia, the wound should be examined, and a meticulous search made for subeschar abscesses. If no abscesses are found, multiple incisions through the eschar are made, to provide open drainage and to allow the antibacterial cream access to the deeper tissues.

General supportive measures should include evaluation of other sources of invasion (urinary tract infection, thrombophlebitis, pneumonia, etc.) as indications for intravenous fluid therapy and ventilatory assistance.

Broad-spectrum antibiotics should be administered parenterally until culture reports are available. This includes an aminoglycoside, a fourth-generation cephalosporin effective against *Pseudomonas* such as cefepime for coverage of enteric gram-negative rods, and a synthetic penicillin or cephalosporin for coverage of beta-hemolytic streptococci, enterococci, and *S. aureus*. If anaerobes are suspected, adequate coverage should include one of the agents previously mentioned. Broad-spectrum antimicrobial therapy should be used with caution, as it may have the untoward effect of predisposing to superinfection by yeast, fungi, or resistant organisms. Antibiotics should be used long enough to produce an effect but not long enough to allow for emergence of opportunistic or resistant organisms.

Burn patients have altered antibiotics pharmacokinetics due to the multiple burn-related pathophysiologic changes (29). These differences must be considered in the selection of agent(s) and their optimal dosage. Patients who are not immunized against tetanus should have both active and passive immunization. Intravenous immunoglobulin and hyperimmunoglobulin G against *P. aeruginosa* and *S. aureus* has been used as adjunctive treatment for septicemia in burn patients with beneficial effect (30,31). Viral infections (Herpes simplex and cytomegaloviruses) can complicate burn infections.

REFERENCES

1. Hoyert DL, Kung HC, Smith BL. Deaths: preliminary data for 2003. National Vital Statistic Reports. 50:1–48, 2005.
2. Barrow RE, Przkora R, Hawkins HK, Barrow LN, Jeschke MG, Herndon DN. Mortality related to gender, age, sepsis, and ethnicity in severely burned children Shock 2005; 23:485–7
3. Sharma BR, Harish D, Singh VP, Bangar S. Septicemia as a cause of death in burns: an autopsy study. Burns 2006; 32:545–9
4. Magnotti LJ, Deitch EA. Burns, bacterial translocation, gut barrier function, and failure. J Burn Care Rehab 2005; 26: 383–91.
5. de Macedo JL, Rosa SC, Castro C. Sepsis in burned patients. Rev Soc Bras Med Trop 2003; 36:647–52.
6. Murray PM, Finegold SM. Anaerobes in burn-wound infection. Rev Infect Dis 1984; 6:S184–6.
7. Larkin JM, Moylan JA. Tetanus following a minor burn. J Trauma 1975; 15:546–8.
8. Brook I, Randolph JG. Aerobic and anaerobic bacterial flora of burns in children. J Trauma 1981; 21:313–8.
9. Gorbach SL. Intestinal microflora. Gastroenterology 1971; 60:1110–29.
10. Wang DW, Li N, Xiao GX, Zhan YP. Anaerobic infections of burns. Burns Incl Therm Inj 1985; 11:192–6.
11. Zhang YP. Anaerobic infection of burns. Chung Hua Wai Ko Tsa Chih 1991; 29:240–1.
12. Huang X, Ma E, Gong L. Clinical analysis of anaerobic septicemia in 26 patients with extensive burn. Chung Hua Wai Ko Tsa Chih 1995; 33:752–3.
13. Mousa HA. Aerobic, anaerobic and fungal burn wound infections. J Hosp Infect 1997; 37:317–23.
14. Luterman A, Dacso CC, Currei PW. Infection in burn patients. Am J Med 1986; 81(Suppl. 1A):45.
15. Deitch EA, Bridges RM, Dobke M, et al. Burn wound sepsis may be promoted by a failure of local antibacterial host defenses. Ann Surg 1987; 206:340–6.
16. Alexander JW. Mechanism of immunologic suppression in burn injury. J Trauma 1990; 30:S70–5.
17. Theodorczyk-Injeyan JA, Sparkes BG, Peters WJ. Regulation of IgM production in thermally injured patients. Burns Incl Therm Inj 1989; 15:241–7.
18. Finegold SM. Anaerobic Bacteria in Human Disease. New York: Academic Press, 1977.
19. Kelly ME, Fourney DR, Guzman R, Sadanand V, Griebel RW, Sanche SE. *Propionibacterium acnes* infections after cranial neurosurgery. Can J Neurol Sci 2006; 33:292–5.
20. Moore WEC, Cato EP, Holdeman LV. Anaerobic bacteria of the gastrointestinal flora and their occurrence in clinical infections. J Infect Dis 1969; 119:641–9.
21. Hecht DW. Anaerobes: antibiotic resistance, clinical significance, and the role of susceptibility testing. Anaerobe 2006; 12:115–21.
22. Vindenes H, Bjerknes R. The frequency of bacteremia and fungemia following wound cleaning and excision in patients with large burns. J Trauma 1993; 35:742–9.
23. Piel P, Scarnati S, Goldfarb W, Slater H. Antibiotic prophylaxis in patients undergoing burn wound excision. J Burn Care Rehabil 1985; 6:422–4.
24. Church D, Elsayed S, Reid O, Winston B, Lindsay R. Burn wound infections. Clin Microbiol Rev 2006; 19: 403–34.
25. Atiyeh BS, Costagliola M, Hayek SN, Dibo SA. Effect of silver on burn wound infection control and healing: review of the literature. Burns 2007; 33:139–48.
26. Sheridan R, Remensnyder J, Prelack K, Petras L, Lydon M. Treatment of the seriously burned infant. J Burn Care Rehabil 1998; 19:115–8.

27. Liedberg NC, Kuhn LR, Barnes BA, Reiss E, Amspacher WH. Infection in burns: the problem and evaluation of therapy. Surg Gynecol Obstet 1954; 98:535–40.
28. Ergün O, Çelik A, Ergün G, Özok G. Prophylactic antibiotic use in pediatric burn units Eur J Pediatr Surg 2004; 14:422–6
29. Boucher BA, Kuhl DA, Hickerson WL. Pharmacokinetics of systematically administered antibiotics in patients with thermal injury. Clin Infect Dis 1992; 14:458–63.
30. Shirani KZ, Vaughan GM, McManus AT, et al. Replacement therapy with modified immunoglobulin G in burn patients: preliminary kinetic studies. Am J Med 1984; 76:175–80.
31. Hunt JL, Purdue GF. A clinical trial of IV tetravalent hyperimmune pseudomonas globulin G in burned patients. J Trauma 1988; 28:146–51.

28 | Human and Animal Bite Wound Infection

Animal and human bites and other orally contaminated wounds are common, as more than one million animal bites occur in the U.S.A. each year (1–5). Bite wounds include scratches, punctures, lacerations, and evulsions. Often these wounds can look innocuous initially, but frequently they lead to serious infection and complications (6,7).

MICROBIOLOGY

The organisms that can be recovered from bite wounds generally are aerobic and anaerobic polymicrobial flora that originate from the oral cavity of the biting animal, the victim's own skin flora and the environment. Most infections are polymicrobial synergistic in nature. In studies where adequate methods were employed for the recovery of aerobic and anaerobic bacteria, anaerobes were isolated from over two-thirds of human and animal bite wound infections, especially those associated with abscess formation (8–12). *Streptococcus pyogenes* is generally found in human bites, *Pasteurella multocida* in animal bites (13,14), *Eikenella corrodens* in both animal and human bites (mostly with the latter), *Capnocytophaga canimorsus* (formerly called CDC group DF-2) (15), *Capnocytophaga cynodegmi*, *Neisseria weaveri* (formerly M-5) (16,17), *Weeksella zoohelcum* (formerly IIj) (18), *Neisseria canis* (19), *Staphylococcus intermedius* (20), NO-1 (21), and EO-2 (22) in dog bites, a *Flavobacterium* group (IIb-like organism) in infected pig bite (23), and *Actinobacillus* spp. in horse and sheep bite wounds (24). *Vibrio* spp., *Plesiomonas shigelloides*, *Aeromonas hydrophila*, and *Pseudomonas* spp., have caused infections in bites occurring in marine settings (25–27).

Some serious infections can be transmitted through bites: tularemia from cats (27), herpes B virus from monkeys, rat-bite fever and sodoku from rats, hepatitis B virus from humans (28), leptospirosis from dogs and rodents, and rabies from dogs and other mammals.

Human Bites

Staphylococcus aureus was the most frequent organism isolated, in studies that did not employ anaerobic methodology (29). Penicillin-resistant gram-negative rods alone or in mixed culture have been reported in 24% to 43% of bite wounds cultured (29,30).

Studies that employed anaerobic methodologies reported the recovery of anaerobic bacteria in human bites in adults (31) and children (32). Goldstein et al. (31) recovered anaerobic bacteria in over half of human bite wounds and clenched-fist injuries. The predominant isolates were anaerobic gram-negative bacilli (AGNB) (including pigmented *Prevotella* and *Porphyromonas* spp., and *Bacteroides* spp.), *Fusobacterium nucleatum*, and anaerobic gram-positive cocci. The predominant aerobes recovered were *S. aureus*, group A beta-hemolytic streptococci (GABHS), and *E. corrodens*.

Talan et al. (2) conducted a multicenter prospective study of 50 patients with infected human bites. Fifty-six percent of injuries were clenched-fist injuries and 44% were occlusional bites. The median number of isolates per wound culture was 4 (3 aerobes and 1 anaerobe); aerobes and anaerobes were isolated from 54% of wounds, aerobes alone were isolated from 44%, and anaerobes alone were isolated from 2%. Isolates included *Streptococcus anginosus* (52%), *S. aureus* (30%), *E. corrodens* (30%), *F. nucleatum* (32%), and *Prevotella melaninogenica* (22%). *Candida* spp. were found in 8%. *Fusobacterium*, *Peptostreptococcus*, and *Candida* spp. were isolated more frequently from occlusional bites than from clenched-fist injuries. Many strains of *Prevotella* and *S. aureus* were beta-lactamase producers.

Brook (32) recovered anaerobes in 90% of 18 children with human bites (Table 1). A total of 97 isolates (range, 1–8/specimen) were recovered (5.4/specimen): 44 aerobes (2.4/specimen) and 53 anaerobes (3.0/specimen). Beta-lactamase activity was noted in 13 isolates that were recovered from 11 patients. The majority of these were nine isolates of *S. aureus*, two of the six pigmented *Prevotella* and *Porphynomonas* spp., one of the three *Prevotella oralis*, and the single isolate of *Bacteroides ovatus*.

The results of these studies show the normal oral flora, rather than the skin flora, to be the source of most bacteria isolated from human bite wound cultures.

Animal Bites

Almost any aerobic and anaerobic oral flora isolate is a potential pathogen, and therefore the bacteriology of these bite wounds varies and needs individual study (33–38).

Holst et al. (14) investigated the distribution of 159 *P. multocida* isolates from bite wounds. *P. multocida* accounted for 60% of the isolates and was recovered from all cases of bacteremia. *Pasteurella septica*, accounted for 13% of isolates, was more commonly isolated from cat than from dog bites and caused more central nervous system complications. *Pasteurella canis* (biotype 1) was recovered from 18% of wounds in cases of dog bites. Isolates that were less often recovered, including *Pasteurella stomatis*, *Pasteurella dagmatis*, *Pasteurella gallinarum*, *Pasteurella haemolytica*, and *Pasteurella pneumotropica*, have also been associated with endocarditis and bacteremia. In addition to *Pasteurella* spp., anaerobic bacteria play a prominent role in bite wound infections (8–12,37). They can be isolated from about three-fourths of dog and cat bite wound infections, mostly from those where an abscess is formed (8–12,37). AGNB are the predominant anaerobic isolates. The most frequently isolated strains include *Porphyromonas salivosa*, *Porphyromonas gingivalis*, and *Porphyromonas canoris*. Other isolates

TABLE 1 Predominant Aerobic Facultative and Anaerobic Bacteria Isolated from Patients with Animal Bite and Human Bite Wounds

	Animal bite	Human bite
Aerobic and facultative isolates		
Streptococcus spp.		
Alpha-hemolytic	+	+
Group A beta-hemolytic	+	+
Non-group A beta-hemolytic	+	+
Gamma-hemolytic	+	+
Enterococcus spp.	+	+
Staphylococcus aureus	+	+
Staphylococcus epidermidis	+	+
Neisseria spp.	+	+
Corynebacterium spp.	+	+
Pasteurella spp.	+	
Eikenella corrodens	+	+
Acinetobacter spp.	+	
Weeksella zoohelcum	+	
Haemophilus spp.	+	+
Moraxella spp.	+	
Capnocytophaga spp.	+	
Anaerobic isolates		
Peptostreptococcus spp.	+	+
Veillonella spp.	+	+
Bifidobacterium spp.		+
Eubacterium spp.		+
Fusobacterium spp.	+	+
Bacteroides spp.	+	+
Prevotella spp.	+	+
Fusobacterium spp.	+	+

include *Porphyromonas cangingivalis*, *Porphyromonas cansulci*, *Porphyromonas circumdentaria*, *Porphyromonas levii*-like strains, and some unidentified species (11). Saccharolytic *Bacteroides* and *Prevotella* spp. are also often recovered from dog and cat bite wounds. These include *Bacteroides tectum*, *Prevotella heparinolytica*, *Prevotella zoogleoformans*, *Prevotella buccae*, and *Prevotella oris* (10).

Using aerobic and anaerobic cultural methods, Goldstein et al. (37) evaluated 27 dog bite wounds and isolated 109 organisms, 87 aerobes, and 22 anaerobes. All positive cultures yielded multiple organisms, most were potential pathogens. *P. multocida* was recovered from 7 of 27 wounds (30%), and the most common aerobes were the alpha-hemolytic streptococci and *S. aureus*. Anaerobes were present in 41% of wounds and included *Bacteroides* and *Fusobacterium* spp. Similar data were found in other animal bites (cats, squirrels, other rodents, and rattlesnakes) (17).

Brook evaluated 21 children who had *animal* bites, 17 from *dogs* and four from *cats* (32). Aerobes only were isolated from five children (24%), anaerobic bacteria only from 2 (10%), and mixed aerobic and anaerobic isolates from 14 (66%). A total of 59 isolates (2.8/specimen): 37 aerobes (1.8/specimen) and 22 anaerobes (1.0/specimen) were recovered.

Talan et al. (38) studied wounds of 50 patients with dog bites and 57 patients with cat bites. They recovered a median of five isolates/culture. Aerobes and anaerobes were found in 56% of the wounds, aerobes alone in 36%, and anaerobes alone in 1%. *Pasteurella* spp. were the most common isolates from both dog and cat bites. Other common aerobes included streptococci, staphylococci, moraxella, and neisseria. Common anaerobes included *Fusobacterium*, *Bacteroides*, *Porphyromonas*, and *Prevotella*. Isolates not previously identified as human pathogens included *Riemerella anatipestifer* from two cat bites and *B. tectum*, *P. heparinolytica*, and several *Porphyromonas* spp from dog and cat bites. *Erysipelothrix rhusiopathiae* was isolated from two cat bites.

The microbiology of *monkey* and *simian* bite wounds is similar to that of human bites, where aerobic and anaerobic pathogens are the infecting agents. These include *Streptococcus*, *Enterococcus*, and *Staphylococcus* spp., *E. corrodens*, *Neisseria* spp., Enterobacteriaceae, AGNB and *Fusobacterium* spp.

B virus (also known as *Herpesvirus simiae*; Cercopithecine herpesvirus 1) is a potential pathogen from some monkey bites (39,40). This infection can cause fatal encephalomyelitis. It is enzootic in North African and Asian monkeys and affects the macaque and rhesus monkeys.

The organisms recovered from *horse* bite wounds include *S. aureus*, *Streptococcus* spp., *Neisseria* spp., *Escherichia coli*, *Actinobacillus lignieresii*, *Pasteurella* spp., *Bacteroides ureolyticus*, *Bacteroides fragilis*, other AGNB, *P. melaninogenica*, and *P. heparinolytica* (24,41,42). *Actinobacillus* spp. is associated with *sheep* bites (24).

The organisms recovered from *pig* bite infections are: *Staphylococcus* spp., *Streptococcus* spp. (including *Streptococcus sanguis*, *Streptococcus suis*, and *Streptococcus milleri*), diphtheroids, *P. multocida*, other *Pasteurella* spp., *Haemophilus influenzae*, *Actinobacillus suis*, *Flavobacterium* IIb-like organisms, *B. fragilis*, and other AGNB (23,43–46).

Organisms of marine environment cause *aquatic animal* bite infections (26,47–52). These infections often involve *Vibrio* and *Aeromonas* spp., which can also be recovered from the shark's oral cavity (42,47–49). *Vibrio carchariae* is recovered from shark bite infection (48). *A. hydrophila* was recovered from a cellulitis that occurred after a piranha bite (51) and alligator bites (52). Isolates from catfish bites and injuries (26) were *Vibrio* spp. (as *Vibrio vulnificus*), *Vibrio damsela*, *Pseudomonas* spp., Enterobacteriaceae, *A. hydrophila*, and *Peptostreptococcus* spp.

Bird pecking and bites can induce serious infections. A brain abscess that was caused by *Streptococcus bovis*, *Clostridium tertium*, and *Aspergillus niger* developed in an infant after a rooster pecked his skull (53). An owl attack caused superficial cellulitis due to two non-fragilis *Bacteroides* spp. (54), and a swan bite induced cellulitis due to *Pseudomonas aeruginosa* (55).

Ferrets caused serious facial injuries in three infants, and *S. aureus* was isolated from one patient (56).

DIAGNOSIS

The symptoms that emerge following a bite depend on the type of animal inflicting the insult. The immediate local or systemic symptoms can be severe following venomous animals (snake, lizard, spider, etc.). Human or dog bites generally do not cause immediate symptoms in addition to the laceration injury. However, because of the direct inoculation of oral and skin flora into the wound, if an infection occurs, it can develop rapidly. However, the signs and symptoms of infection may take 24 to 72 hours to develop. The signs of infection include redness, swelling, and clear or pussy discharge. The adjacent lymph nodes may be enlarged, and reduction in range of motion of an extremity can develop. There may be leukocytosis of 15,000 to 30,000 cells/mm^3. The observation of an eschariform lesion in a sick-appearing individual may suggest the presence of *C. canimorsus* infection (57).

Human bites generally are more serious than animal bites. This is especially the case in clenched-fist injury when the skin over the knuckles is penetrated after striking the teeth of another person. The teeth can cause a deep laceration that implant oral and skin organisms into the joint capsules or dorsal tendons, thus causing septic arthritis or osteomyelitis. Radiographs of hands injured by teeth are recommended (58). It is very important to determine the medical status of the source of the human bite (e.g., infections with a hepatitis virus, human immune deficiency status, and other transmittable diseases).

Determination of the sedimentation rate or C-reactive protein can help in the cases of osteomyelitis and septic arthritis to determine the duration of antimicrobial therapy.

About 2% to 5% of all typical dog bite wounds seen in emergency departments become infected (1). However, the rabies status of the dog need to be ascertained in each instance. Wounds that completely penetrated the skin have an infection rate of 6% to 13%, depending on the location. In comparison, the infection rate of clean lacerations repaired in the emergency department is about 5% (59).

Gram stain and culture for both aerobic and anaerobic bacteria should be obtained from human and animal bite wounds. Employing culture and microbiological methods that are adequate for the recovery of anaerobic bacteria is essential. If wounds are contaminated by soil or vegetative debris, culture for mycobacteria and fungi should also be performed.

MANAGEMENT

Management of wounds includes proper local care, and utilization when needed of antimicrobial agent(s). The steps involved in evaluation and wound care for bites include: recording medical history (animal involved, provoked or unprovoked attack, current medications, splenectomy, mastectomy, allergies, chronic disease, and immunosuppression), examination of the wound and related structures (odor of exudates, depth, type, and location of wound, range of motion, joint involvement, edema or crush injury, nerve, and tendon damage, presence of infection), obtaining wound cultures, irrigation of the wound with saline and debridement, X ray (when bone penetration is suspected), wound approximation, administration of antimicrobials and tetanus and rabies (when indicated) immunization, herpes B virus evaluation (in monkey bites), and re-examination at 24 and 48 hours. The incident should be reported to the local health authorities when indicated.

Bites should be managed as any laceration: cleanse, explore, irrigate, debride, drain, and possibly suture. The wounds should be washed vigorously with soap or a quaternary ammonium compound and water. This is of primary importance in reducing the high inoculum of the oral flora of the biting human or animal. The physician should explore for damage to tissues caused by crushing or tearing and search for damaged tendons, blood vessels, joints, and bones. X-ray examination for fractures and foreign bodies should be done when feasible. The wound should be irrigated through a 19-gauge needle with 150 mL or more of sterile normal saline or lactated Ringer's solution. Devitalized tissues should be debrided. Drainage of the wound, when indicated, can be performed in customary fashion or by using gentle suction with a 19-gauge scalp vein tubing connected to a vacuum blood collecting tube (60). A controversy still exists whether or not bite wounds that are clinically uninfected and are seen within 24 hours should be surgically closed (37,61). Margins of puncture wounds should be excised and left open after irrigation. Margins of other wounds should be excised and primary closure carried out, with or without drainage (58,60). The utility of suturing fresh bite wounds less than six hours after the injury is undetermined, except for facial wounds.

Delayed primary closure or edge approximation should be done in wounds associated with crush injury, preexisting edema, and hands and feet injuries.

In caring for bite by a monkey that may be a B virus carrier, the wound should be thoroughly scrubbed with soap or detergent and irrigated for at least 15 minutes (40) and viral cultures should be performed after cleansing. Serum for acute viral B virus-specific serology should be stored at −20°C, and compared with a second sample obtained 21 days later. Antiviral therapy with acyclovir, valcyclovir, or famcyclovir should be given to those with moderate or high-risk wounds (40).

Bites of the hand are at the highest risk of deep damage and severe infection because sharp teeth may penetrate tendon sheaths or the mid-palmar space. Human bites should be treated by widely opening the wound, debriding, and irrigating thoroughly (62), and primary closure and tendon and nerve repair should be delayed. Following debridement and irrigation, dog bites can be considered clean and primary closure can be performed. Hospitalization may be necessary in severe cases, with immobilization by splinting or bulky dressings and elevation.

Facial bites, especially of children, require meticulous management. Nearly all victims do well with careful debridement, ample irrigation and cleansing, and loose closure by suture. Close follow-up for at least five days is required. Subsequent plastic reconstruction may be needed, and consultation with a plastic surgeon at the time of initial repair may be useful.

Early management of all human bites, especially those to the hand, must be thorough and vigorous. Clenched-fist injuries require more intensive care, preferably by a hand surgeon, to evaluate the seriousness of injury to the tendon, sheath, joint capsule, joint, and bone.

Rabies prevention should be given after dog bites that indicate such measures (63). This includes hyperimmune serum and active immunization.

A tetanus toxoid booster should be administered if the patient has been adequately immunized before and has received the last dose within the past 10 years. Tetanus immune globulin (human) is required if tetanus immunization has not taken place or is inadequate.

The infectious complications of dog bites make the concept of prophylactic antibiotics attractive. Using antibiotics may be helpful, particularly in high-risk wounds such as those of the hand. The choice of a particular antibiotic for prophylaxis and/or treatment must be based on bacteriology. Unfortunately, no one antibiotic can be expected to effectively treat infections caused by all the organisms that can be present in an infected bite.

The role of prophylactic antimicrobial therapy in bite wounds presenting early is uncertain (58,62). However, because these wounds are usually contaminated with potential pathogens, preventive treatment of all patients having deep bite wounds with antibiotics is advisable. These include puncture wounds, facial bites, and any wound over a tendon or bone.

Antimicrobial treatment should be administered for all bite wounds, with the exception of those patients who present 72 hours or more after injury and have no clinical signs of infection. Antimicrobial therapy of bite wounds is not usually prophylactic, but rather a therapeutic intervention.

Since no single antimicrobial eradicates all of the major pathogens responsible for bite wound infections, establishing a specific etiologic diagnosis by obtaining cultures is helpful in guiding the therapy (Table 2) (64). Penicillin or ampicillin are the most active agents against *P. multocida* and the other oral flora. However, *S. aureus* and almost half of the AGNB recovered from human bite wounds are resistant to this drug (65). The isolation

TABLE 2   Antimicrobials Effective in the Empiric Treatment of Patients with Animal and Human Bite Wounds

	Animal bite	Human bite
Amoxicillin–clavulanate (PO)	+	+
Ampicillin–sulbactam (IV)	+	+
Cefoxitin (IV)	+	+
Moxifloxacin (PO, IV)	+	+
Gatifloxacin (PO, IV)	+	+
Doxycycline (PO, IV)	+	+

Abbreviations: PO, by mouth; IV, intravenous.

of beta-lactamase-producing organisms from over 40% of bite wounds excludes the use of penicillins for bite infections (32). Although oxacillin is effective against methicillin susceptible *S. aureus*, it has poor activity against many bite isolates; 18% of *P. multocida*, 24% of *Bacteroides* spp., and more than 50% of other aerobic gram-negative strains were found to be resistant to this antimicrobial (65). Doxycycline is a good alternative but should not be used in young children. When *S. aureus* is suspected (based on the Gram stain of aspirate, which is specific but not sensitive), penicillin (to cover streptococci) and a penicillinase-resistant penicillin should be used. Vancomycin or linezolid should be used for methicillin resistant *S. aureus*. The combination of amoxicillin and clavulanic acid has been shown to be effective in therapy of human and dog bites (64,66). This is related to the wide spectrum of activity of the combination against most pathogens isolated from these wounds. First generation cephalosporins are not as effective as the above combination due to resistance of some anaerobic bacteria and *E. corrodens*. Clindamycin and the penicillinase-resistant penicillins should not be administered without penicillin because of their poorer activity against *P. multocida*. Erythromycin is generally ineffective against *P. multocida*, *Moraxella* spp., fusobacteria, and peptostreptococci. Azithromycin is generally more active than clarithromycin against all *Pasteurella* spp. Azithromycin and clarithromycin are only modestly effective against *E. corrodens* and *Peptostreptococcus* spp. Cefoxitin or the combination of penicillin or a first generation cephalosporin plus a beta-lactamase-resistant penicillin or the combination of ticarcillin and clavulanic acid will provide adequate parenteral therapy for animal as well as human bites. The newer quinolones (gatifloxacin and moxifloxacin) (67), and tigecycline (68) are active against all major bite wound pathogens including anaerobic bacteria. However, these agents are not approved for use in children.

   E. corrodens, a capnophilic gram-negative rod that is part of the normal oral flora, can be recovered from 25% of human bite wounds (31). *E. corrodens* is susceptible to penicillin, ampicillin, and the quinolones, but resistant to oxacillin, methicillin, nafcillin, tigecycline, and clindamycin, and some strains are resistant to cephalosporins (64,65,67). Therefore, any isolated *E. corrodens* should have susceptibility testing if cephalosporin therapy is considered.

   When antibiotics are administered in this manner and are combined with good wound toilet, most bite wounds can be sutured with good results and an acceptable infection rate. The duration and route of antibiotic therapy should be individualized based on the site involved, the culture results, and the response to treatment. A 7- to 14-day course is generally adequate for infections limited to soft tissue and a minimum of 21 days therapy is generally required for those involving joints or bones.

COMPLICATIONS

Complications are common in hand wounds, as 30% or more become infected (60). The rate of complications is high because of the presence of avascular tendon and sheath spaces, and the propensity of the infection to spread. The consequence of these infections on function may be disastrous. In addition to local wound infection, other complications include lymphangitis, local abscess, septic arthritis, tenosynovitis, and osteomyelitis (32,58,60). Rare complications include endocarditis, meningitis (69,70), brain abscess (69,71), and sepsis with disseminated intravascular coagulation (72), especially in immunocompromised individuals. Individuals who are especially prone to complications include those receiving systemic corticosteroids, those suffering from lupus erythematosus, and acute leukemia. Rabies must also be considered; and prophylaxis should be administered when indicated (63).

CONCLUSIONS

Animal and human bite wounds can lead to serious infection and complications. The organisms that can be isolated from bite wounds generally represent the oral cavity of the biting animal and the victim's skin flora. When proper techniques for their isolation are employed, anaerobic bacteria can be isolated from over two-thirds of human and animal bite wound infections, especially those associated with abscess formation. Management of the bite wound infections includes the administration of proper local therapy, and utilization when needed of proper antimicrobial agents.

REFERENCES

1. McCaig LF. National hospital ambulatory medical care survey: 1998 emergency department summary. Adv Data 2000; 10:1–23.
2. Talan DA, Abrahamian FM, Moran GJ, et al. Clinical presentation and bacteriologic analysis of infected human bites in patients presenting to emergency departments. Clin Infect Dis 2003; 37:1481–9.
3. Kizer KW. Epidemiologic and clinical aspects of animal bite injuries. JACEP 1979; 8:134–41.
4. Litovitz TL, Klein-Schwartz W, White S, et al. 2000 annual report of the American Association of Poison Control Centers Toxic Exposure Surveillance System. Am J Emerg Med 2001; 19:337–95.
5. Goldstein EJC, Pryor EP, Citron DM. Monkey bites and infection. Clin Infect Dis 1995; 20:1551–2.
6. Farmer CB, Mann RJ. Human bite infections of the hand. South Med J 1996; 59:515–8.
7. Mann RJ, Hoffeld TA, Farmer CB. Human bites of the hand: twenty years of experience. J Hand Surg 1977; 2:97–104.
8. Goldstein EJC. New horizons in the bacteriology, antimicrobial susceptibility and therapy of animal bite wounds. J Med Microbiol 1998; 47:95–7.
9. Goldstein EJC, Citron DM, Finegold SM. Role of anaerobic bacteria in bite wound infections. Rev Infect Dis 1984; 6(Suppl. 1):177–83.
10. Alexander CJ, Citron DM, Gerardo SH, Clams MC, Talan D, Goldstein EJC. Characterization of saccharolytic *Bacteroides* and *Prevotella* isolates from infected dog and cat bite wounds in humans. J Clin Microbiol 1997; 35:406–11.
11. Citron DM, Clams MC, Gerardo SH, Abrahamian F, Talan D, Goldstein EJC. Frequency of isolation of *Porphyronionas* species from infected dog and cat bite wounds in humans and, their characterization by biochemical tests and AP-PCR fingerprinting. Clin Infect Dis 1996; 23(Suppl. 1):78–82.
12. Goldstein EJC, Citron DM, Nesbit C, et al. Prevalence and characterization of anaerobic bacteria from 50 patients with infected cat and dog bite wounds. In: Eley A, Bennett, eds. Anaerobic Pathogens. Sheffield, U.K.: Sheffield Academic Press, 1997:177–85.
13. Weber DJ, Wolfson JS, Swartz MN, Hooper DC. *Pasteurella multocida* infections: report of 34 cases and review of the literature. Medicine 1984; 63:133–54.
14. Holst E, Rollof J, Larsson L, Nielsen JP. Characterization and distribution of *Pasteurella* species recovered from infected humans. J Clin Microbiol 1992; 30:2984–7.
15. Brenner DJ, Hollis DG, Fanning GR, Weaver RE. *Capnocytophaga canimorsus* sp. nov. (formerly CDC group DF-2), a cause of septicemia following dog bite, and *C. cynodegmi* sp. nov., a cause of localized wound infection following dog bite. J Clin Microbiol 1989; 27:231–5.
16. Graham DR, Band JD, Thornsberry C, et al. Infections caused by *Moraxella, Moraxella urethralis, Moraxella*-like groups M-5 and M-6, and *Kingella kingae* in the United States, 1953–1980. Rev Infect Dis 1990; 12:423–31.
17. Andersen BM, Steigerwalt AG, O'Connor SP, et al. *Neisseria weaveri* sp. nov., formerly CDC group M-5, a gram-negative bacterium associated with dog bite wounds. J Clin Microbiol 1993; 31:2456–66.
18. Reina J, Borrell N. Leg abscess caused by *Weeksella zoohelcum* following a dog bite. Clin Infect Dis 1992; 14:1162–3.
19. Guidourdenche M, Lambert T, Riou JY. Isolation of *Neisseria canis* in mixed culture from a patient after a cat bite. J Clin Microbiol 1989; 27:1673–4.
20. Talan DA, Goldstein EJC, Staatz D, Overturf GD. *Staphylococcus intermedius*: clinical presentation of a new human dog bite pathogen. Ann Emerg Med 1989; 18:410–3.
21. Hollis DG, Moss CW, Daneshvar MI, et al. Characterization of Centers for Disease Control group NO-1, a fastidious, nonoxidative, gram-negative organism associated with dog and cat bites. J Clin Microbiol 1993; 31:746–8.
22. Moss CW, Wallace PL, Hollis DG, Weaver RE. Cultural and chemical characterization of CDC groups EO-2, M-5 and M-6, *Moraxella (Moraxella)* species, *Oligella urethralis, Acinetobacter* species, and *Psychrobacter immobilis*. J Clin Microbiol 1988; 26:484–92.
23. Goldstein EJC, Citron DM, Merkin TE, Pickett MJ. Recovery of an unusual *Flavobacterium* group IIb-like isolate from a hand infection following pig bite. J Clin Microbiol 1990; 28:1079–81.
24. Peel MM, Hornidge KA, Luppino M, Stacpoole AM, Weaver RE. *Actinobacillus* spp. and related bacteria in infected wounds of humans bitten by horses and sheep. J Clin Microbiol 1991; 29:2535–8.
25. Erickson T, Vanden Hoek TL, Kuritza A, Leiken JB. The emergency management of moray eel bites. Ann Emerg Med 1992; 21:212–6.
26. Murphey DK, Septimus EJ, Waagner DC. Catfish-related injury and infection: report of two cases and review of the literature. Clin Infect Dis 1992; 14:689–93.

27. Capellan J, Fong IW. Tularemia from a cat bite: case report and review of feline-associated tularemia. Clin Infect Dis 1993; 16:472–5.

28. Hui AY, Hung LC, Tse PC, et al. Transmission of hepatitis B by human bite—confirmation by detection of virus in saliva and full genome sequencing. J Clin Virol. 2005; 33:254–6.

29. Guba AM, Mulliken JB, Hoopes JE. The selection of antibiotics for human bites of the hand. Plast Reconstr Surg 1975; 56:538–41.

30. Shields C, Patzakis MJ, Meyers MH, Harvey JP, Jr. Hand infections secondary to human bites. J Trauma 1975; 15:235–6.

31. Goldstein JC, Citron DM, Wield B, et al. Bacteriology of human and animal bite wounds. J Clin Microbiol 1978; 8:667–72.

32. Brook I. Microbiology of human and animal bite wounds in children. J Pediatr Infect Dis 1987; 6:29–32.

33. Francis DP, Holmes MA, Brandon G. *Pasteurella multocida* infections after domestic animal bites and scratches. JAMA 1975; 233:42–5.

34. Hawkins LG. Local *Pasteurella multocida* infections. J Bone Joint Surg 1969; 51:362–6.

35. Saphir DA, Carter GR. Gingival flora of the dog with special reference to bacteria associated with bites. J Clin Microbiol 1976; 3:344–9.

36. Bailie WE, Stowe EC, Schmitt AM. Aerobic bacterial flora of oral and nasal fluids of canines with reference to bacteria associated with bites. J Clin Microbiol 1978; 7:223–31.

37. Goldstein EJC, Citron DM, Finegold SM. Dog bite wounds and infection: a prospective clinical study. Ann Emerg Med 1980; 9:508–12.

38. Talan DA, Citron DM, Abrahamian FM, Moran GJ, Goldstein EJ, Emergency Medicine Animal Bite Infection Study Group. Bacteriological analysis of infected dog and cat bites. N Engl J Med 1999; 340:85–92.

39. Weigler BJ. Biology of B virus in macaque and human hosts: a review. Clin Infect Dis 1992; 14:555–67.

40. Holmes GP, Chapman LE, Stewart J, et al. Guidelines for the prevention and treatment of B virus infections in exposed persons. Clin Infect Dis 1995; 20:421–39.

41. Bailey GD, Moore LVH, Love DN, Johnson JL. *Bacteroides heparinolyticus*: deoxyribonucleic acid relatedness of strains from the oral cavity and oral—associated disease conditions of horses, cats, and humans. Int J Syst Bacteriol 1988; 38:42–4.

42. Benaoudia F, Escande F, Simonet M. Infection due to *Actinobacillus lignieresii* after a horse bite. J Clin Microbiol Infect Dis 1994; 13:439–40.

43. Barnham M. Pig bite injuries and infection: report of seven human cases. Epidemiol Infect 1988; 101:641–5.

44. Escande F, Bailly A, Bone S, Lemozy J. *Actinobacillus suis* infection after a pig bite. Lancet 1996; 348:888.

45. Rolle U. *Haemophilus influenzae* cellulitis after bite injuries in children. J Pediatr Surg 2000; 35:1408–9.

46. Morgan MS. Treatment of pig bites. Lancet 1996; 348:1246.

47. Auerbach PS, Yajko DM, Nassos PS, et al. Bacteriology of the marine environment: implications for clinical therapy. Ann Emerg Med 1987; 16:643–9.

48. Pavia AT, Bryan JA, Maher KL, Hester R, Jr., Framer JJ, III. *Vibrio carchariae* infections after a shark bite. Ann Intern Med 1989; 111:85–6.

49. Buck JD, Spotte S, Gadbaw JJ, Jr. Bacteriology of the teeth from a great white shark: potential medical implications for shark bite victims. J Clin Microbiol 1984; 20:849–51.

50. Rosenthal SG, Bernhardt HE, Phillips JA, III. *Aeromonas hydrophila* wound infections. Plast Reconstr Surg 1974; 53:77–9.

51. Revord ME, Goldfarb J, Shurin SB. *Aeromonas hydrophila* wound infection in a patient with cyclic neutropenia following a piranha bite. Pediatr Infect Dis J 1988; 7:70–1.

52. Flandry F, Lisecki EJ, Domingue GJ, Nichols RL, Greer DL, Haddad RJ, Jr. Initial antibiotic therapy for alligator bites. South Med J 1989; 82:262–6.

53. Berkowitz FE, Jacobs DWC. Fatal case of brain abscess caused by rooster pecking. Pediatr Infect Dis J 1987; 6:941–2.

54. Davis B, Wenzel RP. Stringes scalp: *Bacteroides* infection after an owl attack. J Infect Dis 1992; 165:975–6.

55. Eberly RJ, Hayek LJ. Antibiotic prophylaxis after a swan bite. Lancet 1997; 350:340.

56. Paisley JW, Lauer BA. Severe facial injuries to infants due to unprovoked attacks by pet ferrets. JAMA 1988; 259:2005–6.

57. Kalb R, Kaplan MH, Tenenbaum MJ, et al. Cutaneous infection at dog bite wounds associated with fulminant DF-2 septicemia. Am J Med 1985; 78:687–90.

58. Bunzli WF, Wright DH, Hoang AT, et al. Current management of human bites. Pharmacotherapy 1998; 18:227–34.

59. Galvin JR, DeSimone D. Infection rate of simple suturing. JACEP 1976; 5:332–3.

60. Morgan M, Palmer J. Dog bites. BMJ 2007; 334:413–7.

61. Maroy SM. Infections due to dog and cat bites. Pediatr Infect Dis 1982; 1:351–4.

62. Stefanopoulos P, Karabouta Z, Bisbinas I, et al. Animal and human bites evaluation and management. Acta orthop Belg 2004; 70:1–10.
63. Update on emerging infections from the Centers for Disease Control and Prevention. Update rabies postexposure prophylaxis guidelines. Ann Emerg Med 1999; 33:590–7.
64. Goldstein EJ. Selected nonsurgical anaerobic infections: therapeutic choices and the effective armamentarium. Clin Infect Dis 1994; 18(Suppl. 4):S273–9.
65. Goldstein EJC, Citron DM, Vagvolgyi AE, Finegold SM. Susceptibility of bite wound bacteria to seven oral antimicrobial agents including RU-285, a new erythromycin: consideration for choosing empiric therapy. Antimicrob Agents Chemother 1986; 29:556–9.
66. Goldstein EJ, Citron DM. Comparative activities of cefuroxime, amoxicillin–clavulanic acid, ciprofloxacin, enoxacin, and ofloxacin against aerobic and anaerobic bacteria isolated from bite wounds. Antimicrob Agents Chemother 1988; 32:1143–8.
67. Goldstein EJ, Citron DM, Merriam CV, Tyrrell K, Warren Y. Activity of gatifloxacin compared to those of five other quinolones versus aerobic and anaerobic isolates from skin and soft tissue samples of human and animal bite wound infections. Antimicrob Agents Chemother 1999; 43:1475–9.
68. Goldstein EJ, Citron DM, Merriam CV, Warren Y, Tyrrell K. Comparative in vitro activities of GAR-936 against aerobic and anaerobic animal and human bite wound pathogens. Antimicrob Agents Chemother 2000; 44:2747–51.
69. Stefanopoulos PK, Tarantzopoulou AD. Facial bite wounds: management update. Int J Oral Maxillofac Surg. 2005; 34:464–72.
70. Bracis R, Seibers K, Jullien RM. Meningitis caused by IIj following a dog bite. West J Med 1979; 131:438–40.
71. Klein DM, Cohen ME. *Pasteurella multocida* brain abscess following perforating cranial dog bite. J Pediatr 1978; 92:588–9.
72. Check W. An odd link between dog bites, splenectomy. JAMA 1979; 241:225–6.

29 | Infection in Solid Tumors

Infection has been recognized as one of the major obstacles to the successful management of patients with malignant tumors (1). Infection is often suspected in patients with solid tumors who develop fever, especially when associated with neutropenia. Although most infections in febrile neutropenic patients with malignancy are related to systemic infections (1), in a large proportion of patients, no obvious source of infection is discovered. It is possible that infection in the tumor mass accounts for a proportion of these febrile episodes. Although the occurrence of infection in necrotic tumor mass has been recognized, the microbiology of infected tumors is not well established.

Aerobic and anaerobic bacteria of endogenous source are a major cause of infections in necrotic tumor, especially when they occur in proximity to a site where these bacteria reside as part of the normal flora. Management of these infections includes directing appropriate antimicrobial therapy against potential bacterial pathogens.

MICROBIOLOGY

Multiple studies provided insight into the etiology of infected tumor mass indirectly through the administration of antimicrobial agents effective against these organisms (2–7). Therapy directed against anaerobes improved or prevented infections in many of these studies. However, the microbiology of infected tumors was not established in these reports.

Several case reports described the microbiology of infected solid tumors (8–11). Lenkey et al. (8) recovered *Bacteroides orchraceus* and *Prevotella melaninogenica* from a necrotic perinephric adenocarcinoma. Braverman et al. (9) reported a patient with *Clostridum welchii* gas gangrene of the uterus that was associated with endometrial adenocarcinoma.

Graham et al. (10) described a case of a large gas-filled clostridial abscess in a previously unrecognized renal cell carcinoma. Trump et al. (11) presented a patient in whom the first recurrence of a carcinoma of the rectum was an intrahepatic metastasis associated with a hepatic abscess caused by *Peptostreptococcus prevotii*. They also reviewed three other reported cases of infection associated with hepatic tumor nodules in which anaerobic bacteria were the primary or only infecting organisms.

Three studies investigated the microbiology of infected tumors (12–14). Rotimi and Durosinmi-Etti (12) studied 70 patients with infected ulcers; 30 of the underlying lesions in these patients were carcinoma of the breast, and 19 were a variety of skin cancers. Most infections were mixed, yielding both anaerobes and aerobes. Anaerobes were the predominant organisms isolated from individual ulcers. There were 282 bacteria isolates, and anaerobic bacteria accounted for 179 (63%). Of the 179 anaerobes isolated, 37 were *Porpyromonas asaccharolytica*, 31 each were *P. melaninogenica* and anaerobic streptococci, 29 *Bacteroides fragilis*, and 17 *Bacteroides ureolyticus*. Among the facultative organisms, *Escherichia coli* was the commonest and was isolated mainly from patients with carcinoma of the breast. Most infections were mixed yielding both anaerobic and aerobic bacteria and this made interpretation of the role of individual pathogens difficult to assess.

Brusis and Luckhaupt (13) reported the microbiology of 15 patients with tumors of the oral cavity, the oropharynx and with recurrent tumors of the hypopharynx and larynx that were infected with anaerobic bacteria. *P. melaninogenica*, *Prevotella oralis*, *Prevotella bivia*, *Peptostreptococcus* spp., and *Fusobacterium* spp. were most frequently represented. Five cases showed mixed aerobic–anaerobic infections. Foul odor was present in most of the tumors and disappeared after a short time by therapy effective against anaerobic bacteria with clindamycin or metronidazole.

Brook (14) reviewed his experience in culturing necrotic tumors for aerobic and anaerobic bacteria over a period of 10 years. Specimens were obtained from 91 patients, 20 of them younger than 18 years. Bacterial growth was present in 63 (69%) specimens. Of these tumors, 14 were abdominal, 5 pelvic, 23 head and neck, 4 lung, 4 mediastinum, 2 lymphatic, 3 breast, and 8 miscellaneous. Aerobic or facultative anaerobic bacteria only were present in 12 (19%) specimens, anaerobes only in 10 (16%), and mixed aerobic and anaerobic bacteria in 41 (65%). The average number of isolates was 2.1/infected tumor. A total of 84 anaerobic and 46 aerobic and facultative anaerobic bacteria were recovered. The predominant anaerobic bacteria were *Bacteroides* spp., anaerobic cocci, and *Propionibacterium acnes*. The most frequently isolated aerobic and facultative bacteria were *Staphylococcus aureus*, alpha-hemolytic streptococci, *E. coli*, *Staphylococcus epidermidis*, *Klebsiella pneumoniae*, and *Pseudomonas aeruginosa* (Table 1).

PATHOGENESIS

The anaerobes recovered from the infected tumors originated most probably from the mucous membranes adjacent to the tumor site (oral, gastrointestinal, and vaginal flora) (Table 2). In most mucus membranes, anaerobes outnumber aerobic and facultative bacteria in ratios ranging from 10:1 to 10,000:1, with anaerobic gram-negative bacilli (AGNB) predominating (15,16). This explains the predominance of *B. fragilis* group in infected abdominal tumors and the predominance of *Prevotella* spp. and *Fusobacterium* spp. in infected tumors of the head and neck. Gram-positive anaerobic cocci that are normal skin inhabitants and part of the normal fecal flora can be recovered from all sites.

Malignancy is often associated with the development of local or systemic infections. Systemic infections may reflect compromises in host defenses at several levels. Infections may be due to alterations in local conditions at the site of the neoplasm, allowing bacteria to gain access to the blood. The humoral immunity, the bactericidal plasma action, and the intracellular killing properties of neutrophils, monocytes, and macrophages may be compromised (17–20).

Local conditions at the neoplasm site can also predispose to infection. The condition in the tumor may predispose for an anaerobic–aerobic infection. Tumors may outgrow their blood supply and become necrotic. The lowered oxygen tension may therefore favor the growth of anaerobic organisms. A tumor can extend into surrounding tissues, causing barrier breakthrough onto mucosal and epithelial surfaces. Alimentary tract inflammatory and focal necrosis can be found in the colonic mucosa in leukemia (21–23) and after cancer chemotherapy (24). Another factor underlying the increased susceptibility of patients with cancer to infection and bacteremia is their overall poor nutritional status (18).

TABLE 1 Predominant Aerobic and Anaerobic Bacteria Recovered from 63 Infected Tumors

Aerobic and facultative organisms	
Staphylococcus aureus	7
Staphylococcus epidermidis	5
Escherichia coli	7
Klebsiella pneumoniae	5
Pseudomonas aeruginosa	5
Total	46
Anaerobic organisms	
Peptostreptococcus spp.	20
Bacteroides fragilis group	17
Prevotella and *Porphyromonas* spp.	8
Total	84

Source: From Ref. 14.

TABLE 2 Predominant Bacterial Isolates in Infected Tumors and Antimicrobials Effective against them

Site	Organisms	Antibiotics
Abdomen	*Bacteroides fragilis* group, *Escherichia coli*, and *Clostridium* spp.	Metronidazole or clindamycin plus gentamicin[a], a penicillin plus a BLI, cefoxitin, a carbapenem[b]
Pelvis	*E. coli*, gram-negative anaerobic bacilli	Metronidazole or clindamycin plus gentamicin[a], a penicillin plus a BLI, cefoxitin, a carbapenem[b]
Head and neck	*Peptostreptococcus* spp., *Prevotella* spp., *Staphylococcus aureus, Streptococcus* spp., and *Pseudomonas* spp.[c]	A penicillin plus a BLI, clindamycin, metronidazole plus dicloxacillin, cefoxitin, a carbapenem[b]
Breast	*Bacteroides* spp., *Prevotella* spp., and *Peptostreptococcus* spp.	Metronidazole plus penicillin, clindamycin, a penicillin plus a BLI, a carbapenem[b]

[a] Cefepime or a quinolone can substitute an aminoglycoside.
[b] Imipenem, meropenem, and ertapenem.
[c] For *Pseudomonas* spp. administer an aminoglycoside.
Abbreviation: BLI, beta-lactamase inhibitor.
Source: From Ref. 14.

Insufficient blood supply of rapidly growing solid tumors can lead to the presence of tissue hypoxia. Vaupel (25) demonstrated that tumor oxygenation, powerfully predicts the prognosis of patients receiving radiotherapy for intermediate and advanced stage cancer of the uterine cervix. Hypoxia is also known to decrease the efficiency of the currently used anticancer modalities like surgery, chemotherapy, and radiotherapy. Therefore, hypoxia seems to be a major limitation in current anticancer therapy.

Clostridium spp. possesses a selective colonization ability of hypoxic/necrotic areas within the tumor. The anaerobic environment within the tumor provided this oxygen-sensitive organism with adequate conditions for proliferation. The use of nonpathogenic *Clostridium* spp. to deliver toxic agents to the tumor cells which is under investigation, takes advantage of this unique physiology (26).

Anaerobic glycolysis is significantly increased in tumor tissue, with a resulting accumulation of lactic acid in this tissue and its environment. Spores of nonpathogenic *Clostridium* spp. can localize and germinate in neoplasms and produce extensive lysis of tumors without concomitant effect on normal tissue (27).

Clostridium septicemia originating from an infection within tumor lesions has been reported (28–31). *C. septicum* infection is highly associated with the presence of a malignancy, either known or occult at the time infection occurs. Occult tumors are mostly situated in the cecal area of the bowel. Predisposing conditions for this type of infection are hematologic malignancies, colon carcinoma, neutropenia, diabetes mellitus, and disruption of the bowel mucosa (32,33).

Bacteremia due to AGNB is also common in patients with infected solid tumors (31). Felner and Dowell (34) reported that 57 out of 250 (23%) patients with AGNB (*B. fragilis* group, *Fusobacterium* spp., and pigmented *Prevotella* spp.) bacteremia had malignancy as a predisposing condition. The most common one were adenocarcinoma of the colon, and uterine or cervical tumors.

Many bacterial infections in children with malignancies are polymicrobial in nature (31). The bacteria isolated from many of these patients originated from the normal flora of the skin or the mucous membrane at or adjacent to the site of the infection.

Aerobic and facultative anaerobic bacteria have also been associated with tumors. *Streptococcus bovis* septicemia and other infections are a relatively uncommon entity that is associated with an increased incidence of colonic neoplasms (35). The organism can be recovered from fecal cultures from patients with carcinoma of the colon (36) and may cause endocarditis in such patients. *Stenotrophomonas maltophilia* has also been associated with infection in patients with solid tumors (37).

DIAGNOSIS

The patient may present with fever. However, because of the depressed immune status, the usual inflammatory signs such as leukocytosis may not be present. Pain, swelling, and enlargement of the lesion may occur. Bleeding into a necrotic tumor can occur and may have deleterious consequences. In tumors adjacent to the skin or oropharynx, a foul odor may be noticed in association with the infection.

Purulent fluid obtained by needle aspiration should be appropriately stained and cultured in media supportive of both aerobically and anaerobic bacteria. Blood and other body fluids and sites should also be cultured to exclude any systemic infection.

Radiological studies may detect localized collections of pus when collections of gas are present or when abnormal tissue density is observed. Ultrasound and computed tomography and magnetic resonance imaging scans, angiography, and radionuclide scans may be helpful.

MANAGEMENT

The polymicrobial aerobic–anaerobic infection in a necrotic tumor may represent a serious threat to the patient, especially when the immune system is suppressed, a common occurrence in those who receive chemotherapy or develop granulocytopenia.

Although surgical removal or evacuation of the purulent fluid is preferred, this is not always feasible in a patient with a malignant tumor. Antimicrobial therapy is often the sole therapy or is used along with surgical drainage or removal of the infected area. Antimicrobial therapy should be continued when there is an associated granulocytopenia until the granulocyte count is increased about 1000/mL.

The choice of antimicrobials should be based whenever possible on the results of culture and susceptibility testing. However, the choice is often empiric. Antimicrobial agents that generally provide coverage for *S. aureus* as well as anaerobic bacteria include cefoxitin, clindamycin, tigecycline, a carbapenem (i.e., imipenem, meropenem, ertapenem), and the combinations of a beta-lactamase inhibitor (i.e., clavulanic acid) and a penicillin (i.e., ticarcillin) and the combination of metronidazole plus a beta-lactamase-resistant penicillin (Table 2). In instances where *S. aureus* is resistant to methicillin, vancomycin, linezolid or tigecycline should be used. Tigecycline, cefoxitin, a carbapenem, and a penicillin plus a beta-lactamase inhibitor also provide coverage against members of the family Enterobacteriaceae. However, agents effective against these organisms as well as *Pseudomonas* spp. (i.e., aminoglycosides, cefepime, and quinolones in adults) should be added to the other agents when treating infections that include these bacteria.

The empiric choice of antimicrobials according to the tumor anatomical site and the predicted causative organisms is presented in Table 2. However, specific choice can be made according to culture results.

CONCLUSIONS

Infection is one of the major obstacles in the management of patients with solid tumors. Aerobic and anaerobic bacteria of endogenous origin are a common source of infections in necrotic tumor, especially when they occur in proximity to a site where these bacteria reside as part of the normal flora. The administration of antimicrobials effective against potential pathogens is often the sole therapy or is used in combination with surgical drainage or removal of the infected tumor. Early removal of solid tumors should be employed whenever possible to prevent them from becoming infected.

REFERENCES

1. Bodey GP. Infection in cancer patients: a continuing association. Am J Med 1986; 81(Suppl. 1A):11–26.
2. Klastersky J, Husson M, Weerts-Ruhl D, Daneau D. Anaerobic wound infection in cancer patients: comparative trials of clindamycin, tinidazole and doxycycline. Antimicrobial Agents Chemother 1977; 12:563–70.
3. Ashby EC, Rees M, Dowding CH. Prophylaxis against systemic infection after transrectal biopsy for suspected prostatic carcinoma. Br Med J 1978; ii:1263–4.
4. Kastersky J, Coppens L, Mombelti G. Anaerobic infections in cancer patients: comparative evaluations of clindamycin and cefoxitin. Antimicrobial Agents Chemother 1979; 16:366–71.

5. Lagast H, Klastersky J. Anaerobic infections in cancer patients: comparative trials of clindamycin, tinidazole, doxycycline, cefoxitin and moxalactam. Infection 1982; 10:144–8.
6. Lagast H, Meunter-Carpenter F, Klasterky J. Moxalactam treatment of anaerobic infections in cancer patients. Antimicrobial Agents Chemother 1982; 22:604–10.
7. Sinkovits JG, Smith JP. Septicaemia with *Bacteroides* in patients with malignant disease. Cancer 1970; 25:663–71.
8. Lenkey JL, Reece GJ, Herbert DL. Gas abscess transformation of a huge hypernephroma. AJR Am J Roentgenol 1979; 133:1174–6.
9. Braverman J, Adachi A, Lev-Gur M, et al. Spontaneous clostridia gas gangrene of uterus associated with endometrial malignancy. Am J Obstet Gynecol 1987; 156:1205–7.
10. Graham BS, Johnson AC, Sawyers JL. Clostridial infection of renal cell carcinoma. J Urol 1986; 135:354–5.
11. Trump DL, Fahnestock R, Cloutier CT, Dickman MD. Anaerobic liver abscess and intrahepatic metastases: a case report and review of the literature. Cancer 1978; 41:682–6.
12. Rotimi VO, Durosinmi-Etti FA. The bacteriology of infected malignant ulcers. J Clin Pathol 1984; 37:592–5.
13. Brusis T, Luckhaupt H. Anaerobic infections in ulcerating tumors of the head and neck. A contribution to the problem of odors. Laryngol Rhinol Otol (Stuttg) 1986; 65:65–8.
14. Brook I. Bacteria from solid tumours. J Med Microbiol 1990; 32:207–10.
15. Gorbach SL. Intestinal microflora. Gastroenterology 1971; 50:1110–6.
16. Finegold SM. Anaerobic Bacteria in Human Disease. New York: Academic Press, Inc., 1977.
17. Maderazo EC, Anton TF, Ward PA. Inhibition of leukocytes in patients with cancer. Clin Immunol Immunopathol 1978; 9:166–76.
18. Phair JP, Riesing KS, Metzger E. Bacteremic infection and malnutrition in patients with solid tumors. Investigation of host defense mechanisms. Cancer 1980; 42:2702–6.
19. Chanock SJ, Pizzo PA. Infectious complications of patients undergoing therapy for acute leukemia: current status and future prospects. Semin Oncol 1997; 24:132–40.
20. Hughes WT, Armstrong D, Bodey GP, et al. 2002 guidelines for the use of antimicrobial agents in neutropenic patients with cancer. Clin Infect Dis 2002; 34:730–51.
21. Dosik GM, Luna M, Valdivieso M, et al. Necrotizing colitis in patients with cancer. Am J Med 1979; 67:646–56.
22. Leach WB. Acute leukemia: a pathological study of the causes of death in 157 proved cases. Can Med Assoc J 1961; 85:345–9.
23. Viola MV. Acute leukemia and infections. JAMA 1967; 201:923–6.
24. Prella JC, Kirsner JB. The gastrointestinal lesions and complications of the leukemias. Ann Intern Med 1964; 61:1084–103.
25. Vaupel P. Oxygen transport in tumors: characteristics and clinical implications. Adv Exp Med Biol 1996; 388:341–51.
26. Nuyts S, Van Mellaert L, Theys J, Landuyt W, Lambin P, Anne J. Clostridium spores for tumor-specific drug delivery. Anticancer Drugs 2002; 13:115–25.
27. Malmgren RA, Flanigan CC. Localization of the vegetation form of *Clostridium tetani* in mouse tumors following intravenous spore administration. Cancer Res 1955; 15:473–8.
28. Alpern RJ, Dowell VR, Jr. *Clostridium septicum* infection and malignancy. J Am Med Assoc 1969; 209:385–8.
29. Cabrera A, Tsukada Y, Pickren JW. Clostridial gas gangrene and septicemia in malignant disease. Cancer 1965; 18:800–6.
30. Caya JG, Farmer SG, Ritch PS, et al. *Clostridia septicemia* complicating the course of leukemia. Cancer 1986; 57:2045–8.
31. Brook I. Bacterial infection associated with malignancy in children. Int J Pediatr Hematol Oncol 1999; 5:379–86.
32. Larson CM, Bubrick MP, Jacobs DM, West MA. Malignancy, mortality, and medicosurgical management of *Clostridium septicum* infection. Surgery 1995; 118:592–7.
33. Prinssen HM, Hoekman K, Burger CW. *Clostridium septicum* myonecrosis and ovarian cancer: a case report and review of literature. Gynecol Oncol 1999; 72:116–9.
34. Felner JM, Dowell VR, Jr. "Bacteroides" bacteremia. Am J Med 1971; 50:787–96.
35. Tabibian N, Clarridge JE. *Streptococcus bovis* septicemia and large bowel neoplasia. Am Fam Physician 1989; 39:227–9.
36. Siegert CE, Overbosch D. Carcinoma of the colon presenting as *Streptococcus sanguis* bacteremia. Am J Gastroenterol 1995; 90:1528–9.
37. Nagai T. Association of *Pseudomonas maltophilia* with malignant lesions. J Med Microb 1984; 20:1003–5.

30 | Joint and Bone Infections

SEPTIC ARTHRITIS

Septic arthritis is defined as a purulent infection in a joint cavity. The infection commonly reaches the joint by hematogenous spread or by direct extension of pathogenic bacteria.

Microbiology

Staphylococcus aureus is a predominant etiologic agent of septic arthritis in all age groups. A history to trauma often is associated with *S. aureus* infection (1,2). This organism is the cause in over three-fourth of infected joints affected by rheumatoid arthritis. *Neisseria gonorrhoeae* is the most frequent pathogen among younger sexually active individuals. *Streptococcus* spp., such as *Streptococcus viridans*, *Streptococcus pneumoniae*, and group B streptococci, account for 20% of cases. Aerobic gram-negative rods cause about 20% to 25% of cases. Most of these infections occur in the very young or old, the immunosuppressed, and intravenous drug abusers (2). In the newborn, however, group B beta-hemolytic streptococci and gram-negative enteric organisms are also involved (1). *Haemophilus influenzae* type b, *S. aureus*, group A streptococci and *pneumoniae* cause arthritis in children younger than five years of age. *H. influenzae* type b infection is, however, now rare in immunized children (3,4). *S. aureus* and group A streptococci are the most common causes of arthritis in children older than five years.

Other organisms reported to cause pyogenic arthritis in children include *Kingella kingae* (5), *Neisseria meningiditis* (6), *Salmonella* spp. (7), and anaerobic bacteria (8,9). Gonococcal arthritis can occur in sexually active adolescents.

In intravenous drug addicts, enteric bacteria, *Pseudomonas aeruginosa* and *Candida* spp. can cause septic arthritis, especially in the sternoclavicular joint and intervertebral disk space (10).

Rare causes of septic arthritis include mycobacteria (11), *Mycoplasma pneumoniae*, *Borrelia burgdorferi*, fungi (11,12) (e.g., *Candida albicans*, *Histoplasma* spp., *Sporothrix schenckii*, *Coccidioides immitis*, *Blastomyces* spp.) (12,13) and viruses (e.g., HIV, lymphocytic choriomeningitis virus, hepatitis A, B, and C viruses, rubella virus) (2).

The timing of prosthetic joint infections (PJI) can be divided into three periods within 3 months of implantation between 3 to 24 months of implantation; and after 24 months following the implantation. Most early PJI is caused by *S. aureus*, while delayed infections are caused by coagulase-negative *S. aureus* and gram-negative aerobes (14). Both of the earlier infections are acquired during the surgical procedure while the late infections are secondary to hematogenous spread from various infectious foci.

Anaerobes rarely have been reported as a cause of septic arthritis in children. Feigin et al. (15) reported two children with septic arthritis caused by clostridia. Nelson and Koontz (16,17) reported three patients of 219 with septic arthritis: one with *Clostridium novyi*, one with *Clostridium bifermentans*, and one with *Bacteroides funduliformis*. Sanders and Stevenson (18) reviewed the literature published before 1968 of *Bacteroides* infections in children, and reported five patients with joint infection, of whom two were their patients, and three were reported by others (19,20). The patients of Sanders and Stevenson also had agammaglobulinemia.

A review of all the adult and pediatric literature by Finegold (21) summarized 1236 joint infections involving anaerobic bacteria. The majority of these cases were reported from the preantimicrobial era, and the most common anaerobe was *Fusobacterium necrophorum*, which accounted for a third of the anaerobes recovered from these patients.

Anaerobic gram-negative bacilli (AGNB, including *Bacteroides fragilis* group) and fusobacteria and gram-positive anaerobic cocci were also recovered from patients with septic arthritis involving anaerobes (22). Sternoclavicular joint infection due to *Prevotella oralis* was reported (23). Hip arthritis due to *F. necrophorum* was described after tonsillectomy in a nine-year-old boy (24). *Propionibacterium acnes* is associated with arthritis in prosthetic joints (25) and following arthroscopy (26). The joints most frequently involved with anaerobic infection were the larger ones, especially the hip and knee, and less frequently the elbow and shoulder.

Most of the cases of anaerobic arthritis, in contrast to anaerobic osteomyelitis, involved one isolate, and approximately 8% involved mixed bacterial flora.

Fitzgerald et al. (27) reported 43 patients ranging in age from 10 to 78 years with anaerobic septic arthritis. Postoperative infection after arthroplasty was present in 23 patients, posttraumatic infection in 12, and arthritis with underlying debilitating diseases in eight patients. Anaerobic gram-positive cocci, especially *Peptostreptococcus magnus*, were the predominant anaerobic isolates in cases of postsurgical and posttraumatic septic arthritis. These organisms probably originate from the skin's normal flora. This is in contrast to the previously recognized association of *Clostridium* spp. with traumatic injuries. However, patients with anaerobic arthritis with underlying debilitating disease were infected with AGNB, especially *B. fragilis*. Fitzerald et al. (27) were also able to recover similar organisms from the blood of seven of their patients. These patients had concomitant distant infections such as intraabdominal sepsis, decubitus ulcers, and osteomyelitis.

Brook and Frazier studied 65 infected joints for aerobic and anaerobic bacteria in adults (28). Seventy-four organisms (1.1 isolates/specimen), consisting of 67 anaerobic bacteria and seven facultative or aerobic bacteria, were isolated from 65 joint specimens. The predominate isolates were *P. acnes* (24 isolates), anaerobic cocci (17), AGNB (10), and *Clostridium* spp. (5).

Pathogenesis

In the initial stages, there is an effusion in the joint cavity, which rapidly becomes purulent. Destruction of cartilage occurs at areas of joint contact. Bone is not affected in the early stages, but the femoral and humeral heads, if involved, may undergo necrosis and subsequent fragmentation and pathologic dislocation. Epiphyses with synchondroses located within the joint capsule are at particularly high risk for infection and necrosis.

During the chronic phase of the disease and the phase of repair, organization of the exudates is present in the joint, and granulation tissue appears and becomes fibrous. This may bind the joint surfaces together, causing fibrous ankylosis. When motion is present, the synovial fluid tends to regenerate, but limitation of motion and associated pain generally remain as a result of the production of residual strong intrasynovial adhesions.

Most of the cases of anaerobic arthritis are secondary to hematogenous spread. Almost all of the isolates of AGNB, including the fusobacteria and the gram-positive anaerobic cocci that were reported, were also involved in a concomitant anaerobic sepsis. In contrast, arthritis secondary to a penetrating wound or foreign body is associated with clostridia (20,27).

Predisposing conditions to joint infection are trauma, prior surgery, presence of a prosthetic joint, and contiguous infection (28). *P. acnes* isolates were associated with PJI, members of the *B. fragilis* group with hematogenous spread, and *Clostridium* spp. with trauma.

The presence of multiple septic joints was common in cases of spread of the organisms from a primary site through the blood stream or in cases of endocarditis (21). The ability of anaerobes to cause tissue destruction is illustrated by the amount of damage they can inflict on the joints, cartilage, capsule, and adjacent periosteum.

Diagnosis

Severe systemic findings such as fever, malaise, and vomiting may be present. Pain may be severe; motion is limited, and the joint is splinted by muscular spasm. In infants this may produce pseudoparalysis. An effusion occurs but may not be palpable at first. The overlying tissues become swollen, tender, and warm. As the infection proceeds, contractures and muscular atrophy may result. Polyarticular arthritis is generally seen in gonococcal disease, viral infections, Lyme disease, reactive arthritis, and various noninfectious processes. Reactive arthritis usually involves a few large joints in an asymmetric fashion. Viral arthritis often exhibits symmetric involvement of the smaller joints, mostly of the hands, with a concurrent rash.

Radiographic examination may reveal distention of the joint capsule and subsequent narrowing of the cartilage space, erosion of the subchondral bone, irregularity and fuzziness of the bone surfaces, bone destruction, diffuse osteoporosis, and associated osteomyelitis. Radiologic examination of the joint also may be useful in detecting unsuspected fracture or chronic bone or joint disease. Plain radiographs can be normal in children with proven pyogenic hip arthritis (29).

Radionuclide scans (i.e., technetium Tc 99m, gallium 67, indium 111 leukocyte scans) are used to nonspecifically localize areas of inflammation and can be valuable in evaluating involvement of the hip or sacroiliac joints. Computed tomography (CT) can be helpful in the diagnosis of arthritis of the shoulder, hip, and sacroiliac joint.

Magnetic resonance imaging (MRI) is very sensitive in the early detection of joint fluid (30). Positive findings include high signal periarticular changes and periarticular abscesses in some cases. MRI can delineate abnormalities of soft tissue, adjacent bone, and the extent of cartilage destruction.

Other helpful tests include sedimentation rate, and C-reactive protein (CRP) which generally are elevated (31,32); peripheral leukocytes count, which is generally increased; and blood cultures, which may recover the causative organisms.

Arthrocentesis can provide a rapid diagnosis of suppurative arthritis. The joint fluid should be examined for glucose (which is generally reduced when compared to serum levels) (32) and leukocytes (which are generally elevated above 50,000 cells/mm^3) (33). Gram's stain should be done, and aerobic, anaerobic, fungal and mycobacterial cultures should be done. At least two blood cultures should be obtained. Polymerase chain reaction (PCR) can assist in detecting infective arthritis due to *Yersinia* spp., *B. burgdorferi*, *Chlamydia* spp., *N. gonorrhoeae*, and *Ureaplasma* spp.

The joint fluid may have a foul odor in the case of anaerobic infection, and, rarely, there may be gas under pressure in the joint. Other clues to purulent arthritis involving anaerobes include failure to obtain organisms on routine culture, Gram stain of the joint fluid showing organisms with the unique morphologic characteristics of anaerobes, and evidence of anaerobic infection elsewhere in the body.

The early and accurate diagnosis of septic arthritis is clinically important. Differentiation of an infectious arthritis from a non-infectious inflammatory synovitis is a frequent diagnostic problem. Synovial fluid analysis often does not yield a diagnosis, despite careful bacteriologic examination and especially in partially treated cases (32,33).

Brook et al. (34) studied 84 patients with acute arthritis. Their data suggest that lactic acid measurements of joint fluid may clearly differentiate between septic arthritis, other than gonococcal arthritis, and other sterile inflammatory and noninflammatory conditions in the joints. Lactic acid levels higher than 65 mg/100 mL should be considered highly suggestive of the presence of a bacterial infection. The synovial fluid also can be studied for bacterial antigens by immunoelectrophoresis or gas liquid chromatography (35,36).

Treatment

Parenteral antibiotic therapy should be initiated immediately after aspiration of the joint, and the choice of therapy should be directed by results of Gram's stain and bacterial cultures. Adequate penetration into the joint is essential.

Therapy of anaerobic arthritis is not different from that required for arthritis caused by aerobes, including treatment of any underlying disease, appropriate drainage and debridement, temporary immobilization of the joint, and antimicrobial therapy pertinent to the bacteriologic characteristics of the individual patient.

Ceftriaxone, or fluroquinolones are generally effective against *N. gonorrhoeae*. Beta-lactamase–resistant penicillin derivative, first-generation cephalosporins, vancomycin or lenizolid should be administered to patients suspected of *S. aureus* infection. Ampicillin with chloramphenicol or a third-generation cephalosporin is administered for *H. influenzae* suppuration, until the antimicrobial susceptibility report is available. Clindamycin, cefoxitin, a carbapenem (e.g., imipenem, meropenem, ertapenem), tigecycline or the combination of amoxicillin or ticarcillin plus clavulanic acid are alternative drugs, affecting *S. aureus* and most anaerobic bacteria. An agent that is effective only against anaerobic bacteria is metronidazole. Because of the recent increase in the isolation, methicillin-resistant *S. aureus* (MRSA), patients with serious staphylococcal infections should therefore be initially started on agents active against MRSA until susceptibility results are available. Vancomycin, daptomycin, linezolid, tigecycline and quinupristin/dalfopristin can be administered to treat these infections.

The exact duration of antimicrobial therapy is not determined; however, it should be given for at least three to four weeks in mild cases. Orally administered antibiotics can be substituted for parenteral treatment after adequate control of infection and inflammation, if compliance and monitoring are possible (37).

Surgical drainage of the joint may be required when rapid reaccumulation of fluid occurs after the initial diagnostic drainage is done, when the appropriate antibiotic and vigorous percutaneous drainage fails to clear the infection after five to seven days, the infected joints are difficult to aspirate (e.g., hip), or the adjacent soft tissue is infected. Drainage of pus may be by intermittent aspiration or by open incision and drainage followed by continuous suction irrigation. Debridement by arthroscopy can be done in some cases of pyogenic arthritis of the knee (38).

OSTEOMYELITIS

Osteomyelitis is an acute or chronic pyogenic inflammatory process that may involve all parts of a bone, although the initial focus usually involves the metaphysis of a bone.

Microbiology

The etiology of acute hematogenous osteomyelitis varies with age: in newborns-*S. aureus*, enteric gram-negative bacteria and group B streptococci predominate; in older children-*S. aureus*, group A streptococci, *H. influenzae*, and enteric gram-negative bacteria are the most frequent isolates. In adult the commonest species are *S. aureus* and occasionally enteric gram-negative bacteria, *Streptococcus* spp. and anaerobes.

S. aureus is the most common organism recovered from infected bones, accounting for more than half of the cases. Other causative agents are beta-hemolytic streptococci and *S. pneumoniae*, *K. kingae*, *Bartonella henselae*, and *Borrelia burgdorferi*. Factors that predispose to the development of osteomyelitis include impetigo, furunculosis, burns, and direct trauma. Rare causes of osteomyelitis are mycobacteria, actinomycosis, and fungi (39–44).

Osteomyelitis caused by direct extension is generally due to *S. aureus*, *Enterobacter* spp., and *Pseudomonas* spp. Wound through sneakers can cause *Pseudomonas* and *S. aureus* infection, while sickle cell disease is associated with *S. aureus* and *Salmonellae* spp.

Specimens from 73 infected bone specimens were studied for aerobic and anaerobic bacteria by Brook and Frazier (28). One hundred and fifty-seven organisms (2.2 isolates/specimen), consisting of 122 anaerobic bacteria (1.7 isolates/specimen) and 35 facultative or aerobic bacteria (0.5 isolate/specimen), were recovered from the 73 bone specimens. Anaerobic bacteria were recovered with aerobe or facultative bacteria in 24 (33%) instances. The predominant anaerobes were *Bacteroides* spp. (49 isolates), anaerobic cocci (45), *Fusobacterium* spp. (11), *P. acnes* (7), and *Clostridium* spp. (6). Conditions predisposing to bone infections are vascular disease, bites, contiguous infection, peripheral neuropathy, hematogenous spread, and trauma. Pigmented *Prevotella* and *Porphyromonas* spp. were mostly isolated in skull and bite infections, members of the *B. fragilis* group in hand and feet infection, and *Fusobacterium* spp. in skull, bite, and hematogenous long bone infections.

Anaerobic bacteria have received increasing recognition in the etiology of osteomyelitis (28,45,46), although the exact prevalence of anaerobes in this disease is unknown. More than 800 cases of bone infection involving anaerobic bacteria have been reported (21).

A few reports describe the recovery of anaerobic organisms from infected bones in children. Raff and Melo (46) reported the recovery of *S. aureus* mixed with *Eubacterium lentum* from osteomyelitis of the right femur of a 13-year-old patient. Schubiner et al. (47) recovered fusobacteria from an infected tibia in a seven-year-old patient with Gaucher's disease. Chandler and Breaks (48) reported the recovery of *Bacteroides* spp. from the hip of a 12-year-old patient with osteomyelitis. Pichichero and Friesen (49) described a nine-year-old female with paronychia and osteomyelitis of the phalanx. Six organisms were recovered from the infected site, including two anaerobes, *Prevotella melaninogenica* and *Veillonella parvula*. Sanders and Stevenson (18) reported a three-year-old patient with Bruton's agammaglobulinemia and septic arthritis of the hip, who had osteomyelitis of the femur caused by *Bacteroides* spp. Beigelman and Rantz (50) recovered *Bacteroides* spp. in an infected osteoma of the mandible in a five-year-old patient. Ogden and Light (51) reported nine cases of anaerobic osteomyelitis in patients ranging from 3 months to 13 years. Four patients were malnourished, and three had sickle cell anemia. Seven patients had infections in the long bones, one had infection in the vertebrae, and one had infection in a metacarpal bone. *Bacteroides* spp. were recovered in six patients, *Clostridium* spp. in two patients, and anaerobic cocci in two patients. Garcia-Tornel et al. (52) described a four-year-old girl with osteoarthritis of the right femur caused by *Bacteroides coagulans*. Numerous anaerobes were recovered from children with infected mastoid bones (53). Chronic osteomyetitis caused by *Clostridium difficile* was absorbed in an adolescent with sickle cell disease (54).

Ten years experience in diagnosis and therapy of osteomyelitis caused by anaerobic bacteria in children was described by Brook (55). Twenty-six pediatric patients with osteomyelitis caused by anaerobic bacteria were presented. The etiologic factors to the infection were chronic mastoiditis (7 patients), decubitus ulcers (5), chronic sinusitis (4), periodontal abscesses (3), bites (3), paronychia (2), trauma (1), and scalp infection after fetal monitoring (1). Seventy-four organisms (2.8 isolates/specimen), 63 anaerobes (2.4/specimen), and 11 facultative and aerobic bacteria (0.4/specimen) were recovered. Anaerobic bacteria that were recovered from all patients were mixed with aerobes in 11 (42%). The predominant organisms were anaerobic cocci (29 isolates), AGNB (21), *Fusobacterium* spp. (8), and *Clostridium* spp. (4). The organisms generally reflected the microbial flora of the mucus surface adjacent to the infected site. Eight beta-lactamase–producing organisms were recovered from seven (27%) patients. These included all isolates of the *B. fragilis* group (4) and of *S. aureus* (3), two of the 12 pigmented *Prevotella* and *Porphyromonas* spp., and one of three *P. oralis*.

Finegold (21) reviewed the world literature on anaerobic osteomyelitis until 1976. He found that most of the cultures that yielded anaerobes also yielded aerobic or facultative organisms, except for infections involving actinomycetes. When anaerobes are present in combination with aerobic organisms, they may act synergistically in producing disease. Over one-third of the isolates were AGNB, mainly *Bacteroides* and *Fusobacterium* spp. Other frequently recovered anaerobes were anaerobic gram-positive cocci, actinomycetes, and *F. necrophorum*. Infections of long bones involved mainly clostridia, and vertebral osteomyelitis involved actinomycetes. Anaerobic gram-positive cocci were recovered mostly from small bones of the extremities.

Two reports summarized more than 300 cases of nonactinomycotic anaerobic osteomyelitis, mostly in adults (45,46). Lewis et al. (45) reported 23 patients and reviewed 260 patients and found an adjacent soft-tissue infection in 49% of the patients. Fractures associated with trauma were a predisposing factor in 28% of the patients, approximately half in the long bones, and one-quarter each in the hands or feet and mandible or maxillae. Raff and Melo (46) reviewed 121 patients and also found fractures to be the most common etiological factor (occurring in 48%), followed by diabetes mellitus (11%), human bites (9%), otitis media (6%), and decubitus ulcers (4%).

These two reports (45,46) found infection in the skull and facial bones in approximately one-third of the cases, generally after chronic otitis media or sinusitis, facial cellulitis, dental abscesses or extractions, fractures, and surgical procedures. Complications of these infections included meningitis, brain abscesses, and septic pulmonary infarctions.

The most common organisms responsible for these infections, as reported by Lewis et al. (45) and Raff and Melo (46), were anaerobic gram-positive cocci, *Bacteroides* spp., and *Fusobacterium* spp., all residents of the oral flora. Similiar organisms were found to be the major pathogens in osteomyelitis of the skull and facial bones in children (55). However, in contrast to adults, osteomyelitis of the skull and facial bones accounted for 15 (57%) of the infections. The higher frequency of this type of infection in children may be related to the common occurrence of chronic otitis and sinusitis in the pediatric age group, compared with adults.

The polymicrobial nature of anaerobic osteomyelitis is apparent from these studies (45,48,55). Mixed aerobic and anaerobic flora was recovered in 11 (42%) of 26 cases presented by Brook (55) and Lewis et al. (45) recovered 2.2 aerobes and 4.0 anaerobes/specimen in the 23 patients they studied.

Pathogenesis

Many patients with osteomyelitis attributed to anaerobic bacteria have evidence of anaerobic infection elsewhere in the body, which is the source of the organisms involved in osteomyelitis. Spread to bone is by contiguous infection extending to the bone or by infection that reaches the bone by way of the bloodstream during the course of sustained or intermittent bacteremia. This infection can be of any type, but often shows characteristic features of anaerobic infection such as abscess formation, septic thrombophlebitis, production of foul odor and gas, and tissue necrosis (55). Some of the patients with anaerobic osteomyelitis will also have arthritis involving anaerobic bacteria, usually in an adjacent joint. A certain number of patients will have positive blood cultures. Blood cultures were obtained from 21 of the 26 patients reported by Brook (55) and were positive in four patients (19%). The microorganisms recovered in these cultures were similar to those isolated from the infected site.

Diabetes mellitus and vascular insufficiency have been incriminated as predisposing factors in anaerobic infection (56). Ischemia and necrotic tissue provide an optimum environment for invasion and proliferation of anaerobes.

Human bites frequently result in anaerobic osteomyelitis. Of patients with anaerobic osteomyelitis of the hand for whom a predisposing factor was given, more than two-thirds had sustained a human bite (46,55).

The bacteria recovered in osteomyelitis after decubitus ulcers generally reflect the normal bacterial flora of the closest mucus membrane and are also recovered from the infected ulcers (57). Infections of the skull related to decubitus ulcers in that area were associated with anaerobes generally found in the oral flora, and infections after decubitus ulcers around the anal area were caused by colonic flora. Similarly, osteomyelitis of the occipital bone after fetal monitoring is caused by organisms that are normal residents of the female genital tract and were introduced by the fetal-monitoring electrodes (58).

Many other conditions may predispose to invasion of bone by anaerobic bacteria. These include chronic otitis media, decubitus ulcers, abscesses, chronic sinusitis, and odontogenic infections (59). Few reports of anaerobic osteomyelitis also show a direct extension of the anaerobic infection for an adjacent sinusitis (57,60), or direct implantation of the organisms from the oral (60,61) or vaginal flora (58).

Diagnosis

Local inflammatory signs may be absent in the early stages. Later, there usually is localized, erythema, warmth, tenderness, swelling, fever, elevated pulse, pain that is severe, constant, and throbbing over the end of the shaft; and limitation of joint motion. Laboratory findings may reveal leukocytosis, and elevated sedimentation rate and CRP (62–64). Blood cultures are generally positive early in the course. Aspirated pus should be Gram stained, and sent for aerobic and anaerobic cultures.

The importance of obtaining adequate specimens for Gram's stain and culture cannot be overemphasized. Many cases of culture-negative osteomyelitis may have been caused by anaerobes that were not detected. Aliquots of bone obtained either by needle biopsy or as surgical specimens immediately should be placed in media under conditions appropriate for isolation of obligate anaerobic pathogens.

Radiographs may show soft-tissue edema at three to five days after infection. A spotty rarefaction can be observed followed shortly by periosteal new bone formation, which is generally absent for the first 10 to 14 days of the disease (65–67). A considerable portion of bone usually is involved, and the bone is demineralized. Radionuclide scanning with 3-phase technetium 99m bone scan may be positive before bony changes are seen on the radiograph (65–67). MRI can be an effective means of imaging bone (68,69), with a sensitivity for early detection of osteomyelitise that ranges from 92% to 100%. It is superior to plain radiography, CT, and radionuclide scanning in selected anatomic locations. MRI can differentiate cellulitis from osteomyelitis, and differentiate acute from chronic osteomyelitis (71). Ultrasonography may demonstrate changes as early as 24 to 48 hours after onset of symptoms. It can detect soft-tissue abscess or fluid collection and periosteal elevation and can guide an aspiration.

There are no significant clinical differences between the patients with and without anaerobes cultured from their bone infections. There is a relative lack of systemic symptoms in the patients with bone infections involving anaerobes (39). Foul odor may be present in approximately half of the patients (46,55).

Although the clinical presentation of anaerobic or mixed aerobic and anaerobic osteomyelitis may not differ markedly from that of aerobic osteomyelitis, anaerobic osteomyelitis should be suspected in particular clinical settings:

1. Hand infections occurring as a result of bites,
2. Osteomyelitis of the pelvis or ilium after intraabdominal sepsis,
3. Osteomyelitis following decubitus ulcers,
4. Patients with osteomyelitis of the skull and facial bones,
5. Chronic nonhealing indolent ulcers of the foot, particularly in diabetics or in patients with associated vascular insufficiency who have underlying foci of bony involvement,
6. Presence of foul-smelling exudates,
7. Presence of sloughing of necrotic tissue, gas in soft tissues, or black discharge from a wound or both,
8. Gram stains of clinical material reveals multiple organisms having different morphologic characteristics,
9. Failure to grow organisms from clinical specimens, particularly but not only when the results of the Gram stain has shown organisms,
10. Presence of sequestra in the bone,
11. Presence of exacerbation of chronic osteomyelitis of long bones.

Treatment

Management of osteomyelitis includes symptomatic therapy, immobilization in some patients, adequate drainage of purulent material, and antibiotic therapy consisting of parenteral administration of antibiotics for at least four to six weeks and in some cases even longer. The average duration of antimicrobial therapy for patients in a previous reported study was 31 days (range 22–58 days) (55). Except for diagnostic aspiration, extensive surgical drainage or debridement was performed in 18 (60%) of the patients (55). This included all patients with mastoiditis, sinusitis, periodontal abscess, fetal monitoring, two of five with decubitus ulcer, and one of two with paronychia.

Although antibiotic therapy most often is started before the results of cultures are available, treatment programs must be adjusted according to the susceptibility of microorganisms recovered from bone cultures obtained by needle, surgery, or from blood cultures. Once cultures are obtained, the need to initiate therapy without delay is important, if treatment failures and structural complications are to be avoided.

In the choice of antibiotic, numerous factors are important. The least toxic agent should be given at doses that yield the optimal inhibitory concentration for a long enough period to inhibit all organisms. Culture information is essential for this choice. In general, the penicillins, cephalosporins, clindamycin, and vancomycin can achieve clinically effective bone concentrations against staphylococci. Clindamycin has especially good bone penetration, attaining a high bone-to-serum ratio (71). Aminoglycosides should be used only when other agents would not be effective.

For the most common isolate, *S. aureus*, the preferred drug is a penicillinase (beta-lactamase)-resistant penicillin. Alternatives are the cephalosporins, clindamycin, and vancomycin. Antimicrobials effective against MRSA, include vancomycin, daptomycin, tigecycline linezolid, and quinupristin/dalfopristin.

Other gram-positive organisms such as groups A and B streptococci, *S. pneumoniae*, clostridia, actinomycetes, and gram-positive anaerobic cocci usually are penicillin sensitive.

Aerobic and facultative gram-negative microorganisms should be treated with third-generation cephalosporins, quinolones (after closure of the epiphyseal line), and aminoglycosides.

Penicillin G seems to be the preferred drug for most anaerobic infections other than those caused by *B. fragilis* (21,72). *B. fragilis* group are known to resist penicillin through production of beta-lactamase. Many AGNB (e.g., pigmented *Prevotella* and *Porphyromonas* spp.) and *Fusobacterium* spp., which formerly were susceptible to penicillins, have shown increased resistance to these drugs by producing beta-lactamase (73,74). This phenomenon was also observed in our report (55) in which five of the AGNB produced beta-lactamase. When such organisms are present, an antimicrobial that is resistant to this enzyme should be used. These include clindamycin, chloramphenicol, cefoxitin, a carbapenem, (i.e., imipenem, meropenem, ertapenem), tigecycline, metronidazole, or the combination of a beta-lactamase inhibitor and a penicillin (74).

Surgical intervention often is required to establish a diagnosis and to remove foreign material. Otherwise, surgery is limited therapeutically to a small number of patients in whom drainage of a subperiosteal collection or debridement of necrotic or devitalized bone is necessary. Failure to respond to appropriate treatment, coupled with continued pain, swelling, fever, and elevated leukocyte count and sedimentation rate are indications for surgery. For vertebral osteomyelitis complicated by neurologic compromise, immediate surgical intervention is required to relieve cord compression. Surgery also should be used to drain a septic hip when it accompanies osteomyelitis.

The usual duration of therapy is four to eight weeks and depends on the etiology, extent of infection, and clinical and laboratory responses.

A change to oral antibiotics can be made when pain, fever, and signs of local inflammation have resolved, and depends on the willingness of the patients to comply and adhere with to the oral regimen.

Hyperbaric oxygen also may be considered as adjunctive therapy for anaerobic osteomyelitis (75). Slack et al. (76) treated five patients with chronic osteomyelitis caused by aerobic organisms and had encouraging results. Other authors (77,78) have reported various degrees of success in the treatment of patients with wound infections caused by aerobic organisms and in experimental treatment of staphylococcal osteomyelitis (79).

Although anaerobic osteomyelitis occurs infrequently, if unrecognized or inappropriately treated, this infection can lead to severe local and systemic complications. Early recognition, use of appropriate diagnostic and laboratory methods, and proper medical and surgical treatment can contribute to rapid resolution of the infection.

REFERENCES

1. Welkon CJ, Long SS, Fisher MC, Alburger PD. Pyogenic arthritis in infants and children: a review of 95 cases. Pediatr Infect Dis J 1986; 5:669–76.
2. Tarkowski A. Infection and musculoskeletal conditions: infectious arthritis. Best Pract Res Clin Rheumatol 2006; 20:1029–44.
3. Broadhurst LE, Erickson RL, Kelley PW. Decreases in invasive *Haemophilus influenzae* diseases in U.S. Army children, 1984–1991. JAMA 1993; 269:227–31.
4. Adams WG, Deaver KA, Cochi SL, et al. Decline of childhood *Haemophilus influenzae* type B (Hib) disease in the Hib vaccine era. JAMA 1993; 269:221–6.

5. Yagupsky P, Dagan R, Howard CB, et al. Clinical features and epidemiology of invasive *Kingella kingae* infection in southern Israel. Pediatrics 1993; 92:800–4.
6. Rompalo AM, Hook EW, Roberts PG, et al. The acute arthritis dermatitis syndrome. The changing importance of *Neisseria gonorrhoeae* and *Neisseria meningitidis*. Arch Intern Med 1987; 147:281–3.
7. Hill Gaston JS, Lillicrap MS. Arthritis associated with enteric infection. Best Pract Res Clin Rheumatol 2003; 17:219–39.
8. Renne JW, Tanowitz HB, Chulay JD. Septic arthritis in an infant due to *Clostridium ghoni* and *Hemophilus parainfluenzae*. Pediatrics 1976; 57:573–4.
9. Yocum RC, McArthur J, Petty BG, et al. Septic arthritis caused by *Propionibacterium acnes*. JAMA 1982; 248:1740–1.
10. Bisbe J, Miro JM, Latorre X, et al. Disseminated candidiasis in addicts who use brown heroin: report of 83 cases and review. Clin Infect Dis 1992; 15:910–23.
11. Harrington JT. Mycobacterial and fungal arthritis. Curr Opin Rheumatol 1998; 10:335–8.
12. Kohli R, Hadley S. Fungal arthritis and osteomyelitis. Infect Dis Clin North Am 2005; 19:831–51.
13. Hansen BL, Andersen K. Fungal arthritis. A review. Scand J Rheumatol 1995; 24:248–50.
14. Anguita-Alonso P, Hanssen AD, Patel R. Prosthetic joint infection. Expert Rev Anti Infect Ther 2005; 3:797–804.
15. Feigin RD, Pickering LK, Anderson D, Keeney RE, Shackleford PG. Clindamycin treatment of osteomyelitis and septic arthritis in children. Pediatrics 1975; 55:213–23.
16. Nelson JD. The bacterial etiology and antibiotic management of septic arthritis in infants and children. Pediatrics 1972; 50:437–40.
17. Nelson JD, Koontz WC. Septic arthritis in infants and children: a review of 117 cases. Pediatrics 1966; 38:966–71.
18. Sanders DY, Stevenson J. *Bacteroides* infection in children. J Pediatr 1968; 72:673–7.
19. Ament ME, Gaal SA. *Bacteroides* arthritis. Am J Dis Child 1967; 114:427–8.
20. McVay LV, Sprunt DH. *Bacteroides* infections. Ann Intern Med 1952; 36:56–9.
21. Finegold SM. Anaerobic Bacteria in Human Disease. New York: Academic Press, 1977.
22. Rosenkranz P, Lederman MM, Gopalakrishna KV, Ellner JJ. Septic arthritis caused by *Bacteroides fragilis*. Rev Infect Dis 1990; 12:20–30.
23. Ramos A, Calabrese S, Salgado R, Alonso MN, Mulero J. Sternoclavicular joint infection due to *Bacteroides oralis*. J Rheumatol 1993; 20:1438–9.
24. Beldman TF, Teunisse HA, Schouten TJ. Septic arthritis of the hip by *Fusobacterium necrophorum* after tonsillectomy: a form of Lemierre syndrome? Eur J Pediatr 1997; 156:856–7.
25. Sulkowski MS, Abolnik IZ, Morris EI, Granger DL. Infectious arthritis due to *Propionibacterium acnes* in a prosthetic joint. Clin Infect Dis 1994; 19:224–5.
26. Kooijmans-Coutinho MF, Markusse HM, Dijkmans BA. Infectious arthritis caused by *Propionibacterium acnes*: a report of two cases. Ann Rheum Dis 1989; 48:851–2.
27. Fitzgerald RH, Rosenblatt JE, Tenney JH, Bourgault AM. Anaerobic septic arthritis. Clin Orthop 1982; 164:141–8.
28. Brook I, Frazier EH. Anaerobic osteomyelitis and arthritis in a military hospital: a 10-year experience. Am J Med 1993; 94:21–8.
29. Volberger FM, Sumner TE, Abramson JS, Winchester PH. Unreliability of radiographic diagnosis of septic hip in children. Pediatrics 1984; 74:118–20.
30. Sanchez RB, Quinn SF. MRI of inflammatory synovial processes. Magn Reson Imaging 1989; 7:529–40.
31. Kunnamo I, Kallio P, Pelkonen P, Hovi T. Clinical signs and laboratory tests in the differential diagnosis of arthritis in children. Am J Dis Child 1987; 141:34–40.
32. Margaretten ME, Kohlwes J, Moore D, Bent S. Does this adult patient have septic arthritis? JAMA 2007; 297:1478–88.
33. Mathews CJ, Kingsley G, Field M, et al. Management of septic arthritis: a systematic review. Ann Rheum Dis 2007; 66:440–5.
34. Brook I, Reza MJ, Bricknell KS, Bluestone R, Finegold SM. Synovial fluid lactic acid: a diagnostic aid in septic arthritis. Arthritis Rheum 1978; 21:774–9.
35. Brooks JB, Kellogg DS, Alley CC, Short HB, Handsfield HH, Huff B. Gas chromatography as a potential means of diagnosing arthritis. I. Differentiation between staphylococcal, streptococcal, gonococcal, and traumatic arthritis. J Infect Dis 1974; 129:660–8.
36. Feldman SA, DuClos T. Diagnosis of meningococcal arthritis by immunoelectrophoresis of synovial fluid. Appl Microbiol 1973; 25:1006–12.
37. Kolyvas E, Ahronheim G, Marks MI, Gledhill R, Owen H, Rosenthall L. Oral antibiotic therapy of skeletal infections in children. Pediatrics 1980; 65:867–71.
38. Siparsky P, Ryzewicz M, Peterson B, Bartz R. Arthroscopic treatment of osteoarthritis of the knee: are there any evidence-based indications? Clin Orthop Relat Res 2007; 455:107–12.
39. Waldvogel FA, Papageorgiou PS. Osteomyelitis: the past decade. N Engl J Med 1980; 303:360–70.
40. Scott RJ, Christoferson MR, Robertson WW, et al. Acute osteomyelitis in children: a review of 116 cases. J Pediatr Orthop 1990; 10:649–52.

41. Faden H, Grossi M. Acute osteomyelitis in children: reassessment of etiologic agents and their clinical characteristics. Am J Dis Child 1991; 145:65–9.
42. Vadheim CM, Greenbery DP, Erikson E, et al. Protection provided by *Haemophilus influenzae* type B conjugate vaccines in Los Angeles County: a case control study. Pediatr Infect Dis J 1994; 13:274–80.
43. Burch KH, Fine G, Quinn EL, Eisses JF. *Cryptococcus neoformans* as a cause of lytic bone lesions. JAMA 1975; 231:1057–9.
44. Arias F, Mata-Essayag S, Landaeta ME, et al. *Candida albicans* osteomyelitis: case report and literature review. Int J Infect Dis 2004; 8:307–14.
45. Lewis RP, Sutter VL, Finegold SM. Bone infections involving anaerobic bacteria. Medicine 1978; 57:279–305.
46. Raff MJ, Melo JC. Anaerobic osteomyelitis. Medicine 1978; 57:83–103.
47. Schubiner H, Letourneau M, Murray DL. Pyogenic osteomyelitis versus pseudo-osteomyelitis in Gaucher's disease: report of a case and review of the literature. Clin Pediatr 1981; 20:607–9.
48. Chandler FA, Breaks VM. Osteomyelitis of femoral neck and head. JAMA 1941; 116:2390–6.
49. Pichichero ME, Friesen AH. Polymicrobial osteomyelitis: report of three cases and review of the literature. Rev Infect Dis 1982; 4:86–96.
50. Beigelman PM, Rantz LA. Clinical significance of *Bacteroides*. Arch Intern Med 1949; 84:605–9.
51. Ogden JA, Light TR. Pediatric osteomyelitis III. Clin Orthop 1979; 145:230–6.
52. Garcia-Tornel S, Marques JC, Gairi Tahull JM, Ullot R, Minguella JM. *Bacteroides coagulans* osteo-arthritis. Pediatr Infect Dis 1983; 2:472–4.
53. Brook I. Aerobic and anaerobic bacteriology of chronic mastoiditis in children. Am J Dis Child 1981; 135:478–9.
54. Gaglani MJ, Murray JC, Morad AB, Edwards MS. Chronic osteomyelitis caused by *Clostridium difficile* in an adolescent with sickle cell disease. Pediatr Infect Dis J 1996; 15:1054–6.
55. Brook I. Anaerobic osteomyelitis in children. Pediatr Infect Dis 1986; 5:550–6.
56. Felner JM, Dowell VR. Anaerobic bacterial endocarditis. N Engl J Med 1970; 283:1188–92.
57. Brook I. Anaerobic and aerobic bacteriology of decubitus ulcers in children. Am Surg 1980; 6:624–6.
58. Brook I. Osteomyelitis and bacteremia caused by *Bacteroides fragilis*: a complication of fetal monitoring. Clin Pediatr 1980; 19:639–40.
59. Calhoun KH, Shapiro RD, Stiernberg CM, Calhoun JH, Mader JT. Osteomyelitis of the mandible. Arch Otolaryngol Head Neck Surg 1988; 114:1157–62.
60. Brook I, Friedman EM, Rodriguez WJ, Controni G. Complications of sinusitis in children. Pediatrics 1980; 66:568–72.
61. Brook I. Bacteriology of paronychia in children. Am J Surg 1981; 141:703–5.
62. Vaughan PA, Newman NM, Rosman MA. Acute hematogenous osteomyelitis in children. J Pediatr Orthop 1987; 7:652–5.
63. Chelsom F, Solberg CO. Vertebral osteomyelitis at a Norwegian University Hospital 1987–97: clinical features, laboratory findings and outcome. Scand J Infect Dis 1998; 30:147–51.
64. Unkila-Kallio L, Kallio MJ, Eskola J, Peltola H. Serum C-reactive protein, erythrocyte sedimentation rate, and white blood cell count in acute hematogenous osteomyelitis of children. Pediatrics 1994; 93:59–62.
65. Sullivan DC, Rosenfield NS, Ogden S, Gottschalk A. Problems in the scintigraphic detection of osteomyelitis in children. Radiology 1980; 135:731–6.
66. Bressler EL, Conway JJ, Weiss SC. Neonatal osteomyelitis examined by bone scintigraphy. Radiology 1984; 152:685–8.
67. Ash JM, Gilday DL. The futility of bone scanning neonatal osteomyelitis: concise communication. J Nucl Med 1980; 21:417–20.
68. Aloui N, Nessib N, Jalel C. Acute osteomyelitis in children: early MRI diagnosis. J Radiol 2004; 85:403–8.
69. Dangman BC, Hoffer JA, Rand FF, O'Rourke EJ. Osteomyelitis in children: adolinium-enhanced MR imaging. Radiology 1992; 182:743–7.
70. Sammak B, Abd El Bagi M, Al Shahed M. Osteomyelitis: a review of currently used imaging techniques. Eur Radiol 1999; 9:894–900.
71. Mandracchia VJ, Sanders SM, Jaeger AJ. Management of osteomyelitis. Clin Podiatr Med Surg 2004; 21:335–51.
72. Finegold SM, Bartlett JG, Chow AW, et al. Management of anaerobic infections. Ann Intern Med 1975; 83:375–89.
73. Brook I, Calhoun L, Yocum P. Beta-lactamase–producing isolates of *Bacteroides* species from children. Antimicrob Agents Chemother 1980; 18:164–6.
74. Hecht DW. Anaerobes: antibiotic resistance, clinical significance, and the role of susceptibility testing. Anaerobe 2006; 12:115–21.

75. Sheridan RL, Shank ES. Hyperbaric oxygen treatment: a brief overview of a controversial topic. J Trauma 1999; 4:426–35.
76. Slack WK, Thomas DA, Perrins D. Hyperbaric oxygenation in chronic osteomyelitis. Lancet 1965; 1:1093–4.
77. Irvin TT, Norman JN, Suwanagel A. Hyperbaric oxygen in the treatment of infections by aerobic microorganisms. Lancet 1966; 1:392–4.
78. Mader JT, Shirtliff ME, Bergquist SC, Calhoun J. Antimicrobial treatment of chronic osteomyelitis. Clin Orthop 1999; 360:47–65.
79. Mendel V, Reichert B, Simanowski HJ, Scholz HC. Therapy with hyperbaric oxygen and cefazolin for experimental osteomyelitis due to *Staphylococcus aureus* in rats. Undersea Hyperb Med 1999; 26:169–74.

31 | Pseudomembranous Colitis

Pseudomembranous colitis (PMC) is commonly associated with hospitalization and prior antibiotic exposure. PMC is currently believed to be caused almost exclusively by toxins produced by *Clostridium difficile*. The clinical spectrum of this disease may range from a mild, nonspecific diarrhea to severe colitis with toxic megacolon, perforation, and death (1). Discontinuation of antibiotics and supportive therapy usually lead to resolution of this disorder (2). PMC may affect all age groups, although a lower incidence was noted in children (3).

MICROBIOLOGY AND PATHOGENESIS

Ampicillin, amoxicillin, the second and third generation cephalosporins, clindamycin, and recently the quinolones are most frequently associated with the development of PMC, although nearly all antimicrobials have been implicated as causes of diarrhea and colitis (4,5). Antibiotics that infrequently cause PMC are other penicillins, first generation cephalosporins, chloramphenicol, macrolides, tetracyclines, and trimethoprim-sulfamethoxazole. Rarely causing PMC are aminoglycosides, fluorouracil, rifampin, methrotrexate, and sulfonamides. The resistance of some clostridia to clindamycin initially led researchers to speculate that clostridia might play a role in clindamycin-associated colitis. The research in the 1970th associated the development of PMC with clindamycin-resistant *C. difficile*. However, this condition was also found to be associated with all other antimicrobials (5–7).

Since 2003, *C. difficile* colitis has become more frequent, severe, and refractory to standard therapy, and more likely to relapse. This pattern is widely distributed in the U.S.A., Canada, and Europe and is attributed to a new strain of *C. difficile*-designated BI, NAP1, or ribotype 027 (synonymous terms). This strain appears more virulent, possibly because of the production of large amounts of toxins. Fluoroquinolones are now major inducing agents along with cephalosporins, which presumably reflects newly acquired in vitro resistance and escalating rates of use (7).

Numerous studies (5–8) implicated *C. difficile* as an etiologic agent of PMC. Other species of *Clostridium* (*Clostridium innocuum*, *Clostridium oroticum*, and *Clostridium ramosum*) were implicated in rare cases in PMC along with *Candida* spp. and aerobic gram-negative bacilli. Some reports have also described infants (5) and adults (8,9) with severe PMC associated with *C. difficile* toxin in the stools without previous antibiotic exposure.

C. difficile can produce at least two toxins both necessary to produce PMC (10), an enterotoxin (toxin A), and a cytotoxin (toxin B). The cytotoxin is potent in tissue culture assays and is a relatively sensitive and specific marker for *C. difficile*-induced disease, whereas toxin A is significantly more potent in biologic assays of enteric toxins when animal models are used, and it may be more important in the clinical expression of gastrointestinal complications. Serum antibodies to *C. difficile* toxins are present in about 2/3 of children and adults in the U.S.A., but their protective nature is not established (11). The immune protection against *C. difficile* toxins requires toxin A-specific secretory antibodies in the intestinal lumen and recombinant polymeric IgA specific for both toxins in the lamina propria (12). Immature enterocyte toxin–binding sites or maternal protective antibody have been postulated to protect neonates from developing disease (13).

Most stools from patients with antibiotic-associated PMC contain the *C. difficile* organism as well as its' cytotoxin (14). Individuals treated with antibiotics can become susceptible to acquire the organism from an environmental source (9). Nearly 30% of healthy newborns harbor *C. difficile* as a component of the fecal flora and some also have detectable toxin in their stool without clinically apparent consequences (15). Carrier rates for *C. difficile* in stool decrease with age, and this microbe is found in more than 5% of children more than one year of age. *C. difficile* is not involved in the etiology of childhood diarrhea (16).

C. difficile can be spread in neonatal nursery, hospital wards, and households (17). The organism is transmitted by the hands of personnel caring for symptomatic or colonized patients (5), and by fomites. A high incidence of asymptomatic carriage of *C. difficile* was found in children less than two years of age, especially those who received antibiotics (18). Even though toxigenic *C. difficile* was recovered in 22% of the cystic fibrosis patients (19), these children rarely suffer from PMC, although they almost continuously receive antimicrobials.

Disruption of the competitive microbial balance in the intestine is an important initiating step of PMC. *C. difficile's* ability to produce PMC mostly in the presence of antibiotic exposure is explained by its enhanced growth in an environment in which there is reduced bacterial competition. Animal studies support this hypothesis.

Most cases of PMC in pediatric patients occur in previously healthy children. PMC has also been rarely described in the neonatal period (20). The incidence of antibiotic-associated diarrhea and colitis seems to rise with increasing age. Certain conditions predispose to *C. difficile* PMC. These include exposure to all antibiotics (within 5–10 days after the initiation of antibiotic therapy and as late as 10 weeks after cessation of therapy), colonization with *C. difficile* (obtained from fomites and people), exposure to agents and interventions that slow gut motility (i.e., enemas, stool softeners, opioids, illeus, Hirschsprung's disease, and colonic stricture), and prematurity (21–25).

The toxin of *C. difficile* has not generally been implicated in the pathogenesis of necrotizing enterocolitis (NEC). It is speculated that infants are generally not susceptible to the toxicity of *C. difficile* toxin as older children (20). Rietra et al. (26) found that 17 of 121 stools (14%) from infants more than five months of age caused cytotoxicity in tissue culture that was consistent with the effect of *C. difficile* toxin. No toxin was, however, identified in stools from 24 patients with NEC examined by Bartlett et al. (27) or from 18 patients studied by Chang and Areson (28). Cashore et al. (29) found toxin in five infants with NEC, suggesting a role for clostridial toxin in some cases of this disease. Hypoxia and circulatory disturbances in small premature infants at risk for NEC may lead to ischemic segments of bowel, in which multiplication of clostridia and toxin production may result in bowel ulceration, infarction, pneumatosis, and the clinical picture of enterocolitis.

Some suggest that *C. difficile* may be responsible for exacerbation of symptoms in patients with inflammatory bowel disease, especially in association with sulfasalazine or other antimicrobial therapy (30,31).

Incidence

C. difficile colitis occurs more frequency in patients who are hospitalized; the rate is reported at one to 10 cases per 1000 discharges. Outside the hospital, the overall risk is less than one case per 10,000 antibiotic prescriptions written or 0.5 to 1 hospital admissions per 100,000 person-years (3,4).

PMC is rare in the pediatric age group (32). Mortality is rare and involves patients with serious coexistent illness, infection, or congenital defects. Antibiotics were previously given to most patients with PMC and usually were administered parenterally (5).

C. difficile cytotoxin was recovered from the stool of 18 of 208 (9%) children whose specimens were sent for routine microbiologic studies (33). Cytotoxin was identified more often in younger patients, those with an associated illness and those with antibiotic-associated condition. Strong evidence exists for nosocomial acquisition of disease, but the frequency of this event and the usefulness of preventive measures in children need to be determined.

Clinical Presentation

Diseases due to *C. difficile* represent a wide spectrum. These ranges from asymptomatic cases, watery diarrhea, dysentery, PMC, complicated colitis and bacterial metastatic infections (7,8). Some degree of watery diarrhea, infrequent with blood or mucus, develops in most patients. The extent of other abdominal complaints or systemic symptoms varies from mild to severe. The disease may be fatal. Abdominal pain, cramps, lower quadrant tenderness, fever, and leukocytosis are common. Other findings include nausea, malaise, anorexia, hypoalbuminemia, anasarca, electrolyte disturbances, occult colonic bleeding, and dehydration. Extraintestinal manifestations are rare and include bacteremia, generally polymicrobial, splenic abscess, osteomyelitis, and reactive arthritis or tenosynovitis.

The duration of symptoms in those with mild disease not requiring specific therapy usually ranges from 7 to 10 days after discontinuation of the instigating antibiotic. More prolonged symptoms or significant toxicity may indicate the need for specific antimicrobial intervention.

The severe form of PMC must be differentiated from other causes of acute intraabdominal pathology (e.g., appendicitis, perforated viscus, intussusception, or ischemic bowel), whereas the mild, selflimited disease can resemble viral gastroenteritis. Blood in stool out of proportion to diarrhea or systemic illness is a clue to *C. difficile* disease. *C. difficile* can also cause extraintestinal infections (34).

Clostridium perfringens, a producer of a potent exotoxin, is an important cause of toxigenic diarrhea (35). *C. perfringens* diarrhea has been associated with the ingestion of contaminated beef, beef products, and poultry. Onset is usually sudden and is characterized by moderately severe colicky abdominal pain. Vomiting is not a feature of *C. perfringens* diarrhea. Generally, the stools are unusually foul but free of blood and mucus. As with other clostridia, the effect of *C. perfringens* is caused by its preformed thermolabile toxin, which is synthesized before ingestion prior to sporulation. Additional toxin is produced in the vegetative phase in the gastrointestinal tract. As with other enterotoxins, it exerts its effect on the proximal small bowel by activating intestinal adenyl cyclase, resulting in increased intestinal fluid secretion and decreased reabsorption.

Diagnosis

The diagnostic test of choice to detect the presence of *C. difficile* toxin B is a tissue culture assay to demonstrate a cytopathic toxin that may be neutralized by clostridial antitoxin (8). No rapid test is completely reliable. Several new enzyme immunoassays approach the accuracy of tissue culture assay and can detect toxin A, B, or both. Latex particle agglutination assay is not as reliable. The immunoblot assay and polymerase chain reaction can detect toxin A only (36).

Stool cultures for *C. difficile* using selective medium should be attempted, accompanied by a reliable toxin assay. Determining the role of *C. perfringes* in diarrhea is difficult. Fluorescent-stained antibodies to *C. perfringes* capsule can be used to identify the organism in stool.

Endoscopy can detect the appearance of 2- to 10-mm raised yellow nodules, which are usually discrete but may become confluent plaques in more advanced cases. The pseudomembranes can be easily removed, revealing an erythematous, inflamed mucosa. Sigmoidoscopy may be sufficient when the distal colon is involved, but if the pseudomembranes are restricted to the right colon, colonoscopy is necessary. Findings range from a normal mucosa through a spectrum of changes including erythema and edema, friability, ulceration, and hemorrhage, as well as PMC. In mild cases, pseudomembranes may not be grossly present, and diagnosis must be confirmed with biopsy (8). The most useful X-ray study is air–contrast barium enema, which is often nonspecific. However, the demonstration of PMC by either X-rays or endoscopy is an anatomic, not an etiologic, diagnosis.

Histologically, earliest findings are patchy necrosis of colonic epithelium with intraluminal exudation of neutrophils and fibrin. Epithelial ulcers become apparent and pseudomembranes, comprised of leukocytes, fibrin, mucus, and cell debris, then cover the diffuse epithelial necrosis. With recovery, normal colonic mucosa returns with minimal abnormality.

Management

The initial management requires discontinuation of antibiotics or other potentially inciting agents and supportive care for the diarrhea, including repletion of fluid and electrolyte losses. Up to a quarter of patients resolve without further treatment. The rest generally require specific therapy for *C. difficile* infection, particularly if antibiotic therapy cannot be discontinued. Those with severe symptoms or persistent diarrhea require aggressive therapy. Vancomycin is effective, but is expensive, tastes bad, and is associated with up to 20% relapse rate.

Anion-exchange resin agents (e.g., cholestyramine, colestipol) that bind both *C. difficile* toxins are an alternative to vancomycin. They are more likely to result in primary treatment failure than vancomycin, but are less likely to be followed by relapse (37). Metronidazole, bacitracin, teicoplanin, and fusidic acid can also be used to treat PMC (37, 38). Metronidazole orally has similar efficacy to vancomycin orally in mild and moderate cases (39), is lower in cost and does not select enterococcal resistance to vancomycin. Disadvantages of metronidazole are occasional resistance of *C. difficile*, rare induction of PMC (37, 39), lack of FDA approval for this indication in children, absence of convenient preparations for children, and its complete absorption at the upper gastrointestinal tract so that bactericidal levels are achieved erratically in the lower gastrointestinal tract. Despite the lack of conclusive clinical trials, intravenous metronidazole is generally recognized as adequate therapy for patients who cannot tolerate oral therapy. Rectal vancomycin as adjunctive therapy with intravenous metronidazole has been anecdotally reported. Concomitant therapy with rifampin has also been used; however, conclusive data are lacking. Anti-motility agents, including loperamide, diphenoxylate hydrochloride with atropine, and opioids, should be avoided because they can adversely affect the ability to clear the toxins.

Fever, systemic manifestations, and severe diarrhea generally improve within one to two days of therapy, but diarrhea may last for four to five days (40). Relapses may be caused by reacquisition or persistence of spores in the colon. Most patients with a relapse respond to the re-treatment, but may experience multiple recurrences.

Options for the management of multiple relapses include vancomycin or metronidazole plus *Saccharomyces boulardii* (41) or Fleischmann's baker's yeast (42); or followed by cholestyramine with or without lactobacilli (43); intravenous immunoglobulin (44); solution of fresh stool from healthy donor (45); and broth culture bacteria (46).

Treatment of *C. perfringens* diarrhea is supportive. The disorder is self-limiting and lasts less than 24 hours.

Surgical intervention may be required in severe cases of PMC unresponsive to medical therapy or to manage complications such as toxic megacolon or colonic perforation. Various approaches can be used, including diverting ostomy of the affected segment or subtotal colectomy. In fulminate PMC, careful vigilance is necessary to detect early signs of peritonitis and abdominal cellulitis that can indicate underlying intestinal perforation. The overall mortality rate after surgery is 30% to 35%.

Complications

Complications include dehydration, electrolyte imbalance, hypotension, hypoalbuminemia with anasarca, toxic megacolon, transverse volvulus, colon perforation, and toxic megacolon. Severe cases of PMC are prone to secondary systemic infection because of acquired malnutrition, hypogammaglobulinemia, lymphopenia, ascites, pleural effusions, and bacteremia from the intestinal inflammatory process.

Recurrent colitis and diarrhea occur in one of five patients two to eight weeks after completion of therapy; occasionally, more than six episodes may occur.

Prevention

Administration of antibiotics associated with PMC to patients with intestinal disease should be avoided. Antibiotic therapy should always be done prudently and be limited to those who unequivocally need it. Patients, who receive antimicrobials, should be warned about this complication and told to contact their physician as soon as symptoms of PMC appear.

Preventive measures against recurrent disease include avoidance of any antimicrobials in the first two months after PMC. Patients with multiple (more than 10) episodes of recurrent diarrhea may benefit from long-term therapy. Innovative strategies with adjunctive agents and probiotics are used in patients with recurrent disease. These include recolonization of the gastrointestinal tract with *Lactobacillus GG* strain, *S. boulardii*, yeast, or feces enemas.

C. difficile can spread within health care institutions with relative ease. Because hospitalized individuals are at a significant risk, the spread of *C. difficile* within the hospital setting should be prevented. The cornerstones of control are strict adherence to handwashing practices and limitations on the use of broadspectrum antimicrobial agents and unnecessary antimicrobial therapy. Strict contact isolation, cohorting patients and personnel in epidemics and, rarely, closing units may be required when an outbreak cannot be aborted (47). Patients with *C. difficile* disease should be cared for in protected areas, where meticulous handwashing technique and proper handling of soiled diapers and fomites are practiced. Children with *C. difficile* disease should be excluded from child care for the duration of diarrhea.

Sigmoidoscopes and colonoscopes should be decontaminated to avoid possible transmission of *C. difficile* to others. The only sporicidal cleaning agents effective against *C. difficile* are sodium hypochlorite and glutaraldehydes (48).

REFERENCES

1. Cleary RK. *Clostridium difficile*-associated diarrhea and colitis: clinic manifestations, diagnosis, and treatment. Dis Colon Rectum 1998; 41:1435–49.
2. McFarland LV, Surawicz CM, Stamm WE. Risk factors for *Clostridium difficile* carriage and *C. difficile*-associated diarrhea in a cohort of hospitalized patients. J Infect Dis 1990; 162:678–84.
3. Samore MH. Epidemiology of nosocomial *Clostridium difficile* diarrhoea. J Hosp Infect 1999; 43(Suppl.):S183–90.
4. Gerding DN, Johnson S, Peterson LR, Mulligan ME, Silva J, Jr. *Clostridium difficile*-associated diarrhea and colitis. Infect Control Hosp Epidemiol 1995; 16:459–77.
5. Zwiener RJ, Belknap WM, Quan R. Severe pseudomembranous enterocolitis in a child: case report and literature review. Pediatr Infect Dis J 1989; 8:876–82.
6. Fekety R, Shah AB. Diagnosis and treatment of *Clostridium difficile* colitis. JAMA 1993; 269:71–5.
7. Bartlett JG. The new epidemic of *Clostridium difficile*-associated enteric disease. Ann Intern Med 2006; 145:758–64.
8. Johnson S, Gerding DN. *Clostridium difficile*-associated diarrhea. Clin Infect Dis 1998; 26:1027–34.
9. Larton HE, Price AB. Pseudomembranous colitis: presence of clostridial toxin. Lancet 1977; 2:1312–4.
10. Kelly CP, Pothoulakis C, LaMont JT. *Clostridium difficile* colitis: current concepts. N Engl J Med 1994; 330:257–62.
11. Kelly CP, Pothoulakis C, Orellana J, et al. Human colonic aspirates containing immunoglobulin A antibody to *Clostridium difficile* toxin A inhibit toxin A-receptor binding. Gastroenterology 1992; 102:35–40.
12. Stubbe H, Berdoz J, Kraehenbuhl JP, et al. Polymeric IgA is superior to monomeric IgA and IgG carrying the same variable domain in preventing *Clostridium difficile* toxin A damaging of T84 monolayers. J Immunol 2000; 164:1952–60.
13. Eglow R, Pothoulakis C, Itzkowitz S, et al. Diminished *Clostridium difficile* toxin: a sensitivity in newborn rabbit ileum is associated with decreased toxin A receptor. J Clin Invest 1992; 90:822–9.
14. Willey S, Bartlett JG. Cultures for *Clostridium difficile* in stools containing a cytotoxin neutralized by *Clostridium sordellii* antitoxin. J Clin Microbiol 1979; 10:880–4.
15. Sherertz RJ, Sarubbi FA. The prevalence of *Clostridium difficile* and toxin in a nursery population: a comparison between patients with necrotizing enterocolitis and an asymptomatic group. J Pediatr 1982; 100:435–9.
16. Cerquetti M, Luzzi I, Caprioli A, et al. Role of *Clostridium difficile* in childhood diarrhea. Pediatr Infect Dis J 1995; 14:598–603.
17. Sutphen JL, Grand RJ, Flores A, et al. Chronic diarrhea associated with *Clostridium difficile* in children. Am J Dis Child 1983; 137:275–8.
18. Vesikari T, Isolauri E, Maki M, et al. *Clostridium difficile* in young children: association with antibiotic usage. Acta Paediatr Scand 1984; 73:86–91.
19. Welkon CJ, Long SS, Thompson CM, Jr., et al. *Clostridium difficile* in patients with cystic fibrosis. Am J Dis Child 1985; 139:805–8.
20. Adler SP, Chandrika T, Berman WF. *Clostridium difficile* associated with pseudomembranous colitis: occurrence in a 12-week-old infant without prior antibiotic therapy. Am J Dis Child 1981; 135:820–2.

21. Brearly S, Armstrong GR, Nairn R. Pseudomembranous colitis: a lethal complication of Hirschsprung's disease unrelated to antibiotic usage. J Pediatr Surg 1987; 22:257–9.
22. Church JM, Fazio VW. A role for colonic stasis in the pathogenesis of disease related to *Clostridium difficile*. Dis Colon Rectum 1986; 29:804–9.
23. Perelman R, Rowe JC, Christie DL, et al. Pseudomembranous colitis following obstruction in a neonate. Clin Pediatr 1981; 20:212–4.
24. Singer DB, Cashore WJ, Widness JA, et al. Pseudomembranous colitis in a preterm neonate. J Pediatr Gastroenterol Nutr 1986; 5:318–20.
25. Han VKM, Sayed H, Chance GW, et al. An outbreak of *Clostridium difficile* necrotizing enterocolitis: a case for oral vancomycin therapy?. Pediatrics 1983; 71:935–41.
26. Rietra PJ, Slaterus KW, Zanen HC, et al. Clostridia toxin in feces of healthy infants. Lancet 1978; 2:319.
27. Bartlett JG, Moon N, Chang TW, et al. Role of *Clostridium difficile* in antibiotic-associated pseudomembranous colitis. Gastroenterology 1978; 75:778–82.
28. Chang TW, Areson P. Neonatal necrotizing enterocolitis: absence of enteric bacterial toxins. N Engl J Med 1978; 299:424.
29. Cashore WJ, Peter G, Lauermann M, et al. Clostridia colonization and clostridial toxin in neonatal necrotizing enterocolitis. J Pediatr 1981; 98:308–11.
30. Meyers S, Mayer L, Bottone E, et al. Occurrence of *Clostridium difficile* toxin during the course of inflammatory bowel disease. Gastroenterology 1981; 80:687–90.
31. Dorman SA, Liggoria E, Winn WC, Jr., et al. Isolation of *Clostridium difficile* from patients with inactive Crohn's disease. Gastroenterology 1982; 82:1348–51.
32. Viscidi RP, Bartlett JG. Antibiotic-associated pseudomembranous colitis in children. Pediatrices 1981; 67:381–6.
33. Thompson CM, Gilligan PH, Fisher MC, et al. *Clostridium difficile* cytotoxin in pediatric population. Am J Dis Child 1983; 137:271–4.
34. Feldman RJ, Kallick M, Weinstein MP. Bacteremia due to *Clostridium difficile*: case report and review of extraintestinal *C. difficile* infections. Clin Infect Dis 1995; 20:1560–2.
35. Bos J, Smithee L, McClane B, et al. Fatal necrotizing colitis following a foodborne outbreak of enterotoxigenic *Clostridium perfringens* type A infection. Clin Infect Dis 2005; 40:e78–83.
36. DeGirolami PC, Hanff PA, Eichelberger K, et al. Multicenter evaluation, of a new enzyme immunoassay for detection of *Clostridium difficile* enterotoxin A. J Clin Microbiol 1992; 30:1085–8.
37. George WL, Rolfe RD, Finegold SM. Treatment and prevention of antimicrobial agents-induced colitis and diarrhea. Gastroenterology 1980; 79:366–72.
38. Young GP, Ward PB, Bayley N, et al. Antibiotic-associated colitis due to *Clostridium difficile*: double blind comparison of vancomycin with bacitracin. Gastroenterology 1985; 89:1038–45.
39. Bartlett JC. *Clostridium difficile*: history of its role as an enteric pathogen and the current state of knowledge about the organism. Clin Infect Dis 1994; 18:S265–72.
40. Owens RC. *Clostridium difficile*-associated disease: changing epidemiology and implications for management. Drugs 2007; 67:487–502.
41. McFarland LV, Surawicz CM, Greenberg RN, et al. A randomized placebo-controlled trial of *Saccharomyces boulardii* in combination with standard antibiotics for *Clostridium difficile* disease. JAMA 1994; 271:1913–8.
42. Chia JKS, Chan SM, Goldstein H. Baker's yeast as adjunctive therapy relapses of *Clostridium difficile* diarrhea. Clin Infect Dis 1995; 20:1581 (letter).
43. Gorbach SL, Chang TW, Goldin B. Successful treatment of relapsing *Clostridium difficile* colitis with *Lactobacillus* GG. Lancet 1987; 2:1519 (letter).
44. Leung DYM, Kelly CP, Boguniewicz M, et al. Treatment with intravenously administered gamma globulin of chronic relapsing colitis induced by *Clostridium difficile*. J Pediatr 1991; 118:633–7.
45. Schwan A, Sjolin S, Trottestam U, et al. Relapsing *Clostridium difficile* enterocolitis cured by rectal infusion of normal faeces. Scand J Infect Dis 1984; 16:211–5.
46. Tvede M, Rask-Madsen J. Bacteriotherapy for chronic relapsing *Clostridium difficile* diarrhea in six patients. Lancet 1989; 1:1156–60.
47. Enad D, Meislich D, Brodsky NL, et al. Is *Clostridium difficile* a pathogen in the newborn intensive care unit? A prospective evaluation. J Perinatol 1997; 17:355–9.
48. Rutala WA, Gergen MF, Weber DJ. Inactivation of *Clostridium difficile* spores by disinfectants. Infect Control Hosp Epidemiol 1993; 14:36–9.

32 | Anaerobic Bacteremia

Anaerobic bacteremia has been most frequently related to an abdominal infection source (50–70% of cases), pelvic infections (5–20% of cases), and skin and soft tissue infections (5–20% of cases). Anaerobes accounted for 10% to 20% of episodes of bacteremia in studies performed up to the 1990s (1). However, in the 1990s the incidence was lowered to approximately 4% (0.5–12%) of all cases of bacteremias (or approximately one case per 1000 admissions), with variation by geographic location, hospital patient demographics, and especially patient age (2). Increased awareness of the importance of anaerobes and enhanced recognition of the types of clinical infection caused by these organisms, along with appropriate prophylaxis and treatment, were postulated as reasons that explain the decrease in the incidence of anaerobic bacteremia during 1974–1988 (2). Recent studies, however, documented a resurgence in bacteremia due to anaerobic bacteria. A study from the Mayo Clinic (Rochester, Minnesota, U.S.A.) has reported that the mean incidence of anaerobic bacteremias increased from 53 cases per year during 1993–1996 to 75 cases per year during 1997–2000 to 91 cases per year during 2001–2004 (an overall increase of 74%). The total number of cases of anaerobic bacteremia per 100,000 patient-days increased by 74% ($p < 0.001$). The number of anaerobic blood cultures per 1000 cultures performed increased by 30% ($p = 0.002$) (3).

There was a greater proportion of patients with anaerobic bacteremia with underlying malignancies in 2004 than during 1993–1994; however, no statistically significant difference was shown (46% vs. 39%, respectively; $p = 0.39$). Hematologic malignancies were most common during both periods, followed by gastrointestinal, gynecological, and urogenital malignancies (3).

MICROBIOLOGY

About 75% of anaerobic bacteremia are due to gram-negative bacilli, mostly *Bacteroides fragilis* group. *B. fragilis* is the most common blood isolate recovered from patients with anaerobic bacteremia; this organism and species of the *B. fragilis* group account for approximately 55% of anaerobic bacteremias. *B. fragilis* bacteremia is associated with a mortality of 19%, with a mortality risk of 3.2; a 16-day increase in hospital stay; and often, intra-abdominal disease. Associated risks for mortality include chronic liver disease and congestive heart failure. The other species of anaerobes causing bacteremia include *Peptostreptococcus* spp., *Clostridium* spp. (10% each), and *Fusobacterium* spp. (5%). Many of these infections are polymicrobial (3,4). *Propionibacterium acnes* is a common isolate, but is often a skin contaminate of blood cultures. However, it can be recovered from the blood of patients with shunt or vascular catheter bacteremia (5).

PATHOGENESIS

Anaerobic bacteremia is almost invariably secondary to a focal primary infection where the strain of anaerobic organisms recovered depended to a large extent on the portal of entry and the underlying disease (1,6).

The gastrointestinal tract accounted for half of anaerobic bacteremias and the female genital tract is source of 20%. The gastrointestinal (GI) tract is the principal source of *B. fragilis* group and clostridial bacteremias, and the female genital tract is the principal source of Peptostreptococcus and Fusobacterium bacteremias (1,6).

The origin of bacteremias due to *B. fragilis* group is the gastrointestinal tract, soft-tissue wound infections, female genitourinary tract, lung infections, and malignancies (genitourinary, gynecological, acute leukemia, and gastrointestinal) (7,8).

The ear, sinus, and oropharynx are the portals of entry for bacteremia with *Peptostreptococcus* spp. and *Fusobacterium* spp. This is not surprising since these organisms are part of the oral flora and are involved in local infections (6).

Predisposing Factors

A review of the suspected portal of entry for 855 episodes of bacteremia involving anaerobes indicated an intraabdominal source in 52%, the female genital tract in 20%, the lower respiratory tract in 6%, the upper respiratory tract in 5%, and soft tissue infections in 8% (8). Elderly persons seem to be at increased risk for developing anaerobic bacteremia, while young children (two to five years of age) are at the least risk.

Predisposing factors to anaerobic bacteremia in adults include malignant neoplasms, hematologic disorders, transplantation of organs, recent GI or obstetric gynecologic surgery, intestinal obstruction, diabetes mellitus, post-splenectomy, use of cytotoxic agents or corticosteroids, an undrained abscess, and use of prophylactic antimicrobial agents for bowel preparation prior to surgery (4,6).

The predisposing conditions in children include chronic debilitating disorders such as malignant neoplasms, hematologic abnormalities, immunodeficiencies, chronic renal insufficiency, decubitus ulcers, and infectious mononucleosis and carries poor prognosis (9–11).

Anaerobic bacteremia in newborns is associated with prolonged labor, premature rupture of membranes, maternal amnionitis, prematurity, fetal distress, and respiratory difficulty. Bacteremia in newborns has also been attributed to *Bacteroides* spp., *Clostridium* spp., and *Fusobacterium nucleatum* (10).

Dental or oral surgery can also predispose to anaerobic bacteremia in adults and children due to oral flora anaerobes (i.e., *Prevotella*, *Eubacterium*, and *Peptostreptococcus* spp.) (1,12).

The recent report of anaerobic bacteremia at the Mayo Clinic (3) observed that the "typical" clinical contexts for anaerobic bacteremia was less predictable than it used to be in the past. The data showed that 38% of patients with anaerobic bacteremia in 2004 had sources other than the genitourinary and GI tracts. Internal review of unpublished data from the Mayo Clinic during 1995–1996 showed that, in 34.3% of patients, anaerobes would not have been suspected as the cause of bacteremia on the basis of typical clinical predictors (3). The authors concluded that the sources of anaerobic bacteremia are now more varied than previously, especially among immunosuppressed patients and patients with complex underlying disease.

DIAGNOSIS AND CLINICAL FEATURES

The clinical features of anaerobic bacteremia are not much different from other types of bacteremia; however, a relatively longer period is generally needed before an etiologic diagnosis can be made. This can be a result of the longer time needed for growth and identification of anaerobic organisms.

Diagnosis should include detection of the primary infection. The clinical presentation of anaerobic bacteremia relates in part to the nature of the primary infection, which will typically include fever, chills, and leukocytosis. Anemia, shock, and intravascular coagulation also may be present. Bacteroides bacteremia is generally characterized by thrombophlebitis, metastatic infection, hyperbilirubinemia, and high mortality rate (up to 50%). *Clostridium perfringens* bacteremia may present with hemolytic anemia, hemoglobinemia, hemoglobinuria, disseminated intravascular coagulation, bleeding tendency, bronze color skin, hyperbilirubinemia, shock, oliguria, and anemia. Clostridial bacteria may, however, be transient and inconsequential. However, *Clostridium septicum* infection may be a marker for a silent colonic or rectal malignancy (10).

Blood culture supporting the growth of anaerobic bacteria should be used routinely in all patients. Inadequate methodology can lead to missing cases of anaerobic bacteremia. Susceptibility testing for the isolated organisms should be performed.

MANAGEMENT

Institution of early and prolonged effective therapy is important. The primary source of infection, such as an abscess, should be drained.

Selection of the appropriate antimicrobial therapy is of great importance. Nguyen et al, (13) who performed a prospective observational study of 128 cases of bacteremia involving the *B. fragilis* group, illustrated that mortality, microbial persistence, and clinical failure occurred more frequently among patients who did not receive an appropriate antibiotic agent(s) to treat infection with resistant members of the *B. fragilis* group.

When anaerobes resistant to penicillin, such as the *B. fragilis* group, are suspected or isolated, antimicrobials such as clindamycin, chloramphenicol, metronidazole, cefoxitin, a carbapenem, or the combination of a penicillin and a beta-lactamase inhibitor should be administered. Local surveillance of antimicrobial susceptibility patterns can provide guidelines as to the choice of the best antimicrobial agent. The development of resistance to all known agents by anaerobes, make the selection of reliable empirical therapy difficult. Many anaerobic species in addition to the *B. fragilis* group have developed beta-lactamase activity. Rarely, resistance to carbapenems, induced by metalloenzymes, and to metronidazole has been reported. Consequently, one is not able to predict the susceptibility of some anaerobic isolates. Performing susceptibility testing is of great importance in treating bacteremia due to anaerobes. In the case of polymicrobial bacteremia, coverage is needed against all pathogens.

Organisms identical to those causing bacteremia often can be recovered from other infected sites. These extravascular sites may serve as a source of persistent bacteremia in some cases; however, most patients recover when prompt treatment with appropriate antimicrobials is instituted.

Preventing bacteremia associated with dental or oral surgery can be accomplished by prophylactic administration of penicillin alone or with metronidazole or clindamycin (14).

COMPLICATIONS

Mortality remains high (15–35%). Risk factors for a fatal outcome include compromised status, advanced age, inadequate or no surgical therapy, and the presence of polymicrobial sepsis. *B. fragilis* group bacteremia contributes significantly to morbidity and mortality. The attributable mortality of bacteremia associated with the *B. fragilis* group was examined in a matched case-control study (15). Patients with *B. fragilis* group bacteremia were matched to a control patient without bacteremia but with the same principal diagnosis or the same major surgical procedure. Those with *B. fragilis* group bacteremia had a significantly higher mortality rate compared to control patients (28% compared to 9%), and an attributable mortality rate of 19% (95% CI, 3.7–6.0).

Certain other serious concomitant sites of infection can be present in patients with anaerobic bacteremia. Most of these sites serve as the source of the infection; however, others may represent a site of secondary hematogenous spread.

REFERENCES

1. Finegold SM. Anaerobic Bacteria in Human Disease. New York: Academic Press, 1977.
2. Dorsher CW, Rosenblatt JE, Wilson WR, Ilstrup DM. Anaerobic bacteremia: decreasing rate over a 15-year period. *Rev Infect Dis* 1991; 13:633–6
3. Lassmann B, Gustafson DR, Wood CM, Rosenblatt JE. Reemergence of Anaerobic Bacteremia. Clin Infec Dis 2007;44:895–900.
4. Brook I, Martin WJ, Cherry JD, Sumaya CV. Recovery of anaerobic bacteria from pediatric patients: a one-year experience. Am J Dis Child 1979; 133:1020–4.
5. Brook I, Frazier EH. Infections caused by propionibacterium species. Rev Infect Dis 1991; 13:319–22.
6. Brook I. Anaerobic bacterial bacteremia: 12-year experience in two military hospitals. J Infect Dis 1989; 160:1071–5.
7. Fainstein V, Elting LS, Bodey GP. Bacteremia caused by non-sporulating anaerobes in cancer patients. A 12-year experience. Medicine (Baltimore) 1989; 68:151–62.
8. Finegold SM, George WL, Mulligan ME. Anaerobic infections. Part I. Dis Mon 1985; 31:1–77.

9. Brook I, Controni G, Rodriguez WJ, Martin WJ. Anaerobic bacteremia in children. Am J Dis Child 1980; 134:1052–6.
10. Caya JG, Farmer SG, Ritch PS, et al. Clostridial septicemia complicating the course of leukemia. Cancer 1986; 57:2045–8.
11. Dagan R, Powell KR. Postanginal sepsis following infectious mononucleosis. Arch Intern Med 1987; 147:1581–3.
12. Rajasuo A, Perkki K, Nyfors S, Jousimies-Somer H, Meurman JH. Bacteremia following surgical dental extraction with an emphasis on anaerobic strains. J Dent Res 2004; 83:170–4.
13. Nguyen MH, Yu VL, Morris AJ, et al. Antimicrobial resistance and clinical outcome of *Bacteroides* bacteremia: findings of a multicenter prospective observational trial. Clin Infect Dis 2000; 30:870–6.
14. Maestre Vera JR, Gomez-Lus Centelles ML. Antimicrobial prophylaxis in oral surgery and dental procedures. Med Oral Pathol Oral Cir Bucal 2007; 12:e44–52.
15. Redondo MC, Arbo MD, Grindlinger J, Snydman DR. Attributable mortality of bacteremia associated with the *Bacteroides fragilis* group. Clin Infect Dis 1995; 20:1492–6.

33 | Endocarditis

Endocarditis, which is an infection of the endocardial surface of the heart, can have intracardiac effects including severe valvular insufficiency leading to intractable congestive heart failure and myocardial abscesses. It can also produce various systemic signs and symptoms through both sterile and infected emboli and various immunological phenomena. Endocarditis due to anaerobic bacteria is uncommon and over the past three decades accounts for 2% to 16% of all cases of infectious endocarditis (1–4).

MICROBIOLOGY

Staphylococcus aureus; *Streptococcus viridans*; groups A, C, and G streptococci; and enterococci are the most common microorganisms that cause endocarditis (5–7).

S. *viridans* accounts for 50% to 60% of subacute diseases; *Streptococcus anginosus* group causes either acute or subacute infection, accounting for 15% of streptococcal cases. Approximately 5% of subacute cases are due to nutritionally variant streptococci. Most cases of *Enterococcus* spp., which is the third most common cause of endocarditis, are subacute and are generally of gastrointestinal or genitourinary tract source and often reflecting underlying abnormalities of the large bowel (e.g., ulcerative colitis, polyps, cancer). Group B streptococci are generally seen in pregnant women and older patients with underlying diseases (e.g., cancer, diabetes, and alcoholism). Groups A, C, and G streptococcal endocarditis resemble that of S. *aureus* (30–70% mortality rate) with suppurative complications. S. *aureus* is the most common cause of all forms of endocarditis, has a high mortality rate of 40% to 50%, is associated with intravascular lines and many of the isolates are currently methicillin resistant. Coagulase-negative Staphylococci causes a subacute disease, and *Pseudomonas aeruginosa* generally induces acute infection where surgery is commonly required for cure. The HACEK organisms (i.e., *Haemophilus aphrophilus*, *Actinobacillus actinomycetemcomitans*, *Cardiobacterium hominis*, *Eikenella corrodens*, *Kingella kingae*) usually cause subacute disease and account for approximately 5% of cases. Fungi (*Candida* and *Aspergillus* spp.) mostly cause subacute disease; and *Bartonella* spp. is common in individuals with extremely substandard hygiene.

Anaerobic bacteria are an uncommon but important cause of endocarditis accounting for 2% to 16% of all cases. Most cases of anaerobic endocarditis are caused by anaerobic cocci, *Propionibacterium acnes*, and *Bacteroides fragilis* (8). Predisposing factors and signs and symptoms of endocarditis caused by anaerobic bacteria are similar to those seen in endocarditis with facultative anaerobic bacteria with the following exceptions: there is a lower incidence of preexisting valvular heart disease, a higher incidence of thromboemboli events and a higher mortality rate with anaerobic endocarditis.

The probable increase in the number of reported cases of anaerobic endocarditis noted in recent years may be explained by: the increased frequency of polymicrobial bacteremias (9), the decreased frequency of "culture-negative" cases (10,11), the increased use of prosthetic intravascular devices, and improvements in microbiological methods. Polymicrobial endocarditis is more common in addicts (2–9% of cases) (2).

In a review of 1046 cases of endocarditis from 1963 to 1969, a total of 14 (1.3%) cases were caused by anaerobes (1): 12 were due to anaerobic streptococci, one was caused by *Bacteroides* species, and one by a diphtheroid. An additional 33 new cases were also presented. Polymicrobial infection was observed in eight (24%) patients—mostly due to *P. melaninogenica* or peptostreptococci together with facultative streptococci. Nastro and Finegold (12) reviewed 37 cases of anaerobic endocarditis; where polymicrobial infections were found in five (13.5%). In another review of 66 cases, seven (10.6%) were caused by anaerobes and three of seven were polymicrobial (2). Cohen et al. (13) described 11 cases of endocarditis due to *Bacteroides* spp., while Kolander et al. (14) reported one case of *Clostridium bifermentans* endocarditis, and reviewed 16 other cases of clostridial endocarditis. None of the patients had conditions predisposing to infection.

The role of *Propionibacterium* spp. in endocarditis in 36 patients was recently summarized (15). In most cases, infection was protracted, with minimal signs in the early stages. Fourteen cases (42.4%) involved native valves, 16 (48.5%) involved prosthetic valves and three (9.1%) were associated with other intracardiac prosthetic material. Intracardiac abscesses were commonly encountered, with Propionibacterium endocarditis occurring in 28.6% of native valve infections and 52.9% of prosthetic valve infections. Most of the cases (70.6%) required surgical intervention. Several factors delayed institution of appropriate therapy and may have contributed to abscess formation, including an indolent clinical course, negative or delayed culture results, and the tendency to consider this organism as a blood-culture contaminant. The data supports careful clinical evaluation before disregarding a blood-culture isolate of *Propionibacterium* spp. as a skin contaminant, and consideration of this bacterium as a potential cause of apparently culture-negative endocarditis.

PATHOGENICITY

The process of causing endocarditis evolves several stages that include bacteremia (nosocomial or spontaneous) that delivers the organisms to the valve's surface, adherence of the organisms to the valves, and invasion of the valvular leaflets.

The origins of organisms causing native valve endocarditis are related to events causing bacteremia as well as the ability of bacteria to adhere to vascular endothelium. The entry portals of bacteroides and clostridia are generally the gastrointestinal and the female genital tracts. The portal of entry of anaerobic cocci is generally the respiratory tract (8). Bacteremia can be induced after numerous procedures (16).

The potential of invasive procedures to produce a bacteremia varies greatly. The rates of bacteremia and causative organisms (in parenthesis) are: in endoscopy a rate of 0% to 20% (coagulase negative staphylococcus. streptococci, diphtheroids), in colonoscopy a rate of 0% to 20% (*Escherichia coli*, *Bacteroides* spp.), in barium enema a rate of 0% to 20% (enterococci, aerobic, and anaerobic gram-negative rods), in dental extractions a rate of 40% to 100% (*S. viridans* and oral flora anaerobes, i.e., *Prevotella*, *Eubacterium* and *Peptostreptococcus* spp.), in transurethral resection of the prostate a rate of 20% to 40% (Enterobacteriacae, Enterococci, *S. aureus*), and in transesophageal echocardiography a rate of 0% to 20% (*S. viridans*, oral flora anaerobes, streptococci) (16).

Antecedent cardiac anomalies can also predispose to endocarditis. Endocarditis can also occur in prosthetic valves or homographs. When recovered from blood cultures, anaerobes that may be considered contaminants should be considered as possible pathogens in patients with a vascular graft, a prosthetic heart valve, or an intravascular prosthesis. In such patients, infections have been caused by *P. acnes*, *Lactobacillus*, *Eubacterium*, *Bifidobacterium* or *Veillonella* spp. (4,16–20).

The gastrointestinal tract was the most common source for *B. fragilis* group endocarditis; the head and neck were the most common origins for *Fusobacterium* and *Bacteroides* spp., and the head and neck or genitourinary tract were the most common sources for peptostreptococci (1,12). The most common gastrointestinal sources were peritonitis, cholecystitis, appendicitis (1,12), and aortoduodenal fistula. Oropharyngeal sources included carious teeth, periodontal abscesses, and suppurative tonsillitis. The most common genitourinary tract source was the female pelvis (1,12).

A lower frequency (43–64%) of preexisting valvular heart disease has been found in anaerobic endocarditis compared to the frequency (75–100%) in endocarditis due to aerobic bacteria (1,12,21). However, the valve involved in patients with anaerobic endocarditis is similar to that in those with endocarditis caused by aerobic organisms. The tricuspid valve is most often infected in anaerobic endocarditis among users of intravenous drugs.

The presence of large vegetations with extensive valvular destruction and congestive heart failure is classically reported, particularly in *B. fragilis* group endocarditis (60–70%). Peripheral embolization is frequently seen (30–54%) and may be related to the production of heparinase by this organism (2,13,22). The high mortality rate observed (64%) might be due to delay in diagnosis or in earlier series to the absence of effective bactericidal antimicrobial agents for the treatment of some anaerobic infections (12,20). Sapico and Sarma (2) observed that no deaths occurred among seven patients with endocarditis due to anaerobic or microaerophilic organisms. In a review of 101 cases of polymicrobial endocarditis (23), the survival rate was higher in patients infected with anaerobes (82%) than in patients infected with aerobes (*Streptococcus* spp. 84%, enterococci 31%, and *S. aureus* 67%). Infections caused by anaerobic gram-positive cocci have a better prognosis than infections due to *B. fragilis* group or *Fusobacterium* spp.

DIAGNOSIS

Patients present with fever, chills, weakness, dyspnea, sweats, malaise, anorexia and weight loss, chest pain, and worsening cardiac function (24). The subtle nature of symptoms may postpone the diagnosis for months. Endocarditis should be suspected in children with congenital heart disease with unexplained fatigue, anemia, and fever, which is not influenced by oral antibiotics, and in those who have sudden onset of sepsis, or vascular lesions in soft tissues or mucous membranes.

Physical examination typically reveals enlargement of the spleen, changing or new heart murmur, clubbing petechiae and evidence of peripheral emboli or vasculitis, especially involving the mucous membranes.

Other findings are rarer but specific: Osler nodes, Janeway lesions, Roth spots and splinter hemorrhages in the nail beds. Several case definitions and diagnostic criteria have been published (25,26).

The course of patients with anaerobic endocarditis is generally subacute. *B. fragilis* endocarditis is associated with the formation of large valve vegetations and peripheral embolization (27). Septic emboli occurred in 60% to 70% of patients with *B. fragilis* (1,2,12). Three of five patients with *B. fragilis* endocarditis had thrombophlebitis, which may be attributed to heparinase production by this organism (19,28).

Laboratory tests can be helpful in supporting the diagnosis of infective endocarditis, although there are no pathognomonic findings. Erythrocyte sedimentation rate is generally elevated, and serum rheumatoid factor and hematuria are present in only 25% to 50% of patients. Hematuria and low serum complement are found in 5% to 40% of patients (24).

Obtaining cultures for aerobic and anaerobic bacteria, using proper blood culture media, is of great importance. More than a single blood culture should be obtained. The clinical significance of a single positive culture for a possible contaminant is difficult to determine. If several cultures are obtained and only one is positive, the diagnosis of endocarditis is uncertain.

Echocardiography is an important diagnostic technique for imaging vegetations. Sensitivity and diagnostic accuracy have improved with the use of Doppler echocardiography (29). Echocardiography is helpful in monitoring regression of vegetations (6). Transesophageal echocardiography increases the sensitivity for imaging vegetations (30).

TREATMENT

The treatment of endocarditis mandates the use of bactericidal antimicrobials. The administration of bactericidal antimicrobials such as metronidazole alone or combined with clindamycin was more effective in preventing experimental endocarditis than were bacteriostatic agents such as clindamycin, chloramphenicol (31), cefoxitin or erythromycin. Similar experiences were noted in a limited number of patients (32).

Carbapenems (i.e., imipenem, merpenem) should be effective for anaerobic endocarditis, including *B. fragilis* group. Patients with endocarditis caused by penicillin-susceptible anaerobic microorganisms such as Peptostreptococci should receive therapy with penicillin G or vancomycin, and those unable to receive penicillin should be treated with metronidazole or clindamycin if the organism is susceptible to these agents.

Presumptive antimicrobial therapy is based on the patient's age, pre-existing cardiac condition, and other risk factors such as intravenous drug use, surgery, and previous episodes of bacteremia or endocarditis.

For therapy of aerobic and facultatives bacteria, a beta-lactamase–resistant penicillin or vancomycin are chosen because of their activity against staphylococci and streptococci. An aminoglycoside is given for synergistic interaction with those agents against enterococci and other streptococcal species and to cover aerobic or facultative gram-negative bacilli. If blood cultures do not show growth but the patient responds to treatment, initially selected antibiotics are not stopped while other methods of diagnosis are continued. If the blood cultures are positive, antibiotic treatment is then based on the susceptibility test results.

Therapy is given intravenously for four to six weeks. Individuals with prosthetic intravascular valves are treated for six weeks.

Surgical intervention may be indicated (33) for abscess of the valve annulus or myocardium, two or more embolic events, rupture of valve leaflet or chordae, valvular insufficiency, rupture of an aneurysm of the sinus of Valsalva, conduction disturbances caused by a septal abscess, deteriorating cardiac failure, and inability to sterilize the blood. Removal of prosthetic valves may be indicated if medical therapy fails.

COMPLICATIONS

Valvular destruction frequency is greater than that associated with viridans streptococcal endocarditis, but less than the destruction that occurs with enterococcal, streptococcal, or gram-negative aerobic bacteria (34,35). Other complications with anaerobic endocarditis include multiple mycotic aneurysms (36), aortic ring abscess and aortitis (37,38), cardiogenic shock, dysrhythmias, and septic shock.

The mortality rate for patients with anaerobes endocarditis is 21% to 43% (1,20). Endocarditis by *B. fragilis* or *Fusobacterium necrophorum* has been associated with the highest mortality—46% and 75%, respectively (1,12). *F. necrophorum* has been associated with acute endocarditis, rapid valve destruction, and death (12). Patients with endocarditis caused by *Peptostreptococcus* spp. or drug addicts with anaerobic endocarditis have a more favorable prognosis than those with endocarditis due to the *B. fragilis* group or *Fusobacterium* (39).

PREVENTION

Antimicrobial prophylaxis for bacterial endocarditis has become standard and routine in most developed countries. The antimicrobial prophylaxis guidelines of the American College of Cardiology (ACC) and the American Heart Association (AHA) were revised in 1997 and updated by the Medical Letter in 2005; (40,41) the recommendations were unchanged in the 2006 ACC/AHA guidelines on the management of valvular heart disease (33).

The cardiac conditions in which antimicrobial prophylaxis is indicated are situations where the risk of endocarditis is considered by most authorities to be high and in which antimicrobial prophylaxis is generally indicated. These include patients with prosthetic heart, a prior history of endocarditis, complex cyanotic congenital heart diseases, and those with surgically constructed systemic or pulmonary conduits. Prophylaxis is also recommended in those with conditions in which the risk of endocarditis is moderate. These include most other congenital cardiac malformations, acquired valvular dysfunction and patients who have undergone valve repair, those with hypertrophic cardiomyopathy with obstruction, mitral valve prolapse with valvular regurgitation on auscultation and/or thickened leaflets on echocardiography, and intracardiac defects that have been repaired within the preceding six months or that are associated with significant hemodynamic instability.

The AHA has listed those dental and nondental procedures in which prophylaxis is generally indicated for patients with high or intermediate risk of endocarditis (40,41).

These include tonsillectomy and/or adenoidectomy, surgical operations that involve the respiratory mucosa, bronchoscopy with a rigid bronchoscope, sclerotherapy for esophageal varices, esophageal stricture dilation, biliary tract endoscopy or surgery, surgery involving the intestinal mucosa, prostatic surgery, cystoscopy, and urethral dilatation.

The prophylactic antimicrobial regimen for dental, oral, or upper respiratory tract procedures is a single dose of amoxicillin, 2 g orally one hour before the procedure (41). Those allergic to penicillins can be treated one hour before the procedure with clindamycin (600 mg), cephalexin or cefadroxil (2 g), or azithromycin (500 mg). To those unable to take oral medications, 2 g of intravenous or intramuscular ampicillin is given 30 minutes before the procedure. Patients allergic to penicillin can be given clindamycin (600 mg IV) or cefazolin (1 g IV) 30 minutes before the procedure.

For genitourinary or gastrointestinal procedures, the antimicrobials given are ampicillin (2 g intravenously or intramuscularly) plus gentamicin (1.5 mg/kg up to a maximum dose of 120 mg) 30 minutes before the procedure followed by ampicillin (1 g IV or IM) or amoxicillin (1 g orally) six hours later. Those allergic to penicillin receive the same dose of gentamicin plus vancomycin (1 g IV) one to two hours prior to the procedure.

A patient with a moderate risk for endocarditis is treated with amoxicillin (2 g orally) or ampicillin (2 g IV or IM) within 30 minutes of starting the procedure. Those allergic to penicillin can be treated with vancomycin (1 gm IV).

CONCLUSIONS

Endocarditis due to anaerobic bacteria is rare, accounting for 2% to 16% of all cases of infectious endocarditis. Most cases of anaerobic endocarditis are caused by anaerobic cocci, *P. acnes*, and *B. fragilis* (8). Predisposing factors and signs and symptoms of endocarditis caused by anaerobic bacteria are similar to those seen in endocarditis with facultative anaerobic bacteria. Complications with anaerobic endocarditis include valvular destruction, multiple mycotic aneurysms, aortic ring abscess, aortitis, cardiogenic shock, dysrhythmias, and septic shock. Treatment of endocarditis involving anaerobic bacteria includes the use of antibiotic therapy effective for these organisms.

REFERENCES

1. Felner JM, Dowell VR, Jr. Anaerobic bacterial endocarditis. N Engl J Med 1970; 283:1188–92.
2. Sapico FL, Sarma RJ. Infective endocarditis due to anaerobic and microaerophilic bacteria. West J Med 1982; 137:18–23.
3. Von Reyn CF, Levy BS, Arbeit RD, et al. Infective endocarditis: an analysis based on strict case definitions. Ann Intern Med 1981; 94:505–18.
4. Wilson WR, Geraci JE. Anaerobic infections of the cardiovascular system. In: Finegold SM, et al. eds. First United States Metronidazole Conference. Biomedical Information Information Corporation, New York. Proceedings from a symposium, Tarpon Springs, Florida, February 19–20, 1982: 319–30.
5. Opie GF, Fraser SH, Drew JH, Drew S. Bacterial endocarditis in neonatal intensive care. J Paediatr Child Health 1999; 35:545–8.
6. Milazzo AS, Jr., Li JS. Bacterial endocarditis in infants and children. Pediatr Infect Dis J 2001; 20:799–801.
7. Bashore TM, Cabell C, Fowler V, Jr. Update on infective endocarditis. Curr Probl Cardiol 2006; 31:274–352.
8. Nord CE. Anaerobic bacteria in septicemia and endocarditis. Scand J Infect Dis Suppl 1982; 31:95–104.
9. Lassmann B, Gustafson DR, Wood CM, Rosenblatt JE, et al. Reemergence of anaerobic bacteremia. Clin Infect Dis 2007; 44:895–900.
10. Griffin MR, Wilson WR, Edwards WD, O'Fallon WM, Kurland LT. Infective endocarditis. Olmstead County, Minnesota, 1950 through 1981. J Am Med Assoc 1981; 254:1199–202.
11. Van Scoy RE. Culture-negative endocarditis. Mayo Clin Proc 1982; 57:149–54.
12. Nastro LJ, Finegold SM. Endocarditis due to anaerobic gram-negative bacilli. Am J Med 1973; 54:482–96.
13. Cohen PS, Maguire JH, Weinstein L. Infective endocarditis caused by gram-negative bacteria: a review of the literature, 1945–1977. Prog Cardiovasc Dis 1980; 22:205–42.
14. Kolander SA, Cosgrove EM, Molavi A. Clostridial endocarditis. Report of a case caused by *Clostridium bifermentans* and review of the literature. Arch Intern Med 1989; 149:455–6.

15. Clayton JJ, Baig W, Reynolds GW, Sandoe JA. Endocarditis caused by *Propionibacterium* species: a report of three cases and a review of clinical features and diagnostic difficulties. J Med Microbiol 2006; 55:981–7.
16. Durack DT. Prevention of infective endocarditis. N Engl J Med 1995; 332:38–44.
17. Loewe L, Rosenblatt P, Alture-Werber E. A refractory case of subacute bacterial endocarditis due to *Veillonella gazogenes* clinically arrested by a combination of penicillin, sodium para-aminohippurate, and heparin. Am Heart J 1946; 32:327–38.
18. Sans MD, Crowder JG. Subacute bacterial endocarditis caused by *Eubacterium acrofaciens*. Report of a case. Am J Clin Pathol 1973; 59:576–80.
19. Watanakunakorn C. Changing epidemiology and newer aspects of infective endocarditis. Adv Intern Med 1977; 22:2147.
20. Wilson WR, Martin WJ, Wilkowske CJ, Washington JA. Anaerobic bacteremia. Mayo Clin Proc 1972; 47:639–46.
21. Kopelman HA, Graham BS, Forman MB. Myocardial abscess with complete heart block complicating anaerobic infective endocarditis. Br Heart J 1986; 56:101–4.
22. Chow AW, Guze LB. *Bacteroidaceae* bacteremia: clinical experience with 112 patients. Medicine 1974; 53:93–126.
23. Baddour LM, Meyer J, Henry B. Polymicrobial infective endocarditis in the 1980s. Rev Infect Dis 1991; 13:963–70.
24. Beynon RP, Bahl UK, Prendergast BD. Infective endocarditis. BMJ 2006; 333:334–9.
25. Durack DT, Lukes AS, Bright DK. Duke endocarditis service: new criteria for diagnosis of infective endocarditis: utilization of specific echocardiographic findings. Am J Med 1994; 96:220–9.
26. Sexton DJ, Spelman D. Current best practices and guidelines. Assessment and management of complications in infective endocarditis. Cardiol Clin 2003; 21:273–82.
27. Finegold SM, George WL, Mulligan ME. Anaerobic infections. Part I. DM Dis Month 1985; 31:1–77.
28. Gesner BM, Jenkin CR. Production of heparinase by *Bacteroides*. J Bacteriol 1965; 81:595–604.
29. Bricker JT, Latson LA, Huhta JC, Gutgesell HP. Echocardiographic evaluation of infective endocarditis in children. Clin Pediatr 1985; 24:312–7.
30. Jassal DS, Weyman AE. Infective endocarditis in the era of intracardiac devices: an echocardiographic perspective. Rev Cardiovasc Med 2006; 7:119–29.
31. Goldman PL, Durack DT, Petersdorf RG. Effect of antibiotics on the prevention of experimental *Bacteroides fragilis* endocarditis. Antimicrob Agents Chemother 1978; 14:755–60.
32. Galgiani JN, Busch DF, Brass C, Rumans LW, Mangels JI, Stevens DA. *Bacteroides fragilis* endocarditis, bacteremia and other infections treated with oral or intravenous metronidazole. Am J Med 1978; 65:284–9.
33. Bonow RO, Carabello BA, Chatterjee K, et al. ACC/AHA 2006 guidelines for the management of patients with valvular heart disease. A report of the American College of Cardiology/American Heart Association Task Force on Practice Guidelines (Writing committee to revise the 1998 guidelines for the management of patients with valvular heart disease). J Am Coll Cardiol 2006; 48:e1–148.
34. Lerner PI, Weinstein L. Infective endocarditis in the antibiotic era. N Engl J Med 1966; 274:199–206 (see also 259–266;388–393).
35. Vogler WR, Dorney ER, Bridges HA. Bacterial endocarditis: a review of 148 cases. Am J Med 1962; 32:910–21.
36. Huynh TT, Walling AD, Miller MA, Leung TK, Leclerc Y, Dragtakis L. *Propionibacterium acnes* endocarditis. Can J Cardiol 1995; 11:785–7.
37. Cohen CA, Almeder LM, Israni A, Maslow JN. Clostridium septicum endocarditis complicated by aortic-ring abscess and aortitis. Clin Infect Dis 1998; 26:495–6.
38. Caballero GJ, Arana R, Calle G, et al. Acute endocarditis of the native aortic valve caused by *Propionibacterium acnes*. Rev Esp Cardiol 1997; 50:906–8.
39. Menda KB, Gorbach SL. Favorable experience with bacterial endocarditis in heroin addicts. Ann Intern Med 1973; 78:25–32.
40. Dajani AS, Taubert KA, Wilson W, et al. Prevention of bacterial endocarditis. Recommendations by the American Heart Association. JAMA 1997; 277:1794–801.
41. Antibacterial prophylaxis for dental, GI, and GU procedures. Med Lett Drugs Ther 2005; 47:59–60.

34 | Pericarditis

Pericarditis can occur as a life-threatening, fulminant condition or as an incidental finding of pericardial fluid in an asymptomatic patient (1). In the acutely ill patient, prompt diagnosis is lifesaving because decreased stroke volume associated with a large effusion (cardiac tamponade) can compromise cardiac function and cause death. Pericarditis is an inflammation of the pericardium and the proximal part of the great blood vessels. It can be associated with an infection, or a systemic noninfectious disorder, or it can also result from local trauma, as in postoperative pericarditis. Infection or noninfectious pericarditis can be the only manifestation of a disease process or may be part of a multisystem disorder.

MICROBIOLOGY

Infectious pericarditis can be purulent, "benign," or granulomatous. Purulent pericarditis is caused by bacteria; benign pericarditis can be due to viruses, and can also occur in postpericardiotomy syndromes, hypersensitivity, or postinfectious; and granulomatous pericarditis is caused by *Mycobacterium tuberculosis* and fungi (1–5).

The list of etiologic agents of infectious pericarditis include bacteria, viruses, fungi, and other organisms (mycobacteria, fungi, and protozoa) (1–5). The bacteria include *Staphylococcus aureus, Neisseria meningitidis, Streptococcus pyogenes, Streptococcus pneumoniae, Haemophilus influenzae, Escherichia coli, Klebsiella* spp., *Salmonella* spp., *Pseudomonas aeruginosa, Staphylococcus epidermidis*, and anaerobic bacteria. The viruses include enteroviruses (coxsackieviruses A, B, and echoviruses), human immunodeficiency virus, influenza virus, mumps virus, adenoviruses, hepatitis B virus, Epstein–Barr virus, cytomegalovirus, and measles virus. The fungi include *Histoplasma capsulatum, Coccidioides immitis, Blastomyces dermatitidis*, and *Aspergillus* spp. Other organisms include *M. tuberculosis, Mycoplasma pneumoniae, Coxiella burnetti*, and protozoa (amoebas and *Toxoplasma gondii*).

While *S. aureus, S. pneumoniae*, and *S. pyogenes* were the predominant isolates recovered before 1961 (2), gram-negative aerobic bacilli, fungi, and, rarely, anaerobic bacteria were recovered in studies performed in the 1970s (2,4). These changes in the etiologic diversity of acute pericarditis were related to advances in medicine that include cardiac surgery, chemotherapy for cancer, organ transplantation, and antimicrobial therapy.

The role of anaerobic bacteria was not well studied in most investigations, as methods for the recovery of these bacteria were inadequate (3,5–8) or not used consistently (4).

We reported our experience in studying the microbiological and clinical characteristics in 15 cases of acute pericarditis treated over a 12-year period (9). Aerobic or facultative bacteria alone were present in seven specimens (47%), anaerobic bacteria alone in six specimens (40%), and mixed aerobic–anaerobic flora in two specimens (13%). In total, there were 21 isolates: 10 aerobic or facultative bacteria and 11 anaerobic bacteria, an average of 1.4/specimen. Anaerobic bacteria predominated in patients with pericarditis who also had mediastinitis that followed esophageal perforation and in patients whose pericarditis was associated with orofacial and dental infections. The predominant aerobic bacteria were *S. aureus* (three isolates) and *Klebsiella pneumoniae* (two), and the predominant anaerobic bacteria were *Prevotella* spp. (four), *Peptostreptococcus* spp. (three), and *Propionibacterium acnes* (two).

Skiest et al. (10) present one case and review 29 cases of anaerobic pericarditis previously reported in the English language literature. In 17 cases, only anaerobic bacteria were isolated, while in 13 anaerobes were isolated mixed with facultative and/or aerobic bacteria. The predominant anaerobes were *Bacteroides* spp. (mostly *B. fragilis* group), anaerobic streptococci, *Clostridium*, *Fusobacterium*, and *Bifidobacterium* spp. Five of the patients were children, two of whom had pneumonia.

Pathogenesis

The inflammation, generates an influx of fibrin, mononuclear cells, polymorphonuclear leukocytes, and fluid exudates into the pericardial space. Proliferation of fibrous tissue, neovascularization, and scarring also occur. These induces loss of elasticity, restriction of cardiac filling, and constrictive pericarditis (11).

Pericarditis often results from contiguous extension of pneumonia, empyema, myocarditis, suppurative mediastinal lymphadenitis, myocardial abscess, and infective endocarditis. Pericarditis can also result from spread during bacteremia, especially in pericarditis due to *S. aureus* and *H. influenzae* in children.

Anaerobic bacteria can be isolated in pericarditis resulting from four known pathogenetic mechanisms (2–7,9,10): (*i*) spread from a contiguous focus of infection, either de novo or after surgery or trauma (pleuropulmonary, esophageal fistula or perforation, and odontogenic), (*ii*) spread from a focus of infection within the heart, most commonly from endocarditis, (*iii*) hematogenous infection, and (*iv*) direct inoculation as a result of a penetrating injury or cardiothoracic surgery.

Diagnosis

Precordial chest pain, exercise intolerance, and fever are the major manifestations along with irritability and a grunting expiratory sound as they splint the thoracic cage (12,13). Pain is felt over the precordium, to the left over the trapezius ridge, and over the scapula; and it sometimes radiates down the arm and can become worse upon movement. Pain also can be referred toward the diaphragm (13). Pain is more common in acute pericarditis than in the indolent forms.

Cardiac examination shows muffled heart sounds, and increasing tachycardia as the effusion reduces the volume of the chambers. A pericardial friction rub may be heard. The rub is most audible during deep inspiration and with the patient kneeling, in the knee–chest position or when leaning forward. Tamponade is manifest by tachycardia, peripheral vasoconstriction, reduced arterial pulse pressure, and pulsus paradoxus.

Diagnosis of pericarditis is based on history, physical examination, and imaging tests. The etiology is best determined by examination of pericardial fluid for cell count and morphology, glucose, and protein concentrations. Serosanguinous or hemorrhagic fluid is often found in trauma, tumor, toxoplasmosis, tuberculosis, and streptococcal infection.

Radiological studies typically shows an increase in the size of the cardiac shadow, mostly in the absence of pulmonary congestion (13). The electrocardiogram usually manifests generalized ST-segment elevations without reciprocal ST-segment depression, except in leads V_1 and aVR. Later this returns to baseline, and there is flattening or inversion of the T waves. Low-voltage QRS complexes can be seen without the pathologic Q waves of myocardial infarction. T-wave abnormalities can persist after recovery.

Ultrasound is the most valuable test when pericardial fluid is present, both M-mode and two-dimensional echocardiography illustrates a sonolucent space between the two layers of pericardium. Two-dimensional echocardiography can assist in direct catheter placement for drainage. Computed tomography can evaluate extracardiac masses and other causes of an enlarged cardiac silhouette: combined studies with flow imaging by magnetic resonance are helpful to define intracardiac masses.

Microbiological evaluation of pericardial fluid retrieved by pericardiocentesis is very important (14). Evaluation of the fluid should include Gram, acid-fast, and silver stains as well as culture for aerobic and anaerobic bacteria, viruses, mycobacteria, and fungi. Latex agglutination tests for bacterial antigens can facilitate diagnosis. Blood cultures should also be performed, as they can be positive in 40% to 70% of instances.

No differences were found in the clinical diagnostic features between cases of pericarditis due to anaerobic bacteria and those due to aerobic and facultative bacteria (9,10). The gram-negative anaerobic bacilli *Prevotella* and *Fusobacterium* spp. have increased their resistance to penicillins and other antimicrobials in the last decade. Complete identification and testing for antimicrobial susceptibility and beta-lactamase production are therefore essential for the management of infections caused by these bacteria.

Viral cultures from a site other than the pericardial fluid, such as the stool or throat, can be used to diagnose the likely cause of concomitant pericarditis. A rise in antibodies to that virus can confirm the infection. Serology is also helpful for the diagnosis of rickettsiae and mycoplasma.

MANAGEMENT

The final choice of antimicrobial agents should be based on isolation of specific organisms, aerobes as well as anaerobes. Although pericardiocentesis for drainage of purulent material may be part of the therapeutic approach in pericarditis, the administration of proper antimicrobial agents is essential. Antimicrobiual agents that generally provide coverage for methicillin-susceptible *S. aureus* as well as for anaerobic bacteria include cefoxitin, clindamycin, carbapenems, tigecycline, and combinations of a penicillin (e.g., ticarcillin) and a beta-lactamase–inhibitor (i.e., clavulanate). A glycopeptide (e.g., vancomycin), daptomycin, line-zolid, tigecycline, or quinupristin/dalfopristin should be administered in cases in which methicillin-resistant *S. aureus* is present or suspected. Cefoxitin, ticarcillin and clavulanate, carbapenems, and tigecycline also provide coverage for Enterobacteriaceae. However, agents that are effective against these organisms (e.g., aminoglycosides and quinolones) should be added to the treatment regimen in cases where the infections include these bacteria. Therapy should be administered for three to four weeks. Fungal infection is treated for several months with amphotericin B.

Large effusions with impending or established tamponade require immediate drainage of fluide by pericardiocentesis or open drainage. In the presence of acute deterioration, ultrasound-guided pericardiocentesis provides instant relief (13). Pericardiectomy is more definitive and is mandated if the fluid is too thick to drain through a small tube, persists after pericardiocentesis, or in a chronic and constrictive process.

Small effusions of viral etiology are managed with bed rest, pain relief, and clinical monitoring. Antiviral therapy may be given for the herpes family of viruses.

COMPLICATIONS

Constrictive pericarditis is prevented by drainage (3). Its presence mandates surgical stripping of the pericardium. Mortality is high (up to 80%) in those who receive antibiotics only, and no drainage, and is reduced to 22% in those who also have surgical drainage (1).

REFERENCES

1. Futterman LG, Lemberg L. Pericarditis. AM J Crit Care 2006; 15:626–30.
2. Boyle JD, Pearce ML, Guze LB. Purulent pericarditis: review of literature and report of eleven cases. Medicine 1961; 40:119–44.
3. Pankuweit S, Ristic AD, Seferovic PM, Maisch B. Bacterial pericarditis: diagnosis and management. Am J Cardiovasc Drugs 2005; 5:103–12.
4. Rubin RH, Moellering RC. Clinical microbiologic and therapeutic aspects of purulent pericarditis. Am J Med 1975; 59:68–78.
5. Klacsmann PG, Bulkley BH, Hutchins GM. The changed spectrum of purulent pericarditis. Am J Med 1975; 59:68–78.
6. Ilan Y, Oren R, Ben-Chetrit E. Acute pericarditis: etiology, treatment and prognosis. Jpn Heart J 1991; 32:315–21.
7. Soler-Soler J, Permanyer-Miralda G, Sagrista-Sauleda J. A systematic diagnostic approach to primary acute pericardial disease: the Barcelona experience. Cardiol Clin 1990; 8:609–20.
8. Connolly DC, Burchell HB. Pericarditis: a 10-year survey. Am J Cardiol 1961; 7:7–14.

9. Brook I, Frazier EH. Microbiology of acute purulent pericarditis. A 12-year experience in a military hospital. Arch Intern Med 1996; 156:1857–60.

10. Skiest DJ, Steiner D, Werner M, Gamer JG. Anaerobic pericarditis: case report and review. Clin Infect Dis 1994; 19:435–40.

11. Aikat S, Ghaffari S. A review of pericardial diseases: clinical, ECG and hemodynamic features and management. Cleve Clin J Med 2000; 67:903–14.

12. Hancock EW. Differential diagnosis of restrictive cardiomyopathy and constrictive pericarditis. Heart 2001; 86:343–9.

13. Fowler NO, Manitsas GT. Infectious pericarditis. Prog Cardiovasc Dis 1973; 16:323–36.

14. Corey GR, Campbell PT, Van Trigt P, et al. Etiology of large pericardial effusions. Am J Med 1993; 95:209–13.

35 | Botulism

Botulism is a rare paralytic disease caused by a neurotoxin produced from the spore-forming bacterium *Clostridium botulinum* and in rare cases, *Clostridium butyricum* and *Clostridium baratii*. Botulism in humans is usually caused by toxin types A, B, and E. Since 1973, a median of 24 cases of foodborne botulism, 3 cases of wound botulism, and 71 cases of infant botulism have been reported annually to the Centers for Disease Control and Prevention (CDC) (1,2). Botulism has four naturally occurring syndromes: foodborne, wound, infant botulism, and adult intestinal toxemia. Inhalational botulism could result from aerosolization of botulinum toxin, and iatrogenic botulism can result from injection of toxin. All of these produce the same clinical syndrome of symmetrical cranial nerve palsies followed by descending, symmetric flaccid paralysis of voluntary muscles, which may progress to respiratory compromise and death. The weaponization of botulinum toxin is of great concern.

MICROBIOLOGY AND TOXINS

C. botulinum is a gram-positive spore-forming obligate anaerobe, present in the soil worldwide, and has been identified in up to 18.5% of the U.S. soil surveyed (3).

C. botulinum is made of four groups of clostridia (groups I–IV), linked by their ability to produce potent neurotoxins which have identical pharmacologic modes of action. *C. botulinum* produces seven closely related serological toxins (A–G). Human illness is usually caused by type A, B, or E toxin, and rarely by type C_1, C_2, D, F, or G (4–8). Types A and B toxins are highly poisonous proteins resistant to digestion by gastrointestinal enzymes. Unexpressed toxin genes can be found in other clostridial species (and more than one toxin type in a single botulinal strain), confounding molecular diagnostics (9).

Each of the four groups of *C. botulinum* are distinguished by its characteristic biochemical activities. The production of each toxin appears to depend on the presence of a plasmid that encodes the toxin gene. All of the toxins are large, single polypeptides of similar structure. Elimination of the plasmid renders the bacteria nontoxigenic. The molecular weights of the toxins, which now are believed to be cellular proteins released during lysis, vary within the range of 130 to 150 kDa. The active moiety of the protein may be as small as 10 kDa. The toxin exerts its action through affecting the transmission at all peripheral cholinergic junctions. It interferes with the normal release of acetylcholine from nerve terminals in response to depolarization (10). The toxin binds irreversibly, and recovery of function depends on ultraterminal sprouting of the nerve to form new motor end plates. Following absorption or dissemination, the toxins give rise to neurologic symptoms by interfering with the release of acetylcholine from the terminal endings of cholinergic nerve fibers (10). Type A toxin may cause more severe disease than types B and E because of differences in amount of ingested toxin, absorption, or receptor affinity (11).

Botulinum toxins are the most potent toxins known. The estimated lethal doses for purified crystalline botulinum toxin type A for a 70-kg man are 0.09 to 0.15 µg when introduced intravenously, 0.80 to 0.90 µg when introduced inhalationally, and 70 µg when introduced orally (12). Botulinal toxin type A has therapeutic value in the treatment of several neurologic and ophthalmologic disorders through chemical denervation (13). It is used as a therapeutic agent through local instillations in strabismus, blepharospasm, and other facial nerve disorders.

C. botulinum sporulates under stress and survives standard cooking and food processing but not industrial canning. The spores are highly heat-resistant; they may survive several hours at 100°C; however, exposure to moist heat at 120°C for 30 minutes will kill the spores. Botulinum toxins are temperature sensitive, and are inactivated by heating to 85°C for five minutes (14). Germination can occur in anaerobic milieu, nonacidic pH, and low salt and sugar content (15). The conditions in the normal human intestine do not support germination, vegetation, and toxin production by *C. botulinum*. However, this can occur in a small number of infants who develop infant botulism or adults who develop adult toxemic infectious botulism (16).

BOTULISM SYNDROMES

Foodborne Botulism

Foodborne botulism is caused by consumption of foods contaminated with botulinum toxin.

Foodborne botulism, the most common form of botulism, usually occurs in small sporadic outbreaks. These are typically small, involving two or three persons (1,2). An average of 9.4 outbreaks involving 24.2 cases occur annually in the U.S.A. Children acquire the disease less often than adults, perhaps reflecting protection or more fastidious eating habits. The disease occurs throughout the U.S.A. In the west, type A intoxications predominate; in the Mississippi valley and Atlantic coast regions, type B intoxications are more common.

C. botulinum multiplies and produces toxin only when the conditions in the food favor its growth. These include an anaerobic milieu, a pH of <4.5, low salt and sugar, and a temperature of 4°C to 121°C (17). Home-canned foods are a major source of intoxication (1,18,19). Most U.S.A. outbreaks of botulism are associated with food products (e.g., home-canned vegetables), which are not heated adequately before consumption and in which spores produce toxins. In the U.S.A., preserved foods in which the toxin is most often found include string beans, corn, mushrooms, spinach, olives, onions, beets, asparagus, seafood, pork products, and beef (1,20). Improperly smoked or canned fish is the source of type E intoxications. Botulinum spores are common in soil, dust, lakes, and other environmental matter and can contaminate fruits, vegetables, meats, and fish. Honey has been recognized as a potential source of *C. botulinum* spores and one of the botulism.

Clinical Findings
There are four cardinal clinical features of botulism (21).

1. Symmetric and descending neurologic manifestations
2. Intact mental processes
3. No sensory disturbances, and intellectual function is preserved, although vision may be impaired because of extraocular muscle involvement
4. Absence of fever unless secondary infectious complications occur

The disease almost always follows ingestion of improperly preserved food in which the toxin has been produced during the growth of the causative organism.

The clinical manifestations of botulism are related in some measure to age, with considerably less specific symptoms in infants than in older patients. At 18 to 48 hours after ingestion of tainted food, patients with botulism typically present with cranial nerve dysfunction manifested by ptosis, diplopia, dysphagia, and difficulty in speaking (dysarthria). Patients remain lucid, although anxiety and agitation may develop. Generally, fever is absent unless superinfection occurs. Additional signs may include pupillary dilation, vertigo, and tinnitus. Prominent autonomic symptoms include anhydrosis with severe dry mouth and mucous membranes and throat and postural hypotension. In some cases, pharyngeal collapse secondary to cranial nerve paralysis may compromise the airway and require intubation in the absence of respiratory muscle compromise. Cranial nerve palsies may be followed by flaccid, descending, symmetric paralysis of voluntary muscles, affecting (in order) the neck muscles, shoulders, the proximal and then distal upper extremities, and the proximal followed by distal lower extremities. Paralysis of the diaphragm and accessory breathing muscles may cause respiratory compromise or arrest. The descending progression of paralysis in botulism occurs at various rates, spreading and involving muscles of respiration and most voluntary musculature. The major manifestation is respiratory embarrassment, which may appear gradually or suddenly. If progression is slow, repeated measurements of tidal volume and other pulmonary function tests may be useful to predict the need for ventilatory support.

Symptoms may be limited to a few cranial nerves or may progress to cause complete paralysis of all voluntary muscles, and symptoms may progress over hours to days.

In cases involving toxin types B and E, the gastrointestinal symptoms of nausea and vomiting may precede neurologic symptoms. Involvement of the gastrointestinal tract varies and is related somewhat to the toxin serotype. Types A and B, the most common causes of botulism in the U.S.A., cause abdominal complaints (e.g., abdominal pain, bloating, cramps, diarrhea) in approximately one-third of patients. These complaints are replaced quickly by constipation or obstipation. Type E produces more significant gastrointestinal complaints than do the other types.

Death in untreated patients results from airway obstruction from pharyngeal muscle paralysis and inadequate tidal volume, due to the diaphragmatic and accessory respiratory muscles paralysis.

Paralysis resolves in weeks to months and often requires extended outpatient rehabilitation therapy. The duration of flaccidity and respiratory embarrassment in all forms of botulism may be fairly prolonged. The chief cause of mortality is respiratory or bulbar paralysis. The typical duration of symptoms exceeds one month, and full recovery from weakness and fatigue may require as long as one year. The nerve terminals regenerate slowly and recovery is complete in 95%. Although no additional specific complications of botulism intoxication are listed, the potential complications of prolonged paralysis, assisted ventilation, and nutritional support are significant. Patients who progress to significant respiratory compromise should be treated in tertiary-care centers where experienced ventilatory support teams are available. The susceptibility to hospital-acquired infections of skin, respiratory tract, urinary tract, and indwelling intravascular devices defines the additional clinical signs and symptoms that may be present in these patients.

Diagnosis

Routine studies of blood, urine, and cerebrospinal fluid usually are normal (22). Diagnosis is suggested by the pattern of neuromuscular disturbances and a likely food source such as recent consumption of home-canned food. It is important to solicit this information early, before the development of respiratory failure and the patient's ability to communicate is compromised. The simultaneous occurrence of two or more cases following ingestion of the same food simplifies the diagnosis. Diagnosis is confirmed by demonstration of botulinum toxin or *C. botulinum* in suspected food, vomitus, and, occasionally, of toxin in the serum. Electromyography is helpful in the diagnosis of botulism. Where affected, muscle findings are neuromuscular junction blockage, normal axonal conduction, and potentiation with rapid repetitive stimulation. Suggestive confirmatory evidence may be derived from the recovery of *C. botulinum* from vomitus, feces, gastric and intestinal contents, and, rarely, from viscera. Pets that have eaten the same contaminated food may also develop botulism.

Suspected cases of botulism must be immediately reported to local and state health authorities and to the CDC [Tel. 770-488-7100], from which trivalent antitoxin for types A, B, and E is available. Blood and stool samples should be obtained and refrigerated for transport to a laboratory (usually state health departments) equipped to determine botulinal toxin. These specimens must be handled with utmost care because percutaneous or mucous membrane exposure to minute quantities of the toxin may cause fatal disease. Stool should be cultured for *Clostridium* because *C. botulinum* is not part of the normal flora, and its identification in stool confirms the clinical diagnosis. All specimens should be refrigerated (preferably not frozen) and examined as soon as possible after collection. Definitive diagnosis can be made by demonstration of preformed toxin in the serum or stool by the mouse inoculation test, in which a patient's specimen is injected into the peritoneal cavity of a mouse. If death is prevented by the preadministration of *C. botulinum* antitoxin, the diagnosis is established

(22). The toxin may routinely be found in the serum seven to nine days after exposure and can be found up to a month later. Forty-five percent of suspected cases will be thus confirmed.

Botulism may be confused with poliomyelitis, viral encephalitis and meningitis, myasthenia gravis, Guillain–Barré syndrome, tick paralysis, stroke syndromes, Eaton–Lambert syndrome, alcohol intoxication, drug overdose, antimicrobial-associated paralysis, and atropine, shellfish, or mushroom poisoning (10,21).

Management

Although the number of outbreaks of botulism remains steady each year, the fatality rate has dropped from 60% to 16%, most likely a result of improvement in critical care management (1,2,23). The mortality rate is lower with type B disease (10%) than with type A or E disease (1,2). The mortality rate is lower in those younger than 20 years of age (10%). The longer the incubation period, the better the prognosis.

Management of botulism involves optimal supportive care and specific therapy directed at neutralizing unbound toxin and eradicating any infection with *C. botulinum*. Speed is essential in establishing the diagnosis with reasonable certainty so that circulating toxin can be neutralized before it binds to nerve endings. Because the only available antitoxin is of equine origin and, therefore, carries a significant risk of serum sickness, every effort should be made to substantiate the diagnosis. Hospitalization is essential in the management of the acute phase. Induced vomiting and gastric lavage should be carried out if exposure has occurred within several hours. An emetic agent should be given, and purgation and enemas are advisable, even after several days, to facilitate the elimination of unabsorbed toxin. Airway control and management of adequate ventilation is of great importance. Endotracheal intubation may be required in serious cases. Supportive care includes proper oxygenation and management of secondary infections.

Oral or parenteral antimicrobial agents such as penicillin have limited value but may destroy some viable *C. botulinum* organisms. No data address the safety or efficacy of oral vancomycin for the eradication of enteric *C. botulinum*, despite its demonstrated efficacy in *Clostridium difficile* enteric infections. Additional systemic antibiotic therapy is warranted only if superinfection occurs. Because aminoglycosides can affect the neuromuscular junction and potentiate the effect of botulinal toxin, they should be avoided. Bowel purges have been suggested as a mode of eliminating unabsorbed toxin from the intestine.

The CDC recommends administration of trivalent equine botulism antitoxin for adult patients with botulism as soon as diagnosis is made, without waiting for laboratory confirmation. Before administration of antitoxin, skin testing for sensitivity to serum or antitoxin should be done as hypersensitivity is reported to be 9% to 20%. A regimen for desensitization is included in the package. The standard dose is one vial IV and one vial IM. A single vial of the antitoxin administered IV results in serum levels of type A, B, and E antibodies capable of neutralizing serum toxin concentrations in excess of those reported for botulism patients. This need not be repeated even though the insert package recommends repeated doses in four hours in severe cases, as circulating antitoxins have a half-life of five to eight days. Antitoxin packages, including instructions for skin or conjunctival testing for hypersensitivity to horse serum and a regimen for desensitization, are available through the CDC (emergency assistance number 770-488-7100). Antitoxin packages can be obtained through state health departments. Antitoxin that neutralizes toxin not yet bound to nerve terminals has circulating half-life of five to eight days and patients who do not receive antitoxin treatment show free toxin in serum for up to 28 days (10,21,24).

Antitoxin should also be given to those who consumed the food that has been incriminated in the disease, even in the absence of illness. Several forms of equine botulism antitoxin are available: monovalent type E, bivalent AB, trivalent ABE, and polyvalent ABCDEF. If the causative toxigenic type is unknown, or if type-specific antitoxin is not available, the trivalent ABE preparation should be used. Monovalent antitoxins should be used only for type established disease. The polyvalent ABCDEF preparation is reserved for established cases of C, D, or F disease (25). Human-derived immune globulin preparation is currently under investigation (26). If found effective, this preparation will offer the advantage of not inducing reactions to foreign protein and of having a prolonged, effective half-life.

The use of guanidine has been suggested because it enhances the release of acetylcholine from nerve terminals and may help in mild cases; however, guanidine is less effective in overcoming respiratory muscle paralysis (27).

Prevention

Prevention of the disease is of utmost importance. Proper home and commercial canning and adequate heating of food before serving are essential. Food showing any evidence of spoilage should be discarded.

Because the commercial food industry is attentive to appropriate temperatures and aseptic conditions, few cases of botulism are traced to such sources. In the home preparation of food, all hot foods should be brought to the appropriate temperature before consumption, with particular attention to canning and preserving foods. The elimination of viable *C. botulinum* spores is ensured by the use of sterile containers and pressure cookers in which temperatures of 120°C can be reached and maintained for 30 minutes. Boiling home-preserved foods for 10 minutes before consumption inactivates the toxin. Neither microwaves nor the temperatures commonly achieved in microwave ovens are adequate to kill *C. botulinum* spores or to inactivate the toxin. Home-preserved foods should be cooked in traditional equipment.

Although botulinal toxoid is immunogenic and presumably protective, the rarity of this disease makes active immunization impractical. The best preventive measure is to ensure adequate care of food products and infant feedings. After a case has been recognized, health authorities must be notified so that other potential cases can be identified and treated expectantly.

Wound Botulism

Wound botulism occurs as a result of wound contamination with *C. botulinum* spores that germinate and produce toxin within the anaerobic milieu of the wound.

Wound botulism has been associated with major soil contamination through compound fractures, severe trauma, lacerations, puncture wound, and hematoma. Of the pediatric cases in the U.S.A. more than half have been associated with compound fracture (10,21,28). Wound botulism was rare in the U.S.A. until the early 1990s. Since that time the incidence increased mostly in the western U.S.A. among deep tissue injectors (skin popping) of "black tar heroin" (29–32). Minor skin abscesses and paranasal sinusitis (in a heavy user of intranasal cocaine) were the speculated or proved sources of infection and toxin production. Spores may be a contaminant of the drug or from skin (in infection-related cases). The disease has occurred primarily in young males between March and November, the period of maximum outdoor activity. Most cases have been associated with type A toxin–producing organism, although some cases have been associated with type B.

Clinical Signs and Diagnosis

Because wound botulism symptoms result from infection with *C. botulinum* organisms and subsequent in vivo production of toxin, the incubation period is longer (4–18 days) than for foodborne illness (six hours to eight days) (10,21,22). The clinical manifestations are similar to those of foodborne botulism except for the lack of early gastrointestinal symptoms. Early symptoms can include appearance of lethargy owing to muscle weakness, ptosis, blurred or double vision, dry, sore throat (21), and a subsequent descending weakness of the respiratory muscles. Fever, which usually is absent in foodborne botulism, may be present in wound botulism.

The wound can look benign, with minimal erythema, induration or discharge, but the organism and toxin are usually present. Wound botulism has been reported in parenteral drug abusers (31,32). Therefore, botulism should be considered in any patient with typical neurologic symptoms, even if gastrointestinal symptoms are not present.

The diagnosis of wound botulism is suggested by clinical findings and the presence of an apparent wound source. Diagnostic methods are the same as for other forms of botulism and also include unroofing of lesions to obtain specimens for culture and toxin assay. Confirmation of the diagnosis is made by demonstration of toxin in serum or by isolation of *C. botulinum* and/or toxin from the wound in association with appropriate clinical findings. Electromyogram can be helpful in diagnosis when lowered amplitude action potentials following low-frequency stimulation and posttetanic facilitation of the muscle action potential can be demonstrated.

Differential diagnosis in a patient without a suggestive food ingestion history and sudden onset of neurologic symptoms includes Guillain–Barré syndrome, myasthenia gravis, cerebrovascular accident, tick paralysis, intoxications, and infectious diseases of the central nervous system.

Management

Treatment of wound botulism must include debridement, drainage, and irrigation of the wound. Good supportive care, primarily respiratory support, is also an important aspect of management for patients with botulism. Although antitoxin will not improve paralysis from toxin already bound at the neuromuscular junction, antitoxin will bind circulating toxin.

Experience from infant botulism has suggested a potentiation of neuromuscular weakness by aminoglycosides (33). Aminoglycosides should be avoided if possible in a patient with botulism. The role of guanidine hydrochloride therapy in the treatment of botulism is controversial (27).

The efficacy of treatment with systemic antimicrobials such as penicillin or vancomycin is unclear; moreover, antimicrobials have not prevented the development of wound botulism in several cases (34).

Adult Intestinal Toxemia Botulism

Adult intestinal toxemia botulism occurs rarely and sporadically, and it results from the absorption of toxin produced in situ by botulinum toxin–producing *Clostridia* that colonizes the intestine. Generally, patients have an anatomical or functional bowel abnormality or are using antimicrobials, which may select fastidious *Clostridium* species from the normal bowel flora (30,35,36). The symptoms may be protracted and relapsed even after treatment with antitoxin because of the ongoing intraluminal production of toxin. Typically, there is no known food or wound source and prolonged excretion of organisms and toxin is present in the stool.

Inhalational Botulism

Inhalational botulism is iatrogenic and described only once among laboratory workers in 1962, with symptoms similar to foodborne botulism (37). Deliberate dissemination of botulinum toxin by aerosol is a potential biological weapon that could produce an outbreak of inhalational botulism (12).

Iatrogenic Botulism

Iatrogenic botulism occurs after injection of botulinum toxin for therapeutic or cosmetic purposes. The doses recommended for cosmetic treatment are too low to cause systemic disease. However, higher doses injected for treatment of muscle movement disorders have caused systemic botulism-like symptoms in patients (38). Injection of highly concentrated botulinum toxin has caused severe botulism in some patients who received it for cosmetic purposes.

Infant Botulism (See Chapter 9)

Infant botulism results from absorption of heat-labile neurotoxin toxin produced in situ by *C. botulinum* that can colonize the intestines of infants younger than one year of age (39). It is an age-limited neuromuscular disease that is distinct from classic botulism, in that the toxin is elaborated by the organism in the infant's intestinal lumen and is then absorbed.

Honey and environmental exposure are the main sources of acquisition of the organism (40). Clinical manifestations are due to progressive neuromuscular blockade, initially of muscles innervated by cranial nerves and later of the trunk, extremities, and diaphragm.

Presynaptic autonomic nerves are also affected. The diagnosis is made on clinical grounds and is confirmed by recovery of the organism or by detection of toxin in stool. Management includes meticulous supportive intensive care that may include mechanical ventilation and administration of human botulinum immunoglobulin in severe cases (41).

REFERENCES

1. Shapiro RL, Hatheway C, Swerdlow DL. Botulism in the United States: a clinical and epidemiologic review. Ann Intern Med 1998; 129:221–8.
2. Centers for Disease Control and Prevention (CDC). Jajosky RA, Hall PA, et al. Summary of notifiable diseases—United States, 2004. MMWR Morb Mortal Wkly Rep 2006; 53:1–79.
3. Smith LDS. The occurrence of *Clostridium botulinum* and *Clostridium tetani* in the soil of the U.S. Health Lab Sci 1978; 15:74–80.
4. Oguma K, Yokota K, Hayashi S, et al. Infant botulism due to *Clostridium botulinum* type C toxin. Lancet 1990; 336:1449–50.
5. Aureli P, Fenicia L, Pasolini B, et al. Two cases of type E infant botulism caused by neurotoxigenic *Clostridium butyricum* in Italy. J Infect Dis 1986; 154:207–11.
6. McCroskey L, Hatheway C, Fenicia L, et al. Characterization of an organism that produces type E botulinal toxin but which resembles *Clostridium buryricum* from the feces of an infant with type E botulism. J Clin Microbiol 1986; 23:201–2.
7. Hall J, McCroskey L, Pincomb B, Hatheway CL. Isolation of an organism resembling *Clostridium berati* which produces type F botulinal toxin from an infant with botulism. J Clin Microbiol 1985; 21:654–5.
8. Hoffman R, Pincomb B, Skeels M, et al. Type F infant botulism. Am J Dis Child 1982; 136:270–1.
9. Franciosa G, Ferreira JL, Hatheway CL. Detection of type A, B, and E botulism neurotoxin genes in *Clostridium botulinum* and other *Clostridium* species by PCR: evidence of unexpressed type B toxin genes in type A toxigenic organisms. J Clin Microbiol 1994; 32:1911–6.
10. Horowitz BZ. Botulinum toxin. Crit Care Clin 2005; 21:825–39.
11. Brin MF. Botulinum toxin: chemistry, pharmacology, toxicity, and immunology. Muscle Nerve Suppl 1997; 6:S146–68.
12. Arnon SS, Schechter R, Inglesby TV, et al. Botulism toxin as a biological weapon: medical and public health management. JAMA 2001; 285:1059–70.
13. Lew MF. Review of the FDA-approved uses of botulinum toxins, including data suggesting efficacy in pain reduction. Clin J Pain 2002; 18(6):S142–6.
14. Centers for Disease Control and Prevention (CDC). Botulism in the United States, 1899–1996. Handbook for Epidemiologists, Clinicians and Laboratory Workers. Atlanta, GA: CDC, 1998.
15. Meyer K. The protective measures of the state of California against botulism. Am J Prev Med 1931; 5:261–93.
16. Paton JC, Lawrence AJ, Steven IM. Quantities of *Clostridium botulinum* organisms and toxin in feces and presence of *Clostridium botulinum* toxin in the serum of an infant with botulism. J Clin Microbiol 1983; 17:13–5.
17. International Commission on Microbiological Specifications for Foods. *Clostridium botulinum*. Micro-Organisms in Foods 5: Characteristics of Microbial Pathogens. New York: Blackie Academic & Professional, 1996:68–111.
18. Cengiz M, Yilmaz M, Dosemeci L, Ramazanoglu A. A botulism outbreak from roasted canned mushrooms. Hum Exp Toxicol 2006; 25:273–8.
19. Gangarosa EA. Botulism in the U.S., 1899–1969. Am J Epidemiol 1971; 93:93–101.
20. Sobel J, Tucker N, Sulka A, McLaughlin J, Maslanka S. Foodborne botulism in the United States, 1990–2000. Emerg Infect Dis 2004; 10:1606–11.
21. Sobel J. Botulism. Clin Infect Dis 2005; 41:1167–73.
22. Lindstrom M, Korkeala H. Laboratory diagnostics of botulism. Clin Microbiol Rev 2006; 19:298–314.
23. Varma JK, Katsitadze G, Moiscrafishvili M, et al. Signs and symptoms predictive of death in patients with foodborne botulism—Republic of Georgia, 1980–2002. Clin Infect Dis 2004; 39:357–62.
24. Cherington M. Botulism: update and review. Semin Neurol 2004; 24:155–63.
25. Jones RG, Corbel MJ, Sesardic D. A review of WHO International Standards for botulinum antitoxins. Biologicals 2006; 34:223–6.
26. Metzger JF, Lewis GE, Jr. Human-derived immune globulins for the treatment of botulism. Rev Infect Dis 1979; 1:689–92.
27. Dock M, Ben Ali A, Karras A, et al. Treatment of severe botulism with 3,4-diaminopyridine. Presse Med 2002; 31:601–2.
28. Mechem CC, Walter FG. Wound botulism. Vet Hum Toxicol 1994; 36:233–7.
29. Chia JK, Clark JB, Ryan CA, Pollack M. Botulism in an adult associated with food-borne intestinal infection with *Clostridium botulinum*. N Engl J Med 1986; 315:239–54.

30. Arnon S. Botulism as an intestinal toxemia. In: Blaser MJ, Smith PD, Ravdin JI, Greenberg HB, Guerrant RL, eds. Infections of the Gastrointestinal Tract. New York: Raven Press, 1995:257–71.

31. Passaro DJ, Werner SB, McGee J, MacKenzie W, Vugia D. Wound botulism associated with black tar heroin among injecting drug users. JAMA 1998; 279:859–63.

32. Werner SB, Passaro DJ, McGee J, Schechter R, Vugia DJ. Wound botulism in California, 1951–1998: a recent epidemic in heroin injectors. Clin Infect Dis 2000; 31:1018–24.

33. Santos JI, Swensen P, Glasgow LA. Potentiation of *Clostridium botulinum* toxin aminoglycoside antibiotics: clinical and laboratory observations. Pediatrics 1981; 68:50–4.

34. Keller MA, Miller VH, Berkowitz CD, Yoshimori RN. Wound botulism in pediatrics. Am J Dis Child 1982; 136:320–2.

35. Fenicia L, Franciosa G, Pourshaban M, Aureli P. Intestinal toxemia botulism in two young people, caused by *Clostridium butyricum* type E. Clin Infect Dis 1999; 29:1381–7.

36. Griffin PM, Hatheway CL, Rosenbaum RB, Sokolow R. Endogenous antibody production to botulinum toxin in an adult with intestinal colonization botulism and underlying Crohn's disease. J Infect Dis 1997; 175:633–7.

37. Middlebrook JL, Franz DR. Botulinum toxins. In: Sidell FR, Takafuji TE, Franz DR, eds. Medical Aspects of Chemical and Biological Warfare. Washington, DC: Borden Institute, Walter Reed Army Medical Center, 1997:643–54.

38. Bakheit AM, Ward CD, McLellan DL. Generalized botulism-like syndrome after intramuscular injections of botulinum toxin type A: a report of two cases. J Neurol Neurosurg Psychiatry 1997; 62:198 (Letter).

39. Long SS. Infant botulism. Pediatr Infect Dis J 2001; 20:707–9.

40. Long SS, Gajewski JL, Brown LW, Gilligan PH. Clinical, laboratory, and environmental features of infant botulism in Southeastern Pennsylvania. Pediatrics 1985; 75:935–41.

41. Centers for Disease Control and Prevention (CDC). Infant botulism—New York City, 2001–2002. MMWR Morb Mortal Wkly Rep 2003; 52:21–4.

36 | Tetanus

Tetanus is an acute toxemic illness caused by *Clostridium tetani* infection at a laceration or break in the skin. It can also complicate burns, puerperal infections, umbilical stump infections (tetanus neonatorum), and surgical sites (due to contaminated sutures, dressings, or plaster).

Tetanus is an intoxication manifested mainly by neuromuscular dysfunction and caused by tetanal exotoxin (tetanospasmin), a potent exotoxin elaborated by *C. tetani*. It begins with tonic spasms of the skeletal muscles and is followed by paroxysmal contractions. The muscle stiffness involves first the jaw (lockjaw) and neck and later becomes generalized. The disease can be prevented by immunization with tetanal toxoid.

EPIDEMIOLOGY

C. tetani is distributed worldwide and has been isolated from diverse sites including soil, feces, house dust, and contaminated heroin. Tetanus ranks high among the infectious diseases as a cause of death throughout the world, and in developing countries it is an important cause of neonatal death. The percentage of natural immunity in isolated, unimmunized communities averages 30% and increases with age (1). Beyond the neonatal period, the attack rate and age-related mortality rate are especially higher in males.

The incidence of tetanus varies widely throughout the world; in the United States, there has been a sharp decline in the rate of tetanus, although 50 to 100 cases are reported annually (average incidence of 0.03 cases per 100,000 persons) (2,3). Neonatal tetanus is rare in the United States. This decline reflects the efficacy of the intensive immunization program in the United States, compared with developing countries where mortality is still high. Unhygienic childbirth, non-medical abortion practices, inadequate immunization of mothers, and lack of attention to penetrating wounds explain most cases of neonatal and adult tetanus in the developing world. Additionally, climate and soil pH in the tropics probably contribute to the prevalence of *C. tetani* and its availability to contaminate wounds (4).

Approximately 50% of cases of tetanus in the United States occur after injuries. Infected wounds (both traumatic and surgical), abscesses, surgical wounds, parenteral drug abuse, major trauma, and animal-related injuries account for 25% of the tetanus-associated injuries; about 20% of wounds are from unknown circumstances and in 5% no source can be identified (2).

Because immunization is effective in preventing tetanus, the disease is most frequently noted in countries or in ethnic groups in which effective immunization is less likely to be accomplished. In the U.S.A., inadequate tetanus protection was found in rural elderly individuals as compared to the entire population (5). Tetanus remains a major cause of death in those areas of the world without appropriate hygiene and immunization programs.

ETIOLOGY AND PATHOPHYSIOLOGY

The tetanus bacillus is a gram-positive anaerobic rod that may develop a terminal spore, giving it a drumstick appearance. The spores resist heat and the usual antiseptics and can persist in tissues for many months. They can survive in soil for years and may be found in house dust, soil, salt, fresh water, and the feces of many animal species (6).

The portal of entry is usually the site of minor puncture wounds or scratches. Deep puncture wounds, burns, crushing, and other injuries that promote favorable growth conditions for anaerobic organisms may lead to the development of tetanus. Occasionally, no apparent portal of entry can be established. Sources of infection that have been incriminated include the alimentary tract, tonsils, ear lesions, as well as contaminated vaccines, sera, and catgut (7,8).

Following introduction into tissues, spores convert to vegetative forms, multiply, and elaborate tetanospasmin. In many cases, there is no associated inflammation or apparent local infection. Tetanospasmin enters the peripheral nerve at the site of entry and travels to the central nervous system (CNS) through the nerves or is transferred by the lymphocytes to the CNS (9–13). The toxin affects the nervous system centrally and peripherally. The toxin binds to gangliosides at the presynaptic nerve ending in the neuronal membrane, prevents release of neurotransmitters, and affects polarization of postsynaptic membranes in complex poly-synaptic reflexes. The lack of inhibitory impulses that result is manifested in the characteristic spasms, seizures, and sympathetic overactivity of tetanus. The toxin has no effect on the mental status, and consciousness is not impaired directly by this illness.

Tetanospasmin also becomes bound to gangliosides within the CNS where it suppresses the motor neurons and interneurons without directly enhancing synaptic excitatory action. Additional actions of tetanospasmin are evident in the neurocirculatory, neuroendocrine, and vegetative nervous systems (10). Once it binds to tissue, toxin cannot be dissociated or neutralized by tetanus antitoxin. Antitoxin may prevent binding in the CNS if binding has taken place in the periphery.

The length and course of the illness are determined by the location and amount of the bound toxin. The complete course of tetanus takes usually from two to four weeks and is influenced by patient age and the development of complications.

CLINICAL MANIFESTATION

In addition to neonatal tetanus, tetanus can present in one of three clinical forms: localized, generalized, or cephalic.

Generalized Tetanus

This is the most common form of clinical tetanus. It may occur after relatively minor injuries and often follows non-tetanus–prone wounds. The onset may be insidious; however, the typical initial findings of trismus due to spasms of the parapharyngeal and masseter muscles are seen in 50% of cases (2,7,8). Common complaints are pain, swallowing difficulty, and unilateral or bilateral stiffness of the neck and other muscle groups, such as those of the abdomen or thorax (11,14). Persistent trismus accounts for the "risus sardonicus," which is considered a classic finding of tetanus.

As the illness progresses, additional muscle groups become involved. One of the most striking findings occurs with spasm of the paraspinal musculature, which may result in severe opisthotonos; in young infants, the soles of the feet may touch the head. Vertebral fractures are common in this situation. The tetanic contractions progress over the course of several days, with recruitment of additional muscle groups and significant worsening of symptoms. Painful spasms and contraction further contort and distort the patient's posture. These spasms are extraordinarily painful and are not true seizures. All voluntary muscles can be affected and the disease may involve the larynx, which can be fatal. Fractures of vertebrae or other bones and hemorrhage into muscles can occur. Minor stimuli including light, drafts, noises or voices, and light touch may trigger spasms. Since patients remain fully conscious throughout these spasms, anxiety and pain further complicate management and contribute to the severity of the untreated disease.

The effect of tetanospasmin on the autonomic nervous system can induce cardiovascular instability. Labile hypertension and episodes of tachycardia or other tachyarrhythmias are common (12,13,15). The sympathetic overactivity or superinfections such as pneumonia can cause fever (14). Cardiovascular complications are the primary problem in management in the modern intensive care setting, where ventilatory support and therapeutic paralysis are available. Spasms and cardiovascular complications occur most commonly during the first week and resolve slowly during the ensuing two to four weeks.

Localized Tetanus

This unusual presentation of tetanus occurs when circulating antitoxin prevents general spread of the toxin but is insufficient to stop local uptake at a wound site (11). This results in prolonged, steady, and painful muscle contraction in the region of the wound, lasting several weeks, with subsequent complete resolution. Localized tetanus may be unrecognized or be mistaken for pain-induced muscle spasms.

Cephalic Tetanus

This is a rare manifestation of tetanus which exclusively involves the cranial nerves after entry of *C. tetani* into wounds or chronic infections of the head and neck. Although any of the cranial nerves may be affected, singly or in combination, cranial nerve VII is most frequently involved. Cephalic tetanus may precede generalized disease, and isolated cephalic tetanus can occur and follow a chronology similar to generalized disease.

Neonatal Tetanus

This is a generalized form of the disease that often develops in infants delivered vaginally to mothers who have not been immunized. Birth practices in developing countries, such as applying mud or feces to the umbilical stump, increase the risk of acquiring this illness and are responsible for a large proportion of cases. The mortality rate is high, with infants dying of complications such as CNS hemorrhage, pneumonia, pulmonary hemorrhage, and laryngeal spasms.

Complications

Complications of tetanus include those due to direct toxic effect (laryngeal and phrenic nerves palsy and cardiomyopathy), and those that are secondary to spasms (respiratory compromise, rhabdomyolysis, myositis ossificans circumscripta, and vertebral compressed fracture), respiratory compromise (hypoxic cerebral injury), and rhabdomyolysis (acute renal failure), as well as the psychological impact.

DIAGNOSIS AND DIFFERENTIAL DIAGNOSIS

Tetanus is rare in developed nations, where immunization and appropriate hygienic practices have eliminated the disease. The classic presenting complaints in tetanus of muscle spasms, trismus, stiffness, and pain with dysphagia and cranial nerve weakness can be seen in other conditions.

Conditions that can mimic some manifestations of tetanus include parapharyngeal and peritonsillar abscesses, poliomyelitis and other forms of viral encephalomyelitis, meningoencephalitis (including rabies), Bell's palsy, hypocalcemic tetany, and dystonic reactions to phenothiazines. These conditions can be differentiated from tetanus by specific laboratory or radiographic evaluations or by the clinical findings. The lack of altered consciousness in tetanus is an important point of differentiation from CNS infections, and a parapharyngeal inflammation can be diagnosed by clinical examination and/or radiographs of the airway (16).

Specific diagnosis of tetanus by routine laboratory tests is difficult. Blood counts are normal or slightly elevated; cerebrospinal fluid indexes are normal; and electroencephalogram and electromyogram are normal and nonspecifically abnormal, respectively. Gram stains and anaerobic cultures of wounds reveal the characteristic gram-positive bacilli with terminal spores in as many as one-third of tetanus patients. Even though a positive wound culture can support the clinical diagnosis, a positive culture in the absence of symptoms does not indicate that tetanus intoxication will develop.

MANAGEMENT AND PROGNOSIS

Appropriate treatment based on the clinical diagnosis is warranted even without specific confirmatory laboratory tests. The goals of therapy are to eradicate *C. tetani*, neutralize its toxin, and provide appropriate supportive care. Specific therapy includes intramuscular administration of tetanus immune globulin (TIG) to neutralize circulating toxin before it binds to neuronal cell membranes. Early administration of antitoxin may prevent spread of the toxin within the CNS. The recommended dosage of TIG ranges from 500 to 3000 U. Although a dosage recommendation based on body weight is not available, it is reasonable to give a newborn a smaller dose, of a single vial of TIG (250 U). The efficacy of concomitant intrathecal administration of TIG has not been proven (11,14).

Additionally, specific therapy includes antimicrobial agents for *C. tetani* such as penicillin-G administered as 200,000 U/kg/day in four divided intravenous doses for 10 days. Alternatives for those allergic to penicillin include oral tetracycline (40 mg/kg/day, maximum of 2 g) or intravenous vancomycin (30–40 mg/kg/day). The cephalosporins are not reliably active against *C. tetani*.

Local wound care, including surgical debridement, is essential. Foreign bodies should be removed and wounds irrigated well and left open. Excision of necrotic tissue may be required, but excision of the umbilical stump is no longer recommended in cases of neonatal tetanus. Local antibiotic or TIG instillation is not needed.

Patients should be managed in an intensive care setting of a tertiary-care center whenever possible. Facilities and equipment that should be available include a quiet darkened room, suction equipment and oxygen, cardiac and respiratory monitors, a ventilator, and tracheostomy equipment. The patients must be managed by experienced caregivers skilled in ventilatory support and maintenance of cardiovascular stability. Minimizing external stimuli and maintaining intravenous hydration may be sufficient in the initial days of the illness. Sedation and muscle relaxation should be instituted, usually with diazepam (0.1–0.2 mg/kg intravenously every four to six hours). Additional sedation with phenothiazines may be needed. If spasms are not adequately controlled, therapeutic paralysis may be necessary (4).

Neuromuscular blockade can be achieved with curariform drugs. The agents used most often are pancuronium and vecuronium. Vecuronium, an intermediate-acting neuromuscular blocking agent is given in an initial dose of 0.08 to 0.1 mg/kg intravenously, with maintenance doses of 0.01 to 0.15 mg/kg every 30 to 60 minutes, as needed. Doxacurium, a long-acting agent of the same class with similar cardiovascular safety profile, offers more prolonged effect with each dose. The recommended initial dose is 0.03 to 0.05 mg/kg intravenously, followed by 0.01 mg/kg in 60 to 90 minutes, as needed. The intervals between maintenance doses may be adjusted by the administration of smaller or larger doses. Patients who undergo therapeutic paralysis must be sedated to avoid the associated anxiety.

The hypertension that results from sympathetic overactivity may require treatment. Beta-blocking agents are the most useful. Propranolol is administered most commonly (usual dose: 0.01–0.10 mg/kg every six to eight hours). Additionally, this agent may be helpful for the control of tachyarrhythmias. The duration of these therapies ranges from two to three weeks.

Maintenance of adequate nutrition and hydration is of outmost importance. Parenteral nutrition is usually required because of the likely length of the disease and the undesirability of oral or nasogastric feedings. Adequate nutritional support can minimize weight loss, maintain electrolyte balance, and improve management of arrhythmias. Attention must be paid to skin care, and excretory functions must be monitored closely for urinary retention or serious constipation. Patients must be immunized with tetanus toxoid to prevent further disease. Tracheostomy may be required to prevent laryngospasm, which greatly increases the mortality rate of the disease.

The worldwide mortality rate for generalized tetanus ranges from 45% to 55%; it is about 1% in localized tetanus and more than 60% in tetanus neonatorum (2). Although survivors generally experience no neurologic sequelae, prolonged convalescence with residual muscle rigidity is seen for several months.

The main predictors of prognosis are the rapidity of symptom onset and the rate of progression from trismus to severe spasms. Poor outcome is predicted by an interval between

TABLE 1 Tetanus Prophylaxis in Routine Wound Management

Immunization history	Type of wound	
	Clean, mirror	All others
Three or more doses of tetanus toxoid	No TIG; toxoid only if >10 yr since last dose	No TIG; toxoid only if >5 yr since last dose
Fewer than three doses or uncertain history	No TIG; toxoid, 0.5 mL	TIG, 500 units; toxoid, 0.5 mL

Immune globulin intravenous or equine tetanus antitoxin should be used when TIG is not available.
Abbreviations: TIG, tetanus immune globulin.
Source: From Ref. 18.

injury and trismus shorter than seven days or by progression from trismus to spasms in less than three days (4).

PREVENTION

Active immunization with tetanus toxoid is the most effective means of protection (17). The primary series of tetanus toxoid, administered as DTP vaccine at two, four, and six months and a booster 12 months later, ensures protection in childhood. Additional boosters of tetanus toxoid should be given each decade throughout life with further tetanus prophylaxis after acute wounds, as advocated by the American Academy of Pediatrics Advisory Committee on Immunization Practices (Table 1) (18).

Individuals who have documentation of full primary immunization and appropriate boosters need no tetanus prophylaxis beyond appropriate local wound care for clean minor wounds, but should receive a toxoid booster after a dirty, tetanus-prone injury if the most recent dose was received more than five years before. Patients who are not known to have completed the primary series require a tetanus toxoid booster after any penetrating wound and TIG after a tetanus-prone injury. The prophylactic dose of TIG is 250 to 500 U, given intramuscularly. A human gammaglobulin product, TIG, does not carry the risk of serum sickness seen with equine antitoxin, and skin testing for hypersensitivity is unnecessary.

REFERENCES

1. Matzkin H, Regev S. Naturally acquired immunity to tetanus in an isolated community. Infect Immun 1985; 48:267–8.
2. Mallick IH, Winslet MC. A review of the epidemiology, pathogenesis and management of tetanus. Int J Surg 2004; 2:109–12.
3. Pascual FB, McGinley EL, Zanardi LR, et al. Tetanus surveillance—United States, 1998–2000. MMWR Surveill Summ 2003; 52:1–8.
4. Sanders RK. The management of tetanus. Trop Doct 1996; 26:107–15.
5. Scher KS, Baldera A, Wheeler WE, et al. Inadequate tetanus protection among the rural elderly. South Med J 1985; 78:153–6.
6. LaForce FM, Young LS, Bennett JV. Tetanus in the United States (1965–1966): epidemiologic and clinical features. N Engl J Med 1969; 280:569–74.
7. Fischer MGW, Sunakorn P, Duangman C. Otogenous tetanus: a sequelae of chronic ear infections. Am J Dis Child 1977; 131:445–6.
8. Nourmand A. Clinical studies on tetanus: notes on 42 cures in southern Iran with special emphasis on portal of entry. Clin Pediatr 1973; 12:652–3.
9. Montecucco C, Schiuvo G. Mechanism of action of tetanus and botulinium neurotoxin. Mol Microbiol 1994; 13:1–8.
10. Turton K, Chaddock JA, Acharya KR. Botulinum and tetanus neurotoxins: structure, function and therapeutic utility. Trends Bicochem Sci 2002; 27:552–8.
11. Weinstein L. Tetanus. N Engl J Med 1973; 289:293–6.
12. Kerr JH, Corbett JL, Prys-Roberts C, et al. Involvement of the sympathetic nervous system in tetanus: studies on 82 cases. Lancet 1968; 2:236–41.
13. Turton K, Chaddock JA, Acharya KR. Botulinum and tetanus neurotoxins: structure, function and therapeutic utility. Trends Biochem Sci 2002; 27:552–8.
14. Edmondson RS, Flowers MWW. Intensive care in tetanus: management, complications and mortality in 100 patients. BMJ 1979; 1:1401–4.

15. Tseuda K, Oliver PB, Richter RW. Cardio-vascular manifestations of tetanus. Anesthesiology 1974; 40:588–92.
16. Henderson S, Mody T, Groth DE, et al. The presentation of tetanus in an emergency department. J Emerg Med 1998; 16:705–8.
17. Thayaparan B, Nicoll A. Prevention and control of tetanus in childhood. Curr Opin Pediatr 1998; 10:4–8.
18. American Academy of Pediatrics. Tetanus (lockjaw). In: Pickering LK, ed. Red Book: Report of the Committee on Infectious Diseases. 27th ed. Elk Grove Village, IL: American Academy of Pediatrics, 2006:650.

37 | Antibiotic Resistance of Anaerobic Bacteria and Its Effect on the Management of Anaerobic Infections

INFECTIONS CAUSED BY ANAEROBIC BACTERIA

Infections caused by anaerobic bacteria are common and may be serious and life-threatening. Anaerobes as the predominant components of the bacterial flora of normal human skin and mucous membranes (1) are a common cause of bacterial infections of endogenous origin. Because of their fastidious nature, they are difficult to isolate from infectious sites and are often overlooked. Failure to direct therapy against these organisms often leads to clinical failures. Their isolation requires appropriate methods of collection, transportation, and cultivation of specimens (2–4). Treatment of anaerobic bacterial infection is complicated by the slow growth of these organisms, which makes diagnosis in the laboratory only possible after several days, by the often polymicrobial nature of the infection and by the growing resistance of anaerobic bacteria to antimicrobial agents.

The inadequate isolation, identification, and subsequent performance of susceptibility testing of anaerobes from an infected site can prevent detection of antimicrobial resistance and correlation of resistance with clinical outcome (1,2). Correlation of the results of in vitro susceptibility and clinical and bacteriological response is not always possible. This discrepancy occurs because of a variety of reasons: individuals may improve without antimicrobial or surgical therapy and others can get better because of adequate drainage. In some instances of polymicrobial infection, eradication of the aerobic component may be adequate; although it is well established, it is important to eliminate the aerobic pathogens as well in most cases. Infections vary in duration, severity and extent; failure can occur because of lack of needed surgical drainage; response depends on individual patients status such as underlying condition, age and nutritional status; and the antimicrobial may not be effective because of enzymatic inactivation or a low Eh or pH at the infection site, low levels at the site of infection, and because of variations or imperfections in the susceptibility testing.

Microbiological quantitation of all the infecting flora is important; it is not necessary to eliminate all the infecting organisms because reduction in counts or modification of the metabolism of certain isolates alone may be sufficient to achieve a good clinical response. Synergy between two or more infecting organisms, which is a common event in anaerobic infections, may confuse the clinical picture.

A correlation between the antibiotic susceptibility of anaerobes and poor clinical outcome has been reported in several retrospective studies (5,6). A prospective study of *Bacteroides* bacteremia reported the adverse clinical outcomes in 128 individuals who receiving an antibiotic to which the organism was not susceptible (7). Clinical outcome was correlated with results of in vitro susceptibility testing of *Bacteroides* isolates recovered from blood and/or other sites, and was determined with use of three end points: mortality at 30 days, clinical response (cure vs. failure), and microbiological response (eradication vs. persistence). The mortality rate among those who received inactive therapy (45%) was higher than among patients who received active therapy (16%; $p = 0.04$). Clinical failure (82%) and microbiological persistence (42%) were higher for those who received inactive therapy than for patients who received active therapy (22% and 12%, respectively; $p = 0.0002$ and 0.06, respectively). In vitro activity of agents directed at *Bacteroides* spp. reliably predicts outcome (specificity 97%, and positive predictive value 82%). The authors conclude that the antimicrobial susceptibility testing may be indicated for patients whose blood specimens yield *Bacteroides* spp. (7). All these observations reinforce the recommendation that susceptibility testing of anaerobic bacteria should be performed in selected cases (8,9).

These findings emphasize that is important, to perform susceptibility testing to isolates recovered from sterile body sites, those that are isolated in pure culture or those that are clinically important and have variable or unique susceptibility (see Table 4, chapter 3). Screening of anaerobic gram-negative bacteria (AGNB) isolates (particularly *Prevotella, Bacteroides*, and *Fusobacterium* spp.) for beta-lactamase (BL) activity is also helpful. However, occasional resistance is through other mechanisms. Recent standardization of testing methods by the Clinical and Laboratory Standard Institute (CLSI), previously called National Committee for Clinical Laboratory Standards (NCCLS), allows for comparison of resistance trends among various laboratories (8,9). Organisms that should be considered for individual isolate testing include highly virulent pathogens for which susceptibility cannot be predicted, such as *Bacteroides, Prevotella, Fusobacterium*, and *Clostridium* spp., *Bilophila wadsworthia*, and *Sutterella wadsworthensis* (3,8,9).

The routine susceptibility testing of all anaerobic isolates is extremely time-consuming and in many cases unnecessary. Therefore, susceptibility testing should be limited to selected anaerobic isolates. Antibiotics tested should include penicillin, a broad-spectrum penicillin, a penicillin plus a BL inhibitor, clindamycin, chloramphenicol, cefoxitin, a third-generation cephalosporin, metronidazole, a carbapenem (i.e., imipenem) tigecycline, and an extended spectrum quinolone (i.e., moxifloxacin).

The antimicrobial resistance among anaerobes has consistently increased in the past three decades and the susceptibility of anaerobic bacteria to antimicrobial agents has become less predictable. The most commonly isolated antibiotic-resistant anaerobe is the *Bacteroides fragilis* group. Resistance to several antimicrobial agents by *B. fragilis* group and other AGNB has increased over the past decade (3,8,9). Antimicrobial resistance has also increased among other anaerobes such as *Clostridium* spp. that were previously very susceptible to antibiotics. This increase made the choice of appropriate empirical therapy more difficult. Even though resistance patterns have been monitored through national and local surveys, susceptibility testing of anaerobic bacteria at individual hospitals is rarely done.

SUSCEPTIBILITY PATTERNS OF ANAEROBIC BACTERIA

The increase in antibiotic resistance among anaerobes generated extensive studies of the mechanisms of resistance and resistance-gene transfer. These investigations brought about more insight into the causes of the rapid development of resistance. The observed resistance patterns to different antibiotics vary among the different groups of organisms as variations in the mechanisms of resistance exist.

AGNB which are among the most important anaerobic pathogens recovered from infectious sites also possess the broadest spectrum of recognized resistances to antimicrobials. Their resistance and its transfer mechanisms were extensively investigated. Studies that monitor the development of antimicrobial resistance in specific organisms are routinely conducted in many countries. The antimicrobial agents that are studied include those that have been extensively used to treat anaerobic infections (beta-lactams, clindamycin, metronidazole, and chloramphenicol), as well as newer agents.

B. fragilis group as well as many other AGNB and *Fusobacterium* spp. are resistant to the penicillins and the ureidopenicillin (i.e., piperacillin) through the production of BL. However, the addition of a BL inhibitor enables penicillins to overcome this mechanism of resistance. Cefoxitin, a second generation cephalosporin formerly very active against anaerobes, has lost potency in most recent surveys. The carbapenems are the most effective beta-lactam agents. Tigecycline, a glycycline, is very active against AGNB as well as anaerobic gram positive bacteria.

Metronidazole as well as clindamycin are active against the *B. fragilis* group. However, resistance to clindamycin of up to 25% has been noted in localized areas such as Southern Europe, Japan and some regions of the U.S.A. (10–12). Penicillins are still effective against other anaerobes including *Clostridium* and *Propionibacterium* spp., and most *Fusobacterium* spp. Resistance to metronidazole have been observed in a few strains of *Clostridium perfringens*, and is common in *Propionibacterium* spp. (12).

As a guide to the efficacy of available antibiotics effective against anaerobic bacteria, the susceptibility results from the Wadsworth Anaerobic Bacteriology Laboratory at Los Angeles are presented in Tables 1 and 2 (13).

SUSCEPTIBILITY TESTING AND THEIR INTERPRETATION (SEE CHAPTER 3)

There are currently three susceptibility testing methods for anaerobic bacteria that provide reproducible results that correlate with a reference standard: the agar dilution, the broth micro dilution, and the the E-test (AB Biodisk, soloans, Sweden) (4,8,14). At present, there are no automated methods. The CLSI currently recommends that for surveillance purposes to monitor for resistance trends, the agar dilution method is used to test at least 100 anaerobic isolates per year at individual hospitals. The agar dilution method is reproducible, labor-intensive, and allows for batch testing of up to 30 anaerobic isolates at one time against a single antibiotic.

The broth micro dilution panel is a convenient, user-friendly method that determines susceptibilities of a single anaerobic isolate to several antibiotics at the same time. This panel provides results that correlate well with those of the agar dilution standard for anaerobes that grow well in broth supplemented with CLSI-recommended *Brucella* blood agar. Both methods are equivalent for determining antimicrobial susceptibilities of *B. fragilis* group isolates, but the CLSI does not recommend the broth micro dilution for non-bacteroides anaerobes unless the laboratory validates their results against the agar dilution standard.

The E-test (AB Biodisk, soloans, Sweden) is a simple user-friendly, gradient method that delivers accurate results. However, the limitation of this test is that each test strip is used only for a single isolate. Both the broth micro dilution and the the E-test methods are adequate for testing individual isolates and can provide guidance in selection of therapy on the basis of positive culture results.

The susceptibility results are considered when antibiotic treatment is chosen. The results are expressed as the minimal inhibitory concentration (MIC) or by providing degrees of susceptibility as sensitive (S), intermediate (I), and resistant (R). These sensitivity breakpoints are established by the CLSI and the U.S. Food and Drug Administration (FDA). The MIC value obtained by any of the methods does not represent an absolute number because the accurate MIC is actually between the obtained MIC and the next-lower or -higher test concentration. Also a two-fold difference on successive testing is allowed in all dilution-based susceptibility methods (8). The phenotypic interpretation of the results of the MIC tests as sensitive, intermediate, and resistant are based on the MIC distribution of the bacterial population, the antibiotic pharmacokinetics and pharmacodynamics, and the verification of antibiotic efficacy in clinical studies. The dosages of antibiotics administered for infections caused by anaerobic organisms whose MICs are at or near the S or I breakpoints, should be maximal to overcome their lower penetration and instability at the site of most infections (8).

RESISTANCE MECHANISMS OF ANAEROBIC BACTERIA

Antimicrobial susceptibility test results may depend on the methods and media used, the study size (single vs. numerous hospitals), the geographic location, and the antibiotic utilization. Whenever the susceptibility of an individual isolate is not available, the most clinically relevant antibiotic susceptibility information can be provided by longitudinal surveys that use the same methodology over time.

TABLE 1 Susceptibility of Gram-Positive Anaerobic Bacteria

Anaerobe	Percentage susceptible to[a]						
	Less than 50	50–69	70–84	85–95	More than 95		
Bacteroides fragilis	PEN[b]	CFP	MOX	CTT	PIP	FOX	SIT
	CIP	CTX	CRO	ZOX	AMC	BIA	LVX
	FLE	CAZ	CLR	CLI	SAM	IPM	OFX
	LOM	SPX		MIN	CPS	MEM	TVA
	AZM				TZP	CHL	MND
	ERY				TIM	CLX	
	ROX						
	TET						
Other *B. fragilis group*[c]	PEN	CFP	LVX	AMC	SAM	IPM	SIT
	CTX	CTT	CLR	PIP	CPS	MEM	TVA
	CAZ	MOX	CLI	FOX	TZP	CHL	MND
	CRO	OFX		ZOX	TIM	CLX	MIN
	CIP	SPX			BIA		
	FLE						
	LOM						
	AZM						
	ERY						
	ROX						
Other *Bacteroides* spp.	FLE	CIP	PEN	CTT	PIP	CTX	CLX
	LOM	TET	MOX	CAZ	AMC	FOX	SIT
			OFX	CRO	SAM	ZOX	LVX
			SPX	CLR	TIM	BIA	TVA
			AZM	ERY	CFP	IPM	MND
				ROX	CPS	CHL	CLI
				MIN			
Prevotella spp.	FLE	TET	CIP	CRO	PIP	ZOX	CLX
	LOM		OFX	AZM	AMC	BIA	SIT
			SPX	CLR	SAM	IPM	TVA
			MIN	ERY	TZP	MEM	MND
				ROX	TIM	CHL	CLI
				FOX			
Porphyromonas spp.	FLE	TET		CIP	PIP	IPM	SPX
	LOM			CLR	AMC	MEM	TVA
				CLI	FOX	CHL	MND
				ERY	ZOX	CLX	AZM
				ROX	CRO	SIT	MIN
					BIA		
Fusobacterium nucleatum	FLE			CIP	PIP	BIA	OFX
	LOM			AZM	AMC	IPM	SPX
	CLR				TZP	MEM	TVA
	ERY				TIM	CHL	CLI
	ROX				FOX	CLX	MND
					ZOX	SIT	MIN
					CRO	LVX	TET
Fusobacterium mortiferum and *Fusobacterium varium*	FLE	CIP	CLI	AMC	PIP	IPM	SIT
	LOM	SPX	TET	ZOX	TZP	MEM	TVA
	AZM	TEM		CRO	TIM	CHL	MND
	CLR				FOX	CLX	MIN
	ERY				BIA		
	ROX						
Other *Fusobacterium* spp.	FLE		CAZ	PIP	PEN		
	LOM		MOX	AMC	SAM	IPM	MND
	CLR		CIP	TIM	TZP	MEM	CLI
	ERY		SPX	CPS	FOX	CHL	MIN
	ROX		AZM	CTX	BIA	CLX	TET
				CTT		SIT	
				ZOX			
				CRO			

TABLE 1 (*Continued*) Susceptibility of Gram-Positive Anaerobic Bacteria

[a] The order of listing of drugs within percent susceptible categories is not significant. According to the national committee for clinical laboratory standards -approved breakpoints (M11-A3), using the intermediate category as susceptible.

[b] The national committee for clinical laboratory standards approved breakpoint is 4 μg/mL. However, the breakpoint should probably be lowered to 1 μg/mL, which will considerably lower the values for percentage susceptible. For example, at 1 μg/ml, no strains of the *B. fragilis* group were susceptible.

[c] Excluding *B. fragilis*.

Abbreviations: AMC, amoxicilin/clavulanate; AZM, azithromycin; BIA, biapenem; CAZ, ceftazidime; CFP, cefoperazone; CHL, chloramphenicol; CIP, ciprofloxacin; CLI, clindamycin; CLR, clarithromycin; CLX, clinafloxacin; CPS, cefoperazone/sulbactam; CRO, ceftriaxone; CTT, cefotetan; CTX, cefotaxime; ERY, erythromycin; FLE, fleroxacin; FOX, cefoxitin; IPM, imipenem; LOM, lomefloxacin; LVX, levofloxacin; MEM, meropenem; MIN, minocycline; MND, metronidazole; MOX, moxalactam; OFX, ofloxacin; PEN, penicillin; PIP, piperacillin; ROX, roxithromycin; SAM, ampicillin/sulbactam; SIT, sitafloxacin; SPX, sparfloxacin; TEM, temafloxacin; TET, tetracycline; TIM, ticarcillin/clavulanate; TVA, trovafloxacin; TZP, piperacillin/tazobactam; ZOX, ceftizoxime.

Source: From Ref. 13.

Clindamycin Resistance

Clindamycin has been used for the treatment of anaerobic infection since the 1960s. Resistance to clindamycin among anaerobes has slowly increased over time. The frequencies of resistance among anaerobes in the *B. fragilis* group in the U.S.A. was 3% in 1987, and increased to 16%, 26%, and 43% in 1996, 2000, and 2003, respectively (15–18). However, resistance at some locations reached 44% (19). Results from one medical center cannot predict those at other centers as resistance to clindamycin in individual site varies. Surveillance of local resistance is essential in assessing the utility of clindamycin at a certain location. Resistance to clindamycin among *Prevotella Porphyromonas, Fusobacterium*, and *Peptostreptococcus* spp. is generally lower and is often less than 10% (20). The anaerobe, most resistant to clindamycin is *Clostridium difficile* with up to 67% of isolates resistant (21).

These are three mechanisms of resistance: inactivation of the drug, altered permeability, and changed ribosomal target site (22,23). Several genetic clindamycin resistance determinants were identified in the *B. fragilis* group (*ermF, ermG*, and *ermS*), *C. perfringens* (*ermQ* and *ermP*), *C. difficile* (*ermZ, ermB*, and *ermBZ*), and *Porphyromonas, Prevotella, Peptostreptococcus*, and *Eubacterium* spp. (*ermF*) (24). These determinants are located on the chromosome, plasmids, or transposons and are transferable by conjugation for both *B. fragilis* and *C. difficile*. Resistance is mediated by a macrolide–lincosamide–streptogramin (MLS) type 23S RNA methylase at one of two adenine residues (25,26), which prevents binding of clindamycin to the ribosomes and makes them resistant. The same mechanism of resistance was detected in *Bacteroides* spp. Ribosomes isolated from a clindamycin resistance *Bacteroides vulgatus* strain, induced with either clindamycin or erythromycin, decreased susceptibility to clindamycin compared with ribosomes isolated from a clindamycin-susceptible strain or a strain with clindamycin resistance that was not induced (25,27). These data illustrate that resistance to clindamycin is at the ribosomal level and probably occurs via methylation of the rRNA.

Three different, but closely related, MLS resistance genes were cloned from various *Bacteroides* strains. These genes exist within a transposon or on a conjugal element: *ermF* is encoded on Tn*4351, ermFS* is encoded on Tn*4551*, and *ermFU* is encoded on a *B. vulgatus* conjugal element (28–30). Their encoded proteins have sequence identities similar to those of the MLS resistance genes from gram-positive organisms (28–30). Most clindamycin-resistant *Bacteroides* harbor an *erm* gene related to one these genes. However, not all clindamycin-resistant *Bacteroides* contain DNA sequences that crosshybridize with the *ermF* gene (31–33), suggesting that another unrelated MLS resistance gene or another mechanism of resistance also exists.

Clindamycin resistance can be inducible and also constitutive. Conjugal transfer of clindamycin resistance is plasmid-mediated with a frequent cotransfer of tetracycline resistance (34–36). These plasmids are mostly self-transmissible and vary in size from 14.6 kilobases (kb; pBFTM 10) to 41 kb (pIP411 and pBF4; 35) to −82 kb (pBI136) (37). These clindamycin resistance genes are carried on transposons Tn*4400* and Tn*4351* (38,39). Chromosomal resistance to clindamycin has identified and was also linked with resistance to tetracycline; and the clindamycin resistance gene was found to exist within the tetracycline resistance transfer element (39–41).

Because of the rapid increase in the prevalence of clindamycin resistance, especially among the *B. fragilis* group, it is no longer considered to be a first-line agent for anaerobic infections

TABLE 2　Susceptibility of Gram-Negative Anaerobic Bacteria

Anaerobe	Percentage susceptible to[a]						
	Less than 50	50–69	70–84	85–95	More than 95		
Peptostreptococcus spp.	LOM	FLE	CIP	LVX	PEN	CTT	MEM
		TET	OFX	CLI	PIP	FOX	CHL
		ROX	AZM	MIN	AMC	CAZ	CLX
			CLR		SAM	ZOX	SIT
			ERY		TZP	CRO	SPX
					TIM	BIA	TVA
					CFP	IPM	MND
					CPS		
Clostridium difficile[b]	FOX	CLI		CRO	AMP	TZP	CLX
	ZOX	MIN		BIA	PIP	TIM	SIT
	CIP	TET		CHL	TIC	CTT	TVA
	FLE	AZM			AMC	IPM	MND
	LOM	CLR			SAM	MEM	
	SPX	ERY					
		ROX					
Clostridium ramosum	CIP	SPX	FOX	AMP	AMC	ZOX	SIT
	FLE	MIN		PIP	TZP	IPM	MND
	LOM	TET		SAM	TIM	CLX	
	AZM			CHL			
	CLR			TVA			
	ERY			CLI			
	ROX						
Clostridium perfringens		TET	MIN	LOM	AMP	ZOX	SPX
				CLI	PIP	BIA	TVA
					TIC	IPM	MND
					SAM	CHL	AZM
					AMC	CIP	CLR
					TZP	CLX	ERY
					TIM	SIT	ROX
					CTT	FLE	
Other *Clostridium* spp.	CAZ	CFP	LVZ	MOX	AMX	TIC	CLX
	FLE	CTX	OFX		AMP	SAM	SIT
	LOM	FOX	SPX		CAR	AMC	TVA
		ZOX	CLI		PEN	BIA	MND
		CRO	TET		PIP	IPM	MIN
		CIP				CHL	
		AZM					
		CLR					
		ERY					
		ROX					
Non-spore-forming gram-positive rod	FLE	CIP	CFP	CTT	PEN	FTX	CLI
	LOM	OFX	MOX	FOX	PIP	ZOX	CLX
		MND	SPX	CRO	AMC	BIA	SIT
			TET	CPS	SAM	IPM	LVX
				TVA	TZP	MEM	MIN
				AZM	TIM	CHL	
				CLR			
				ERY			
				ROX			

[a] The order of listing of drugs within percent susceptible categories is not significant. According to the national committee for clinical laboratory standards -approved breakpoints (M11-A3), using the intermediate category as susceptible.

[b] Breakpoint is used only as a reference point. *Clostridium difficile* is primarily of interest in relation to antimicrobial induced pseudomembranous colitis. These data must be interpreted in the context of level of drug achieved in the colon and impact of agent on indigenous colonic flora.

Abbreviations: AMC, amoxicilin/clavulanate; AMP, ampicillin; AMX, amoxicillin; AZM, azithromycin; BIA, biapenem; CAZ, ceftazidime; CFP, cefoperazone; CHL, chloramphenicol; CIP, ciprofloxacin; CLI, clindamycin; CLR, clarithromycin; CLX, clinafloxacin; CPS, cefoperazone/-sulbactam; CRO, ceftriaxone; CTT, cefotetan; CTX, cefotaxime; ERY, erythromycin; FLE, flerofloxacin; FOX, cefoxitin; IPM, imipenem; LOM, lomefloxacin; LVX, levofloxacin; MEM, meropenem; MIN, minocycline; MND, metronidazole; MOX, moxalactam, OFX, ofloxacin; PEN, penicillin; PIP, piperacillin; ROX, roxithromycin; SAM, ampicillin/sulbactam; SIT, sitafloxacin; SPX, sparfloxacin; TEM, temafloxacin; TET, tetracycline; TIC, ticarcillin; TIM, ticarcillin/clavulanate; TVA, trovafloxacin; TZP, piperacillin/tazobactam; ZOX, ceftizoxime.

Source: From Ref. 13

due to these organisms (42). Clindamycin can still be considered when treating AGNB with known susceptibilities or other mixed infections that do not harbor or are not likely to harbor these bacteria, such as oral, upper and lower respiratory tract infections (URTIs) and lower.

Beta-Lactam Resistance

Beta-lactams are still useful agents for the treatment of anaerobic infections, even though significant resistance has been noted. The *B. fragilis* group has the highest prevalence of resistance to beta-lactams as almost all (more than 97%) of *B. fragilis* group isolates resist penicillin G. In contrast, the cephamycins (e.g., cefoxitin cefotetan) have better activity, although the prevalence of resistance among *B. fragilis* group has increased. During 1987–2000, resistance to cefoxitin was observed in 8% to 14% of *B. fragilis* group (15,17). However, variations were noted among individual medical centers, with higher resistance at some (15).

Cefotetan is as active as cefoxitin against *B. fragilis*, but is much less effective against other members of the *B. fragilis* group with resistance rates of 30% to 87%, depending on the species. This high prevalence of resistance resulted in recent recommendations against the use of both cephamycins as empirical therapy for intra-abdominal infections (42). However, they, can still be used when susceptible testing shows them to be active. Piperacillin resistance has also increased from less than 10% in 1980 to 25% with significant variability among the *B. fragilis* group (15,24). This agent is not currently recommended for empirical therapy for intra-abdominal infections.

The most active beta-lactam agents against anaerobic bacteria are the carbapenems (imipenem, meropenem, and ertapenem) with resistance of less than 0.2% of *B. fragilis* group isolates (15,20,43), and the combinations of a beta-lactam agent with a BL inhibitor (ampicillin/sulbactam, ticarcillin/clavulanate, and piperacillin/tazobactam) where less than 4% of *B. fragilis* group strains were resistant in 2003 (18). When organisms are resistant to penicillins through the production of BL, the addition of a BL inhibitor usually makes them effective against these isolates. However, strains of non-BL-resistant *Bacteroides distasonis* frequently have higher MICs for all beta-lactam–BL inhibitor combinations.

Resistance to beta-lactam agents among non-Bacteroides anaerobes is variable but is generally lower than the *B. fragilis* group. In one multicenter study 83% of *Prevotella* isolates were resistant to penicillin G, whereas resistance was lower for *Porphyromonas* (21%), *Fusobacterium* (9%), and *Peptostreptococcus* (6%) (20). All isolates were susceptible to cefoxitin, beta-lactam/BL inhibitor combinations, and carbapenems, except for *Peptostreptococcus* isolates (4% were resistant to ampicillin/sulbactam) and *Porphyromonas* (5% were resistant to cefoxitin) (20).

Resistance to beta-lactam antibiotics is mediated by at least one of three resistance mechanisms: inactivating enzymes (BL); reduced-affinity penicillin-binding proteins; or decreased antimicrobial permeability. The production of BLs is the most common mechanism and mediates the most diverse mechanisms of resistance.

Production of Beta Lactamase

BL hydrolyzes the cyclic amide bond of the penicillin or cephalosporin nucleus, causing its inactivation. A variety of BLs which are produced by different organisms and can be exoenzymes, inducible or constitutive; and can be of either chromosomal or plasmid origin (44). There are different classifications of the enzymes. A classification based on amino-acid sequence has created by Ambler (45,46), and a classification based upon substrate of inhibition profiles, molecular weight, and isoelectric points was made by Richmond and Sykes (47,48).

Most *B. fragilis* group produce constitutive BLs that are primarily cephalosporinases (49,50). Pigmented *Prevotella* and *Porphyromonas*, *Prevotella bivia*, *Prevotella disiens*, and *Fusobacterium nucleatum* produce primarily penicillinases (51).

Over 97% of *Bacteroides* isolates in the U.S.A. (45–48) and 76% in Great Britain (49,50) produce BLs. Of other AGNB, 65% produce BLs (51). Most enzymes produced by *Bacteroides* are constitutive and are chromosomally mediated. They include enzymes with serine at the active site as well as metalloenzymes that require an active site with Zn(II).

Other anaerobes capable of producing BL include *Clostridium butyricum* (52,53), *Clostridium clostridioforme* (54), *Clostridium ramosum* (55), and *Prevotella*, *Porphyromonas* (56), and

Fusobacterium spp. (56,57). Although only rare Clostridium strains can produce BLs, *Prevotella*, *Porphyromonas*, and *Fusobacterium* spp. produce these enzymes more often (71, 30, and 41%, respectively) (47,48,52). Enzymes produced by clostridia are usually inducible except the one produced by *C. ramosum* which is a plasmid-mediated TEM-1 enzyme (55).

Acidic isoelectric points are present in most enzymes produced by the anaerobes. Most of the *B. fragilis* group enzymes are group 2e cephalosporinases (58,59) which can be inhibited by BL inhibitors. This makes *Bacteroides* strains susceptible to the combinations of a beta-lactam agent with a BL inhibitor. Cefoxitin-hydrolyzing proteins encoded by *cepA* and *cfxA* that are less common were found in the *B. fragilis* group (60).

Sequencing of several of these enzymes illustrated that they belong to the molecular class A serine cephalosporinases (60–62), that have a smaller molecular size than the inducible group 1 (molecular class C) cephalosporinases from gram-negative bacteria. Only one *Prevotella intermedia* strain produced a group 1 cephalosporinase not inhibited by clavulanic acid (63).

An uncharacterized cefoxitin-hydrolyzing enzymes, which probably belong to the group 2e, was detected in several members of the *B. fragilis* group (64,65). Although high-performance liquid chromatography revealed that the group 2e (class A) CfxA BL from *B. vulgatus* degraded cefoxitin slowly, the hydrolysis was undetected in spectrophotometric assays (62). The slow enzymatic hydrolysis may be coupled with decreased permeability as the organisms were clinically resistant to cefoxitin.

Fusobacteria and clostridia produce BLs that is usually inhibited by clavulanic acid (54,66). BLs produced by fusobacteria and *C. butyricum* are inhibited by clavulanic acid, whereas the BL from *C. clostridioforme* was not inhibited by any BL inhibitors (54). This suggests that these enzymes belonging to molecular class D BLs, which are the group 2d cloxacillin-hydrolyzing enzymes.

B. fragilis group that produce zinc metallo-BLs are the most capable of producing clinical resistance to beta-lactam agents. These enzymes, encoded by the *ccrA* or *cfiA* genes, hydrolyze carbapenems, as well as all beta-lactam agents that are active against anaerobes except the monobactams (64,65). These BLs are not inactivated by current BL inhibitors. Although these enzymes are generally chromosomally mediated, a plasmid mediated metallo-BL has been reported (67). Even though this resistance mechanism was first reported in 1986 in *B. fragilis* (68), it remains relatively rare. As many as 4% of *Bacteroides* spp. harbor the *ccrA* or *cfiA* genes, the proteins are not usually highly expressed to classify the strains as resistant (less than 0.8%) (69). However, high-level expression of this enzyme can occur following in vitro selection with imipenem (70). These resistant strains contain insertion sequences, that are mobile genetic elements with divergent promoters inserted immediately upstream of the *ccrA* or *cfiA* genes, causing an increased expression of the enzymes leading to resistance (71,72). These in-vitro findings were supported by the recovery of an imipenem-resistant clinical isolates that also contained this insertion sequence and gene (70). For patients infected with these resistant strains, treatment with antiinfective other than beta-lactams may be mandated.

The rate of recovery of anaerobic beta-lactamase–producing bacteria (BLPB) in clinical infections and their clinical and therapeutic implications have been extensively investigated and are presented later in this chapter.

Penicillin Binding Proteins

Penicillin binding to the penicillin binding proteins (PBPs) determines the efficacy of beta-lactam antimicrobial. Maintaining PBPs function in the final stage of cell wall synthesis is essential for bacterial growth. Beta-lactams work by binding to the active site of the essential PBP, causing cell death. Three to five PBPs can be found in *Bacteroides* strains: a PBP 1 complex with one to three different enzymes, PBP 2, and PBP 3. These PBPs are most likely similar to the high-molecular-weight PBPs present in aerobic gram-negative bacteria. Other low molecular-weight PBPs may also exist, but their number vary among strains, and may not be essential for bacterial growth (73).

Alteration in PBP are not a major mechanism of resistance in anaerobes as the binding of most beta-lactam agents to PBP 1 complex and PBP 2 is adequate. An exception are the monobactams (i.e., aztreonam) who are not active against *B. fragilis* because they do not have good affinity for their PBPs (74). Decreased affinity of cephalosporins for PBP 3 was demonstrated in *B. fragilis* G-232 recovered in Japan (75). Cefoxitin resistance in some

Bacteroides strains has also been attributed to decreased binding to the PBP 1 complex or the PBP 2 (76,77). This resistance was also inducable in vitro (78).

Permeability

Increased BL production was associated with decreased permeability in gram-negative bacteria. Permeability can vary among strains of *B. fragilis* (68,79,80), and in some *B. fragilis* strains, resistance was associated with both reduced permeability and BL production (80). Cefoxitin resistance correlated with a decrease in outer-membrane permeability and the loss of an outer-membrane protein with a molecular size of 49 to 50 kid (77).

Studies of pore-forming proteins of *Bacteroides, Porphyromonas,* and *Fusobacterium* spp. identified and cloned outer-membrane proteins from these organisms. The absence of at least one outer-membrane protein correlated in some strains with resistance to ampicillin/ sulbactam (81).

Selective pressure similar to that observed for many aerobic species most likely also plays a role in the development and selection of resistance to beta-lactams among anaerobes. Although the prevalence of resistance of anaerobes to beta-lactams has increased, several of these antibiotics are still clinically useful. However, their use should be determined according to the local resistance patterns or the susceptibility of individual isolates.

Metronidazole (5-Nitroimidazoles) Resistance

Metronidazole resistance is common among gram-positive anaerobic bacteria, and includes most isolates of *Propionibacterium acnes* and *Actinomyces* spp., and some lactobacilli and *Peptostreptococcus* spp. strains (43). Resistance of gram-negative anaerobes to metronidazole is rare. Although resistant strains of *B. fragilis* (MICs more than 16 µg/mL) were reported in Europe (82,83), these were not detected in the U.S.A.

Metronidazole, the first 5-nitroimidazole, was used clinically since 1960. Other 5-nitroimidazoles include tinidazole and ornidazole. A metronidazole resistant isolate of *B. fragilis* was first recovered in 1978 from a patient who had received prolonged therapy (84). Even though the rates of metronidazole resistance remain minimal (less than 1%) (10,85–93), and the agent remains very effective as treatment of bacteroides infections, metronidazole resistant *Bacteroides* isolates were subsequently isolated from patients who had not received metronidazole therapy (94–96). It was suggested that in mixed infection metronidazole can be inactivated by another bacteria such as *Enterococcus faecalis* thus protecting *B. fragilis* (97).

The 5-nitroimidazoles have to be reduced to form the active antibacterial agent which is stable only under anaerobic conditions (99,100). The development metronidazole resistance generally occur with the simultaneous decrease in nitroreductase activity and reduction of uptake of the drug (98,99).

Two genes, *nimA* and *nimB,* that can confer moderate to high-level nitroimidazole resistance were identified in strains with high MICs of metronidazole (i.e., more than 4 µg/mL) (101). *nim* genes encode a nitroimidazole reductase, which reduces 4- or 5-nitroimidazole to 4- or 5-aminoimidazole thus preventing the formation of toxic nitroso residues that are required for the agents' activity (102). Six related chromosomal or plasmid-based *nim* genes (*nim A–F*) were found in *Bacteroides* spp. (101). Elements of insertion sequence, that are identical or similar to those present in imipenem-resistant strains, are also located upstream of the *nim* genes, and possibly increasing their expression (103). All metronidazole-resistant *B. fragilis* isolates harbored DNA sequences that hybridized with either an *nimA* or *nimB* DNA probe. In contrast none of the metronidazole-susceptible isolates contained DNA sequences that cross-hybridized with an *nimA* or *nimB* DNA probe (104). The DNA sequence of the *nimA* and *nimB* genes is −73% similar, and may represent two classes of genes generating resistance through the same mechanism (101).

Both the *nimA* and *nimB* genes were present in the chromosome and various plasmids (105,106). The plasmids containing these genes were not self-transmissible, but were mobilized by other conjugal elements or were acquired by transformation (82). The transcriptional information for both genes is provided by an insertion sequence (IS) element integrated 12 to 14 bases upstream from the protein-coding region. For the *nimA* gene, this element is *IS1168*

(106) and a related IS element delivers the transcriptional start information for the *nimB* gene (101). The *IS1168* is almost similar to an IS element, *IS1186*, that provide transcriptional initiation signals for the *Bacteroides* metallo BL gene (101,107).

Because only few anaerobic isolates resist metronidazole, it is still the mainstay for treatment of anaerobic infections. However, the presence of transferable resistance determinants may lead to the development of resistance in the future (108).

Fluoroquinolones Resistance

Fluoroquinolones (FQ) were initially not considered to be active against anaerobic bacteria because they are bacteriostatic under anaerobic conditions (109,110). However, two broad-spectrum FQ are effective against *Bacteroides* spp. and most other anaerobes (temafloxacin and trovafloxacin) were approved by the FDA for treatment of anaerobic infections. However temafloxacin was withdrawan because of toxicity in the early 1990s and trovafloxacin that was approved in 1997 was also severely curtailed because of toxicity. Resistance to trovafloxacin was present in 3% to 8% of *B. fragilis* group in 1994–1996, even before the introduction of the drug, and rose to 13% in 1997, and 15% in 1998, when the drug was launched and reached 25% in 2001 (16,111). This increase in resistance may be due to the result of the use of other FQ. A similar pattern of increase in Bacteroides resistance was also noted with moxifloxacin (111).

Several resistance mechanisms to the FQ are expressed by anaerobes. FQ inhibit the DNA gyrase and topoisomerase IV, both of which are essential for bacterial replication. Resistance in *B. fragilis* emerges by mutations in the gyrase (*gyrA*) and topoisomerase IV (*parC*) genes and by increased expression of efflux pump. Cloning of both *gyrA* and *gyrB* from *B. fragilis*, by stepwise selection with levofloxacin, creates a mutation at residue Ser-82-Phe of GyrA (112). Three mutants with high MICs of levofloxacin had the identical Ser-82-Phe substitutions and cross-resistance to other FQ.

The administration of clinafloxacin induced mutations which selected for in vitro resistance against other FQ (113,114). An efflux pumps mediated resistance to all quinolones was dectected in *B. fragilis* (115,116). These findings illustrate the risk for emergence of resistance among anaerobes to newer FQ by a combination of mutations.

Aminoglycosides Resistance

Anaerobes resist aminoglycosides because they are unable to penetrate these bacteria. Anaerobes do not inactivate aminoglycosides and streptomycin and gentamicin are able to bind and inhibit protein synthesis in both *B. fragilis* and *C. perfringens* ribosomes in vitro (117).

Since anaerobes do not possess the electron transport system needed to allow for aminoglycoside uptake, they are incapable of importing aminoglycosides (116,118).

Chloramphenicol Resistance

No resistance has been noted chloramphenicol which is active against most anaerobes (86,87,91,93). However, clinical failures using this agent have been reported (119). The lack of resistance can be due to its infrequent use.

Bacteroides spp. possess two chloramphenicol resistance genes that generate drug inactivation, by either nitroreduction at the *p*-nitro group on the benzene ring (120) or by acetylation (121,122). The acetylation resistance is transferable and associated with the transfer of a 39.5-kb plasmid, pRYC3373 (121).

Tetracycline Resistance

Bacteroides resistance, to tetracycline is over 80% to 90% (93,123). Because of the high rate of resistance, it is no longer considered as first-line an timicrobial for the empirical treatment of bacteroides infections. Susceptibility testing is needed for the use of tetracycline.

Tetracycline resistance in *Bacteroides* spp. is through changes or protection of the target site. The *tetQ* gene encodes a protein that makes the ribosomal protein synthesis resistant to the inhibitory effects of tetracyclines (33,124,125). The DNA sequences of *Bacteroides tetQ* genes was found to be 40% homologous with TetM and TetO proteins which represent, a new class of ribosomal protection proteins (124,125).

The *tetQ* or *tetQ* related gene are found in most tetracycline-resistant *Bacteroides* isolates (33). Because some tetracycline resistant isolates do not contain *tetQ* DNA sequences other mechanisms (i.e., efflux) or other classes of ribosomal protection proteins may also contribute to resistance (126).

Two tetracycline resistance genes: the *tetA(P)* and *tetB(P)* that create an operon that encodes two unrelated proteins which conveys resistance by two unique mechanisms can be detected in *C. perringens* (127). The *tetA(P)* gene is a tetracycline efflux pump, and the *tetB(P)* is a protein producing ribosomal resistance (127).

Bacteroides spp. may contain two other genes of tetracycline resistance. One is generating oxidation of tetracycline by the product of *tetX* gene that is active only under aerobic conditions (128–130). The second gene encodes produces tetracycline efflux in *Bacteroides* but not in *E. coli* (131,132).

The *tetQ* gene is inducible (124,133) and transferable (34,134), by conjugation through the tetracycline resistance transfer element (133,135,136). The frequency of transfer is usually low but can be increased when the organisms are preexposed to tetracycline (85–87). The transfer is controlled by a prokaryotic two-component regulatory system (133,136). The two regulatory genes, *rteA* and *rteB*, are present in the *tetQ* operon downstream from the *tetQ* gene (136), and are expressed in the presence of tetracycline.

The cytoplasmic membrane protein component of the system RteA, is encoded by the *rteA* gene, and the RteB is encoded by the *rteB* gene (136). RteB assists in the transfer and mobilization of the tetracycline resistance transfer element. The *rteC* gene, produces RteC, can participate in the self-transfer of tetracycline resistance (133).

The regulation of the transfer of unlinked chromosomal elements termed nonreplicating *Bacteroides* units (NBUs) is through RteA and RteB (33,137,138). Even though most NBUs do not harbor an identifiable phenotype, a cefoxitin-hydrolyzing, BL gene [*cfxA* (55)] can be placed on an NBU (139). The transfer of the cefoxitin hydrolyzing BL is facilitated by pretreatment with tetracycline (139,140).

Tetracycline resistance transfer elements are chromosomal placed and are similar to the conjugal transposon *Tn916* in *E. faecalis* (33,141–143).

TRANSFER OF ANTIBIOTIC RESISTANCE

Anaerobes acquire and disseminate mobile DNA transfer factors by conjugation, that can harbor antibiotic resistance genes. Opportunities for the rapid disseminate of antibiotic resistance determinants are in the gut flora, as well as in polymicrobial infections.

Transfer of resistance genes has been found in the *B. fragilis* group and in *Prevotella*, *Clostridium*, and *Fusobacterium* spp. (24). Bacterial conjugation, is the most common method of antibiotic resistance genes transmission in anaerobes. The resistance genes are located in DNA transfer factors that can harbor mobile transposons, plasmids and chromosomal elements (144,145). The transfer from one cell to cell of the DNA requires a connector bridge that is encoded by much larger transferable conjugative transposons (144). Two biochemical processes are required for horizontal transmission of the transmissible DNA (145, 146).

B. fragilis group resisting tetracycline after harbor conjugative transposons. The most thoroughly investigated conjugative transposone, CTnDoT, has a tetracycline resistance determinant and genes involved in the formation of the mating bridge (148).

The conjugative transposons are called Tet elements, because of their ability to harbor a tetracycline resistance gene that confers ribosomal protection (149). They encode the conjugative transfer apparatus that forms the physical conduit through which antibiotic resistance genes are transferred from cell to cell (146,147). Exposure to sub-inhibitory concentration of tetracycline upregulates the expression of transfer apparatus proteins in *Bacteroides* spp. (132), and increases the conjugative transfer frequency of the intracellular Tet elements (150). During conjugation multiple resistance genes can be transfered which can result in the rapid rise in antibiotic resistance among different genera of anaerobic bacteria (151). The conjugative transposon CTnGERM1 that carries an erythromycin resistance gene in gram-positive bacteria, was also found in *Bacteroides* spp. (152). Transposon transfer by conjugation can be demonstrated in vitro, within *Bacteroides* spp. and from *Bacteroides* spp. to *E. coli* and other bacteria.

Human colonic bacteria may acquire resistance determinants from bacteria of animal sources (153). The extensive use of antibiotic in livestock has contributed to the increase in the spread of resistant determinants among their gut flora, many of which may also be acquired by humans.

THE ROLE OF BETA-LACTAMASE-PRODUCING BACTERIA IN MIXED INFECTIONS

Penicillins have been the agents of choice for the therapy of a variety of anaerobic infections at different anatomical locations. However, within the last 50 years, an increased resistance to these drugs has been observed especially in AGNB (*B. fragilis* group, pigmented *Prevotella* and *Porphyromonas*, *P. bivia*, and *P. disiens*) and *Fusobacterium* spp. (2,3,154).

BLPB may have an important clinical role in infections. Not only can these organisms cause the infection, they may also have an indirect effect through their ability to produce the BLs. BLPB may not only survive penicillin therapy but also may protect other penicillin-susceptible bacteria from penicillins by releasing the free enzyme into their environment (155).

Anaerobic BLPB were isolated in a variety of mixed infections. These include respiratory tract, skin, soft tissue, and surgical infections and other infections. The clinical in vitro and in vivo evidence supporting the role of these organisms in the increased failure rate of penicillins in eradication of these infections and the implication of that increased rate on the management of infections is discussed below.

Mixed Infections Involving Anaerobic BLPB

Anaerobic BLPB can be isolated from a variety of infections in adults and children, sometimes as the only isolates and sometimes mixed with other flora (Table 3). Table 4 summarizes our experience in the recovery of these organisms from skin and soft tissue infections (157–166), upper respiratory tract (167–179), lower respiratory tract (180–183), obstetric and gynecologic (184), intra-abdominal (184–186), and miscellaneous infections (187–190).

The rate of isolation of these organisms varies in each infection entity (Table 4) (156). BLPB were present in 288 (44%) of 648 patients with skin and soft tissue infections, 75% harbored aerobic and 36% had anaerobic BLPB. The infections in which BLPB were most frequently recovered were vulvovaginal abscesses (80% of patients), perirectal and buttock abscesses (79%), decubitus ulcers (64%), human bites (61%) and abscesses of the neck (58%). The predominant BLPB were *Staphylococcus aureus* (68% of patients with BLPB) and the *B. fragilis* group (26%).

BLPB were found in 262 (51%) of 514 patients with upper respiratory tract infections 72% URTI had aerobic BLPB and 57% had anaerobic. The infections in which these organisms were most frequently recovered were adenoiditis (83% of patients), tonsillitis in adults (82%) and children (74%), and retropharyngeal abscess (71%). The predominant BLPB were *S. aureus* (49% of patients with BLPB), pigmented *Prevotella* and *Porphyromonas* (28%) and the *B. fragilis* group (20%).

BLPB were isolated in 81 (59%) of 137 patients with *pulmonary infections*; 75% had aerobic BLPB, and 53% had anaerobic BLPB. The largest number of patients with BLPB was found in patients with cystic fibrosis (83% of patients), followed by pneumonia in intubated patients (78%) and lung abscesses (70%). The predominant BLPB was *B. fragilis* group (36% of patients with BLPB), *S. aureus* (35%), pigmented *Prevotella* and *Porphyromonas* spp. (16%), *Pseudomonas aeruginosa* (14%), *Klebsiella pneumoniae* (11%) and *E. coli* (10%).

BLPB were recovered in 104 (92%) of 113 patients with surgical infections; 5% of the patients had aerobic BLPB and 98% had anaerobic BLPB (Table 4). The most predominant BLPB was the *B. fragilis* group (98% of patients with BLPB).

BLPB were recovered in 16 (28%) of 57 patients with miscellaneous infections, which included periapical and intracranial abscesses and anaerobic osteomyelitis; 25% had aerobic

TABLE 3 Infections Involving Beta-Lactamase-Producing Bacteria (BLPB)

Infections	Predominant BLPB
Respiratory tract	
Acute sinusitis and otitis	*Haemophilus influenzae*, *Moraxella catarrhalis*
Chronic sinusitis and otitis	*Staphylococcus aureus*, anaerobic gram-negative bacilli
Tonsillitis	*S. aureus*, anaerobic gram-negative bacilli
Bronchitis, pneumonia	*H. influenzae*, *M. catarrhalis*, *Legionella pneumophila*
Aspiration pneumonia, lung abscesses	*S. aureus*, anaerobic gram-negative bacilli, *Enterobacteriaceae*
Skin and soft tissue	
Abscesses, wounds, and burns in the oral areas, paronychia, bites	*S. aureus*, pigmented *Prevotella* and *Porphyromonas*
Abscesses, wounds, and burns in the rectal area	*Escherichia coli*, *Bacteroides fragilis* group, *Pseudomonas aeruginosa*
Abscesses, wounds, and burns in the trunk and extremities	*S. aureus*, *P. aeruginosa*
Obstetric and gynecologic	
Vaginitis, endometritis, salpingitis, pelvic inflammatory disease	*Neisseria gonorrhoeae*, *E. coli*, *Prevotella* spp.
Intra-abdominal	
Peritonitis, chronic cholangitis, abscesses	*E. coli*, *B. fragilis* group
Miscellaneous	
Periapical and dental abscesses	Pigmented *Prevotella* and *Porphyromonas*
Intracranial abscesses	*S. aureus*, anaerobic gram-negative bacilli
Osteomyelitis	*S. aureus*, anaerobic gram-negative bacilli

Anaerobic gram-negative bacilli = *Bacteroides*, *Prevotella*, and *Porphyromonas*.

BLPB and 80% had anaerobic BLPB. The rate of recovery of BLPB was not significantly different in these infections. The most frequently recovered BLPB were pigmented *Prevotella* and *Porphyromonas* spp. (37% of patients with BLPB), *S. aureus* and *B. fragilis* groups (25% each).

Pelvic inflammatory disease (PID) is a polymicrobial infection (191–193) involving in most cases numerous isolates, including *Neisseria gonorrhoeae*, *Chlamydia trachomatis*, Enterobacteriaceae, and AGNB (*B. fragilis*, *P. bivia*, and *P. disiens*). All of the above organisms (except for *C. trachomatis*) are capable of producing BL. In a summary of 36 studies published from 1973 to 1985, Eschenbach found BLPB in 1483 (22%) of 6637 specimens obtained from obstetric and gynecologic infections (191). The predominant BLPB were Enterobacteriaceae, *S. aureus*, *B. fragilis* group and pigmented *Prevotella* and *Porphyromonas* spp. The increase in the failure rate of penicillin in eradicating these infections is an indirect proof of their importance (192–194).

We have recovered 2052 isolates from 736 patients with obstetrical and gynecological infections (194). Of these isolates, 355 (17%) were BLPB, 211 (59%) were anaerobes, and 144 (41%) were aerobes and facultatives. These BLPB were recovered from 276 (37%) of all 736 patients. The most frequently recovered BLPB were AGNB. Among them *B. fragilis* group accounted for 129 (36%) of all 355 BLPB. Ninety-nine percent of *B. fragilis* group were BLPB. Others were *P. bivia* (49 of 151 isolates, or 32%, were BLPB), *P. disiens* (6 of 17, or 35%), and *Prevotella melaninogenica* (23 of 110, or 21%). *S. aureus* was the second most common BLPB isolated in 21% of patients.

Production of BL by Anaerobic Gram-Negative Bacilli in Clinical Infections

B. fragilis group, the predominant AGNB present in intra-abdominal infections (185) and anaerobic bacteremias (195) produce the enzyme BL. Within the last decade, however, other AGNB previously not recognized as capable of producing BL have acquired this ability. These include the pigmented *Prevotella* and *Porphyromonas* (*P. intermedia*, *P. melaninogenica*, *Porphyromonas asacchanolytica*, and *Porphyromonas gingivalis*), *Prevotella oralis* and *Prevotella oris-buccae*

TABLE 4 Recovery Rate of Anaerobic Beta-Lactamase–Producing Bacteria from Various Sites

Infection	Number of patients with BLPB/total number of patients	Total number of BLPB	Pigmented Prevotella and Porphyromonas spp.	Prevotella oralis	Prevotella oris and buccae	Bacteroides fragilis group	Bacteroides and other anaerobic gram-negative bacilli
Skin/subcutaneous	288/648 (44%) Percentage of patients	332	19/87[a] 7%[b]	2/9 1%	2/3 0.6%	75/75 26%	8/63 3%
Upper respiratory tract	262/514 (51%) Percentage of patients	344	73/191 28%	19/45 7%	2/14 1%	52/52 20%	3/98 1%
Pulmonary	81/137 (59%) Percentage of patients	104	13/59 16%	0/1 0%	1/9 1%	29/29 36%	0/11 0%
Surgical	104/113 (92%) Percentage of patients	113	0/26 0%			102/102 98%	5/23 5%
Other infections	16/57 (28%) Percentage of patients	17	6/24 37%	2/7 12%		4/4 25%	1/10 6%
All patients	744/1469 (51%) Percentage of patients	910	111/387 15%	23/62 3%	5/26 1%	262/262 35%	17/205 2%

[a] Number of strains producing beta-lactamase/total number of strains.
[b] Percentage of the number of patients with the specific BLPB/total number of patients with BLPB.
Abbreviations: BLPB, beta-lactamase–producing bacteria.
Source: From Ref. 156.

(all are the most common AGNB in respiratory tract infections), and *P. disiens* and *P. bivia* (the most prominent AGNB in pelvic and other obstetrical and gynecological infections) (192).

All 262 isolates of *B. fragilis* group that we recovered from our patients produced BL (Table 5). These isolates accounted for 29% of the BLPB and were isolated in 35% of the patients with BLPB. *B. fragilis* was recovered in 98% of patients with BLPB with surgical infections, 36% of those with pulmonary infections, 26% of those with skin and soft tissue infections, and 20% of those with URTI.

One-hundred and eleven of 387 (29%) pigmented *Prevotella* and *Porphyromonas* spp., which accounted for 12% of BLPB, were isolated in 15% of the patients with BLPB. The highest frequency of recovery of BL-producing pigmented *Prevotella* and *Porphyromonas* spp. isolates was found in URTI (38% of all pigmented *Prevotella* and *Porphyromonas* spp. isolates); the isolates were recovered in 28% of patients with URTI, mostly in those with recurrent tonsillitis and chronic otitis media. In pulmonary infections, 22% of the pigmented *Prevotella* and *Porphyromonas* spp. isolates produced BL and they were isolated in 16% of the patients. Although 22% of the isolates of the pigmented *Prevotella* and *Porphyromonas* spp. produced BL in skin and soft tissue infections, these organisms were isolated only in 7% of patients with these infections, mostly in those that were in close proximity or originated from the oral cavity.

Although 37% of isolates of *P. oralis* produced BL, they were isolated in 3% of the patients. Smaller percentages of *P. oris-buccae* and other AGNB were also detected. Their distribution among the infectious processes was similar to the distribution of pigmented *Prevotella* and *Porphyromonas* spp.

Penicillin resistance through production of BL is increasingly seen in Fusobacteria. This is most commonly seen in *F. nucleatum*, but also in other member of the genus such as in *Fusobacterium varium* and *Fusobacterium mortiferum* (196,197). Since *Fusobacterium* spp. predominat in oral infection, it is not surprising that their presence was associated with failure of therapy of respiratory infections (198).

Evidence for Indirect Pathogenicity of Anaerobic BLPB

The production of the enzyme BL is an important mechanism of indirect pathogenicity of aerobic and anaerobic bacteria that is especially apparent in polymicrobial infection. Not only are the organisms that produce the enzyme protected from the activity of penicillins, but other penicillin-susceptible organisms can also be shielded. This protection can occur when the enzyme BL is secreted into the infected tissues or abscess fluid in sufficient quantities to break the penicillin's beta-lactam ring before it can kill the susceptible bacteria (Fig. 1) (199–203).

Clinical and laboratory studies will be described that provide support for this hypothesis.

In Vivo and In Vitro Studies
Animal studies demonstrated the ability of the enzyme BL to influence polymicrobial infections. Hackman and Wilkins (204) showed that penicillin-resistant strains of *B. fragilis*,

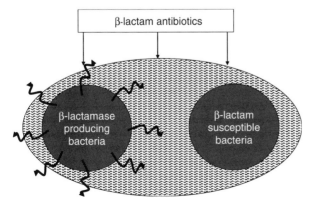

FIGURE 1 Protection of penicillin-susceptible bacteria from penicillin by beta-lactamase–producing bacteria.

pigmented *Prevotella* and *Porphyromonas* spp., and *P. oralis* protected a penicillin-sensitive *Fusobacterium necrophorum* from penicillin therapy in mice. Brook et al. (199–203), using a subcutaneous abscess model in mice, demonstrated protection of group A beta-hemolytic streptococci (GABHS) from penicillin by *B. fragilis* and *P. melaninogenica*. Clindamycin or the combination of penicillin and clavulanic acid (a BL inhibitor), which are active against both GABHS and AGNB, were effective in eradicating mixed infection caused by these organisms. Similarly, BL-producing facultative bacteria protected a penicillin-susceptible *P. melaninogenica* from penicillin (200). O'Keefe et al. (205) demonstrated inactivation of penicillin-G in an experimental *B. fragilis* infection model in the rabbit peritoneum.

In vitro studies have also demonstrated this phenomenon. A 200-fold increase in resistance of GABHS to penicillin was observed when it was inoculated with *S. aureus* (201). An increase in resistance was also noted when GABHS was grown with *Haemophilus parainfluenzae* (202). When mixed with cultures of *B. fragilis*, the resistance of GABHS to penicillin increased 8500-fold (203).

BL in Clinical Infections

Several studies demonstrate the activity of the enzyme BL produced by anaerobic bacteria in polymicrobial infections. De Louvois and Hurley (206) demonstrated degradation of penicillin, ampicillin, and cephaloridine by purulent exudates obtained from 4 of 22 patients with abscesses. Studies by Masuda and Tomioka (207) demonstrated BL activity in empyema fluid. Most infections were polymicrobial and involved both *K. pneumoniae* and *P. aeruginosa*.

The presence of the enzyme BL in clinical specimens was also reported. Bryant et al.(208) detected enzyme activity in 4 of 11 pus specimen obtained from 12 patients with polymicrobial intra-abdominal abscess or polymicrobial empyema.

Brook measured BL activity in 40 (55%) of 109 abscesses (184). One hundred BLPB were recovered in 88 (77%) specimens. These included all 28 isolates of *B. fragilis* group, 18 of 30 pigmented *Prevotella* and *Porphyromonas* spp., 42 of 43 *S. aureus*, and 11 of 14 *E. coli*.

BL activity was detected in 46 of 88 (55%) ear aspirates that contained BLPB (184). Brook et al. found BL activity in ear aspirates of 30 of 38 (79%) children with chronic otitis media (209), in 17 of 19 (89%) ear aspirates of children with acute otitis media who failed amoxicillin (AMX) therapy (210), and in 12 sinus aspirates (three acute and nine chronic infection) of the 14 aspirates that contained BLPB. The predominant BLPBs in acute sinusitis were *H. influenzae*, and *Moraxella catarrhalis*; those in chronic sinusitis were *S. aureus*, *Prevotella* spp., *Fusobacterium* spp., and *B. fragilis* (see Table 5, chapter 14) (211).

A study investigated the monthly changes in the rate of recovery of aerobic and anaerobic penicillin-resistant bacteria in the oropharynx of children (212). Each month over a period of two years, 30 children who presented with URTI were studied. The highest number of aerobic and anaerobic BLPB and number of patients with BLPB was in April (about 60% of patients) and the lowest was in September (11–13%). A gradual increase of BLPB and penicillin-resistant *Streptococcus pneumoniae* occurred from September to April, and a slow decline took place from April to August. These changes correlated directly with the intake of beta-lactam antibiotics. The crowding and the increase use of antibiotics that are more common in the winter might have also contributed to the spread of BLPB. Monitoring the local seasonal variation in the rate of BLPB may be helpful in the empiric choice of antimicrobials. Judicious use of antimicrobials may control the increase of BLPB.

Clinical Studies Illustrating Failure of Penicillins Due to Anaerobic BLPB

The recovery of penicillin-susceptible bacteria mixed with BLPB in patients who have failed to respond to penicillin or cephalosporin therapy suggests the ability of BLPB to protect a penicillin-susceptible or cephalosporin-susceptible organism from the activity of those drugs.

Selection of BLPB following antimicrobial therapy may account for many of the clinical failures after penicillin therapy. Heimdahl et al. (213) described five adults with clinical failures after penicillin therapy associated with the isolation of anaerobic BLPB. In a study of 185 children with orofacial and respiratory infections who failed to respond to penicillin, BLPB were recovered in 75 (40%) (214). The predominant BLPB were *S. aureus*, pigmented *Prevotella* and *Porphyromonas* spp., *B. fragilis* group, and *P. oralis*.

Increased failure rate of penicillins in the therapy of PID has also been noticed and these agents are no longer recommended for this infection. Treatment failure has been noticed in as many as 33% of patients and increased frequency of abscess formation has been observed (215). Therapy with penicillin, either alone or with an aminoglycoside or tetracycline, failed in 15% to 25% of cases (193). This increased failure rate may be due to the increased resistance to penicillin of AGNB and *N. gonorrhoeae* as well as that of the Enterobacteriaceae involved in PID.

The URTI in which the phenomenon of indirect pathogenicity was most thoroughly studied is recurrent tonsillitis due to GABHS (see chapter 16). Penicillin was considered the drug of choice for the therapy of this infection. However, the frequently reported inability of penicillin to eradicate GABHS is of concern. GABHS persists in the pharynx despite treatment with intramuscular penicillin in 21% of the patients after the first course of therapy and in 83% of the remainder of the patients after retreatment (216). Two randomized, single-blind, trials illustrated that either oral penicillin V or intramuscular penicillin failed to eradicate GABHS in pharyngitis in 35% children treated with oral penicillin V and 37% of intramuscular penicillin (217).

Various theories have been offered to explain this penicillin failure. One theory is that repeated penicillin administration results in a shift in the oral microflora with selection of BL-producing strains of *Haemophillus* spp., *S. aureus*, *M. catarrhalis*, and AGNB (201,203,213,218, 219). It is possible that these BLPB can protect the GABHS from penicillin by inactivation of the antibiotic (155).

Clinical evidence supporting the ability of a BLPB to protect a penicillin-susceptible pathogen was reported in numerous studies (201,202,220).

The role of anaerobic BLPB in persistence of GABHS was suggested by Brook et al. (155, 176,177) who studied core tonsillar cultures recovered from children and young adults suffering from recurrent tonsillitis. One or more strains of aerobic and/or anaerobic BLPB were recovered in over three-fourths of the tonsils. The anaerobic BLPB included strains of *B. fragilis* group, pigmented *Prevotella* and *Porphyromonas* spp. and *P. oralis*, and the aerobic bacteria were *S. aureus*, *Haemophilus* spp., and *M. catarrhalis*. This observation was confirmed by Reilly et al. (221), Chagollan et al. (222), and Tuner and Nord (223). Assays of the free enzyme in the tissues demonstrated its presence in 33 of 39 (85%) tonsils that harbored BLPB, while the enzyme was not detected in any of the 11 tonsils without BLPB (224).

Tuner and Nord (225) and Brook and Gober (226) have demonstrated the rapid emergence of aerobic and anaerobic BLPB following penicillin therapy. Tuner and Nord (225) studied the emergence of BLPB in the oropharynx of 10 healthy volunteers treated with penicillin for 10 days. A significant increase in the number of beta-lactamase producing strains of *Bacteroides* spp. *F. nucleatum*, and *S. aureus* was observed. BL activity in saliva increased significantly in parallel to the increase of BLPB.

Brook and Gober isolated BLPB in 3 of 21 (14%) children prior to penicillin therapy, and in 10 of 21 (48%) following one course of penicillin (226). These organisms were also isolated from household contacts of children repeatedly treated with penicillin, suggesting their possible transfer within a family. The organisms were pigmented *Prevotella* and *Porphyromonas* spp., *S. aureus*, *M. catarrhalis*, and *H. influenzae*. In a study of 26 children who received seven days' therapy with penicillin, prior to therapy 11% harbored BLPB in their oropharyngeal flora (227). This increased to 45% at the conclusion of therapy, and the incidence was 27% three months later. These data suggest that it is easy to induce BL production in the upper respiratory tract by penicillin therapy.

Certain groups of children are at greater risk for developing penicillin-resistant flora. The daily administration of AMX chemoprophylaxis selected for colonization with aerobic and anaerobic BLPB in all 20 children studied by Brook and Gober (228).

An association has been noted between the presence of BLPB even prior to therapy of acute GABHS tonsillitis and the outcome of 10-day oral penicillin therapy (229). Of 98 children with acute GABHS tonsillitis, 36 failed to respond to therapy (Table 5). Prior to therapy, 18 isolates of BLPB were detected in 16 (26%) of those cured and following therapy, 30 such

TABLE 5 Beta-Lactamase–Producing Organisms Isolated from Tonsillar Cultures of 98 Children with Group A Streptococci (GABHS) Tonsillitis

	Prior to penicillin therapy		Following 10 days of penicillin therapy	
	Group A (62 patients)	Group B (36 patients)	Group A (62 patients)	Group B (36 patients)
Aerobic and facultative	6	20	11	30
Anaerobic	12	20	19	32
Total	18	40	30	62

Group A = Children who responded to penicillin therapy, and GABHS was eradicated.
Group B = Children who did not respond to penicillin therapy and GABHS persisted in their tonsils.
Abbreviations: GABHS, Group-A beta-hemolytic streptococcus.
Source: From Ref. 229.

organisms were recovered in 19 (31%) of these children. In contrast, prior to therapy, 40 BLPB were recovered from 25 (69%) of the children who failed, and following therapy, 62 such organisms were found in 31 (86%) of the children in that group.

Roos et al. (230) observed high levels of BL in saliva reflecting colonization with numerous BLPB. These investigators also demonstrated that patients with recurrent GABHS tonsillitis had detectable amounts of BL in their saliva compared to patients with tonsillitis that did not recur.

Therapeutic Implications of Indirect Pathogenicity

The presence of BLPB in mixed infection warrants administration of drugs that will be effective in eradication of BLPB as well as the other pathogens. The high failure rate of penicillin therapy associated with the recovery of BLPB in a growing number of cases of mixed aerobic–anaerobic infections highlights the importance of this therapeutic approach (213,214).

One infection in which this therapeutic approach has been successful is recurrent tonsillitis (216,231–244). Antimicrobial agents active against BLPB as well as GABHS were effective in the eradication of this infection. Studies demonstrated the superiority of lincomycin (231–234), clindamycin (235–240), amoxicillin-clavulanate (AMX-C) (244), and penicillin plus rifampin (241,242), over penicillin alone. The superiority of these drugs compared to penicillin is due to their efficacy against GABHS, *S. aureus* as well as AGNB.

Over 83% of the adenoids in children with chronic adeno-tonsillitis are colonized with aerobic and anaerobic BLPB (245) (see chapter 16). The existence of BLPB within the adenoids core may explain the persistence of many pathogens including *S. pneumoniae* where they may be shielded from the activity of penicillins. The effect on the adenoid bacterial flora of 10 day therapy with either AMX, AMX-C (246) or clindamycin (247) prior to adenoidectomy for recurrent OM was recently studied. The total number of isolates and bacteria per gram of tissue were lower in those treated with any of the antibiotics. However, the number of potential pathogens and BLPB was lower in those treated with AMX-C (246) and clindamycin (247) as compared to amoxicillin and controls ($p < 0.001$).

A similar study evaluated the effects of AMX-C and AMX therapy on the nasopharyngeal flora of 50 children with acute otitis media (248). After therapy, 16 (64%) of the 25 patients treated with AMX and 23 (92%) of the 25 patients treated with AMX-C were considered clinically cured. A significant reduction in the number of both aerobic and anaerobic isolates occurred after therapy in those treated with either agent. The number of all isolates recovered after therapy in those treated with AMX-C was significantly lower (60 isolates) than in those treated with AMX (133 isolates, $p < 0.001$). The recovery of known aerobic pathogens (e.g., *S. pneumoniae*, *S. aureus*, GABHS, *Haemophilus* spp., and *M. catarrhalis*) and penicillin-resistant bacteria after therapy was lower in the AMX-C group than in the AMX group ($p < 0.005$).

The superiority of AMX-C and clindamycin over AMX in eradicating penicillin susceptible pathogens such as *S. pneumoniae* and GABHS may be due to their activity against aerobic and anaerobic BLPB. The elimination of both potential pathogenic and non-pathogenic BLPB may be beneficial, as these organisms might "shield" penicillin susceptible pathogens from penicillins. This phenomenon might explain the survival of penicillin susceptible bacteria such as *S. pneumoniae* in children treated with AMX.

Two studies compared the efficacy of clindamycin to penicillin in the therapy of lung abscesses (249,250). Clindamycin was superior to penicillin in treating the infection. The superiority of clindamycin over penicillin was postulated to be due to its ability to eradicate the BL-producing AGNB present in lung abscess.

Antimicrobials effective against anaerobic BLPB (ticarcillin-clavulanate or clindamycin) were superior to an antibiotic without such coverage (ceftriaxone) in the therapy of aspiration or tracheostomy-associated pneumonia in children (93% vs. 46%, $p < .05$) (251).

REFERENCES

1. Hentges DJ. The anaerobic microflora of the human body. Clin Infect Dis 1993; 16(4):S175–80.
2. Finegold SM. Anaerobic infections in humans: an overview. Anaerobe 1995; 1:3–9.
3. Hecht DW. Anaerobes: antibiotic resistance, clinical significance, and the role of susceptibility testing. Anaerobe 2006; 12:115–21.
4. Jousimies-Somer HR, Summanen P, Baron EJ, Citron DM, Wexler HM, Finegold SM. Wadsworth-KTL Anaerobic Bacteriology Manual. 6th ed. Belmont, CA: Star Publishing, 2002.
5. Snydman DR, Cuchural GJ, Jr., McDermott L, Gill M. Correlation of various in vitro testing methods with clinical outcomes in patients with *Bacteroides fragilis* group infections treated with cefoxitin: a retrospective analysis. Antimicrob Agents Chemother 1992; 36:540–4.
6. Finegold SR. National Committee for Clinical Laboratory Standards Working Group on Anaerobic Susceptibility Testing. Susceptibility testing of anaerobic bacteria. J Clin Microbiol 1988; 26:1253–6.
7. Nguyen MH, Yu VL, Morris AJ, et al. Antimicrobial resistance and clinical outcome of *Bacteroides* bacteremia: findings of a multicenter prospective observational trial. Clin Infect Dis 2000; 30:870–6.
8. NCCLS. Methods for Antimicrobial Susceptibility Testing of Anaerobic Bacteria. 6th ed. Villanova, PA: NCCLS, 2004 (Document no. M11-A6).
9. Citron DM, Hecht DW. Susceptibility test methods: anaerobic bacteria. In: Murray PR, Baron EJ, Jorgensen JH, Pfaller MA, Yolken RH, eds. Manual of Clinical Microbiology. 8th ed. Washington, DC: American Society for Microbiology Press, 2003:1141–8.
10. Betriu C, Cabronero C, Gomez M, Picazo JJ. Changes in the susceptibility of *Bacteroides fragilis* group organisms to various antimicrobial agents 1979–1989. Eur J Clin Microbiol Infect Dis 1992; 11:352–6.
11. Watanabe K, Ueno K, Kato N, et al. In vitro susceptibility of clinical isolates of *Bacteroides fragilis* and *Bacteroides thetaiotaomicron* in Japan. Eur J Clin Microbiol Infect Dis 1992; 11:1069–73.
12. Tuner K, Nord CE. Antibiotic susceptibility of anaerobic bacteria in Europe. Clin Infect Dis 1993; 16(Suppl. 4):S387–9.
13. Wexler HM, Finegold SM. Current susceptibility patterns of anaerobic bacteria. Yonsei Med J 1998; 39:495–501.
14. NCCLS. Methods for Antimicrobial Susceptibility Testing of Anaerobic Bacteria. 4th ed. Villanova, PA: NCCLS, 1997 (Document no. M11-A4).
15. Snydman DR, Jacobus NV, McDermott LA, et al. National survey on the susceptibility of *Bacteroides fragilis* group: report and analysis of trends for 1997–2000. Clin Infect Dis 2002; 35:S126–34.
16. Cornick NA, Cuchural GJ, Jr., Snydman DR, et al. The antimicrobial susceptibility patterns of the *Bacteroides fragilis* group in the United States, 1987. J Antimicrob Chemother 1990; 25:1011–9.
17. Snydman DR, Jacobus NV, McDermott LA, et al. Multicenter study of in vitro susceptibility of the *Bacteroides fragilis* group, 1995 to 1996, with comparison of resistance trends from 1990 to 1996. Antimicrob Agents Chemother 1999; 43:2417–22.
18. Jacobus NV, Mc Dernott LA, Golan Y, et al. U.S. survey on the susceptibility of the *B. fragilis* group, report: 2002–2003. In: Abstract of the 7th Biennial Congress of the Anaerobe Society of the Americas. Annapolis, Maryland, July 19–21, 2004 (PII-18).
19. Hecht DW, Osmolski JR, O'Keefe JP. Variation in the susceptibility of *Bacteroides fragilis* group isolates from six Chicago hospitals. Clin Infect Dis 1993; 16(Suppl. 4):S357–60.
20. Aldridge KE, Ashcraft D, Cambre K, Pierson CL, Jenkins SG, Rosenblatt JE. Multicenter survey of the changing in vitro antimicrobial susceptibilities of clinical isolates of *Bacteroides fragilis* group, *Prevotella*, *Fusobacterium*, *Porphyromonas*, and *Peptostreptococcus* species. Antimicrob Agents Chemother 2001; 45:1238–43.
21. Drummond LJ, McCoubrey J, Smith DG, Starr JM, Poxton IR. Changes in sensitivity patterns to selected antibiotics in *Clostridium difficile* in geriatric in-patients over an 18-month period. J Med Microbiol 2003; 52:259–63.
22. Leclercq R, Courvalin P. Bacterial resistance to macrolide, lincosamide, and streptogramin antibiotics by target modification. Antimicrob Agents Chemother 1991; 35:1267–72.

23. Leclercq R, Courvalin P. Intrinsic and unusual resistance to macrolide, lincosamide, and streptogramin antibiotics in bacteria. Antimicrob Agents Chemother 1991; 35:1273–6.

24. Hecht DW, Vedantam G. Anaerobe resistance among anaerobes: what now? Anaerobe 1999; 5:421–9.

25. Jimenez-Diaz A, Reig M, Baquero F, Ballesta JP. Antibiotic sensitivity of ribosomes from wild-type and clindamycin resistant *Bacteroides vulgatus* strains. J Antimicrob Chemother 1992; 30:295–301.

26. Lai CJ, Weisblum B. Altered methylation of ribosomal RNA in an erythromycin-resistant strain of *Staphylococcus aureus*. Proc Natl Acad Sci USA 1971; 68:856–60.

27. Reig M, Fernandez MC, Ballesta JPG, Baquero F. Inducible expression of ribosomal clindamycin resistance in *Bacteroides vulgatus*. Antimicrob Agents Chemother 1992; 36:639–42.

28. Rasmussen JL, Odelson DA, Macrina FL. Complete nucleotide sequence and transcription of *ermF*, a macrolide–lincosamide–streptogramin B resistance determinant from *Bacteroides fragilis*. J Bacteriol 1986; 168:523–33.

29. Smith CJ. Nucleotide sequence analysis of Tn4551: use of *ermFS* operon fusions to detect promoter activity in *Bacteroides fragilis*. J Bacteriol 1987; 169:4589–96.

30. Halula MC, Manning S, Macrina FL. Nucleotide sequence of *ermFU*, a macrolide–lincosamide–streptogramin (MLS) resistance gene encoding an RNA methylase from the conjugal element of *Bacteroides fragilis* V503. Nucleic Acids Res 1991; 19:3453.

31. Marsh PK, Malamy MH, Shimell MJ, Tally FP. Sequence homology of clindamycin resistance determinants in clinical isolates of *Bacteroides* spp. Antimicrob Agents Chemother 1983; 23:726–30.

32. Callihan DR, Young FE, Clark VL. Presence of two unique genes encoding macrolide–lincosamide–streptogramin resistance in members of the *Bacteroides fragilis* group as determined by DNA–DNA homology. J Antimicrob Chemother 1984; 14:329–38.

33. Fletcher HM, Macrina FL. Molecular survey of clindamycin and tetracycline resistance determinants in *Bacteroides* species. Antimicrob Agents Chemother 1991; 35:2415–8.

34. Privitera G, Dublanchet A, Sebald M. Transfer of multiple antibiotic resistance between subspecies of *Bacteroides fragilis*. J Infect Dis 1979; 139:97–101.

35. Welch RA, Jones KR, Macrina FL. Transferable lincosamide–macrolide resistance in *Bacteroides*. Plasmid 1979; 2:261–8

36. Tally FP, Snydman DR, Gorbach SL, Malamy MH. Plasmid-mediated transferable resistance to clindamycin and erythromycin in *Bacteroides fragilis*. J Infect Dis 1979; 139:83-8.

37. Smith CJ, Macrina FL. Large transmissible clindamycin resistance plasmid in *Bacteroides ovatus*. J Bacteriol 1984; 158:739–41.

38. Robillard NJ, Tally FP, Malamy MH. *Tn4400*, a compound transposon isolated from *Bacteroides fragilis*, functions in *Escherichia coli*. J Bacteriol 1985; 164:1248–55.

39. Shoemaker NB, Guthrie EP, Salyers AA, Gardner JF. Evidence that the clindamycin–erythromycin resistance gene of *Bacteroides* plasmid pBF4 is on a transposable element. J Bacteriol 1985; 162:626–32.

40. Shoemaker NB, Barber BD, Salyers AA. Cloning and characterization of a *Bacteroides* conjugal tetracycline-erythromycin resistance element by using a shuttle cosmid vector. J Bacteriol 1989; 171:1294–302.

41. Mays TD, Smith CJ, Welch RA, Delfini C, Macrina FL. Novel antibiotic resistance transfer in *Bacteroides*. Antimicrob Agents Chemother 1982; 21:110–8.

42. Solomkin JS, Mazuski JE, Baron EJ, et al. Guidelines for the selection of anti-infective agents for complicated intra-abdominal infections. Clin Infect Dis 2003; 37:997–1005.

43. Goldstein EJ, Citron DM, Vreni MC, Warren Y, Tyrrell KL. Comparative in vitro activities of ertapenem (MK-0826) against 1001 anaerobes isolated from human intra-abdominal infections. Antimicrob Agents Chemother 2000; 44:2389–94.

44. Bush K. Beta-lactamases of increasing clinical importance. Curr Pharm Des 1999; 5:839–45.

45. Ambler RP. The structure of beta-lactamases. Philos Trans R Soc Lond (Biol) 1980; 289:321–31.

46. Aldridge KE, Henderberg A, Schiro DD, Sanders CV. Susceptibility of *Bacteroides fragilis* group isolates to broad spectrum beta-lactams, clindamycin and metronidazole: rates of resistance, cross-resistance, and importance of, Q-lactamase production. Adv Ther 1988; 5:273–82.

47. Richmond MH, Sykes RB. The beta-lactamases of gram-negative bacteria and their possible physiological role. Adv Microb Physiol 1973; 9:31–88.

48. Jacobs MR, Spangler SK, Appelbaum PC. Beta-lactamase production and susceptibility of U.S. and European anaerobic gram-negative bacilli to beta-lactams and other agents. Eur J Clin Microbiol Infect Dis 1992; 11:1081–93.

49. Mastrantonio P, Cardines R, Spigaglia P. Oligonucleotide probes for detection of cephalosporinases among Bacteroides strains. Antimicrob Agents Chemother 1996; 40:1014–6.

50. Edwards R, Greenwood D. An investigation of beta-lactamases from clinical isolates of *Bacteroides* species. J Med Microbiol 1992; 36:89–95.

51. Appelbaum PC, Spangler SK, Jacobs MR. Beta-lactamase production and susceptibilities to amoxicillin, amoxicillin-clavulanate, ticarcillin, ticarcillin-clavulanate, cefoxitin, imipenem and metronidazole of 320 *non-Bacteroides fragilis Bacteroides* isolates and 129 fusobacteria from 28 U.S. centers. Antimicrob Agents Chemother 1990; 34:1546–50.

52. Nord CE. Mechanisms of beta-lactam resistance in anaerobic bacteria. Rev Infect Dis 1986; 8(Suppl. 5):S543–8.
53. Hart CA, Barr K, Makin T, Brown P, Cooke RWI. Characteristics of a beta-lactamase produced by *Clostridium butyricum*. J Antimicrob Chemother 1982; 10:31–5.
54. Appelbaum PC, Spangler SK, Pankuch GA, et al. Characterization of a beta-lactamase from *Clostridium clostridioforme*. J Antimicrob Chemother 1994; 33:33–40.
55. Matthew M. Plasmid-mediated beta-lactamases of gram-negative bacteria: properties and distribution. J Antimicrob Chemother 1979; 5:349–58.
56. Appelbaum PC, Spangler SK, Jacobs MR. Evaluation of two methods for rapid testing for beta-lactamase production in *Bacteroides* and *Fusobacterium*. Eur J Clin Microbiol Infect Dis 1990; 9:47–50.
57. Tuner K, Lennart L, Nord CE. Purification and properties of a novel beta-lactamase from *Fusobacterium nucleatum*. Antimicrob Agents Chemother 1985; 27:943–7.
58. Appelbaum PC, Philippon A, Jacobs MR, Spangler SK, Gutmann L. Characterization of β-lactamases from non-*Bacteroides fragilis* group *Bacteroides* spp. belonging to seven species and their role in β-lactam resistance. Antimicrob Agents Chemother 1990; 34:2169–76.
59. Giraud-Morin C, Madinier I, Fosse T. Sequence analysis of cfxA2-like β-lactamases in *Prevotella* species. J Antimicrob Chemother 2003; 51:1293–6.
60. Rogers MB, Parker AC, Smith CJ. Cloning and characterization of the endogenous cephalosporinase gene, *cepA*, from *Bacteroides fragilis* reveals a new subgroup of Ambler class A beta-lactamases. Antimicrob Agents Chemother 1993; 37:2391–400.
61. Smith CJ, Bennett TK, Parker AC. Molecular and genetic analysis of the *Bacteroides uniformis* cephalosporinase gene *cblA*, encoding the species-specific beta-lactamase. Antimicrob Agents Chemother 1994; 38:1711–5.
62. Parker AC, Smith CJ. Genetic and biochemical analysis of a novel Ambler class A beta-lactamase responsible for cefoxitin resistance in *Bacteroides* species. Antimicrob Agents Chemother 1993; 37:1028–36.
63. Tajima M, Sawa K, Watanabe K, Ueno K. The beta-lactamase of genus *Bacteroides*. J Antibiot (Tokyo) 1983; 36:423–8.
64. Rasmussen BA, Bush K, Tally FP. Antimicrobial resistance in *Bacteroides*. Clin Infect Dis 1993; 16(Suppl. 4):S390–400.
65. Yang Y, Rasmussen BA, Bush K. Biochemical characterization of the metallo-beta-lactamase CcrA from *Bacteroides fragilis* TAL3636. Antimicrob Agents Chemother 1992; 36:1155–7.
66. Rasmussen BA, Bush K, Tally FP. Antimicrobial resistance in anaerobes. Clin Infect Dis 1997; 24(Suppl. 1):S110–20.
67. Bandoh K, Watanabe K, Muto Y, Tanaka Y, Kato N, Ueno K. Conjugal transfer of imipenem resistance in *Bacteroides fragilis*. J Antibiot (Tokyo) 1992; 45:542–7.
68. Cuchural GJ, Jr., Malamy MH, Tally FP. Beta-lactamase-mediated imipenem resistance in *Bacteroides fragilis*. Antimicrob Agents Chemother 1986; 30:645–8.
69. Podglajen I, Breuil J, Casin I, Collatz E. Genotypic identification of two groups within the species *Bacteroides fragilis* by ribotyping and by analysis of PCR-generated fragment patterns and insertion sequence content. J Bacteriol 1995; 177:5270–5.
70. Podglajen I, Breuil J, Bordon F, Gutmann L, Collatz E. A silent carbapenemase gene in strains of *Bacteroides fragilis* can be expressed after a one-step mutation. FEMS Microbiol Lett 1992; 70:21–9.
71. Podglajen I, Breuil J, Collatz E. Insertion of a novel DNA sequence, 1S1186, upstream of the silent carbapenemase gene *cfiA*, promotes expression of carbapenem resistance in clinical isolates of *Bacteroides fragilis*. Mol Microbiol 1994; 12:105–14.
72. Edwards R, Read PN. Expression of the carbapenemase gene (*cfiA*) in *Bacteroides fragilis*. J Antimicrob Chemother 2000; 46:1009–12.
73. Piddock LJV, Wise R. Properties of the penicillin-binding proteins of four species of the genus *Bacteroides*. Antimicrob Agents Chemother 1986; 29:825–32.
74. Georgopapadakou NH, Smith SA, Sykes RB. Mode of action of azthreonam. Antimicrob Agents Chemother 1982; 21:950–6.
75. Yotsuji A, Mitsuyama J, Hori R, et al. Mechanism of action of cephalosporins and resistance caused by decreased affinity for penicillin-binding proteins in *Bacteroides fragilis*. Antimicrob Agents Chemother 1988; 32:1848–53.
76. Wexler HM, Halebian S. Alterations to the penicillin-binding proteins in the *Bacteroides fragilis* group: a mechanism for non-beta-lactamase mediated cefoxitin resistance. J Antimicrob Chemother 1990; 26:7–20.
77. Piddock LJV, Wise R. Cefoxitin resistance in *Bacteroides* species: evidence indicating two mechanisms causing decreased susceptibility. J Antimicrob Chemother 1987; 19:161–70.
78. Fang H, Edlund C, Nord CE, Hedberg M. Selection of cefoxitin-resistant *Bacteroides thetaiotaomicron* mutants and mechanisms involved in β-lactam resistance. Clin Infect Dis 2002; 35:S47–53.
79. Hurlbut S, Cuchural GJ, Tally FP. Imipenem resistance in *Bacteroides distasonis* mediated by a novel beta-lactamase. Antimicrob Agents Chemother 1990; 34:117–20.

80. Rasmussen BA, Yang Y, Jacobus N, Bush K. Contribution of enzymatic properties, cell permeability, and enzyme expression to microbiological activities of beta-lactams in three *Bacteroides fragilis* isolates that harbor a metallo-beta-lactamase gene. Antimicrob Agents Chemother 1994; 38:2116–20.

81. Wexler HM. Outer-membrane pore-forming proteins in gram-negative anaerobic bacteria. Clin Infect Dis 2002; 35:S65–71.

82. Breuil J, Dublanchet A, Truffaut N, Sebald M. Transferable 5-nitroimidazole resistance in the *Bacteroides fragilis* group. Plasmid 1989; 21:151–4.

83. Urban E, Soki J, Brazier JS, Nagy E, Duerden BI. Prevalence and characterization of *nim* genes of *Bacteroides* sp. isolated in Hungary. Anaerobe 2002; 8:175–9.

84. Ingham HR, Eaton S, Venables CW, Adams PC. *Bacteroides fragilis* resistant to metronidazole after long-term therapy. Lancet 1978; 1:214 (letter).

85. Dubreuil L, Breuil J, Dublanchet A, Sedallian A. Survey of the susceptibility patterns of *Bacteroides fragilis* group strains in France from 1977 to 1992. Eur J Clin Microbiol Infect Dis 1992; 11:1094–9.

86. Chen SCA, Gottlieb T, Palmer JM, Morris G, Gilbert GL. Antimicrobial susceptibility of anaerobic bacteria in Australia. J Antimicrob Chemother 1992; 30:811–20.

87. Bourgault AM, Lamothe F, Hoban DJ, et al. Survey of *Bacteroides fragilis* group susceptibility patterns in Canada. Antimicrob Agents Chemother 1992; 36:343–7.

88. Horn R, Lavallee J, Robson HG. Susceptibilities of members of the *Bacteroides fragilis* group to 11 antimicrobial agents. Antimicrob Agents Chemother 1992; 36:2051–3.

89. Suata K, Watanabe K, Ueno K, Homma M. Antimicrobial susceptibility patterns and resistance transferability among *Bacteroides fragilis* group isolates from patients with appendicitis in Bali, Indonesia. Clin Infect Dis 1993; 16:561–6.

90. Hill GB, Ayers OM, Everett BQ. Susceptibilities of anaerobic gram-negative bacilli to thirteen antimicrobials and beta-lactamase inhibitor combinations. J Antimicrob Chemother 1991; 28:855–67.

91. Cuchural GJ, Jr., Snydman DR, McDermott L, et al. Antimicrobial susceptibility patterns of the *Bacteroides fragilis* group in the United States, 1989. Clin Ther 1992; 14:122–36.

92. Aldridge KE, Gelfand M, Reller LB, et al. A five-year multicenter study of the susceptibility of the *Bacteroides fragilis* group isolates to cephalosporins, cephamycins, penicillins, clindamycin, and metronidazole in the United States. Diagn Microbiol Infect Dis 1994; 18:235–41.

93. Phillips I, King A, Nord CE, Hoffstedt B. European Study Group. Antibiotic sensitivity of the *Bacteroides fragilis* group in Europe. Eur J Clin Microbiol Infect Dis 1992; 11:292–304.

94. Lamothe F, Fijalkowski C, Malouin F, Bourgault A-M, Delorme L. *Bacteroides fragilis* resistant to both metronidazole and imipenem. J Antimicrob Chemother 1986; 18:642–3 (letter).

95. Brogan O, Garnett PA, Brown R. *Bacteroides fragilis* resistant to metronidazole, clindamycin and cefoxitin. J Antimicrob Chemother 1989; 23:660–2 (letter).

96. Rotimi VO, Duerden BI, Ede V, MacKinnon AE. Metronidazole-resistant *Bacteroides* from untreated patient. Lancet 1979; 1:833

97. Nagy E, Foldes J. Inactivation of metronidazole by *Enterococcus faecalis* chromosomal determinant coding for 5-nitroimidazole resistance. FEMS Microbiol Lett 1992; 95:1–6.

98. Edwards DI. Nitroimidazole drugs-action and resistance mechanisms. I. Mechanisms of action. J Antimicrob Chemother 1993; 1:9–20.

99. Edwards DI. Nitroimidazole drugs-action and resistance mechanisms. II. Mechanisms of resistance. J Antimicrob Chemother 1993; 31:201–10.

100. Narikawa S, Suzuki T, Yamamoto M, Nakamura M. Lactate dehydrogenase activity as a cause of metronidazole resistance in *Bacteroides* of a tetracycline resistance determinant related to *tetM*. J Antimicrob Chemother 1991; 27:721–31.

101. Haggoud A, Reysset G, Azeddoug H, Sebald M. Nucleotide sequence analysis of two 5-nitroimidazole resistance determinants from *Bacteroides* strains and of a new insertion sequence upstream of the two genes. Antimicrob Agents Chemother 1994; 38:1047–51.

102. Carlier JP, Sellier N, Rager MN, Reysset G. Metabolism of a 5-nitroimidazole in susceptible and resistant isogenic strains of *Bacteroides fragilis*. Antimicrob Agents Chemother 1997; 41:1495–9.

103. Trinh S, Haggoud A, Reysset G, Sebald M. Plasmids pIP419 and pIP421 from *Bacteroides*: 5-nitroimidazole resistance genes and their upstream insertion sequence elements. Microbiology 1995; 141:927–35.

104. Reysset G, Haggoud A, Sebald M. Genetics of resistance of *Bacteroides* species to 5-nitroimidazole. Clin Infect Dis 1993; 16(Suppl. 4):5401–3.

105. Haggoud A, Reysset G, Sebald M. Cloning of a *Bacteroides fragilis* chromosomal determinant coding for 5-nitroimidazole resistance. FEMS Microbiol Lett 1992; 95:1–6.

106. Reysset G, Haggoud A, Su WJ, Sebald M. Genetic and molecular analysis of pIP417 and pIP419: *Bacteroides* plasmids encoding 5-nitroimidazole resistance. Plasmid 1992; 27:181–90.

107. Podglajen I, Breuil J, Collatz E. Insertion of a novel DNA sequence, *IS1186*, upstream of the silent carbapenemase gene, *cfiA*, promotes expression of carbapenem resistance in clinical isolates of *Bacteroides fragilis*. Mol Microbiol 1994; 12:105–14.

108. Brazier JS, Stubbs SL, Duerden BI. Metronidazole resistance among clinical isolates belonging to the *Bacteroides fragilis* group: time to be concerned? J Antimicrob Chemother 1999; 44:580–1.

109. Lewin CS, Morrissey I, Smith JT. Role of oxygen in the bactericidal action of the 4-quinolones. Rev Infect Dis 1989; 11(Suppl. 5):S913–4.

110. Lewin CS, Morrissey I, Smith JT. The mode of action of quinolones: the paradox in activity of low and high concentrations and activity in the anaerobic environment. Eur J Clin Microbiol Infect Dis 1991; 10:240–8.

111. Golan Y, McDermott LA, Jacobus NV, et al. Emergence of fluoroquinolone resistance among *Bacteroides* species. J Antimicrob Chemother 2003; 52:208–13.

112. Onodera Y, Sato K. Molecular cloning of the *gyrA* and *gyrB* genes of *Bacteroides fragilis* encoding DNA gyrase. Antimicrob Agents Chemother 1999; 43:2423–9.

113. Bachoual R, Dubreuil L, Soussy CJ, Tankovic J. Roles of *gyrA* mutations in resistance of clinical isolates and in vitro mutants of *Bacteroides fragilis* to the new fluoroquinolone trovafloxacin. Antimicrob Agents Chemother 2000; 44:1842–5.

114. Oh H, El Amin N, Davies T, Appelbaum PC, Edlund C. *gyrA* mutations associated with quinolone resistance in *Bacteroides fragilis* group strains. Antimicrob Agents Chemother 2001; 45:1977–81.

115. Oh H, Hedberg M, Edlund C. Efflux-mediated fluoroquinolone resistance in the *Bacteroides fragilis* group. Anaerobe 2002; 8:277–82.

116. Ricci V, Piddock L. Accumulation of garenoxacin by *Bacteroides fragilis* compared with that of five fluoroquinolones. J Antimicrob Chemother 2003; 52:605–9.

117. Bryan LE, Kowand SK, Van Den Elzen HM. Mechanism of aminoglycoside antibiotic resistance in anaerobic bacteria: *Clostridium perfringens* and *Bacteroides fragilis*. Antimicrob Agents Chemother 1979; 15:7–13.

118. Bryan LE, Van Den Elzen HM. Streptomycin accumulation in susceptible and resistant strains of *Escherichia coli* and *Pseudomonas aeruginosa*. Antimicrob Agents Chemother 1976; 9:928–38.

119. Salzer W, Pegram PS, Jr., McCall CE. Clinical evaluation of moxalactam: evidence of decreased efficacy in gram-positive aerobic infections. Antimicrob Agents Chemother 1983; 23:565–70.

120. Onderdonk AB, Kasper DL, Mansheim BJ, Louie TJ, Gorbach SL, Bartlett JG. Experimental animal models for anaerobic infections. Rev Infect Dis 1979; 1:291–301.

121. Britz ML, Wilkinson RG. Chloramphenicol acetyltransferase of *Bacteroides fragilis*. Antimicrob Agents Chemother 1978; 14:105–11.

122. Martinez-Suarez JV, Baquero F, Reig M, Perez-Diaz JC. Transferable plasmid-linked chloramphenicol acetyltransferase conferring highlevel resistance in *Bacteroides uniformis*. Antimicrob Agents Chemother 1985; 28:113–7.

123. Martinez-Suarez JV, Baquero F. Molecular and ecological aspects of antibiotic resistance in the *Bacteroides fragilis* group. Microbiologia Sem 1987; 3:149–62.

124. Nikolich MP, Shoemaker NB, Salyers AA. A *Bacteroides* tetracycline resistance gene represents a new class of ribosome protection tetracycline resistance. Antimicrob Agents Chemother 1992; 36:1005–12.

125. Lepine G, Lacroix J-M, Walker CB, Progulske-Fox A. Sequencing of a *tet*(Q) gene isolated from *Bacteroides fragilis* 1126. Antimicrob Agents Chemother 1993; 37:2037–41.

126. de Barbeyrac B, Dutilh B, Quentin C, Renaudin H, Bebear C. Susceptibility of *Bacteroides ureolyticus* to antimicrobial agents and identification of a tetracycline resistance determinant related to tetM. J Antimicrob Chemother 1991; 27:721–31.

127. Sloan J, McMurry LM, Lyras D, Levy SB, Rood JI. The *Clostridium perfringens* TetP determinant comprises two overlapping genes: *tetA*(P), which mediates active tetracycline efflux, and *tetB*(P), which is related to the ribosomal protection family of tetracycline-resistance determinants. Mol Microbiol 1994; 11:403–15.

128. Speer BS, Bedzyk L, Salyers AA. Evidence that a novel tetracycline resistance gene found on two *Bacteroides* transposons encodes an NADP-requiring oxidoreductase. J Bacteriol 1991; 173:176–83.

129. Speer BS, Salyers AA. Novel aerobic tetracycline resistance gene that chemicallymodifies tetracycline. J Bacteriol 1989; 171:148–53.

130. Speer BS, Salyers AA. Characterization of a novel tetracycline resistance that functions only in aerobically grown *Escherichia coli*. J Bacteriol 1988; 170:1423–9.

131. Park BH, Hendricks M, Malamy MH, Tally FP, Levy SB. Cryptic tetracycline resistance determinant (class F) from *Bacteroides fragilis* mediates resistance in *Escherichia coli* by actively reducing tetracycline accumulation. Antimicrob Agents Chemother 1987; 31:1739–43.

132. Speer BS, Salyers AA. A tetracycline efflux gene on *Bacteroides* transposon Tn4400 does not contribute to tetracycline resistance. J Bacteriol 1990; 172:292–8.

133. Stevens AM, Shoemaker NB, Li L-Y, Salyers AA. Tetracycline regulation of genes on *Bacteroides* conjugative transposons. J Bacteriol 1993; 175:6134–41.

134. Privitera G, Sebald M, Fayolle F. Common regulatory mechanism of expression and conjugative ability of a tetracycline resistance plasmid in *Bacteroides fragilis*. Nature 1979; 278:657–9.

135. Bedzyk LA, Shoemaker NB, Young KE, Salyers AA. Insertion and excision of *Bacteroides* conjugative chromosomal elements. J Bacteriol 1992; 174:166–72.

136. Stevens AM, Sanders JM, Shoemaker NB, Salyers AA. Genes involved in production of plasmidlike forms by a *Bacteroides* conjugal chromosomal element share amino acid homology with two-component regulatory systems. J Bacteriol 1992; 174:2935–42.
137. Privitera G, Fayolle F, Sebald M. Resistance to tetracycline, erythromycin, and clindamycin in the *Bacteroides fragilis* group: inducible versus constitutive tetracycline resistance. Antimicrob Agents Chemother 1981; 20:314–20.
138. Shoemaker NB, Wang G-R, Stevens AM, Salyers AA. Excision, transfer, and integration of NBUI, a mobilizable site-selective insertion element. J Bacteriol 1993; 175:6578–87.
139. Li L-Y, Shoemaker NB, Salyers AA. Characterization of the mobilization region of a *Bacteroides* insertion element (NBU1) that is excised and transferred by *Bacteroides* conjugative transposons. J Bacteriol 1993; 175:6588–98.
140. Smith CJ, Parker AC. Identification of a circular intermediate in the transfer and transposition of Tn4555, a mobilizable transposon from *Bacteroides* spp.. J Bacteriol 1993; 175:2682–91.
141. Rashtchian A, Dubes GR, Booth SJ. Tetracycline-inducible transfer of tetracycline resistance in *Bacteroides fragilis* in the absence of detectable plasmid DNA. J Bacteriol 1982; 150:141–7.
142. Smith CJ, Welch RA, Macrina FL. Two independent conjugal transfer systems operating in *Bacteroides fragilis* V479-1. J Bacteriol 1982; 151:281–7.
143. Franke AE, Clewell DB. Evidence for a chromosome-borne resistance transposon (Tn916) in *Streptococcus faecalis* that is capable of "conjugal" transfer in the absence of a conjugative plasmid. J Bacteriol 1981; 145:494–502.
144. Whittle G, Shoemaker NB, Salyers AA. The role of *Bacteroides* conjugative transposons in the dissemination of antibiotic resistance genes. Cell Mol Life Sci 2002; 59:2044–54.
145. Smith CJ, Tribble GD, Bayley DP. Genetic elements of *Bacteroides* species: a moving story. Plasmid 1998; 40:12–29.
146. Whittle G, Hund BD, Shoemaker NB, Salyers AA. Characterization of the 13-kilobase *ermF* region of the *Bacteroides* conjugative transposon CTnDOT. Appl Environ Microbiol 2001; 67:3488–95.
147. Vedantam G, Hecht DW. Isolation and characterization of BTF-37: chromosomal DNA captured from *Bacteroides fragilis* that confers self-transferability and expresses a pilus-like structure in *Bacteroides* spp. and *Escherichia coli*. J Bacteriol 2002; 184:728–38.
148. Bonheyo GT, Hund BD, Shoemaker NB, Salyers AA. Transfer region of a *Bacteroides* conjugative transposon contains regulatory as well as structural genes. Plasmid 2001; 46:202–9.
149. Salyers AA, Shoemaker NB, Li LY, Stevens AM. Conjugative transposons: an unusual and diverse set of integrated gene transfer elements. Microbiol Rev 1995; 59:579–90.
150. Valentine PJ, Shoemaker NB, Salyers AA. Mobilization of *Bacteroides* plasmids by *Bacteroides* conjugal elements. J Bacteriol 1988; 170:1319–24.
151. Shoemaker NB, Vlamakis H, Hayes K, Salyers AA. Evidence for extensive resistance gene transfer among *Bacteroides* spp. and among *Bacteroides* and other genera in the human colon. Appl Environ Microbiol 2001; 67:561–8.
152. Wang Y, Wang GR, Shelby A, Shoemaker NB, Salyers AA. A newly discovered *Bacteroides* conjugative transposon, CTnGERM1, contains genes also found in gram-positive bacteria. Appl Environ Microbiol 2003; 69:4595–603.
153. Nikolich MP, Hong G, Shoemaker NB, Salyers AA. Evidence for natural horizontal transfer of *tetQ* between bacteria that normally colonize humans and bacteria that normally colonize livestock. Appl Environ Microbiol 1994; 60:3255–60.
154. Brook I, Calhoun L, Yocum P. Beta-lactamase-producing isolates of *Bacteroides* species from children. Antimicrob Agents Chemother 1980; 18:264–6.
155. Brook I. The role of beta-lactamase-producing bacteria in the persistence of streptococcal tonsillar infection. Rev Infect Dis 1984; 6:601–7.
156. Brook I. Recovery of beta-lactamase producing bacteria in pediatric patients. Can J Microbiol 1987; 33:888–95.
157. Brook I. Microbiology of abscesses of head and neck in children. Ann Otol Rhinol Laryngol 1987; 96:429–33.
158. Brook I, Finegold SM. Aerobic and anaerobic bacteriology of cutaneous abscesses in children. Pediatrics 1981; 67:891–5.
159. Brook I, Martin WJ. Aerobic and anaerobic bacteriology of perirectal abscess in children. Pediatrics 1980; 66:282–4.
160. Brook I, Anderson KD, Controni G, Rodriguez WJ. Aerobic and anaerobic bacteriology of pilonidal cyst abscess in children. Am J Dis Child 1980; 134:629–30.
161. Brook I. Aerobic and anaerobic bacteriology of cervical adenitis in children. Clin Pediatr 1980; 19:693–6.
162. Brook I, Randolph J. Aerobic and anaerobic flora of burns in children. J Trauma 1981; 21:313–8.
163. Brook I. Bacteriology of paronychia in children. Am J Surg 1981; 141:703–5.
164. Brook I. Anaerobic and aerobic bacteriology of decubitus ulcers in children. Am Surg 1980; 6:624–6.
165. Brook I. Microbiology of human and animal bites in children. Pediatr Infect Dis 1987; 6:29–32.

166. Brook I. Bacteriology of neonatal omphalitis. J Infect 1982; 5:127–31.
167. Brook I. Aerobic and anaerobic bacterial isolates of acute conjunctivitis in children: a prospective study. Arch Ophthalmol 1980; 98:833–5.
168. Brook I, Finegold SM. Bacteriology of chronic otitis media. JAMA 1979; 241:487–8.
169. Brook I. Microbiology of chronic otitis media with perforation in children. Am J Dis Child 1980; 130:564–6.
170. Brook I. Prevalence of beta-lactamase-producing bacteria in chronic suppurative otitis media. Am J Dis Child 1985; 139:280–4.
171. Brook I, Yocum P, Shah K, Feldman B, Epstein S. The aerobic and anaerobic bacteriology of serous otitis media. Am J Otolaryngol 1983; 4:389–92.
172. Brook I. Aerobic and anaerobic bacteriology of cholesteatoma. Laryngoscope 1981; 91:250–3.
173. Brook I. Aerobic and anaerobic bacteriology of chronic mastoiditis in children. Am J Dis Child 1981; 135:478–9.
174. Brook I. Bacteriological features of chronic sinusitis in children. JAMA 1981; 246:567–9.
175. Brook I. Aerobic and anaerobic bacteriology of adenoids in children: comparison between patients with chronic adenotonsillitis and adenoid hypertrophy. Laryngoscope 1981; 91:377–82.
176. Brook I, Yocum P, Friedman EM. Aerobic and anaerobic flora recovered from tonsils of children with recurrent tonsillitis. Ann Otol Rhinol Laryngol 1981; 90:261–3.
177. Brook I, Yocum P. Bacteriology of chronic tonsillitis in young adults. Arch Otolaryngol 1984; 110:803–5.
178. Brook I. Aerobic and anaerobic bacteriology of peritonsillar abscess in children. Acta Paediatr Scand 1981; 70:831–5.
179. Brook I. Microbiology of retropharyngeal abscesses in children. Am J Dis Child 1987; 141:202–3.
180. Brook I, Finegold SM. Bacteriology of aspiration pneumonia in children. Pediatrics 1980; 65:1115–20.
181. Brook I, Finegold SM. The bacteriology and therapy of lung abscess in children. J Pediatr 1979; 94:10–4.
182. Brook I. Bacterial colonization, trachitis, tracheobronchitis and pneumonia following tracheostomy and long-term intubation in pediatric patients. Chest 1979; 70:420–4.
183. Brook I, Fink R. Transtracheal aspiration in pulmonary infection in children with cystic fibrosis. Eur J Respir Dis 1983; 64:51–7.
184. Brook I. Presence of beta-lactamase-producing bacteria and beta-lactamase activity in abscesses. Am J Clin Pathol 1986; 86:97–101.
185. Brook I. Bacterial studies of peritoneal cavity and postoperative surgical wound drainage following perforated appendix in children. Ann Surg 1980; 192:208–12.
186. Brook I, Altman RP. The significance of anaerobic bacteria in biliary tract infections following hepatic porto-enterostomy for biliary atresia. Surgery 1984; 95:281–3.
187. Brook I, Grimm S, Kielich RB. Bacteriology of acute periapical abscess in children. J Endod 1981; 7:378–80.
188. Brook I. Aerobic and anaerobic bacteriology of intracranial abscesses. Pediatr Neurol 1992; 8:210–4.
189. Brook I. Anaerobic osteomyelitis in children. Pediatr Infect Dis 1986; 5:550–6.
190. Brook I. Recovery of anaerobic bacteria from clinical specimens in 12 years at two military hospitals. J Clin Microbiol 1988; 26:1181–8.
191. Eschenbach DA. A review of the role of beta-lactamase producing bacteria in obstetric-gynecologic infection. Am J Obstet Gynecol 1987; 156:495–503.
192. Martens MG, Faro S, Maccato M, Hammill HA, Riddle G. Prevalence of beta-lactamase enzyme production in bacteria isolated from women with postpartum endometritis. J Reprod Med 1993; 38:795–8.
193. Quentin R, Lansac J. Pelvic inflammatory disease: medical treatment. Eur J Obstet Gynecol Reprod Biol 2000; 92:189–92.
194. Brook I, Frazier EH, Thomas RL. Aerobic and anaerobic microbiologic factors and recovery of beta-lactamase producing bacteria from obstetric and gynecologic infection. Surg Gynecol Obstet 1991; 172:138–44.
195. Brook I. Anaerobic bacterial bacteremia: 12-year experience in two military hospitals. J Infect Dis 1989; 160:1071–5.
196. Brook I. Infections caused by beta-lactamase-producing *Fusobacterium* spp. in children. Pediatr Infect Dis J 1993; 12:532–3.
197. Kononen E, Kanervo A, Salminen K, Jousimies-Somer H. Beta-lactamase production and anti-microbial susceptibility of oral heterogenous *Fusobacterium nucleatum* populations in young children. Antimicrob Agents Chemother 1999; 43:1270–3.
198. Goldstein EJ, Summanen PH, Citron DM, Rosove MH, Finegold SM. Fatal sepsis due to a beta-lactamase-producing strain of *Fusobacterium nucleatum* subspecies polymorphum. Clin Infect Dis 1995; 20:797–800.
199. Brook I, Pazzaglia G, Coolbaugh JC, Walker RI. In vivo protection of group A beta-hemolytic streptococci by beta-lactamase producing *Bacteroides* species. J Antimicrob Chemother 1983; 12:599–606.

200. Brook I, Pazzaglia G, Coolbaugh JC, Walker RI. In vivo protection of penicillin susceptible *Bacteroides melaninogenicus* from penicillin by facultative bacteria which produce beta-lactamase. Can J Microbiol 1984; 30:98–104.

201. Simon HM, Sakai W. Staphylococcal anatagosim to penicillin group therapy of hemolytic strepto-coccal pharyngeal infection: effect of oxacillin. Pediatrics 1963; 31:463–9.

202. Scheifele DW, Fussell SJ. Frequency of ampicillin resistant *Haemophilus parainfluenzae* in children. J Infect Dis 1981; 143:495–8.

203. Brook I, Yocum P. In vitro protection of group A beta-hemolytic streptococci from penicillin and cephalothin by *Bacteroides fragilis*. Chemotherapy 1983; 29:18–23.

204. Hackman AS, Wilkins TD. In vivo protection of *Fusobacterium necrophorum* from penicillin by *Bacteroides fragilis*. Antimicrob Agents Chemother 1975; 7:698–703.

205. O'Keefe JP, Tally FP, Barza M, Gorbach SL. Inactivation of penicillin-G during experimental infection with *Bacteroides fragilis*. J Infect Dis 1978; 137:437–42.

206. De Louvois J, Hurley R. Inactivation of penicillin by purulent exudates. Br Med J 1977; 2:998–1000.

207. Masuda G, Tomioka S. Possible beta-lactamase activities detectable in infective clinical specimens. J Antibiot (Tokyo) 1977; 30:1093–7.

208. Bryant RE, Rashad AL, Mazza JA, Hammond D. Beta-lactamase activity in human plus. J Infect Dis 1980; 142:594–601.

209. Brook I. Quantitative cultures and beta-lactamase activity in chronic suppurative otitis media. Ann Otol Rhinol Laryngol 1989; 98:293–7.

210. Brook I, Yocum P. Bacteriology and beta-lactamase activity in ear aspirates of acute otitis media that failed amoxicillin therapy. Pediatr Infect Dis J 1995; 14:805–8.

211. Brook I, Yocum P, Frazier EH. Bacteriology and beta-lactamase activity in acute and chronic maxillary sinusitis. Arch Otolaryngol Head Neck Surg 1996; 122:418–22.

212. Brook I, Gober AE. Monthly changes in the rate of recovery of penicillin-resistant organisms from children. Pediatr Infect Dis J 1997; 16:255–7.

213. Heimdahl A, Von Konow L, Nord CE. Isolations of beta-lactamase-producing *Bacteroides* strains associated with clinical failures with penicillin treatment of human orofacial infections. Arch Oral Biol 1980; 25:288–92.

214. Brook I. Beta-lactamase-producing bacteria recovered after clinical failures with various penicillin therapy. Arch Otolaryngol 1984; 110:228–31.

215. Ross J. Pelvic inflammatory disease. Br Med J 2001; 322:658–9.

216. Smith TD, Huskins WC, Kim KS, Kaplan EL. Efficacy of beta-lactamase-resistant penicillin and influence of penicillin tolerance in eradicating streptococci from the pharynx after failure of penicillin therapy for group A streptococcal pharyngitis. J Pediatr 1987; 110:777–82.

217. Kaplan EL, Johnson DR. Unexplained reduced microbiological efficacy of intramuscular benzathine penicillin G and of oral penicillin V in eradication of group A streptococci from children with acute pharyngitis. Pediatrics 2001; 108:1180–6.

218. Campos J, Roman F, Perez-Vazquez M, et al. Infections due to *Haemophilus influenzae* serotype E: microbiological, clinical, and epidemiological features. Clin Infect Dis 2003; 37:841–5.

219. Jacobs MR. Worldwide trends in antimicrobial resistance among common respiratory tract pathogens in children. Pediatr Infect Dis J 2003; 22(Suppl. 8):S109–19.

220. Kovatch AL, Wald ER, Michaels RH. Beta-lactamase-producing *Branhamella catarrhalis* causing otitis media in children. J Pediatr 1983; 102:260–3.

221. Reilly S, Timmis P, Beeden AG, Willis AT. Possible role of the anaerobe in tonsillitis. J Clin Pathol 1981; 34:542–7.

222. Chagollan JR, Macias JR, Gil JS. Flora indigena de las amigalas. Invest Med Int 1984; 11:36–43.

223. Tuner K, Nord CE. Beta lactamase-producing microorganisms in recurrent tonsillitis. Scand J Infect Dis Suppl 1983; 39:83–5.

224. Brook I, Yocum P. Quantitative measurement of beta-lactamase levels in tonsils of children with recurrent tonsillitis. Acta Otolaryngol Scand 1984; 98:456–9.

225. Tuner K, Nord CE. Emergence of beta-lactamase producing microorganisms in the tonsils during penicillin treatment. Eur J Clin Microbiol 1986; 5:399–404.

226. Brook I, Gober AE. Emergence of beta-lactamase-producing aerobic and anaerobic bacteria in the oropharynx of children following penicillin chemotherapy. Clin Pediatr 1984; 23:338–41.

227. Brook I. Emergence and persistence of β-lactamase-producing bacteria in the oropharynx following penicillin treatment. Arch Otolaryngol Head Neck Surg 1988; 114:667–70.

228. Brook I, Gober AE. Prophylaxis with amoxicillin or sulfisoxazole for otitis media: effect on the recovery of penicillin-resistant bacteria from children. Clin Infect Dis 1996; 22:143–5.

229. Brook I. Role of beta-lactamase-producing bacteria in penicillin failure to eradicate group A streptococci. Pediatr Infect Dis 1985; 4:491–5.

230. Roos K, Grahn E, Holn SE. Evaluation of beta-lactamase activity and microbial interference in treatment failures of acute streptococcal tonsillitis. Scand J Infect Dis 1986; 18:313–8.

231. Breese BB, Disney FA, Talpey WB. Beta-hemolytic streptococcal illness: comparison of lincomycin, ampicillin and potassium penicillin-G in treatment. Am J Dis Child 1966; 112:21–7.
232. Breese BB, Disney FA, Talpey WB, et al. Beta-hemolytic streptococcal infection: comparison of penicillin and lincomycin in the treatment of recurrent infections or the carrier state. Am J Dis Child 1969; 117:147–52.
233. Randolph MF, DeHaan RM. A comparison of lincomycin and penicillin in the treatment of group A streptococcal infections: speculation on the "L" forms as a mechanism of recurrence. Del Med J 1969; 41:51–62.
234. Howie VM, Plousard JH. Treatment of group A streptococcal pharyngitis in children: comparison of lincomycin and penicillin G given orally and benzathine penicillin G given intramuscularly. Am J Dis Child 1971; 121:477.
235. Randolph MF, Redys JJ, Hibbard EW. Streptococcal pharyngitis III. Streptococcal recurrence rates following therapy with penicillin or with clindamycin (7-chlorlincomycin). Del Med J 1970; 42:87–92.
236. Stillerman M, Isenberg HD, Facklan RR. Streptococcal pharyngitis therapy: comparison of clindamycin palmitate and potassium phenoxymethyl penicillin. Antimicrob Agents Chemother 1973; 4:516–20.
237. Massell BF. Prophylaxis of streptococcal infection and rheumatic fever: a comparison of orally administered clindamycin and penicillin. JAMA 1979; 241:1589–94.
238. Brook I, Leyva F. The treatment of the carrier state of group A beta-hemolytic streptococci with clindamycin. Chemotherapy 1981; 27:360–7.
239. Brook I, Hirokawa R. Treatment of patients with recurrent tonsillitis due to group A beta-hemolytic streptococci: a prospective randomized study comparing penicillin, erythromycin and clindamycin. Clin Pediatr 1985; 24:331–6.
240. Orrling A, Stjernquist-Desatnik A, Schalen C. Clindamycin in recurrent group A streptococcal pharyngotonsillitis—an alternative to tonsillectomy? Acta Otolaryngol 1997; 117:618–22.
241. Chaudhary S, Bilinsky SA, Hennessy JL, et al. Penicillin V and rifampin for the treatment of group A streptococcal pharyngitis: a randomized trial of 10 days penicillin vs. 10 days penicillin with rifampin during the final 4 days of therapy. J Pediatr 1985; 106:481–6.
242. Tanz RR, Shulman ST, Barthel MJ, Willert C, Yogev R. Penicillin plus rifampin eradicate pharayngeal carrier of group A streptococci. J Pediatr 1985; 106:876–80.
243. Tanz RR, Poncher JR, Corydon KE, Kabat K, Yogev R, Shulman ST. Clindamycin treatment of chronic pharyngeal carriage of group A streptococci. J Pediatr 1991; 119:123–8.
244. Brook I. Treatment of patients with acute recurrent tonsillitis due to group A beta-haemolytic streptococci: a prospective randomized study comparing penicillin and amoxycillin/clavulanate potassium. J Antimicrob Chemother 1989; 24:227–33.
245. Brook I, Shah K, Jackson W. Microbiology of healthy and diseased adenoids. Laryngoscope 2000; 110:994–9.
246. Brook I, Shah K. Effect of amoxycillin with or without clavulanate on adenoid bacterial flora. J Antimicrob Chemother 2001; 48:269–73.
247. Brook I, Shah K. Effect of amoxicillin or clindamycin on the adenoids bacterial flora. Otolaryngol Head Neck Surg 2003; 129:5–10.
248. Brook I, Gober AE. Effect of amoxicillin and co-amoxiclav on the aerobic and anaerobic nasopharyngeal flora. J Antimicrob Chemother 2002; 49:689–92.
249. Levison ME, Mangura CT, Lorber B, et al. Clindamycin compared with penicillin for the treatment of anaerobic lung abscess. Ann Intern Med 1983; 98:466–71.
250. Gudiol F, Manresa F, Pallares R, et al. Clindamycin vs. penicillin for anaerobic lung infections. High rate of penicillin failures associated with penicillin-resistant *Bacteroides melaninogenicus*. Arch Intern Med 1990; 150:2525–9.
251. Brook I. Treatment of aspiration or tracheostomy-associated pneumonia in neurologically impaired children: effect of antimicrobials effective against anaerobic bacteria. Int J Pediatr Otorhinolaryngol 1996; 35:171–7.

38 | Treatment of Anaerobic Infections

MANAGEMENT

The recovery from an anaerobic infection depends on prompt and proper management. The principles of managing anaerobic infections include neutralizing toxins produced by anaerobes, preventing their local proliferation by changing the environment, and hampering their spread into healthy tissues.

Toxin neutralization by specific antitoxins may be employed, especially in infections caused by *Clostridium* spp. (tetanus and botulism). Controlling the environment is achieved by debriding of necrotic tissue, draining the pus, improving circulation, alleviating the obstruction, and increasing the tissue oxygenation. Certain types of adjunct therapy such as hyperbaric oxygen (HBO) may also be useful (1). Antimicrobials' primary role is in limiting the local and systemic spread of the organisms. In many patients, antimicrobial therapy is the only form of therapy required, whereas in others it is an important adjunct to a surgical approach.

Hyperbaric Oxygen

HBO is at best adjunctive to prevent or reduce gangrene at an early stage (1). HBO benefits are clearer in clostridial myonecrosis than in other necrotizing infections, because HBO is toxic to *Clostridium perfringens* (2) but only bacteriostatic for other bacteria (3). HBO therapy for clostridial myonecrosis is controversial (1). No controlled studies were done, and the published reports do not provide evidence of beneficial effect (1). The use of HBO should be considered when the involved tissue cannot be completely excised surgically, as may be the case in paraspinal or abdominal wall sites. Topical application of oxygen-releasing compounds may be useful as an adjunct to other procedures.

Contraindication

Using HBO in conjunction with other therapeutic measures is not contraindicated except when it may delay the execution of other essential procedures. The most important limitation of utilizing HBO therapy is the lack of availability of appropriate hyperbaric chambers in most hospitals. Transportation of a seriously ill patient to a facility possessing a hyperbaric unit may be hazardous, and the separation from immediate care for the unstable patient is risky. HBO should be limited to specialized centers where complications can be kept to a minimum. Transportation should not be done prior to extensive surgical debridement.

Standard Therapy

Treatment is most commonly provided in a single-patient chamber in which the oxygen atmosphere is 100%. A less commonly used chamber is the multiplace type, which can accommodate several persons and in which the atmosphere is air, with oxygen administered by mask. Larger chambers, which can be used for major surgery, can be found only at a few large medical centers (4).

Treatment exposures are usually at a pressure between 2.0 and 2.8 atm abs for 60 to 90 minutes. Frequency and total number of treatments vary with the disorder and the response of the patient. The treatment pressure is not greater than 2.8 atm abs because of the danger of acute oxygen toxicity at higher pressure, and the length and frequency of treatments are constrained by the need to avoid chronic oxygen toxicity.

Main Side Effect

The potential toxicity of HBO is also of concern. Acute oxygen toxicity occurs only when oxygen is breathed at high pressure and is characterized by the sudden onset of epileptic-like seizures. Chronic oxygen toxicity, on the other hand, can occur at normal atmospheric pressure if 100% oxygen is breathed long enough. Onset is gradual, with premonitory symptoms of cough on inspiration, tracheal burning, and substernal pain. If oxygen administration is not interrupted, pulmonary atelectasis, edema, and hemorrhage may occur, and the patient may die of asphyxia. Both the acute and chronic forms of toxicity are well recognized and treatment schedules are designed to prevent their occurrence, so these complications are rare.

Surgical Therapy

In many cases, surgical therapy is the most important and sometimes the only form of treatment required, whereas in others surgical therapy is an important adjunct to a medical approach.

Surgery is important in draining abscesses, debriding necrotic tissues, decompressing closed space infections, and relieving obstructions. Drainage of pleuropulmonary abscesses, except empyema, is usually contraindicated because the abscesses may spread to other lung tissues during the procedure. Percutaneous or catheter drainage of intra-abdominal abscess, under ultrasound or computed tomography guideline as a substitute to surgery, has been employed with increased frequency.

Drainage of intracranial abscess is generally mandatory (5). The urgency in performing the surgery depends on whether intracranial pressure has increased. However, in the early stages of the disease where only cerebritis exists and a capsule around the abscess has not yet been formed, antimicrobial therapy may be curative. Antimicrobial therapy only may be indicated in patients with multiple abscesses. This approach has been found to be curative by itself (6) and may be considered in high-risk patients or those with multiple abscesses.

In treatment of such lesions, antibiotics are indicated whenever systemic manifestations of infection are present or when suppuration has either extended or threatened to spread into surrounding tissues. Antibiotics are needed in the majority of cases, however.

Antimicrobial Therapy

Appropriate management of mixed aerobic and anaerobic infections requires the administration of antimicrobials that are effective against both aerobic and anaerobic components of the infection (7) in addition to surgical correction and drainage of pus. When such therapy is not given, the infection may persist, and more serious complications may occur (8,9).

A number of factors should be considered when choosing appropriate antimicrobial agents. They should be effective against all target organism(s), induce little or no resistance, achieve sufficient levels in the infected site, have minimal toxicity, and have maximum stability and longevity.

Antimicrobials often fail to cure the infection. Some of the reasons they do not work are the development of bacterial resistance, achievement of insufficient tissue levels, incompatible drug interaction, and the development of an abscess. The environment of an abscess is detrimental for many antimicrobials. The abscess fibrotic capsule interferes with the penetration of antimicrobial agents, and the low pH and the presence of binding proteins or inactivating enzymes (i.e., beta-lactamases) may impair the activity of many antimicrobials. The low pH and the anaerobic environment within the abscess are especially deleterious toward the aminoglycosides (10). It should be remembered that an acidic environment, high osmolarity, and presence of an anaerobic environment can develop in an infection site without the presence of an abscess (11).

When choosing antimicrobials for the therapy of mixed infections, the physician should consider their aerobic and anaerobic antibacterial spectrum and their availability in oral or parenteral form (Table 1). Some antimicrobials have a limited range of activity. Metronidazole is active against only anaerobes and therefore cannot be administered as a single agent for the therapy of mixed infections. Other antimicrobials, such as cefoxitin and the carbapenem

TABLE 1 Antimicrobial Agents Effective Against Mixed Infection

Antimicrobial agent	Anaerobic bacteria		Aerobic bacteria	
	Beta-lactamase–producing bacteroides	Other anaerobes	Gram-positive cocci	Enterobac-teriacea
Penicillin[a]	0	+ + +	+	0
Chloramphenicol[a]	+ + +	+ + +	+	+
Cephalothin	0	+	+ +	+/–
Cefoxitin	+ +	+ + +	+ +	+ +
Imipenem/meropenem/ ertapenem	+ + +	+ + +	+ + +	+ + +
Clindamycin[a]	+ +	+ + +	+ + +	0
Ticarcillin	+	+ + +	+	+ +
Amoxicillin + clavulanic acid[a]	+ + +	+ + +	+ +	+ +
Piperacillin + tazobactam	+ + +	+ + +	+ +	+ +
Metronidazole[a]	+ + +	+ + +	0	0
Moxifloxacin[a]	+ +	+ +	+ +	+ + +
Tigecycline	+ +	+ + +	+ + +	+ +

Degrees of activity: 0 to + + +.
[a] Available also in oral form.

(i.e., imipenem, meropenem), have a wider spectrum of activity against Enterobacteriaceae and anaerobes.

Selecting antimicrobial agents is simplified when a reliable culture result is available. However, this may be particularly difficult in anaerobic infections because of the problems in obtaining appropriate specimens. For this reason, many patients are treated empirically on the basis of suspected, rather than established, pathogens. Fortunately, the types of anaerobes involved in many anaerobic infections and their antimicrobial susceptibility patterns tend to be predictable (12,13). However, some anaerobic bacteria have become resistant to antimicrobial agents, and many can become resistant while a patient is receiving therapy (14,15).

The susceptibility of the *Bacteroides fragilis* group, the most commonly recovered group of anaerobes, to the commonly used antimicrobial drugs was studied systemically over the past several years by collecting strains each year from several medical centers across the U.S.A. (16) and Canada (17). Similar surveys are also available from other countries (Table 2) (18–20). These surveys have shown no resistant strains to chloramphenicol and metronidazole, and resistance to other agents varies. Resistance differs among the contributing centers and generally increases with the extensive use of some of the antimicrobial agents such as penicillins, cephalosporins, and clindamycin.

The results of a multicenter USA survey using the National Committee for Clinical Laboratory Standards evaluated the in vitro susceptibility of 2673 isolates of *B. fragilis* group species from 1997 to 2000 (16). Declines in the geometric mean minimum inhibitory concentrations (MICs) were seen with imipenem, meropenem, ampicillin–sulbactam, and cephamycins. Increased geometric means were observed with the fluoroquinolones and were usually accompanied by an increase in resistance rates. *Bacteroides distasonis* shows the highest resistance rates among beta-lactam antibiotics, whereas *Bacteroides vulgatus* shows the highest resistance levels among fluoroquinolones. *B. fragilis* shows the lowest resistance rates for all antibiotics. All strains were susceptible to chloramphenicol and metronidazole concentrations less than 8 µg/mL (Table 2). The data underscore the need for species identification and continued surveillance to monitor resistance patterns.

Aside from susceptibility patterns, other factors influencing the choice of antimicrobial therapy include the pharmacologic characteristics of the various drugs, their toxicity, their effect on the normal flora, and bactericidal activity (21). Although identification of the infecting organisms and their antimicrobial susceptibility may be needed for selection of optimal therapy, the clinical setting and Gram stain preparation of the specimen may indicate the types of anaerobes present in the infection as well as the nature of the infectious process.

TABLE 2 Percentage of Antimicrobial Resistance in a National Susceptibility Testing of 589 *Bacteroides fragilis* Group Isolates in 2000 (in parenthesis—number of tested strains)

Antibiotic	Bacteroides fragilis (288)	Bacteroides distasonis (36)	Bacteroides thetaiotaomicron (136)	Bacteroides ovatus (61)	Bacteroides vulgatus (35)	Bacteroides uniformis (11)	Other[a] (22)	Bacteroides fragilis group (589)
Imipenem	0.0	2.8	0.0	0.0	0.0	0.0	0.0	0.2
Meropenem	0.0	2.8	0.0	0.0	0.0	0.0	0.0	0.2
Ertapenem	1.0	2.8	0.7	0.0	0.0	0.0	0.0	0.9
Piperacillin/tazobactam	0.0	0.0	0.0	0.0	0.0	0.0	0.0	0.0
Ampicillin/sulbactam	1.4	5.6	2.2	0.0	2.9	0.0	0.0	1.7
Ticarcillin/clavulanate	0.4	2.8	1.5	0.0	0.0	0.0	0.0	0.7
Cefoxitin	3.5	25.0	18.4	14.8	8.6	0.0	13.6	10.0
Cefotetan	13.2	66.7	75.7	77.0	28.6	27.3	59.1	40.4
Cefmetazole	6.6	55.6	69.1	59.0	14.3	18.2	31.8	31.1
Clindamycin	16.3	38.9	33.1	44.3	37.1	36.4	18.2	26.1
Trovafloxacin	20.1	33.3	23.5	14.8	62.9	54.5	18.2	24.3
Clinafloxacin	7.6	27.8	16.2	14.8	45.7	18.2	27.3	14.8

[a] Includes *Bacteroides caccae, Bacteroides eggerthii, Bacteroides merdae,* and *Bacteroides tercoris.*
Source: From Ref. 16.

Because anaerobic bacteria generally are recovered mixed with aerobic organisms, selection of proper therapy becomes more complicated. In the treatment of mixed infection, the choice of the appropriate antimicrobial agents should provide for adequate coverage of most of the pathogens. Some broad-spectrum antibacterial agents possess such qualities, while for some organisms additional agents should be added to the therapeutic regimen.

Antimicrobial therapy for anaerobic infections usually should be given for prolonged periods because of their tendency to relapse.

EFFECTIVE ANTIMICROBIAL AGENTS

Penicillin G

Penicillin G is the drug of choice when the infecting strains are susceptible to this drug in vitro. This includes the vast majority of strains other than those belonging to the *B. fragilis* group (13). Only about 42% of clinical isolates of the *B. fragilis* group are susceptible to 16 units/mL penicillin G, and 10% require up to 256 units/mL for inhibition of growth (13). Therefore, penicillin G should not be used for the treatment of infections by the *B. fragilis* group. Other strains that may show resistance to penicillins are growing numbers of anaerobic gram-negative bacilli (AGNB), such as the pigmented *Prevotella* and *Porphyromonas* spp. and *Prevotella oralis*, *Prevotella bivia*, *Bacteroides disiens*, strains of clostridia, *Fusobacterium* spp. (*F. varium* and *F. mortiferum*), and microaerophilic streptococci. Some of these strains show MIC of 8 to 32 units/mL to penicillin G. In these instances, administration of very high dosage of penicillin G may eradicate the infection. Most *Clostridium* strains (with the exception of some strains of *Clostridium ramosum*, *Clostridium clostridiiforme*, and *Clostridium innocuum*) and *Peptostreptococcus* spp. remain susceptible to penicillin. Clinical experience with penicillin G in the management of susceptible anaerobic bacterial infections has been good. Ampicillin, amoxicillin, and penicillin generally are equally active, but the semisynthetic penicillins are less active than the parent compound. Methicillin, nafcillin, and the isoxazolyl penicillins (oxacillin, cloxacillin, and dicloxacillin) have unpredictable activity and are frequently inferior to penicillin G against anaerobes (22).

Clavulanic acid, sulbactam, and tazobactam are a beta-lactamase inhibitors that resemble the nucleus of penicillin but differs in several ways. They irreversibly inhibit beta-lactamase enzymes produced by some Enterobacteriaceae, staphylococci, and beta-lactamase–producing *Fusobacterium* spp. and AGNB (22–24). When used in conjunction with beta-lactam antibiotic (ampicillin, amoxicillin, ticarcillin, and piperacillin) they are effective in treating anaeroboic infections caused by beta-lactamase–producing bacteria.

Carbenicillin, Ticarcillin, Piperacillin, and Mezlocillin

The semisynthetic penicillins, the carboxypenicillins (carbenicillin and ticarcillin), and ureido-penicillins (piperacillin, azlocillin, and mezlocillin) are generally administered in large quantities to achieve high serum concentration. These drugs are effective against Enterobacteriaceae and have good activity against most anaerobes in these concentrations. However, they are not absolutely resistant to beta-lactamase produced by AGNB, and up to 30% of the *B. fragilis* group are resistant to these agents (13).

Carbenicillin has good in vitro activity against most strains of the *B. fragilis* group, as well as against other penicillin-sensitive anaerobes (13,21), and is effective in the treatment of clinical infections (25). Ticarcillin is similar in structure to carbenicillin and has also good in vitro activity against many anaerobic organisms (13) and was found to be effective in the treatment of anaerobic infections.

Carbenicillin was effective in the treatment of pulmonary and intra-abdominal anaerobic infections in adults (26,27) and active alone or in combination with an aminoglycoside in treatment of aspiration pneumonia (28) and chronic otitis media (29) in children. Carbenicillin has a particular advantage in these infections because of its synergistic quality with aminoglycosides against *Pseudomonas aeruginosa*, which was also present in these infections.

It was shown to be effective in vitro as well as in the treatment of *B. fragilis* infections (22,27,28,30).

Ticarcillin also has been shown to be active against *B. fragilis* (31), and clinical trials suggest that it is effective in the treatment of anaerobic infections. Ticarcillin is similar in pharmacology and spectrum of activity to carbenicillin, and it is effective at only half of the daily dose of carbenicillin. Because of the high sodium content in both of these drugs, the ability to give ticarcillin disodium at a lower dose is an advantage. Another adverse effect of these drugs is the induction of a thrombocytic malfunction noted especially with carbenicillin.

Because of the need to achieve high serum levels, the daily dosage of these drugs is high.

Cephalosporins

The activity of cephalosporins against the beta-lactamase–producing *Bacteroides* spp. varies. The antimicrobial spectrum of the first-generation cephalosporins against anaerobes is similar to penicillin G, although on a weight basis, they are less active. Most strains of the *B. fragilis* group and many *Prevotella, Porphyromonas*, and *Fusobacterium* spp. are resistant to these agents by virtue of cephalosporinase production (13,21). Cefoxitin, a second-generation cephalosporin, is relatively resistant to this enzyme and is, therefore, the most effective cephalosporin against the *B. fragilis* group. Cefoxitin is active in vitro against at least 95% of the *B. fragilis* strains at a level of 32 µg/mL (12). However, increased resistance has been noted in some centers. Cefoxitin is relatively inactive against most species of *Clostridium*, including *Clostridium difficile*; *Clostridium perfringens* is an exception (13,21).

Clinical experience with cefoxitin in the treatment of anaerobic infections effective demonstrated its efficacy in the eradication of these infections (32). Cefoxitin has often been used for surgical prophylaxis at most body sites that evolve mucous membrane because of its activity also against gram-positive falcultative cocci and enteric gram-negative rods. With the exception of moxalactam, the third-generation cephalosporins are not as active against *B. fragilis* as cefoxitin. However, these agents have improved activity against Enterobacteriaceae. The third-generation cephalosporins do not possess any advantage over cefoxitin in antimicrobial prophylaxis and therapy of surgical infections.

Confusion remains regarding the therapy of *B. fragilis* group by the cephalosporins. The members of the *B. fragilis* group are the most important anaerobic pathogens recovered from intra-abdominal infections. The *B. fragilis* group is composed of several *Bacteroides* spp. that were promoted to a genus level (33). Among the *B. fragilis* group, *B. fragilis* accounts for 40% to 54% of the *Bacteroides* isolates recovered from intra-abdominal as well as other infections (12,34–36). However, another important pathogen that belongs to the *B. fragilis* group is *Bacteroides thetaiotaomicron*, which accounts for 13% to 23% of the isolates. Other members of the *B. fragilis* group account for 33% to 39% (Table 3). The antimicrobial susceptibility of some members of the *B. fragilis* group varies, especially to the second- and third-generation cephalosporins. *B. fragilis* is generally the most susceptible, and *B. thetaiotaomicron* and *B. distasonis* are generally more resistant (8,39,40). Among the cephalosporins, cefoxitin is the most effective against *B. fragilis* group (Table 2) (8,39,40).

Carbapenems: Imipenem, Meropenem, and Ertapenem

Imipenem, a thienamycin, is a beta-lactam antibiotic that is effective against a wide variety of aerobic and anaerobic gram-positive and gram-negative organisms including normally multiresistant species such as *P. aeruginosa, Serratia* spp., *Enterobacter* spp., *Acinetobacter* spp., and enterococcus (41,42). It also possesses excellent activity against beta-lactamase–producing *Bacteroides*. It has the lowest MIC for *B. fragilis* group and is also most effective against Enterobacteriaceae. About 10–25% of *Pseudomonas* spp. have shown resistance. The pharmacokinetics of imipenem are characterized by poor absorption from the gastrointestinal tract, high plasma concentration after intravenous administration, a small degree of systemic metabolism, and renal excretion. In the kidney, imipenem is metabolized by breakage of the beta-lactamase bond in the proximal tubular cells. The result is low urinary excretion of active imipenem, which may

TABLE 3 Incidence of *Bacteroides fragilis* Group in Intra-abdominal Infection in Adults (185 isolates) and Children (100 isolates)

	Incidence (%)	
	Adults	**Children**
Bacteroides fragilis	40	54
Bacteroides thetaiotaomicron	23	13
Bacteroides distasonis		
Bacteroides vulgatus	37	33
Bacteroides ovatus		
Bacteroides uniformis		

Source: From Refs. 2, 24, 37, 38.

impair its ability to inhibit certain urinary pathogens. To overcome the problem of renal metabolism of imipenem, it is combined at a 1:1 ratio with an inhibitor of the renal dipeptidase, cilastatin. This increases the urinary excretion of the active drug and its half-life in the serum. This agent is an effective single agent for the therapy of mixed aerobic–anaerobic infections.

Meropenem is a carbapenem antibiotic that has a very broad-spectrum of activity against aerobic and anaerobic bacteria, similar to that of imipenem. Imipenem has more activity than meropenem against staphylococci and enterococci, but meropenem provides better coverage of gram-negative bacteria such as *Pseudomonas, Enterobacter, Klebsiella, Providencia, Morganella, Aeromonas, Alcaligenes, Moraxella, Kingella, Actinobacillus, Pasteurella,* and *Haemophilus* spp. (43,44). Meropenem has been effective in abdominal infections, meningitis in children and adults, community-acquired and nosocomial pneumonia, and neutropenic fever (45).

Ertapenem is a new 1-beta-methyl carbapenem, stable to dehydropeptidase. It has a broad antibacterial spectrum for penicillin-susceptible *Streptococcus pneumoniae, Streptococcus pyogenes,* methicillin-sensitive *Staphylococcus aureus, Haemophilis influenzae, Moraxella catarrhalis, Escherichia coli, Citrobacter* spp., *Klebsiella* spp., *Serratia* spp., *Proteus* spp., *C. perfringens, Fusobacterium* spp., *Peptostreptococcus* spp., and AGNB (46).

In comparison to other available carbapenems, ertapenem has a long half-life of 4.5 hours and is given in a single daily dose. It is less effective than other carbapenems for *P. aeruginosa, Enterococcus* spp., and *Acinetobacter* spp.

Chloramphenicol

Although it is a bacteriostatic agent, chloramphenicol is one of the antimicrobial agents most active against all anaerobic bacteria (13,21,47). Resistance to this drug is rare, although it has been reported in some *Bacteroides* spp. (47). Although several failures to eradicate anaerobic infections, including bacteremia, with chloramphenicol have been reported (48), this drug has been used for over 50 years for treatment of anaerobic infections. Chloramphenicol is regarded as the drug of choice for treatment of serious anaerobic infections when the nature and susceptibility of the infecting organisms are unknown and in infections of the *central nervous system* (CNS). However, the drug's toxicity must be remembered. The risk of fatal aplastic anemia is estimated to be approximately 1 per 25,000 to 40,000 patients treated. This serious complication is unrelated to the reversible, dosage-dependent leukopenic side effect. Other side effects are the production of the potentially fatal "gray baby syndrome" when given to neonates, hemolytic anemia in patients with G6PD deficiency, and optic neuritis in individuals who take the drug for a prolonged time.

Serum level measurements are often advocated for infants, young children, and occasionally for adults, owing to wide variations noted (49). The usual objective is therapeutic levels of 10 to 25 µg/mL. Levels exceeding 25 µg/mL are commonly considered potentially toxic in terms of reversible bone marrow suppression, and levels of 40 to 200 µg/mL have been associated with the gray syndrome in neonates or encephalitis in adults (49).

Chloramphenicol is widely distributed in body fluids and tissue, with a mean volume distribution of 1.4 L/kg (49). The drug has unique property of lipid solubility to permit penetration across lipid barriers. A consistent observation is the high concentrations achieved in the CNS, even in the absence of inflammation. Levels in the cerebrospinal fluid, with or without meningitis, usually are one-third to three-fourths the serum concentrations. Levels in brain tissue may be substantially higher than serum levels (50). The drug also shows unique properties for penetration across the blood–ocular barrier. Joint fluid levels are generally low in the absence of inflammation, but are relatively high—50% or more of serum concentration—in the presence of septic arthritis (51). It readily crosses the placenta to provide cord blood levels. Studies in experimental animals with subcutaneous abscesses show peak levels within abscesses that approximate 15% to 20% of the peak serum concentration (52). This is comparable to the levels achieved with multiple other antimicrobials, including virtually all beta-lactam compounds, and it is substantially lower compared with abscess levels achieved with clindamycin.

Macrolides: Erythromycin, Azithromycin, Clarithromycin, and Spiramycin

The macrolides, which possess low human or animal toxicity, have moderate to good in vitro activity against anaerobic bacteria other than *B. fragilis* and fusobacteria (13,53). Macrolides are active against pigmented *Prevotella* and *Porphyromonas* and microaerophilic streptococci, gram-positive non-spore–forming anaerobic bacilli, and certain clostridia. They are less effective against *Fusobacterium* and *Peptostreptococcus* spp. (53). They show relatively good activity against *C. perfringens* and poor or inconsistent activity against AGNB.

Clarithromycin is the most active of the macrolides against gram-positive oral cavity anaerobes, including *Actinomyces* spp., *Propionibacterium* spp., *Lactobacillus* spp., and *Bifidobacterium dentium*. Clarithromycin showed similar activity to erythromycin against most AGNB (54). Azithromycin is slightly less active than erythromycin against these species (54). Azithromycin is, in general, the most active macrolide against AGNB: *Fusobacterium* spp., *Bacteroides* spp., *Wolinella* spp., and *Actinobacillus actinomycetemcomitans*, including those isolates which were insusceptible to erythromycin.

Emergence of erythromycin-resistant organisms during therapy has been documented (55). Erythromycin is effective in the treatment of mild to moderately severe anaerobic soft-tissue and pleuropulmonary infections when combined with adequate debridement or drainage of infected tissue. Phlebitis is reported to develop in one-third of the patients receiving intravenous erythromycin, but the oral preparation is well tolerated.

Lincomycin and Clindamycin

The in vitro susceptibility of various anaerobic bacteria to lincomycin was initially demonstrated in 1965 (56). Subsequently, the 7-chloro-7-deoxylincomycin analog, clindamycin, was found to be even more active against anaerobes than the parent compound (13). Lincomycin is highly active against a variety of anaerobic bacteria; however, clostridia, *B. fragilis*, and *F. varium* are relatively resistant to lincomycin (13).

Clindamycin has a broad range of activity against anaerobic organisms and has proven its efficacy in clinical trials. Approximately 96% of anaerobic bacteria isolated in clinical practice were susceptible to easily achievable levels of clindamycin (13,21). *B. fragilis* is generally sensitive to levels below 3 µg/mL. There are, however, increasing reports and surveys of an increase in resistant strains associated with clinical infections. Among the other resistant anaerobes are various species of clostridia. Approximately 20% of *C. ramosum* are resistant to clindamycin, as are a smaller number of *C. perfringens*. Many strains of *F. varium* are resistant, but this organism is uncommon in clinical infections. Recently, a few strains of peptostreptococci were found to be resistant (57).

Clindamycin is rapidly removed from serum to body tissues and fluids and it penetrates well into saliva, sputum, respiratory tissue, pleural fluid, soft tissues, prostate, semen, bones, and joints (62), as well as into fetal blood and tissues. No data exist to show that significant concentrations are achievable in the human brain, cerebrospinal fluid, or eye.

Several reports (58–63) described the successful use of this drug in the treatment of anaerobic infection. Clindamycin does not cross efficiently the blood–brain barrier and should not be administered in CNS infections (61,62). Because of the effectiveness of its activity against anaerobes, it is frequently used in combination with aminoglycosides for the treatment of mixed aerobic–anaerobic infection of the abdominal cavity and obstetric infection (63). The side effect of most concern with clindamycin is colitis (64). It should be noted that colitis has been associated with a number of other antimicrobial agents, and has been described in seriously ill patients in the absence of previous antimicrobial therapy. Colitis following clindamycin therapy was associated with recovery of *C. difficile* strains in adults and children (65). The occurrence of colitis in pediatric patients is very rare, however (66). Clinical studies using clindamycin in a pediatric population showed it to be effective in the treatment of intra-abdominal infections (67), aspiration pneumonia (68), chronic otitis media (69), and chronic sinutis (70). Clindamycin has also an important role in treating dental infections (71).

Metronidazole

Metronidazole possess excellent in vitro activity against most obligate anaerobic bacteria, such as *B. fragilis* group, other species of *Bacteroides*, fusobacteria, and clostridia (13,47,72). Occasional strains of anaerobic gram-positive cocci and nonsporulating bacilli are highly resistant. Microaerophilic streptococci, *Propionibacterium acnes*, and *Actinomyces* spp. are almost uniformly resistant (13,72). Aerobic and facultative anaerobes, such as coliforms, are usually highly resistant. Over 90% of obligate anaerobes are susceptible to less than 2 µg/mL metronidazole (72). Metronidazole is active against anaerobic protozoa, including *Trichomonas vaginalis*, *Entamoeba histolytica*, and *Giardia lamblia* (47).

For anaerobic bacterial infections, the most frequently employed oral doses for older children and adults are 250 to 750 mg two or three times daily (47,73). Peak serum levels following a single dose of 250 or 500 mg are approximately 6 µg/mL or 12 µg/mL, respectively. Multiple 500-mg oral doses given four times daily result in peak serum levels of 20 to 30 µg/mL. The recommended dose of the intravenous preparation for serious anaerobic infections is 15 mg/kg infused over one hour (approximately 1 g for a 70-kg adult) with maintenance dosage of 7.5 mg/kg every six hours (approximately 500 mg for a 70-kg adult). The peak blood levels achieved with intravenous administration approximate those noted with oral administration, indicating that the oral formulation is nearly completely absorbed (46,73). Thus, parenteral administration appears to offer no additional benefit for patients who can receive oral treatment; furthermore, the intravenous form is substantially more expensive. The serum half-life is approximately eight hours. The drug diffuses well into nearly all tissues, including the CNS, abscesses, bile, bone, pelvic tissue, breast milk, and placenta. Metronidazole is extensively metabolized in the liver by oxidation, hydroxylation, or conjugation of side chains on the imidazole ring. The major metabolic products are the acid or alcohol metabolites that have antibacterial and mutagenic potential (47,73). The kidney is the major excretory route for the parent compound and its metabolites in the presence of normal renal function. The clearance of metronidazole is not altered in renal failure, but accumulation of metabolites may be noted with repeated doses. The usual dose is recommended in anuric patients. Reduced dosage is recommended in patients with severe hepatic disease, but precise recommendations are not available.

Adverse reactions to metronidazole therapy are rare and include CNS toxicity symptoms of peripheral neuropathy, ataxia, vertigo, headaches, and convulsions. Gastrointestinal side effects include nausea, vomiting, metallic taste, anorexia, and diarrhea. Other adverse reactions include neutropenia, which is reversible with discontinuation of the drug, phlebitis at intravenous infusion sites, and drug fever. The tolerance of metronidazole in patients is generally very good.

Some studies in mice (74) have shown possible mitogenic activity associated with administration of large doses of this drug. It should be noted that in these animal toxicity studies, the drug has generally been administered for the lifetime of the animal, a situation that may not be relevant for humans. Other studies (75) have shown that administration of metronidazole to rats and hamsters does not induce any pathology. Furthermore, evidence of mutagenicity was never found in humans despite metronidazole use for over four decades for other diseases (76). Despite this perplexing issue, the Food and Drug Administration (FDA) approved the use of metronidazole for the treatment of serious anaerobic infections in adults. Clinical experiences in adults (77) indicate it to be a promising agent in the treatment of infections caused by anaerobes, especially CNS infections (78,79).

There is limited experience at present in the use of metronidazole in pediatric patients, and only a few cases are reported in the literature (78–81). Brook (82) studied the tolerance and efficacy of metronidazole in 15 pediatric patients who had anaerobic infection. Five patients had soft-tissue abscess, four had aspiration pneumonia, three had chronic sinusitis, and three had intracranial abscess. No local or systemic adverse reactions were noted. A good response to therapy with a complete cure occurred in 14 of the 15 children.

Metronidazole has not been approved by the FDA for use in children. There are, however, several anaerobic infections in children for which the use of metronidazole seems advantageous. This is especially true in CNS infections because of the excellent penetration of the drug into the CNS (81). Other serious infections for which this drug would be advantageous are anaerobic endocarditis or infections in a compromised host, where the bactericidal activity of the drug is important.

Tetracyclines

Tetracycline, once the drug of choice for anaerobic infections, is presently of limited usefulness because of the development of resistance to it by all types of anaerobes. Only about 45% of all *B. fragilis* strains are presently susceptible to this drug (13,21). The newer tetracycline analogs, doxycycline and minocycline, are more active than the parent compound. There is still significant resistance to these drugs, however, so that they are useful only when susceptibility tests can be done or in less severe infections in which a therapeutic trial is feasible. The use of tetracycline is not recommended before eight years of age because of the adverse effect on teeth.

Tigecycline

Tigecycline is the first antibiotic approved in a new class called glycylcyclines. Glycylcyclines are tetracycline antibiotics containing a glycylamido moiety attached to the 9-position of a tetracycline ring; tigecycline is a direct analog of minocycline with a 9-glycylamide moiety. It has activity against both gram-negative and gram-positive bacteria, anaerobes, and certain drug-resistant pathogens (83). These include methicillin-resistant *Staphylococcus aureus*, penicillin-resistant *S. pneumoniae*, vancomycin-resistant enterococci, *Acinetobacter baumannii*, beta-lactamase–producing strains of *H. influenzae* and *M. catarrhalis*, and extended-spectrum beta-lactamase–producing strains of *E. coli* and *Klebsiella pneumoniae*. In contrast, MICs for *Pseudomonas* and *Proteus* spp. are markedly elevated. It is active against *Streptococcus anginosus* group (includes *Streptococcus anginosus*, *Streptococcus intermedius*, and *Streptococcus constellatus*), *B. fragilis*, *B. thetaiotaomicron*, *Bacteroides uniformis*, *B. vulgatus*, *C. perfringens*, and *Peptostreptococcus micros* (84).

It is indicated for the empiric monotherapy of a variety of complicated intra-abdominal and complicated skin and skin structure infections. The most frequent side effect associated with its administration to date has been nausea and/or vomiting.

Quinolones

The first generation of fluoroquinolones such as ciprofloxacin and ofloxacin are inactive against most anaerobic bacteria. However, some broad-spectrum quinolones, which have recently become clinically available or are under active development, have significant antianaerobic activity (85). Quinolones with low activity against anaerobes include ciprofloxacin, ofloxacin, levofloxacin, fleroxacin, pefloxacin, enoxacin, and lomefloxacin. Compounds with intermediate antianaerobic activity include sparfloxacin and grepafloxacin. Trovafloxacin, gatifloxacin, and moxifloxacin yield low MICs against most groups of anaerobes. Moxifloxacin was recently approved by the FDA for the treatment of complicated intra-abdominal infections in adults. Quinolones with the greatest in vitro activity against anaerobes include clinafloxacin and sitafloxacin (86). However, the use of the quinolones is restricted in growing children because of their possible adverse effects on the cartilage.

Other Agents

Bacitracin is active against pigmented *Prevotella* and *Porphyromonas* spp. but is inactive against *B. fragilis* and *Fusobacterium nucleatum* (13,21).

Vancomycin and teicoplanin are effective against all gram-positive anaerobes but is inactive against gram-negative ones. Quinupristin/dalfopristin shows antibacterial activity against gram positive anaerobic organisms, including *C. perfringens*, *Clostridium* spp., Propionibacterium spp., *Lactobacillus* spp., and *Peptostreptococcus* spp. (87). Linezolid is active against *F. nucleatum*, other fusobacteria, *Porphyromonas* spp., *Prevotella* spp., and *Peptostreptococcus* spp. (53). Little clinical experience has been, however, gained in the treatment of anaerobic bacteria using these agents.

CHOICE OF ANTIMICROBIAL AGENTS

The suggested choice of the different antimicrobials according to the bacteria or infection site and the susceptibility of the predominant anaerobes at the suggested dose are summarized in Tables 4–7. Prophylactic therapy before surgery is generally administered when the area of surgery is expected to be contaminated by the normal mucous membrane at the operated site. Cefazolin, a first-generation cephalosporin, that has poor activity against anaerobes is generally effective in surgical prophylaxis in sites distant from the oral or rectal areas. Cefoxitin is the drug of choice in surgical prophylaxis in procedures that involve the mucous surfaces (oral, rectal, or vulvovaginal) because of its efficacy against the aerobic and anaerobic flora that reside on most mucous surfaces. The parenteral antimicrobials that can be used in most infectious sites are clindamycin, metronidazole, chloramphenicol, cefoxitin, a penicillin (i.e., ticarcillin, ampicillin) and a beta-lactamase inhibitor (i.e., clavulanic acid sulbactam), and a carbapenem (e.g., imipenem, meropenem, ertapenem). Aminoglycosides are generally added to clindamycin, metronidazole, and, occasionally, cefoxitin when treating intra-abdominal infections to provide coverage for enteric bacteria. Failure of therapy in intra-abdominal infections has been noticed more often with chloramphenicol (47), and therefore, this drug is not recommended for these infections. Penicillin is added to metronidazole in the therapy of intracranial and dental infections to cover for microaerophilic streptococci, *Actinomyces* spp., and *Arachnia* spp. A macrolide (i.e., erythromycin) is added to metronidazole in upper respiratory infections to treat *S. aureus* and aerobic streptococci. Penicillin is added to clindamycin to supplement its coverage against *Peptostreptococcus* spp. and other gram-positive anaerobic organisms.

Doxycycline is added to most regimens in the treatment of pelvic infections to provide therapy for chlamydia and mycoplasma. Penicillin is still the drug of choice for bacteremia caused by non-beta-lactamase–producing bacteria. However, other agents should be used for the therapy of bacteremia caused by beta-lactamase–producing bacteria.

Because the duration of therapy for strict anaerobic infections, which are often chronic, is generally longer than for infections due to aerobic and facultative anaerobes, oral therapy is often substituted for parenteral therapy. The agents available for oral therapy are limited and include clindamycin, amoxicillin plus clavulanic acid, chloramphenicol, and metronidazole.

Clinical judgment, personal experience with the antimicrobial agents, safety and patient compliance should direct the physician in the choice of the appropriate antimicrobial agents. The recommended antimicrobials for specific infections are discussed in each of the book's chapters.

Single-Agent vs. Combined Antimicrobial Therapy

The principles of using antimicrobial coverage effective against both aerobic and anaerobic offenders involved in polymicrobial infections have become the cornerstone of practice (8,9,88) and have been confirmed by numerous studies especially in intra-abdominal infections (89,90). The success rate in curing mixed infections varies between studies but the difference between various therapeutic regimens was not statistically significant as long as the therapies adequately covered both Enterobacteriaceae and the *B. fragilis* group. A few of these studies used single-agent antimicrobial therapy, with a cephalosporin (cefoxitin or moxalactam), and demonstrated comparable success with combination therapy of either clindamycin or

TABLE 4 Antimicrobial Drugs of Choice for Anaerobic Bacteria

	First	Alternate
Peptostreptococcus spp.	Penicillin	Clindamycin, chloramphenicol, cephalosporins
Clostridium spp.	Penicillin	Metronidazole, chloramphenicol, cefoxitin, clindamycin
Clostridium difficile	Vancomycin	Metronidazole, bacitracin
Fusobacterium spp.	Penicillin	Metronidazole, clindamycin, chloramphenicol
Bacteroides (BL −)	Penicillin	Metronidazole, clindamycin, chloramphenicol
Bacteroides (BL +)	Metronidazole, a carbapenem, a penicillin and BL inhibitor, clindamycin	Cefoxitin, chloramphenicol, piperacillin, tigecycline

Abbreviation: BL, beta-lactamase.

TABLE 5 Antimicrobial Recommended for the Therapy of Site-Specific Anaerobic Infections

	Surgical prophylaxis	Parenteral	Oral
Intracranial	1. Penicillin 2. Vancomycin	1. Metronidazole[4] 2. Chloramphenicol	1. Metronidazole[4] 2. Chloramphenicol
Dental	1. Penicillin 2. Erythromycin	1. Clindamycin 2. Metronidazole[4], chloramphenicol	1. Clindamycin, amoxicillin + CA 2. Metronidazole[4]
Upper respiratory tract	1. Cefoxitin 2. Clindamycin	1. Clindamycin 2. Chloramphenicol, metronidazole[4]	1. Clindamycin, amoxicillin + CA 2. Metronidazole[5]
Pulmonary	N/A	1. Clindamycin[5] 2. Ticarcillin + CA, ampicillin + SU[6], imipenem or meropenem	1. Clindamycin[8] 2. Metronidazole[5], amoxicillin + CA
Abdominal	1. Cefoxitin 2. Clindamycin[3]	1. Clindamycin[3], cefoxitin[3], metronidazole[3] 2. Imipenem, meropenem, ertapenem, piperacillin-tazobactam, tigecycline	1. Clindamycin[8], metronidazole[8] 2. Amoxacillin + CA
Pelvic	1. Cefoxitin 2. Doxycycline	1. Cefoxitin[6], clindamycin[3] 2. Piperacillin-tazobactam[6], ampicillin + SU[6], metronidazole[6]	1. Clindamycin[6] 2. Amoxacillin + CA[6], metronidazole[6]
Skin and soft tissue	1. Cefazolin[7] 2. Vancomycin	1. Clindamycin, cefoxitin 2. Metronidazole + vancomycin 3. Tigecycline	1. Clindamycin, amoxicillin + CA 2. Metronidazole + linezolid
Bone and joint	1. Cefazolin[7] 2. Vancomycin	1. Clindamycin, imipenem or meropenem 2. Metronidazole + vancomycin, piperacillin-tazobactam	1. Clindamycin 2. Metronidazole + linezolid
Bacteremia with BLPB	N/A	1. Imipenem, meropenem, metronidazole 2. Cefoxitin, piperacillin-tazobactam	1. Clindamycin, metronidazole 2. Chloramphenicol, amoxacillin + CA
Bacteremia with non-BLPB	N/A	1. Penicillin 2. Clindamycin, metronidazole, cefoxitin	1. Penicillin 2. Metronidazole, chloramphenicol, clindamycin

Note: 1, drug(s) of choice; 2, alternative drugs; 3, plus aminoglycoside; 4, plus a penicillin; 5, plus a macrolide (i.e., erythromycin); 6, plus doxycycline; 7, in location proximal to the rectal and oral areas use cefoxitin; 8, plus a quinolone (only in adults).
Abbreviations: BLPB, Beta-lactamase–producing bacteria; CA, clavulanic acid; N/A, not applicable; SU, sulbactam.

TABLE 6 Susceptibility of Anaerobic Bacteria to Antimicrobial Agents

Bacteria	Penicillin	A penicillin and a beta-lactamase inhibitor	Ureido- and carboxypenicillin	Cefoxitin	Chloram-phenicol	Clindamycin	Erythromycin	Metronidazole	Carbapenem	Tigecycline
Peptostreptococcus spp.	4	4	3	3	3	3	2–3	2	3	3
Fusobacterium spp.	3–4	3–4	3	3	3	2–3	1	3	3	3
Bacteroides fragilis group	1	4	2–3	3	3	3–4	1–2	4	4	3
Pigmented *Prevotella* and *Porphyromonas* spp.	1–3	4	2–3	3	3	3–4	2–3	4	4	3
Bacteroides spp.	2–3	4	3	3	3	3	2–3	4	4	3
Clostridium perfringens	4	4	3	3	3	3	3	3	3	3
Clostridium spp.	3	3	3	2–3	3	2	2	3	3	3
Actinomyces spp.	4	4	3	3	3	3	3	1	3	3

Degrees of activity: 1, minimal; 2, moderate; 3, good; and 4, excellent.

TABLE 7 Antimicrobial Agents Effective for the Therapy of Anaerobic Infections

Antimicrobials	Route of administration	Dose (interval) newborn (mg/kg per day)	Dose (interval) children <40 kg (mg/kg per day)	Dose (interval) adults and children >40 kg
Penicillin G	IV, IM	50,000–100,000 units (q.8–12 hr)	100,000–250,000 units (q.4 hr)	10–20 million units/day
Piperacillin	IV, IM	N/A	200–300 (q.4–6 hr)	3–4 g (q.4–6 hr)
Ticarcillin	IV, IM	150–225 (q.8–12 hr)	200–300 (q.4–6 hr)	3–4 g (q.4–6 hr)
Ticarcillin *plus* clavulanic acid	IV	150–225 (q.8–12 hr)	200–300 (q.4–6 hr)	3.1 g (q.4–8 hr)–6.2 g (q.6 hr)
Amoxicillin plus clavulanic acid	Oral	N/A	20–40 (q.8 hr)	250–500 mg (q.8 hr)
Ampicillin plus sulbactam	IV	N/A	50–100 (q.6 hr)	1.5–3.0 g (q.6 hr)
Piperacillin *plus* tazobactam	IV	N/A	75 (q.12 hr)	3.375 g (q.6 hr)
Cefoxitin	IM, IV	N/A	80–160 (q.4–6 hr)	1–2 g (q.4–6 hr)
Chloramphenicol	IV or Oral	25 mg once a day	50–75 (q.6 hr)	1 g (q.6 hr)
Clindamycin	IM, IV	10–15 (q.8–12 hr)	25–40 (q.6–8 hr)	600 mg (q.6 hr), 900 mg (q.8 hr)
	Oral	10–15 (q.8–12 hr)	10–30 (q.6 hr)	150–450 mg (q.6 hr)
Metronidazole	IV	15 (q.12 hr)	30 (q.6 hr)	500–1000 mg
	Oral	15 (q.12 hr)	15–35 (q.8 hr)	500 mg (q.6 hr)
Imipenem	IV	N/A	40–60 (q.6 hr)	250–500 mg (q.4–6 hr)
Meropenem	IV	N/A	60–120 (q.8 hr)	500–1000 mg (q.8 hr)
Ertapenem	IM, IV	N/A	15 (q.12 hr)	1.0 g q.24 hr
Moxifloxacin	IV or Oral	N/A	N/A[a]	400 mg q.24 hr
Tigecycline	IV	N/A	1.5 initially, than 1 (q.12 hr)[a]	100 mg initially, than 50 mg (q.12 hr)

[a] Not approved under the age of 18 years.
Abbreviations: g, gram; IM, intramuscular; IV, intravenous; N/A, not available.

metronidazole plus an aminoglycoside (91–95). Other single drugs or drug combinations that have shown the potential of being effective in the therapy of intra-abdominal infection are the carbapenem (e.g., imipenem, meropenem, ertapenem) (42,91,96–98), the fluoroquinolones (i.e., moxifloxacin, trovafloxacin) (86) and the combination of ticarcillin and clavulanic acid (99) and ampicillin and sulbactam (98).

Single-agent therapy provides the advantage of avoiding the ototoxicity and nephrotoxicity of aminoglycosides, and it is less expensive. But a single agent may not be effective against hospital-acquired resistant bacterial strains, and the use of a single agent is devoid of antibacterial synergy (100) which may be important in immunocompromised hosts. However, for otherwise healthy individuals, when therapy is initiated without a long delay, single agents may provide adequate therapy.

Synergistic Antimicrobial Combinations

Combinations of antibiotics are continually being studied in attempts to discover more effective therapy for serious infections. Combined therapy might delay emergence of antimicrobial resistance, provide broad-spectrum coverage for infections of unknown or mixed etiology, or generate a greater antibacterial effect against specific pathogens than is achievable with a single drug. The improved killing, as expressed by effective bactericidal activity, of the offending anaerobic organisms is especially important in the treatment of endocarditis and bacteremia. Another situation in which combination therapy may be valuable is the treatment of closed space infections, such as brain or lung abscesses, that cannot be surgically drained either because of location or the patient's clinical condition. Combination therapy should not be used indiscriminately: risks of adverse reactions are increased when multiple drugs are administered, and combination therapy is sometimes less effective than a single drug against a specific pathogen (101). Of the antimicrobial agents effective in vitro against *B. fragilis*, only metronidazole has been consistently inhibitory and bactericidal at achievable concentrations (102). Thus, the possibility of synergistic combinations against *B. fragilis* and other anaerobic organisms is clinically important (103).

Most studies on synergistic combinations of anaerobic bacteria were done on *B. fragilis* group (Table 8). Metronidazole has been recognized as one of the most effective antimicrobial agents, consistently inhibitory and bactericidal at achievable in vivo concentrations (72,73). Because of this finding, this agent has been most frequently studied in combination with other antibiotics (100,104–107,111–115) such as clindamycin (105,106), spiramycin (107), trovafloxacin (109), and levofloxacin (110) some of which proved to be synergistic. Metronidazole was synergistic with levofloxacin in 7 of 12 (58%) combinations (110). These included 5 AGNB, and one isolated each of *C. perfringens* and peptosteptococci. The combination of clindamycin and gentamicin has been found to be synergistic by some (111,112) but not all investigators. Clindamycin was synergistic with levofloxacin in 3 of 12 (25%) instances (110). The synergy occurred in 2 AGNB, and one *C. perfringens*. There is general agreement that gentamicin by itself is relatively ineffective (13). Against pigmented *Prevotella* and *Porphyromonas* the effective combinations were penicillin or clindamycin with gentamicin (100), and metronidazole with a macrolide (107) or gentamicin (100).

Synergy was found between trovafloxacin at or below the MIC and both clindamycin and metronidazole at or below the MIC in one strain each of *B. fragilis*, *B. thetaiotaomicron*, *Prevotella intermedia*, *F. varium*, *Peptostreptococcus asaccharolyticus*, and *Clostridium bifermentans* (109). Synergy between trovafloxacin and metronidazole alone was seen in one strain each of *B. distasonis*, *P. bivia*, *F. mortiferum*, *P. asaccharolyticus*, and *C. bifermentans*.

Although rare, in vitro and more often in vivo synergy between penicillin, clindamycin, or metronidazole and gentamicin against *Clostridium* spp. and anaerobic cocci can be found. Although the occurrence of such synergy is less likely to occur with gram-positive anaerobic organisms than with gram-negative anaerobic bacilli (113), when present it may offer significant clinical advantages.

The in vitro and in vivo synergism between penicillin and gentamicin against pigmented *Prevotella* and *Porphyromonas* spp. is of particular interest. Synergistic interaction between aminoglycosides and penicillins have been noted and studied with certain aerobic or facultative anaerobic organisms (101). For example, this combination was found to be effective in the treatment of enterococcal and staphylococcal diseases. It has been postulated that the penicillins, which inhibit cell wall synthesis, enhance the penetration of aminoglycosides, which are capable of interacting with the ribosomes. There is circumstantial evidence that such a mechanism may prevail in pigmented *Prevotella* and *Porphyromonas* spp. Bryan et al. (116) demonstrated that cell-free amino acid incorporation by *B. fragilis* ribosomes was inhibited by gentamicin to about the same extent as by *E. coli* ribosomes. Furthermore, there was no evidence of inactivation of the antibiotic by *B. fragilis* cell extracts. Whole cells of *B. fragilis*, however, did not show any time-dependent accumulation of the antibiotic. This failure was attributed to the lack of proper electron transport system for the transport of the aminoglycoside. The mechanism by which penicillin presumably permits the transport of aminoglycosides in *Bacteroides* spp. has not been investigated.

Some of the combinations that showed synergy are used routinely for the therapy of mixed aerobic–anaerobic infections. These include the combination of clindamycin or metronidazole plus an aminoglycoside used for the therapy of intra-abdominal and pelvic infections, and the combination of metronidazole and a macrolide for the therapy of upper respiratory tract infections. The synergistic effect against some anaerobic strains noticed by the above studies (Table 8) is a valuable additional asset.

The only data available so far are laboratory data of in vitro susceptibility testing and animal studies. Clinical studies in patients are warranted to evaluate the efficacy of synergistic therapy of anaerobic infections.

PREVENTION

Because most anaerobic infections are caused by endogenous flora, usually prevention through isolation techniques or immunization is not possible. Prophylactic use of antimicrobials is indicated in elective intra-abdominal or oropharyngeal surgery. Cefoxitin has been used for

TABLE 8 Summary of Studies Evaluating Synergistic Combination of Antimicrobial Agents Effective Against Anaerobic Bacteria

Agents in combination	Effective synergy	Reference
***Bacteroides fragilis* group**		
Metronidazole (plus)		
Ampicillin	13/16 (80%)[a]	104
Rifampin	17/22 (77%)	105
Clindamycin	29/38 (76%)	105,106
Nalidixic acid	14/19 (74%)	105
Erythromycin	26/54 (67%)	105,106
Spiramycin	3/5 (60%)	107
Gentamicin	7/15 (47%)	106,111,112
Carbenicillin	4/28 (14%)	106
Cefoxitin	3/30 (10%)	106
Levofloxacin	3/4 (75%)	110
Clindamycin (plus)		
Gentamicin	12/26 (46%)	100,111,112
Chloramphenicol	6/19 (32%)	106
Levofloxacin	1/3 (33%)	110
Cefuroxime (plus)		
Penicillin	2/3 (66%)	114
Carbenicillin (plus)	2/3 (66%)	114
Mecillinam		
Carbenicillin	12/29 (41%)	115
Pigmented *Prevotella* and *Porphyromonas* spp.		
Metronidazole (plus)		
Gentamicin	3/15 (20%)[a]	100
Spiramycin	2/3 (66%)	107
Levofloxacin	2/3 (66%)	110
Clindamycin (plus)		
Gentamicin	10/15 (66%)	100
Penicillin (plus)		
Gentamicin	11/15 (73%)	100
***Clostridium* spp.**		
Clindamycin (plus)		
Gentamicin	1/12 (8%)	113
Levofloxacin	1/1 (100%)	110
***Peptostreptococcus* spp.**		
Metronidazole (plus)		
Spiramycin	7/16 (43%)	108
Clindamycin (plus)		
Gentamicin	1/7 (14%)	113

[a] Number of isolates where synergy was demonstrated/number of bacterial strains tested (% synergy).

such prophylaxis. Often, severe anaerobic infections caused by bowel flora after gastrointestinal compromise or perforation can be prevented by early, judicious surgery combined with appropriate antibiotic coverage for *B. fragilis* group and for any aerobic pathogens involved. This therapy constitutes early treatment for infection rather than prophylaxis. Similar management of other potentially contaminated sites may prevent the development of severe infection.

Superficial wounds thought to be contaminated by anaerobes should be irrigated copiously and allowed to heal by secondary intention, particularly if they are ragged lacerations caused by animal or human bites. Appropriate antibiotics may help to prevent severe infection.

CONCLUSIONS

Polymicrobial infections are generally due to aerobic and anaerobic flora that act synergistically with each other. Proper antimicrobial therapy is an important adjunct to surgical management. It should be started as soon as possible and include either combined or single therapy of antimicrobials effective against the aerobic and anaerobic pathogens.

REFERENCES

1. Shupak A, Halpern P, Ziser A, Melamed Y. Hyperbaric oxygen therapy for gas gangrene casualties in Lebanon War, 1982. Isr J Med Sci 1984; 20:323–6.
2. Altemeier WA, Fullen WD. Prevention and treatment of gas gangrene. JAMA 1971; 217:806–13.
3. Fredette V. Effects of hyperbaric oxygen on anaerobic bacteria and toxins. Ann NY Acad Sci 1965; 117:700–5.
4. Kindwall EP. Use of hyperbaric oxygen therapy in the 1990s. Cleve Clin J Med 1992; 59:517–28.
5. Nakajima H, Iwai Y, Yamanaka K, Kishi H. Successful treatment of brainstem abscess with stereotactic aspiration. Surg Neurol 1999; 52:445–8.
6. Pruitt AA. Infections of the nervous system. Neurol Clin 1998; 16:419–47.
7. Brook I, Walker RI. Significance of encapsulated *Bacteroides melaninogenicus* and *Bacteroides fragilis* groups in mixed infections. Infect Immun 1984; 44:12–4.
8. Cinat ME, Wilson SE. New advances in the use of antimicrobial agents in surgery: intra-abdominal infections. J Chemother 1999; 11:453–63.
9. Finegold SM, George WL, Mulligan ME. Anaerobic Infections. Disease a Month., Vol. 31. Chicago, IL: Yearbook Medical Publisher, Inc., 1985:11–7.
10. Verklin RM, Mandell GL. Alteration of antibiotics by anaerobiosis. J Lab Clin Med 1977; 89:65–71.
11. Gorbach SL, Bartlett JG. Anaerobic infections. N Engl J Med 1974; 290:1177–84.
12. Aldridge KE, Sanders CV. Susceptibility trending of blood isolates of the *Bacteroides fragilis* group over a 12-year period to clindamycin, ampicillin-sulbactam, cefoxitin, imipenem, and metronidazole. Anaerobe 2002; 8:301–5.
13. Sutter VL, Finegold SM. Susceptibility of anaerobic bacteria to 23 antimicrobial agents. Antimicrob Agents Chemother 1976; 10:736–52.
14. Brook I, Gober AE. Emergence of beta-lactamase-producing aerobic and anaerobic bacteria in the oropharynx of children following penicillin chemotherapy. Clin Pediatr 1984; 23:338–42.
15. Tuner K, Nord CE. Emergence of beta-lactamase-producing microorganisms in the tonsils during penicillin treatment. Eur J Clin Microb 1986; 5:399–404.
16. Snydman DR, Jacobus NV, McDermott LA, et al. National survey on the susceptibility of *Bacteroides fragilis* group: report and analysis of trends for 1997–2000. Clin Infect Dis 2002; 35(Suppl. 1):S126–34.
17. Labbe AC, Bourgault AM, Vincelette J, Turgeon PL, Lamothe F. Trends in antimicrobial resistance among clinical isolates of the *Bacteroides fragilis* group from 1992 to 1997 in Montreal, Canada. Antimicrob Agents Chemother 1999; 43:2517–9.
18. Bianchini H, Fernandez Canigia LB, Bantar C, Smayevsky J. Trends in antimicrobial resistance of the *Bacteroides fragilis* group: a 20-year study at a medical center in Buenaos Aires, Argentina. Clin Infect Dis 1997; 25:S268–9.
19. Garcia-Rodrigues JE, Garcia-Sanchez JE. Evolution of antimicrobial susceptibility in isolates of the *Bacteroides fragilis* group in Spain. Clin Infect Dis 1990; 12:S142–51.
20. Lee K, Chuong Y, Jeong SH, Xu X-S, Kwon OH. Emerging resistance of anaerobic bacteria to antimicrobial agents in South Korea. Clin Infect Dis 1996; 23:S73–7.
21. Finegold SM. Anaerobic Bacteria in Human Disease. New York: Academic Press, 1977.
22. Busch DF, Kureshi LA, Sutter VL, Finegold SM. Susceptibility of respiratory tract anaerobes to orally administered penicillins and cephalosporins. Antimicrob Agents Chemother 1976; 10:713–20.
23. Finegold SM. In vitro efficacy of beta-lactam/beta-lactamase inhibitor combinations against bacteria involved in mixed infections. Int J Antimicrob Agents 1999; 12(Suppl. 1):S9–14.
24. Acuna C, Rabasseda X. Amoxicillin-sulbactam: a clinical and therapeutic review. Drugs Today (Barc) 2001; 37:193–210.
25. Sutter VL, Finegold SM. Susceptibility of anaerobic bacteria to carbenicillin, cefoxitin, and related drugs. J Infect Dis 1975; 131:417–22.
26. Fiedelman W, Webb CD. Clinical evaluation of carbenicillin in the treatment of infection due to anaerobic bacteria. Curr Ther Res 1975; 18:441–51.
27. Thadepalli H, Huang JT. Treatment of anaerobic infections: carbenicillin alone compared with clindamycin and gentamicin. Curr Ther Res 1977; 22:549–57.
28. Brook I. Carbenicillin in treatment of aspiration pneumonia in children. Curr Ther Res 1978; 23:136–47.
29. Brook I. Anaerobic isolates in chronic recurrent suppurative otitis media: treatment with carbenicillin alone and in combination with gentamicin. Infection 1979; 5:247–51.
30. Tally FP, Jacobus NV, Bartlett JG, Gorbach SL. In vitro activity of penicillins against anaerobes. Antimicrob Agents Chemother 1975; 7:413–4.
31. Roy I, Bach V, Thadepalli H. In vitro activity of ticarcillin against anaerobic bacteria compared with that of carbenicillin and penicillin. Antimicrob Agents Chemother 1977; 11:258–61.
32. Goldstein EJ, Citron DM, Vaidya SA, et al. In vitro activity of 11 antibiotics against 74 anaerobes isolated from pediatric intra-abdominal infections. Anaerobe 2006; 12:63–6.

33. Jousimies H, Summanen P. Recent taxonomic changes and terminology update of clinically significant anaerobic gram-negative bacteria (excluding spirochetes). Clin Infect Dis 2002; 35(Suppl. 1):S17–21.

34. Jousimies-Somer HR, Summanen P, Baron EJ, Citron DM, Wexler HM, Finegold SM. Wadsworth-KTL Anaerobic Bacteriology Manual. 6th ed. Belmont, CA: Star Publishing, 2002.

35. Brook I. Intra-abdominal, retroperitoneal, and visceral abscesses in children. Eur J Pediatr Surg 2004; 14:265–73.

36. Goldstein EJ. Intra-abdominal anaerobic infections: bacteriology and therapeutic potential of newer antimicrobial carbapenem, fluoroquinolone, and desfluoroquinolone therapeutic agents. Clin Infect Dis 2002; 35(Suppl. 1):S106–11.

37. Sutter VL, Citron DM, Edelstein MAC, Finegold SM. Anaerobic Bacteriology Manual. 4th ed. Belmont, CA: Star Publishing Company, 1985.

38. Brook I. Bacterial studies of peritoneal cavity and postoperative surgical wound drainage following perforated appendix in children. Ann Surg 1980; 192:208.

39. Hedberg M, Nord CE. ESCMID Study Group on antimicrobial resistance in anaerobic bacteria. Antimicrobial susceptibility of *Bacteroides fragilis* group isolates in Europe. Clin Microbiol Infect 2003; 9:475–88.

40. Snydman DR, Jacobus NV, McDermott LA, et al. Multicenter study of in vitro susceptibility of the *Bacteroides fragilis* group, 1995 to 1996, with comparison of resistance trends from 1990 to 1996. Antimicrob Agents Chemother 1999; 43:2417–22.

41. Rodloff AC, Goldstein EJ, Torres A. Two decades of imipenem therapy. J Antimicrob Chemother 2006; 58:916–29.

42. Hellinger WC, Brewer NS. Carbapenems and monobactams: imipenem, meropenem, and aztreonam. Mayo Clin Proc 1999; 74:420–34.

43. Edwards JR. Meropenem: a microbiological overview. J Antimicrob Chemother 1995; 36:1–17.

44. Jorgensen JH, Maher LA, Howell AW. Activity of meropenem against antibiotic-resistant or infrequently encountered gram-negative bacilli. Antimicrob Agents Chemother 1991; 35:2410–4.

45. Abramowicz M. Meropenem—a new parenteral broad-spectrum antibiotic. Med Lett 1996; 38:88–90.

46. Keating GM, Perry CM. Ertapenem: a review of its use in the treatment of bacterial infections. Drugs 2005; 65:2151–78.

47. Kasten MJ. Clindamycin, metronidazole, and chloramphenicol. Mayo Clin Proc 1999; 74:825–33 (Review).

48. Thadepalli H, Gorbach SL, Bartlett JG. Apparent failure of chloramphenicol in anaerobic infections. Obstet Gynecol Surg 1978; 35:334–5.

49. Balbi HJ. Chloramphenicol: a review. Pediatr Rev 2004; 25:284–8.

50. Nau R, Sorgel F, Prange HW. Pharmacokinetic optimisation of the treatment of bacterial central nervous system infections. Clin Pharmacokinet 1998; 35:223–46.

51. Drutz DJ, Schaffner W, Hillman JW, Koenig MG. The penetration of penicillin and other antimicrobials into joint fluid. J Bone Joint Surg 1967; 49:1415–21.

52. Joiner KA, Lowe BR, Dzink JL, Bartlett JG. Antibiotic levels in infected and sterile subcutaneous abscesses in mice. J Infect Dis 1981; 143:487–94.

53. Goldstein EJ, Citron DM, Merriam CV. Linezolid activity compared to those of selected macrolides and other agents against aerobic and anaerobic pathogens isolated from soft tissue bite infections in humans. Antimicrob Agents Chemother 1999; 43:1469–74.

54. Williams JD, Maskell JP, Shain H, et al. Comparative in-vitro activity of azithromycin, macrolides (erythromycin, clarithromycin and spiramycin) and streptogramin RP 59500 against oral organisms. J Antimicrob Chemother 1992; 30:27–37.

55. Werner H, Boehm M, Kunstek-Santos H, Lohner C, Jordan T. Susceptibility to erythromycin of anaerobes of the genera *Bacteroides, Fusobacterium, Sphaerophorus, Veillonella, Clostridium, Corynebacterium, Peptococcus, Peptostreptococcus*. Arzneimittelforschung 1977; 27:2263–5.

56. Finegold SM, Harada NE, Miller LG. Lincomycin activity against anaerobes and effect on normal human fecal flora. Antimicrob Agents Chemother 1965; 5:659–67.

57. Klainer AS. Clindamycin. Med Clin North Am 1987; 71:1169–75.

58. LeFrock JL, Molavi A, Prince RA. Clindamycin. Med Clin North Am 1982; 66:103–20.

59. Paap CM, Nahata MC. Clinical pharmacokinetics of antibacterial drugs in neonates. Clin Pharmacokinet 1990; 19:280–318.

60. Feigin RD, Pickering LK, Anderson D, Keeney RE, Shackleford PG. Clindamycin treatment of osteomyelitis and septic arthritis in children. Pediatrics 1975; 55:213–23.

61. Novak E, Wagner JG, Lamb DJ. Local and systemic tolerance, absorption and excretion of clindamycin hydrochloride after intramuscular administration. Int Z Klin Pharmakol Ther Toxikol 1970; 3:201–8.

62. Panzer JD, Brown DC, Epstein WL, Lipson RL, Mahaffey HW, Atkinson WH. Clindamycin levels in various body tissues and fluids. J Clin Pharmacol 1972; 12:259–62.

63. Gorbach SL, Thadepalli H. Clindamycin in the treatment of pure and mixed anaerobic infections. Arch Intern Med 1974; 134:87–92.
64. Gorbach SL. Antibiotics and *Clostridium difficile*. N Engl J Med 1999; 341:1690–1.
65. Mylonakis E, Ryan ET, Calderwood SB. *Clostridium difficile*—associated diarrhea: a review. Arch Intern Med 2001; 161:525–33.
66. Devenyi AG. Antibiotic-induced colitis. Semin Pediatr Surg 1995; 4:215–20.
67. Berlatzky Y, Rubin SZ, Michel J, Sacks T, Schiller M. Use of clindamycin and gentamicin in pediatric colonic surgery. J Pediatr Surg 1976; 11:943–8.
68. Brook I. Clindamycin in treatment of aspiration pneumonia in children. Antimicrob Agents Chemother 1979; 15:342–4.
69. Brook I. Bacteriology and treatment of chronic otitis media in children. Laryngoscope 1979; 89:1129–34.
70. Brook I, Yocum P. Antimicrobial management of chronic sinusitis in children. J Laryngol Otol 1995; 109:1159–62.
71. Brook I, Lewis MA, Sandor GK, Jeffcoat M, Samaranayake LP, Vera Rojas J. Clindamycin in dentistry: more than just effective prophylaxis for endocarditis? Oral Surg Oral Med Oral Pathol Oral Radiol Endod 2005; 100:550–8.
72. Chow AW, Patten V, Guze LB. Susceptibility of anaerobic bacteria to metronidazole: relative resistance of non-spore forming gram-positive bacilli. J Infect Dis 1975; 131:182–5.
73. Freeman CD, Klutman NE, Lamp KC. Metronidazole. A therapeutic review and update. Drugs 1997; 54:679–708.
74. Rustia M, Shubik P. Experimental induction of hematomas, mammary tumors and other tumors with metronidazole in noninbred Sas: WRC (WT)BR rats. J Natl Cancer Inst 1979; 63:863–8.
75. Cohen SM, Erturk E, Von Esch AM, Crovetti AJ, Bryan GT. Carcinogenicity of 5-nitro-furans 5-nitromidazoles, 4-nitrobenzenes and related compounds. J Natl Cancer Inst 1973; 51:403.
76. Beard CM, Noller KL, O'Fallon WM, Kurland LT, Dockerty MB. Lack of evidence for cancer due to use of metronidazole. N Engl J Med 1979; 301:519–22.
77. Tally FP, Gorbach SL. Therapy of mixed anaerobic-aerobic infections. Lessons from studies of intra-abdominal sepsis. Am J Med 1985; 78:145–53.
78. Berman BW, King FH, Jr., Rubenstein DS, Long SS. *Bacteroides fragilis* meningitis in a neonatal successfully treated with metronidazole. J Pediatr 1979; 93:793–5.
79. Rom S, Flynn D, Noone P. Anaerobic infections in a neonate. Early detection by gas liquid chromatography and response to metronidazole. Arch Dis Child 1977; 52:740–1.
80. Brook I. Microbiology and management of brain abscess in children. J Pediatr Neurol 2004; 2:125–30.
81. Law BJ, Marks MI. Excellent outcome of *Bacteroides* meningitis in a newborn treated with metronidazole. Pediatrics 1980; 66:463–5.
82. Brook I. Treatment of anaerobic infections in children with metronidazole. Dev Pharmacol 1983; 6:187–98.
83. Townsend ML, Pound MW, Drew RH. Tigecycline: a new glycylcycline antimicrobial. Int J Clin Pract 2006; 60:1662–7.
84. Goldstein EJ, Citron DM, Merriam CV, Warren YA, Tyrrell KL, Fernandez HT. Comparative in vitro susceptibilities of 396 unusual anaerobic strains to tigecycline and eight other antimicrobial agents. Antimicrob Agents Chemother 2006; 50:3507–13.
85. Appelbaum PC. Quinolone activity against anaerobes. Drugs 1999; 58:60–4.
86. Goldstein EJ. Possible role for the new fluoroquinolones (levofloxacin, grepafloxacin, trovafloxacin, clinafloxacin, sparfloxacin, and DU-6859a) in the treatment of anaerobic infections: review of current information on efficacy and safety. Clin Infect Dis 1996; 23:S25–30.
87. Finch RG. Antibacterial activity of quinupristin/dalfopristin. Rationale for clinical use. Drugs 1996; 51:31–7.
88. Brook I. Pathogenicity and management of polymicrobial infections due to aerobic and anaerobic bacteria. Med Res Rev 1995; 15:73–82.
89. Bartlett JG. Recent developments in the management of anaerobic infection. Rev Infect Dis 1983; 5:235–45.
90. Holzheimer RG, Dralle H. Antibiotic therapy in intra-abdominal infections—a review on randomised clinical trials. Eur J Med Res 2001; 6:277–91.
91. Rodloff AC, Goldstein EJ, Torres A. Two decades of imipenem therapy. J Antimicrob Chemother 2006; 58:916–29.
92. Sanabria A. Decision-making analysis for selection of antibiotic treatment in intra-abdominal infection using preference measurements. Surg Infect (Larchmt) 2006; 7:453–62.
93. Laterre PF, Colardyn F, Delmee M, et al. Antimicrobial therapy for intra-abdominal infections: guidelines from the Infectious Disease Advisory Board (IDAB). Acta Chir Belg 2006; 106:2–21.
94. Marshall JC. Intra-abdominal infections. Microbes Infect 2004; 6:1015–25.

95. Giamarellou H, Kanellakopoulou K. Bacteriologic and therapeutic considerations in intra-abdominal surgical infections. Anaerobe 1997; 3:207–12.

96. Verwaest C, Belgian Multicenter Study Group. Meropenem versus imipenem/cilastatin as empirical monotherapy for serious bacterial infections in the intensive care unit. Clin Microbiol Infect 2000; 6:294–302.

97. Burkhardt O, Derendorf H, Welte T. Ertapenem: the new carbapenem 5 years after first FDA licensing for clinical practice. Expert Opin Pharmacother 2007; 8:237–56.

98. Powell LL, Wilson SE. The role of beta-lactam antimicrobials as single agents in treatment of intra-abdominal infection. Surg Infect (Larchmt) 2000; 1:57–63.

99. Munckhof WJ, Carney J, Neilson G, et al. Continuous infusion of ticarcillin-clavulanate for home treatment of serious infections: clinical efficacy, safety, pharmacokinetics and pharmacodynamics. Int J Antimicrob Agents 2005; 25:514–22.

100. Brook I, Coolbaugh JC, Walker RI, Weiss E. Synergism between penicillin, clindamycin or metronidazole and gentamicin against species of *Bacteroides melaninogenicus* and *fragilis* groups. Antimicrob Agents Chemother 1984; 25:71–7.

101. Acar JF. Antibiotic synergy and antagonism. Med Clin North Am 2000; 84:1391–406.

102. Snydman DR, Jacobus NV, McDermott LA, et al. National survey on the susceptibility of *B. fragilis* group: report and analysis of trends for 1997–2004: a U.S. survey. Antimicrob Agents Chemother 2007; 51:1649–55.

103. Brook I. Synergistic combinations of antimicrobial agents against anaerobic bacteria. Pediatr Infect Dis 1987; 6:332.

104. Bergan T, Fotland MH. In vitro interactions between metronidazole or tinidazole and co-trimoxazole on the effect against anaerobic bacteria. Scand J Gastroenterol 1984; 19:95.

105. Ralph ED, Amatnieks YE. Potentially synergistic antimicrobial combinations with metronidazole against *Bacteroides fragilis*. Antimicrob Agents Chemother 1980; 17:379.

106. Busch DF, Sutter VL, Finegold SM. Activity of combinations of antimicrobial agents against *Bacteroides fragilis*. J Infect Dis 1976; 133:321–8.

107. Brook I. Metronidazole and spiramycin in abscesses caused by *Bacteroides* sp. *Staphylococcus aureus* in mice. J Antimicrob Chemother 1987; 20:713–8.

108. Videau D, Blanchard JC, Sebald M. Bucco-dental flora. Sensitivity to antibiotics and value of the spiramycin-metronidazole combination. Ann Microbiol 1973; 1248:505–16.

109. Ednie LM, Credito KL, Khantipong M, Jacobs MR, Appelbaum PC. Synergic activity, for anaerobes, of trovafloxacin with clindamycin or metronidazole: chequerboard and time-kill methods. J Antimicrob Chemother 2000; 45:633–8.

110. Credito KL, Jacobs MR, Appelbaum PC. Anti-anaerobic activity of levofloxacin alone and combined with clindamycin and metronidazole. Diagn Microbiol Infect Dis 2000; 38:181–3.

111. Fass RJ, Rotilie CA, Prior RB. Interaction of clindamycin and gentamicin in vitro. Antimicrob Agents Chemother 1974; 6:582–7.

112. Okubadejo OA, Allen J. Combined activity of clindamycin and gentamicin on *Bacteroides fragilis* and other bacteria. J Antimicrob Chemother 1975; 1:403–9.

113. Brook I, Walker RI. Interaction between penicillin, clindamycin or metronidazole and gentamicin against species of clostridia and anaerobic and facultative anaerobic gram-positive cocci. J Antimicrob Chemother 1985; 15:31–7.

114. Thadepalli H, White DW, Bach VT. Antimicrobial activity and synergism of cefuroxime on anaerobic bacteria. Chemotherapy 1981; 27:252–8.

115. Trestman I, Kaye D, Levinson ME. Activity of semisynthetic penicillins and synergism with mecillinam against *Bacteroides* species. Agents Chemother 1979; 16:283–6.

116. Bryan LE, Kowand SK, Den Elzen HM. Mechanisms of aminoglycoside antibiotic resistance in anaerobic bacteria: *Clostridium perfringens* and *Bacteroides fragilis*. Antimicrob Agents Chemother 1979; 15:7–13.

Index

About the Author

ITZHAK BROOK is Professor of Pediatrics and Medicine at Georgetown University, Washington, D.C.; and Attending Physician at Georgetown University Medical Center, Washington, D.C. The author, coauthor, or editor of over 600 journal articles, book chapters, and books on the role of anaerobic infections in children and adults, he is considered a world leader in the field. A member of more than 20 professional organizations and a Fellow of the Infectious Disease Society of America, the Society for Pediatric Research, and the Pediatric Infectious Disease Society, as well as a member of several consensus and Advisory Boards on the management of pediatric infection, he is on the editorial board of several medical journals and the USA Editor of the *Journal of Pediatric Infectious Diseases* and a Section Editor on head and neck infections in *Current Infectious Disease Reports*. He is a past chairman of the Anti-infective Drugs Advisory Board for the Food and Drug Administration. He received the M.D. degree (1968) from Hebrew University, Hadassah School of Medicine, Jerusalem, Israel, where he completed his pediatric residency (1974), and the Diploma of Pediatrics (1972), and the M.Sc. degree (1973) in pediatrics from the University of Tel-Aviv, Israel. He completed a Fellowship (1976) in pediatric and adult infectious diseases at the University of California School of Medicine, Los Angeles.